ANATOMY OF THE DOG
An Illustrated Text

FOURTH EDITION

Professor Klaus-Dieter Budras
Institute of Veterinary Anatomy
Free University of Berlin

Professor em. Patrick H. McCarthy
Dept. of Veterinary Anatomy, University of Sydney

Wolfgang Fricke
Science Illustrator

Renate Richter
Science Illustrator

with
Professor Aaron Horowitz
Professor Rolf Berg
Dept. of Structure and Function
School of Veterinary Medicine
Ross University, St. Kitts, West Indies

With the assistance of co-workers
Dr Anita Wünsche *and* **Dr Sven Reese**

With Contributions to Clinical and Functional Anatomy by
Dr Sven Reese, Dr Klaus Gerlach *and* **Professor Klaus-Dieter Budras**

Introduction to Radiographic Technique and Ultrasound Diagnosis
Professor Cordula Poulsen Nautrup

schlütersche

CO-WORKERS ON THE ATLAS OF THE ANATOMY OF THE DOG

Fourth Edition

Title Figure:
Renate Richter

Editor:
Prof. Dr. Klaus-Dieter Budras, Institut für Veterinär-Anatomie, Freie Universität Berlin

Contributions:
Dr. Klaus Gerlach PhD, Tierärztliche Praxis, Berlin
Prof. Horst E. König, Institut für Anatomie, Veterinärmedizinische Universität Wien
Prof. Dr. Dr. h. c. Hans-Georg Liebich, Institut für Tieranatomie, Ludwig-Maximilians-Universität München
Dr. Sven Reese, Institut für Tieranatomie, Ludwig-Maximilians-Universität München
Dr. Anita Wünsche, Institut für Veterinär-Anatomie, Freie Universität Berlin
Prof. Dr. Paul Simoens, Faculteit Diergeneeskunde, Gent, Belgium

Editorial contribution:
Dr. Silke Buda, Institut für Veterinär-Anatomie, Freie Universität Berlin

Labelling of figures:
Christina Braun, Institut für Veterinär-Anatomie, Freie Universität Berlin
Claudia Nöller, Institut für Veterinär-Anatomie, Freie Universität Berlin

Index:
Thilo Voges, Institut für Veterinär-Anatomie, Freie Universität Berlin

An index of earlier co-workers and of the sources for illustrations, radiographs, and photographs can be obtained from the previous edition.

© 2002 Schlütersche GmbH & Co. KG, Verlag und Druckerei,
Hans-Böckler-Allee 7, 30173 Hannover, Germany
E-Mail: info@schluetersche.de

Printed in Germany

ISBN 3-87706-619-4   1004927206

A CIP catalogue record for this book is available from Deutsche Bibliothek, Frankfurt — Germany.

TABLE OF CONTENTS

How to use this book:

The framed introductions at the beginning of the text-pages dealing with topographical anatomy give information with respect to the dissection of the areas shown in the figures. At the same time, they can be used as abbreviated dissection instructions. Boldface terms of anatomical structures serve for emphasis and, insofar as they are identified by numbers, they are represented on the neighboring illustration-page where they are identified by the same number. Numbers on the margin of the text-pages refer to the 'Clinical and Functional Anatomy.' The numbers in the clinical anatomy part refer to the corresponding page in the topographical anatomy; e.g., '8.2' refers to the part numbered '2' on page 8. The anatomical/medical terms and expressions occurring in the text are explained and interpreted in 'Anatomical Terms.' Abbreviations of anatomical terms follow the abbreviations as employed in the Nomina Anatomica Veterinaria (1994). Other abbreviations are explained in the appertaining text, and in the titles and legends for the illustrations. A few abbreviations that are not generally employed are listed here:

The **cranial nerves** *(Nervi craniales)* are designated with roman numerals I – XII.

Spinal nerves *(Nervi spinales)*:

n   — Nervus spinalis
nd   — Ramus dorsalis n. spinalis
ndl — Ramus dorsolateralis
ndm — Ramus dorsomedialis
nv   — Ramus ventralis
nvl — Ramus ventrolateralis
nvm — Ramus ventromedialis
nC   — Nervus cervicalis (*e.g.*, nC1 – first cervical nerve)
nCy — Nervus coccygeus s. caudalis
nL   — Nervus lumbalis
nS   — Nervus sacralis
nT   — Nervus thoracicus

Vertebrae

vC   — Vertebra cervicalis (*e.g.*, vC3 – third cervical vertebra)
vL   — Vertebra lumbalis
vS   — Vertebra sacralis
vT   — Vertebra thoracica

PREFACE TO THE FOURTH ENGLISH EDITION

This work, designated a "Fourth Edition", is an edited English translation of the sixth German edition of *Atlas der Anatomie des Hundes* by Professor Budras, author (with collaborators), and Herr W. Fricke and Frau R. Richter, science illustrators. The purpose of the work is to place before the English-speaking world an up-to-date written and illustrated anatomy of the dog substantially integrated with the clinical sciences of radiology, ultrasound, medicine and surgery. It is the aim of the authors, by textual description and by the numerous illustrations, to provide the student with a good working knowledge and understanding of the anatomy of the dog. The summarizing tables in the mid-section of the book, furnish a concise source of canine anatomy for future use. For the practicing veterinarian, the book remains a current, "quick" source of reference for anatomical information on the dog at the preclinical, diagnostic, clinical and surgical levels. For the specialist, the book will serve to deepen one's knowledge at that level of expertise.

The authors wish to thank all collaborators featured on the title page of this present volume as well as those mentioned for their contributions in the prefaces to previous German and English editions. This English edition is a contribution of veterinary anatomists and clinicians, illustrators and technicians from several continents. It is our wish that the book will find a treasured and useful place in the library.

Finally, the authors acknowledge with gratitude the excellent work of the publisher in the reproduction of the figures and the preparation of the entire work. We extend particular recognition to the contribution of Dr. Ulrike Oslage, Veterinary Editor.

Berlin, St. Kitts, Sydney
Summer 2001

Klaus-D. Budras
Rolf Berg
Aaron Horowitz
Patrick H. McCarthy

PREFACE TO THE THIRD ENGLISH EDITION

This English edition of *Atlas der Anatomie des Hundes* by Professor Dr. K.-D. Budras and collaborators will place their work before a wider scientific community than previously.

To reiterate what has been stated in the prefaces of previous German editons, this volume should rightfully be called a book-atlas. Its main thrust has been a closer integration of theoretical and practical knowledge of the anatomy of the dog and its further integration with clinical, surgical, radiographic and ultrasonographic correlative anatomy. Not only is such applied anatomy of intrinsic importance; it also demonstrates the importance of the basic subject and why one has to persevere with a discipline of great complexity. This is of psychological benefit to students. Indeed, this volume is a blue-print upon which integrated courses of veterinary anatomy can be fashioned according to the requirements of the veterinary course being served.

This book-atlas with its abundance of illustrations, is not only the result of patient, detailed research and design on the part of the authors. Constructive student criticism has been sought and tested over several years. Synoptic tables in the mid-section of the book-atlas provide summarized data on each of the anatomical systems dealt with in lectures and seen in detail in dissection laboratory classes. Such inforamtion has proved invaluable in achieving an overall view of the subject and also serves to encapsulate data prior to examinations.

For the practising veterinarian the book-atlas is a quick source of reference for anatomical information on the dog at the preclinical, diagnostic, clinical and surgical levels. It will also serve to deepen one's knowledge at a specialist level. The authors wish to thank all collaborators featured on the title page of the present volume as well as those mentioned for their contributions in the prefaces to previous German editions. The present edition is a contribution of veterinary anatomists, illustrators and technicians from three continents.

Special thanks should be given to Ms L. Hicks of the Department of Veterinary Anatomy, University of Sydney, Autralia for her secretarial help and skills in word processing and Professor Dr. A. Horowitz, University of Zimbabwe and Professor Dr. R. L. Hullinger, Purdue University, Indiana, U.S.A. for their translation of parts of the General Anatomy. Without such assistance this volume could not have reached fruition.

Berlin, summer 1994

The authors

PREFACE TO THE SIXTH GERMAN EDITION

The topographical anatomy, presented in the main part of our work, achieves an unexpected significance owing to the just completed new order of approval (Approbationsordnung) for veterinarians and with that the dramatic decrease in teaching time in the area of anatomy. The topographical anatomical way of proceeding still makes it possible at the earliest to adequately provide a very comprehensive and important subject matter in the short time available. It is for this reason that we worked continuously for many years toward the improvement of our work. After an extensive revision and completion of the fifth edition there remained still the reorganization, completion and realization of the 'Contributions to Clinical and Functional Anatomy' in the sixth edition. For that important task we obtained our colleagues Dr. Reese, Munich, and Privat Dozent Gerlach, Berlin. The Tierklinik Krüger in Hamburg supported our project by their generous preparation of high quality computer tomographic illustrations. The following colleagues deserve our thanks for having made available to us special exposures: Frau Dr. Allgöwer/Berlin, Professor Dr. Berens v. Rautenfeld/Hannover, Dr. Dr. Fahrenkrug/Quickborn, Frau Professor Dr. Grevel/Leipzig, Professor Dr. W. Kraft/Munich, Dr. Maierl/Munich, Professor Dr. Poulsen Nautrup/Munich, Frau Dr. v. Ruedorffer/Essen.

After completed revision of the fifth and sixth editions we are obliged to give great thanks to the Berlin student body for their constructive suggestions. This holds also for the engaged cooperation of the student and scientific coworkers of our department. For professional suggestions we thank Professors Dr. R. Berg, Dr. G. Böhme, Dr. K. Dämmrich, Dr. K. Donat, Dr. H. Martens and Dr. H.-J. Risse. Of special value were the suggestions of Professor Hashimoto (Sapporo), Professor Horowitz (St. Kitts, West Indies, and U.S.A) and Dr. McCarthy (Sydney), who have brought about the Japanese or, respectively, English translation of our book. We regard as very valuable the cooperation of our internationally highly reputed colleagues, Professor Liebich from Munich, Professor König from Vienna and Professor Simoens from Ghent. Our thanks goes also to Schlütersche for their support and cooperation furnished at all times in the development of this complet-ed and improved edition.

Berlin, spring 2000   The author

PREFACE TO THE SECOND GERMAN EDITION (abridged)

With the publication of the second edition, we had the opportunity to revise completely a concept that had been successful, to improve it decisively, and to bring it up to date. The advantages of the newly developed concept lay clearly at hand as shown by the necessity for a new edition only a few years after the appearance of the first.

The newly added clinical-functional contributions will provide the practical relationship to medically relevant facts and will promote the integration of preclinical and clinical education as well as contribute to the understanding of the connection between medicine and anatomy. The forty or so radiographs document predominantly 'cases from practice', by which the study of anatomy is enhanced. Moreover, they can also be used for the radiographic anatomical study of the normal situation for which the colored illustrations can be used also as a comparison and for orientation.

A special goal for us was to consider the desires of the students with respect to streamlining the content and weighting the priority of the extremely numerous anatomical details. The topographical anatomy main part of the book, with its concept of the text-atlas, is in itself a compression of anatomical description. By plac-ing the figures opposite the text with a close relationship of the content of illustration and text, and with use of corresponding symbols, the essentials can be described in the least space. Especially since many details can be 'read off' directly from the illustrations. In the illustrations and the pertinent description, attention was given to the anatomical 'norm.' To avoid exceeding an appropriate amount of space, we have greatly limited the giving of anatomical variations. Medically important data is emphasized also by the concept of labeling the illustrations with indication lines, numbers and letters which relate to the appropriate text page and by explanations in the clinical-functional contributions; whereas, less important details were mentioned only in the legend or table without a detailed explanation.

The present text-atlas offers to the student clear illustrative material and at the same time an abbreviated textbook for anatomical study and for clinically coordinated study of applied anatomy. Beyond this the text-atlas will help in reviewing and for preparation for examinations. For the teaching of anatomical terminology there is also offered a vocabulary of anatomical-medical terms.

For the practicing veterinarian the present book is intended to be a source of rapid information and refreshment, deepening and complementing the material formerly learned. Especially the list of anatomical-medical technical terms with explanations of their significance, grammar and derivation, as well as the clinical-functional contributions, can be employed of course as a lexicon. Since a valid nomenclature is used, the present book can also serve as an illustrated nomenclature.

Berlin, summer 1987   The author

PREFACE TO THE FIRST GERMAN EDITION (abridged)

The *Atlas of the Anatomy* of the Dog was conceived as a compendium and at the same time as an introduction to the topographical anatomical dissection as well as for teaching. The subject matter of anatomy was prepared from a topographical point of view with separation into systems. To do that, the osteology, myology, angiology, neurology and splanchnology of the different parts of the body were dealt with in sequence in their reciprocal relationship to one another and demonstrated by topographical colored plates with complementary schematic diagrams. The methods of presentation emphasize the mutual topographical relationships of the vessels and nerves considered, laying stress on their nomenclatural agreement. In that way, the concern for the multiplicity, the breadth, and the complexity of the material should be minimized. The concept chosen here, with its close relationship of content and apposition of illustration and pertinent description, has the advantage of being able to deal with the essential in the smallest space.

The present book offers to the students a clearly arranged illustrative material and an abbreviated reading supplementing textbook study and classroom material as well as an aid for review, especially for preparation for examinations. For the practising veterinarian, it is drawn up as a source of quick information and to refresh and deepen what was previously learned. The breadth, division and sequence of the subject matter according to the preceding are coordinated with the topographical dissection that is offered to the students at the Free University of Berlin as the teaching program in their first semester of study. Upon the foundation achieved, the subsequent study of comparative and clinically applied anatomy is con-tinued. Topographical anatomy is the foundation and the key to understanding the associated medicine. It is of special value to the surgeon and pathologist.

Professor Fritz Preuss introduced the whole-animal topographical anatomy in Berlin, and his dissection instructions directed the way for teaching up to the dras-tinc shortening and repositioning of the dissection exercises. The successful and exacting method of dissection with the short time available places high demands on the students and requires a multisided support by the instructors. With its true to nature rendition of areas of dissection with accompanying text, the present atlas should serve for this purpose also. Instructions for dissection of the illustrated preparation and guidance to the person carrying out the exercise were placed at the beginning of the described part. Structures to be dissected are specially emphasized in the text by boldface print. To keep the space limitations, anatomical variations are given less attention. The current Nomina Anatomica Veterinaria (HOLZHAUSEN, Vienna 1973) was utilized, which also holds in the main for the applied abbreviations. Moreover, in the written material only vertebrae and nerve branches were abbreviated (*e.g.*: VL 1 for the first lumbar vertebra; nL 1vl for the ventrolateral branch of the first lumbar nerve). In the legends of the figures and the tabular compositions, owing to the limitations of space even more extensive, otherwise uncommon, abbreviations had to be used. Suggestions and wishes of the students, for example with respect to preparing the tables for special myology and for anatomical terms were largely considered.

Dissections from the anatomical collection of the Department of Anatomy, Histology and Embryology (Institute for Veterinary Anatomy, Histology and Embryology) of the Free University of Berlin served as models for the figures. These specimens were prepared by the technical staff of the depart-ment, Mr. Seifert, Mr. Dressel, and Mr. Schneider.

Berlin, summer 1983   The author

INTRODUCTION TO ANATOMY

The term *anatomy* stems from the Greek word, 'anatemnein' which means to dissect, to cut apart. The important anatomist Hyrtl spoke consistently also of the art of dissection. The original meaning is true even today; although the term has gained a wider meaning. Modern anatomy is not limited to mere description but emphasizes the interrelations between form and function as well as the application of anatomical knowledge in the clinic. Then as today the student gains most of his knowledge by dissection of the animal body in the laboratory, where he lays bare the 'naked truth' *(Nudas veritas)*. This practice also serves to obtain a necessary finger-dexterity, which in later professional life, in the first place in surgery, is of immeasurable value. Beyond that there are hardly any limits to investigation by enthusiastic dissection. Even the very best anatomical collection of outstanding demonstration-dissections cannot replace practical work in the laboratory, but can however indeed make it easier and more efficient. The thorough study of anatomical preparations is indispensable like the industrious use of textbooks and atlases. All of these aids are more important today than ever since there is much less time available for practical work in the laboratory than formerly. Shortening the teaching time allotted to anatomy in favor of newer disciplines was unavoidable.

Anatomical study is, unlike any other basic discipline, important in learning the language of medicine, the **terminology**. Many terms for diseases and methods of treatment have their origin in anatomical terms. Centuries-long research and description brought an unforeseen abundance of synonyms. The function of the international nomenclature commission has been to thin out the jungle of terms and to publish a recognized list of official terms with useful synonyms.

In its entirety, anatomy is subdivided into macroscopic (gross) anatomy, microscopic anatomy and developmental anatomy. However, the areas of anatomy flow together without boundary, forming a unit, an understanding constantly and forcefully advocated by the important Berlin veterinary anatomist and, at an earlier time, the professorial chair of our department, Professor Preuss. The oldest and most encompassing area is macroscopic anatomy, often placed equal to the term *anatomy*. Where the accessories to observation in macroscopic anatomy, the bare eye and the dissection hand lens no longer reach, it passes over into the area of microscopic anatomy (histology and cytology), to which the microscope serves as accessory. The boundary between macroscopic and microscopic anatomy is also called mesoscopy, which is gaining more and more in significance. The latter area deals with the same material and pursues the same goals; it is only the technique that is different. The third area, embryology, is concerned with ontogenesis (development of the individual) before and after birth and, in addition to embryological methods, applies also macroscopic, microscopic and mesoscopic methods.

Like the remaining disciplines, macroscopic anatomy can be presented from different points of view with emphasis on special areas of greater difficulty. In so doing, the basic facts remain of course unchanged.

Systematic, descriptive anatomy describes the animal body with all its parts as systems of structure and organ-systems, strictly divided from one another and therefore without attention to their natural interdependence. Expansive descriptions treat many particulars and allow sometimes the view to the important to be missed; nevertheless they are a necessary prerequisite to the remaining, subsequent kinds of observations to which the descriptive anatomy has led.

Systematic anatomy can be subdivided further into general and special anatomy.

General anatomy treats of facts that are generally valid for the entire system of structure or the organ-system.

Special anatomy provides special data for these structure- and organ-systems that hold for individual structures, as for one bone.

Comparative anatomy emphasizes anatomical correlations, similarities and variations between the individual animal species and human beings. Comparisons of anatomy between the individual species are very often informative and helpful for homology and determining the function of anatomical structure. Already Goethe utilized principles of comparative anatomy to good advantage with the discovery of the incisive bone of human beings. This bone occurs regularly in our domestic animals and only occasionally in human beings. With his study of the human skull he encountered a specimen with a developed incisive bone. It was by comparison with the animal skull that he was able to identify the bone and establish its homology.

Topographical anatomy emphasizes the varying position-relationship of anatomical structures and underlines the areas of application for clinical medicine. The relationship of anatomical structures is analyzed step by step and in doing so the whole structural plan of the body is regarded.

Applied anatomy is directed clinically and emphasizes the relationship of anatomical structures from which treatments or diseases of animals can be determined or explained. In that way not only interdisciplinary cooperation and interest for the veterinary profession are promoted but also the learning of anatomy is made easier.

The anatomy of the living dog is undoubtedly a significant part of the whole of anatomy. It presents the body in its natural condition. In that way a significant completion and an adjustment for unavoidable disadvantage becomes imperative in the remaining subjects of the whole of anatomy, which must tolerate postmortem changes such as variations in color, consistency and character as well as artificial changes resulting from fixation. Anatomy of the living dog cannot be given attention here for several reasons. It is adaped even less for rendering in a book, but can be offered to the students better and more successfully in an exercise under the instruction of a clinically experienced anatomist.

Radiographic anatomy and sonography are directly connected to the clinic. In the teaching of anatomy, the first experiences are obtained in analysis of radiographs of the normal animal body. This experience will be utilized and considerably supplemented in the total associated area of study. Presentations of abnormal or even pathological changes should awaken the interest and accordingly add 'spice' to the teaching of anatomy.

The atlas of anatomy presented here is adapted in special measure to significantly combine and coordinate the different methods of presenting anatomy and the manner of viewing it. The textual part can be presented in a very compressed form since the different anatomical circumstances can be 'read off' from time to time from the adjacent color-plate. Beyond that, a good topographical color-plate presents an ideal introduction for topographical dissection, which is then completed only by brief remarks. Also the requisites of comparative veterinary anatomy are taken into account in this atlas insofar as the simply structured (from many points of view) canine body is set out as the 'cornerstone.' Building upon this knowledge, the more complicated (from many points of view) anatomy of the remaining domestic animals can be comprehended from the aspect of comparative anatomy.

Art and anatomy with their mutual interrelations are forcefully impressed on us with each visit to a museum. The artist is inspired by the corporeal beauty, and teachers and students of anatomy enjoy and profit from the talent and painstaking detail in the artistic presentation. Gifted with genius were realized the claims of Leonardo da Vinci, whose abundant anatomical drawings came about after basic studies of anatomy. Aristotle published among other things an anatomical description of senile sexual reversal in the bird as well of the horse hoof in regard to founder. What fascination of anatomy passes over to art, Rembrandt immortalized in his work 'The anatomy lesson of Dr. Nicolaes Tulp.' The greats of world history gifted with genius like Aristotle, Leonardo da Vinci and Goethe show proof of their enthusiasm for anatomy with anatomical illustrations, descriptions and research results. To Goethe's credit was the promotion of educational art and the introduction of plastic wax models in Germany, to which he, himself, was inspired during his journey to Italy, especially in Florence. The good qualities of wax models, which is true to an equal measure for well done true-to-nature illustrations, Goethe expressed in his novel 'Wilhelm Meisters Wanderjahre' with the following excellent formulation: 'If you concede that most physicians and surgeons retain in their minds only a general impression of the dissected human body and believe that to satisfy the purpose; so such models will certainly suffice, which refresh in his mind again little by little pictures that are fading and actively retain for him just the necessary.' His investigative mind held Goethe, who with his discovery of the human incisive bone felt 'unspeakable joy.'

TOPOGRAPHICAL ANATOMY
CHAPTER 1: SURFACE OF THE BODY AND AXIAL SKELETON
1. DIVISION OF THE ANIMAL BODY

a) SUBDIVISION OF THE BODY

The longitudinal lines and planes of the body are useful for the orientation of the body and of the body surface. The **dorsal (a) and ventral midline (b)** are the dorsal and ventral median lines of the body, respectively.

The **median plane (A)** is the plane between the two lines mentioned above. It divides the body into right and left halves. **Sagittal (paramedian) planes (B)** are adjacent planes parallel and lateral to the median plane. They divide the body longitudinally, but into unequal parts. **Transverse planes (C)** are planes that divide the body transversely and are perpendicular to the median and sagittal planes. **Dorsal planes (D)** lie parallel to the dorsal body surface. They divide the body perpendicular to the longitudinal (median and paramedian planes) and transverse planes. In that view, two symmetrical body sides appear and it is for that reason that dorsal planes are also called bilateral planes.

b) TERMS THAT DESCRIBE THE DIRECTION AND TOPOGRAPHICAL RELATIONS OF ORGANS derive partially from body parts, e.g., in direction toward the tail (**caudal** −c), partially from landmarks of the body surface, e.g., parallel to the median plane (**sagittal** −d) or designate with respect to hollow organs *external* or *internal*. Furthermore terms are used as left (*sinister*) and right (*dexter*), short (*brevis*) and long (*longus*) or deep (*profundus*) and superficial (*superficialis*), longitudinal (*longitudinalis*) or transverse (*transversus*) as well as lateral (*lateralis*) and toward the median plane (*medialis*). The term **cranial (e)**, in a direction toward the head, cannot be applied in the head region. Here the term **rostral** is used (f, in a direction toward the tip of the nose). The term **dorsal (g)** relates to the 'back' or *dorsum*

of the body. It may also be used with respect to the proximal parts of the limbs; but has a different meaning on the limb extremities. The term **ventral**, in a direction toward the belly (*venter*), may be used on the proximal parts of the limb, but is not used on the free part of the limbs. The terms **proximal** (i, toward the attached end) and **distal** (m, toward the free end) are related to the axis of the body (vertebral column and spinal cord with the origin of spinal nerves). On the limbs, from the carpus distally, the term **palmar** (l, the surface of the manus that faces caudally in the normal standing attitude) is employed; from the tarsus distally (**m**, the surface of the pes that faces caudally in the normal standing attitude of the animal), the term **plantar**. The term **dorsal** is utilized alike on the thoracic limb from the carpus distally and on the pelvic limb from the tarsus distally. It refers to surface of the manus and pes that is cranial in the normal standing attitude of the animal. Terms like **abaxial** (n, away from the axis) and **axial** (o, toward the axis) are related to the central axis of the hand (manus) or foot (pes), in which the axis lies between the third and fourth digits. In front (anterior), behind (posterior), above (superior) and below (inferior) are terms often used in human anatomy and refer to the human body in the normal upright attitude. To avoid misunderstanding, these terms are not applied to the quadruped animal body. Their use in veterinary anatomy is restricted to certain areas of the head; e.g., upper and lower eyelids, anterior and posterior surfaces of the eye.

c) PARTS OF THE BODY AND BODY REGIONS subdivide the body, including the surface of the body. Parts of the body are head and trunk with neck, rump, and tail, as well as the limbs. The body regions divide the surface of the body and can be subdivided into subregions. In the latter case, they appear indented in the following table.

REGIONS OF THE BODY

Regions of the cranium
1 Frontal region
2 Parietal region
3 Occipital region
4 Temporal region
5 Auricular region

Regions of the face
6 Nasal region
6' Dorsal nasal region
6" Lateral nasal region
6''' Region of the naris
7 Oral region
7' Superior labial region
7" Inferior labial region
8 Mental region
9 Orbital region
9' upper palpebral
9" lower palpebral
10 Zygomatic region
11 Infraorbital region
12 Region of the temporomandibular articulation
13 Masseteric region
14 Buccal region
15 Maxillary region
16 Mandibular region
17 Intermandibular region

Regions of the neck
18 Dorsal neck region
19 Lateral neck region
20 Parotid region
21 Pharyngeal region
22 Ventral neck region

22' Laryngeal region
22" Tracheal region

Regions of the dorsum
23 Thoracic vertebral region
23' Interscapular region
24 Lumbar region

Pectoral regions
25 Presternal region
26 Sternal region
27 Scapular region
28 Costal region
29 Cardiac region

Regions of the abdomen
30 Cranial abdominal region
30' Hypochondriac region
30" Xiphoid region
31 Middle abdominal region
31' Lateral abdominal region
31" Paralumbar fossa
31''' Umbilical region
32 Caudal abdominal region
32' Inguinal region
32" Pubic region and preputial region

Pelvic regions
33 Sacral region
34 Gluteal region
35 Region of the tuber coxae
36 Ischiorectal fossa
37 Region of the tuber ischiadicum
38 Caudal region (tail region)
38' Region of the root of the tail

39 Perineal region
39' Anal region
39" Urogenital region
40 Scrotal region

Regions of the thoracic limb
41 Region of the humeral joint
42 Axillary region
42' Axillary fossa
43 Brachial region
44 Tricipital region
45 Cubital region
46 Region of the olecranon
47 Antebrachial region
48 Carpal region
49 Metacarpal region
50 Phalangeal region
(region of the digits,
digital region)

Regions of the pelvic limb
51 Region of the hip joint
52 Region of the thigh
53 Genual region (region of the knee, region of the stifle joint)
53' Patellar region
54 Popliteal region
55 Region of the crus
(region of the leg)
56 Tarsal region
57 Calcaneal region
58 Metatarsal region
59 Phalangeal region (region of the digits, digital region)

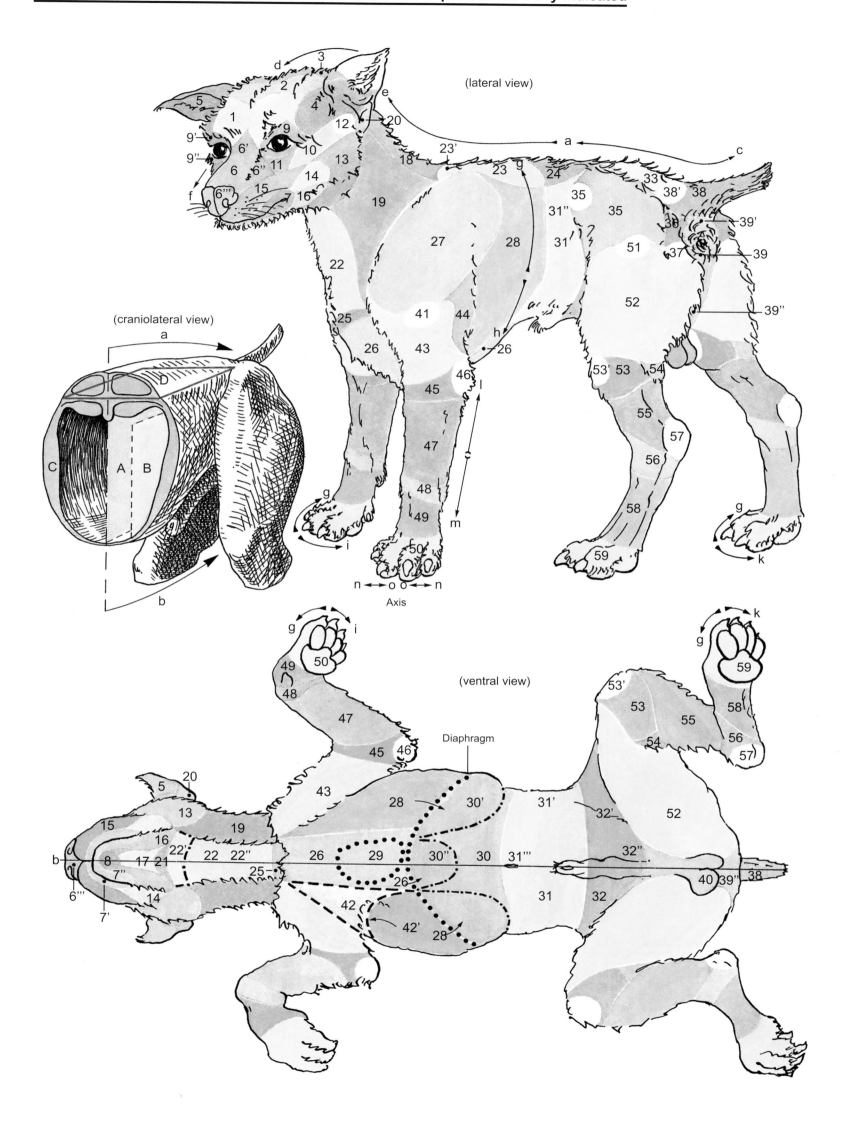

(lateral view)

(craniolateral view)

(ventral view)

Diaphragm

Axis

2. THE SKIN (COMMON INTEGUMENT)

1 a) The **SKIN** forms the external surface of the body and consists of two layers: I. an epithelial layer designated *epidermis* and II. a connective tissue layer designated *dermis* or *corium*. The dermis rests upon an underlying layer of connective tissue, the subcutaneous layer or *subcutis (Tela subcutanea)*. The latter consists of a fatty part, the *panniculus adiposus*, and a supporting fibrous part that, together, constitute the superficial fascia.

I. The **epidermis (1)** is made up of a stratified squamous epithelium that is cornified (keratinized) at its surface. Thickness and degree of keratinization depend on the mechanical stress to which this layer is subject. The epidermis is composed of a deep, still living, layer, (**stratum germinativum = basal layer, −27**) which, by mitotic division, furnishes cell replacement, a **spinous layer (26)**, a cornifying, dying layer (**stratum granulosum, −25**) as well as **2** cornified cell layers, **stratum lucidum (24)** and **stratum corneum (23)**. In addition to the epidermal cells, there are melanocytes, LANGERHANS' cells, and MERKEL'S tactile discs, especially in the stratum germinativum.

'Horn' is cornified epidermis and is of varying quality in the different regions of the body. On the pads and in other regions of the skin there is soft horn. Hard horn is found at the claw. In the skin and at the pads, the cornified cells are shed as scales owing to reduced adhesion of membrane coating materials. At the same time, because of good adhesion as a solid mass, the **horn of the claws** remains restored by distal growth **conical**. The individual horn cell of the claw is distinctly harder than that of the skin. In areas where soft horn is formed, the epidermis exhibits a stratum granulosum be-tween the stratum spinosum and the cornified layers. The stratum granulosum is so-named because of the keratohyalin granules that it contains. The proteins within this layer of cells coat and 'glue' the keratin filaments together. At individual sites additionally a stratum lucidum occurs. It consists of young, not yet differentiated, cornifying cells, the cytoplasm of which appears somewhat transparent when examined under the microscope, hence the name stratum lucidum. In the areas of formation of hard horn, these layers are absent, so that the cells of the stratum spinosum cornify directly without intervening strata granulosum and lucidum.

The **function of the epidermis** consists of the replacement of cornified cells as a protection from radiation (radiation absorbing pigments; see histology), from the loss and entrance of water into the body, from the entrance of parasites and for protection against trauma. With traumatic injury to the skin, healing is furthered by covering the exposed dermis by epidermal cells as soon as possible.

3 II. The **dermis or corium (6)** consists of a thin, loosely arranged **papillary layer (2)**, the papillae of which are seated in corresponding depressions of the epidermis, and a dense **reticular layer (7)**. The papillary layer contains mainly loosely arranged collagenous fibrils. The reticular layer consists of a plexus of coarse nondistensible collagenic fibers with a predominant course direction. Elastic fibers are present in both layers and function to restore the typical texture of the tissue following lacerations or other distortion of the skin (with respect to the cells that are found here, especially fibrocytes, fibroblasts, mast cells, plasma cells, macrophages and pigment cells, see histology).

4 The **subcutis (10)** *(Tela subcutanea)* consists mainly of loose connective and adipose tissue. It is penetrated by connective tissue cords that fix the skin to the underlying fascia or periosteum. The panniculus adiposus is the layer of fat tissue within the subcutis.

Functionally, the subcutis with its subcutaneous fat tissue serves as a cushioning tissue, serves for the storage of calories and water as well as thermoregulation. Its loose connective tissue functions as a gliding layer. Where the subcutis is lacking (lips, cheeks, and eyelids) this gliding function is lacking and the striated musculature ends here directly in the dermis.

The **blood supply** of the skin is provided by larger arteries and veins of the subcutis that, owing to the mobility of the skin, have a tortuous course. They send branches to the dermis that form here two networks. The **arterial network of the dermis (9)** is located at the boundary with the subcutis and the **subpapillary network (3)** lies between the papillary and reticular layers and gives off subepidermal capillary loops into the papillary body. The corresponding venous plexuses have a comparable location. A further subfascial vascular plexus joins the blood supply of the subcutis. The blood flow can be cut short by **arteriovenous anastomoses (4)**, thus avoiding the capillary bed, and in this way the vascularization of the skin is regulated. The papillary layer is especially well supplied with blood. These vessels dilate in order to give off heat and constrict to conserve body temperature. In this way they function like the sweat glands in thermoregulation. The venous plexuses also function as a place to store blood.

The **lymphatic supply** is by lymph capillary networks that begin subepidermally and invest the hair follicles and skin glands.

The **nerve supply** is by sensory and sympathetic neurons (sympathetic nerve plexuses invest the blood vessels and function to regulate the blood pressure and in thermoregulation). The skin can be considered as the largest sensory organ of the body. Numerous **nerve terminals (16)** and terminal end corpuscles (*e.g.,* **MEISSNER'S tactile discs, −17**, and **VATER-PACINIAN lamellar corpuscles, −22**) serve as receptors for sensory stimuli. With loss of their myelin sheaths, free nerve endings penetrate the epidermis at particular sites of the body and serve to mediate the sensation of pain.

b) The **HAIRS** cover nearly the entire body surface, except the *planum nasale*, anus, vulvar lips and limb pads. Hairs are cornified filiform structures that are formed by the skin. The hair is subdivided into the **shaft (15)**, which projects beyond the surface of the skin, the **root (21)**, which is obliquely oriented within the dermis and has at its proximal end an expanded part, the **hair bulb (8)**. Hair root and hair bulb are in a divided epithelial root sheath (*Vagina epithelialis radicularis*). The outer part of the sheath is continuous with the superficial epidermis. Its inner part cornifies above the mouth of the **sebaceous gland (18)** and will be shed. The connective tissue root sheath (*Vagina dermalis radicularis*) is continuous with the surrounding connective tissue. The epidermal and dermal root sheaths together with the bulb of the hair constitute the hair follicle. The parts of the hair are **medulla (12)**, the **cortex (13)** and the **superficial hair cuticle (14)**, which consists of thin scale-like cornified cells and, the same as the medulla, is used for forensic species identification and individual diagnostic procedures. The **arrector pili muscle (5)** terminates below the mouth of the sebaceous gland, attaching obliquely to the dermal sheath of the root of the hair. Its contraction results in erection of the hair (in human beings, this brings about the phenomenon of 'goose pimples'). Contraction of the arrector pili muscle compresses the sebaceous glands and, in erecting the hair, increases the air space between the hairs and the skin sur-face for thermo-isolation.

The **hair coat** depends on the breed and is characterized by the individual and group-like arrangement of the hairs, the different portions of the individual hair types (lead hairs, guard hairs, wool hairs) as well as by the density, length and color of the hairs. There are basically three types of hairs:

5 The **'lead' hair** or 'main' hair is long, stiff, and slightly curved. It is independent of other hairs and in the dog occurs only rarely. **Guard hairs** are shorter than the lead hair, arched near the tip and thickened. Both lead and guard hair types form the **hair coat (Capilli)**. The third and shortest type of hair is the wool hair. It is very thin, pliable and in its course slightly or strongly undulated. Guard and wool hairs pass in a bundle or tuft together from a compound hair follicle, in which case one guard hair is surrounded by the six to twelve wool hairs that accompany it.

5 The **wool hairs (11)** predominate in the coat of the puppy. In most canine breeds they lie under the hair coat and only in a few breeds such as the Puli and Commodore, do they project above the hair coat and form a superficial 'wool coat.'

Sinus or tactile hairs (19) are remarkably long, special forms of hair in the vicinity of the opening of the mouth (*Rima oris*). To receive tactile stimuli, the root of the hair is ensheathed by a **blood sinus (20)** that is contacted by numerous sensory nerve endings. Owing to the great lever action of this long hair even the finest tactile stimuli result in stimulation of this receptor.

The length of the hairs varies considerably and is dependent on breed. In the ancestors of the dog, who lived in the wild, the longest hairs are found on the dorsum and the shorter ones on the belly and head. But this pattern is mostly lost with domestication. In wild Canidae, the thickness of the hairs increases toward the belly (thickness is about 0.1 mm). The color of the hair is effected by the melanin content of the cornified cells as well as the inter- and intracellular air bubbles, especially of the medullary cells.

The **direction of the hairs** characterizes the coat. That part of the coat in which the hairs have a uniform direction is called the *Flumina pilorum*. In a *vortex*, the hairs are arranged divergently or convergently with respect to a central point. By the crossing of converging lines of hairs, hair 'crosses' are formed.

Common integument

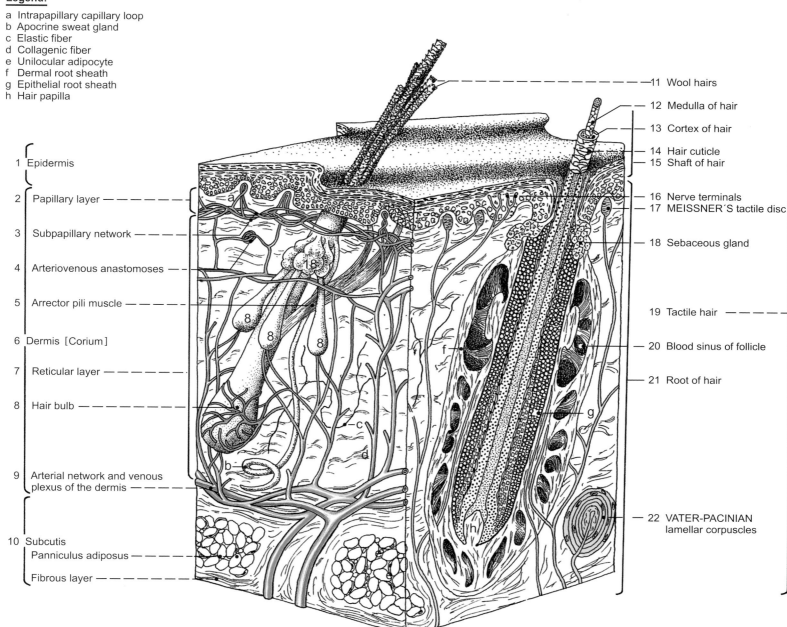

Legend:
a Intrapapillary capillary loop
b Apocrine sweat gland
c Elastic fiber
d Collagenic fiber
e Unilocular adipocyte
f Dermal root sheath
g Epithelial root sheath
h Hair papilla

1 Epidermis

2 Papillary layer

3 Subpapillary network

4 Arteriovenous anastomoses

5 Arrector pili muscle

6 Dermis [Corium]

7 Reticular layer

8 Hair bulb

9 Arterial network and venous plexus of the dermis

10 Subcutis
Panniculus adiposus
Fibrous layer

11 Wool hairs
12 Medulla of hair
13 Cortex of hair
14 Hair cuticle
15 Shaft of hair
16 Nerve terminals
17 MEISSNER'S tactile disc
18 Sebaceous gland
19 Tactile hair
20 Blood sinus of follicle
21 Root of hair
22 VATER-PACINIAN lamellar corpuscles

Epidermis

Epidermis of digital pad

Epidermis of wall of claw

23 Stratum corneum
24 Stratum lucidum
25 Stratum granulosum
26 Spinous layer
27 Stratum germinativum

5

3. CUTANEOUS GLANDS, MODIFICATIONS OF THE SKIN, DIGITAL END-ORGANS

a) The **CUTANEOUS GLANDS** comprise sebaceous and sweat glands as well as the mammary gland, which is a modified sweat gland.

1 I. The **sebaceous glands** (see p. 4) open into the hair follicles and are present at a few sites of the body independent of the presence of hairs as at the transition of the skin to the cutaneous mucous membrane (lips, anus). Sebaceous glands are lobular. The peripheral cells have a high rate of mitosis and the daughter cells are pushed centrally to the lumen of the gland. Here the enlarged and aging cells break down (holocrine secretion) and the sebum thus liberated reaches the lumen of the gland. It passes by way of a short excretory duct to the lumen of the hair follicle and thus to the skin. Sebum makes the skin soft and pliable and gives the hairs a natural sheen.

II. The **sweat or sudoriferous glands** are classified as merocrine (eccrine) and apocrine glands (odor glands). This classification was based on a supposed apocrine secretion of the (apocrine) odor glands; however, this was subsequently disproven. Both types of sweat glands secrete according to the merocrine (eccrine) manner of secretion (see histology).

The **merocrine sweat glands** are usually coiled, unbranched, tubular glands. They occur in the dog only on the pads of the limbs (see below; some authors consider these glands to be apocrine sweat glands). In human beings, real merocrine (eccrine) sweat glands are present in large areas of the skin surface.

Apocrine sweat glands or odor glands (see p. 4) are present over wide areas of the skin surface, but they are comparatively underdeveloped. These tubular glands open usually into the hair follicle. Their thick secretion has an alkaline reaction and is responsible for the individual species odor. In man, the glands are well developed but limited to a few regions of the body: anus, vulva, axilla.

III. **Special modifications of the skin** occur as the glands of the external acoustic meatus, the circumanal glands, glands of the paranal sinus ('anal sac') and glands of the dorsal tail organ, glands of the eyelids and the mammary glands.

2 The **ceruminal glands** of the external acoustic meatus are mainly sebaceous glands with fewer apocrine sweat glands. Their brown, oily secretion is called cerumen.

3 The **circumanal glands** surround the anus in the hairless or nearly hairless region of the anal cutaneous area. In the dog, we are dealing with modified sebaceous glands; in other domesticated animals, with modified apocrine sweat glands. Superficially located individual glands open into the hair follicles. Deep glands are also called hepatoid glands as their secretory cells appear similar to hepatocytes. The glands lack an excretory duct and their function is unclear.

4 The **glands of the wall of the paranal sinus** (see clinical-functional anatomy, 56.5) are apocrine sweat glands and sebaceous glands. The paranal sinus is commonly termed the 'anal sac.'

5 The **dorsal caudal (tail) organ** is composed of sebaceous and apocrine glands and is described more fully in the clinical-functional anatomy (6.5).

Glands of the eyelids are described in the clinical-functional anatomy (see also 118.1)

Mammary gland; see p. 32.

b) **SKIN MODIFICATIONS** are the nasal plane and the limb pads: carpal pad, metacarpal/metatarsal pad, digital pads.

I. The **nasal plane** (see p. 98), depending on breed, varies from unpigmented to its being strongly pigmented. The dermis forms distinct papillae. The epidermis is strikingly thin, and its superficial, cornified layer (stratum corneum) consists of hard 'horn' (hard cornified epidermis) that exhibits a polygonal pattern. The surface pattern is individually specific and for this reason serves to identify the individual animal. Glands are absent. The nose of the dog is kept moist by lacrimal fluid (see p. 98) and the secretion of the lateral nasal gland, which is located deeply in the maxillary recess of the nasal cavity. The evaporation of the fluid lowers the temperature of the nasal plane, which ordinarily feels cold to the touch (hence the saying, 'cold as a dog's nose').

6 II. The **pads** of the dog are the **digital pads (14)** at the level of the distal interphalangeal joints, the **metacarpal (13) or metatarsal pad** at the level of the metacarpophalangeal and metatarsophalangeal joints and the **carpal pad (12)** that is laterodistal at the carpus. The thick subcutis of the pads has much fat tissue und contains sweat glands. It is subdivided into compartments by radiating strands of collagenous and elastic fibers and is very sensitive (painful) if swollen due to increased tissue pressure when inflamed. The connec-

tive tissue strands radiate from the dermis of the pad into the subcutis and fix the pad to the underlying fascia and to the skeleton. Well-developed **connective tissue bands (Tractus tori —15)** are present in the metacarpal and metatarsal pads. They fix the pads proximally to the metacarpal or metatarsal bones, respectively. The dermis has very firm connective tissue bundles and forms a very high papillary body with conical papillae. The epidermis of the pad is up to 2 mm in thickness and forms corresponding depressions in the soft horn (soft cornified epidermis). The pads are richly supplied with blood and lymph vessels as well as nerves.

Cutis of pad

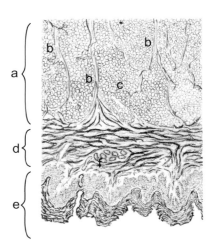

Legend :

a   Subcutaneous tissue of pad [digital cushion] :
b   Retinacula
c   Panniculus adiposus
d   Dermis [Corium] of pad
e   Epidermis of pad
f   Merocrine sweat gland

c) The **DIGITAL END-ORGAN** is the bony end of the digit invested by a highly modified cutis (skin). Except for the digital pad, a subcutis is lacking. The dermis is developed in the form of papillae, villi or laminae or it has a smooth surface. The inner surface of the epidermis has a corresponding configuration: depressions that seat the papillae and villi, narrow furrows adaped to the laminae, or a smooth surface where it contacts the smooth surface of the dermis.

7 The cornified epidermis of the **claw (Unguicula)** is conical in form and invests the **unguicular process (11)**. Dermis and epidermis are segmentally similarly differentiated as on the fingernail of the human being and on the equine hoof. Both, dermis and epidermis, are adapted to one another like the patrix (stamp = dermis) to the matrix (impression = epidermis).

The bony unguicular crest is overlain basally by a prominence of the skin, the **vallum (7)**. The external lamina of the vallum is haired; the unhaired inner lamella is comparable to the limbus (periople) of the horse. It forms a soft horn (**Eponychium, —1**) over the hard cornified epidermis of the claw. The eponychium corresponds to the periople of the horse and, like the periople, is worn off far proximal to the distal end of the claw. (On the human fingernail, the soft eponychium is removed at the manicure.)

In the depth of the unguicular groove is the fold that corresponds to the coronary part of the equine hoof. Its dermis bears **papillae (10)**. Its covering epidermis produces a tubular horn that, as a **mesonychium (2)**, provides a considerable part of the claw. Dorsal on the unguicular process there is a smooth **dorsal swelling of the dermis (Dorsum dermale —8)**, that is particular to the digital end-organ of the dog and that, according to our investigations, is not comparable to the coronary part of the equine hoof. On the epidermis covering it, the **dorsal horn of the wall (dorsal hyponychium —3)** is formed. In the lateral region of the unguicular process lamellae are present, **dermal lamellae (9)** and correspondingly formed noncornified epidermal lamellae that form the lateral wall horn (**Hyponychium laterale, —4**), which is simply layered and forms the internal lining of the conical claw horn.

Palmar (plantar) on the unguicular process is the solear part on which the dermis bears distinct villi. Here, tubular **solear horn (5)** is formed, the cells of which undergo substantial desquamation.

Around the tip of the unguicular process there is present a soft **terminal horn (Hyponychium terminale, —6)** that fills out the distal part of the conical claw horn and serves thus as a 'filling' horn.

Claw and digital pad

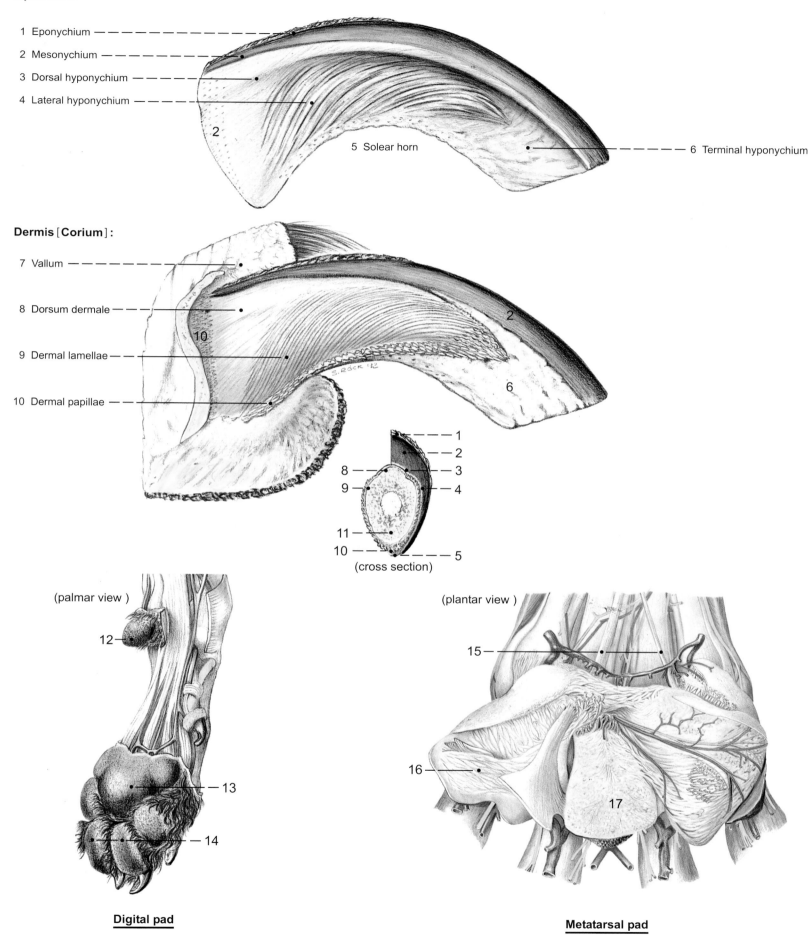

Epidermis:

1 Eponychium
2 Mesonychium
3 Dorsal hyponychium
4 Lateral hyponychium

2

5 Solear horn

6 Terminal hyponychium

Dermis [Corium]:

7 Vallum
8 Dorsum dermale
9 Dermal lamellae
10 Dermal papillae

10

2

6

1
2
3
4
5

8
9

11
10

(cross section)

(palmar view)

12

13

14

Digital pad

(plantar view)

15

16

17

Metatarsal pad

Legend :

11 Unguicular process
12 Carpal pad
13 Metacarpal pad

14 Digital pads
15 Tractus of
   metatarsal pad

Subcutaneous tissue of pad:
16 Retinacula
17 Panniculus adiposus (Fat pad)

(see pp. 19, 81, 83)

4. VERTEBRAL COLUMN AND THORAX

The vertebrae are studied individually and on the mounted skeleton to obtain a total overview of the normal S-shaped curvature with its lordoses (ventral convexities) and kyphoses (ventral concavities). From a forensic view, particular attention is placed on the identification of individual vertebrae, for which reason comparison of the different segments of the vertebral column is done.

1 a) The **VERTEBRAL COLUMN** encloses and protects the spinal cord. It has a supporting function with respect to the statics and dynamics of the animal's body. For that, stability is assured by the individual vertebrae, and elasticity as well as pliability by the intervertebral symphyses and the vertebral joints.

The vertebral column consists of seven cervical vertebrae (vC 1 – 7), thirteen thoracic (vT 1 – 13), seven lumbar (vL 1 – 7), three sacral (vS 1 – 3), which are fused to form the sacrum, and about twenty caudal (coccygeal) vertebrae (vCy 1 – 20).

2 I. The **vertebrae** (see text-illustration) consist of three basic constituents: body and its parts, arch and processes, that are modified in different ways according to the functional requirements of the particular region.

3 The **body of the vertebra (1)** has a **ventral crest (2)**, (distinct in the region of the cervical vertebral column) and **cranial (3)** and **caudal (4)** extremities. On the thoracic vertebrae, both the **caudal (5)** and **cranial costal foveae (6)** form a common articular facet for the head (*Capitulum*) of the rib (see below).

4 The **vertebral foramen (7)** is the space enclosed by the body and arch. The vertebral canal is formed by the serial vertebral foramina and the soft tissues extending between adjacent vertebral arches and bodies. It contains the spinal cord with its cauda equina.

5 The **arch of the vertebra (8)** is made up of a pedicle basally and a flattened lamina dorsally. The **intervertebral foramina (9)** are bounded by the **cranial (10)** and **caudal (11)** vertebral notches of the vertebra of the same and preceding segments. Excepting the first cervical nerve (see below), these foramina are passages for the spinal nerves.

Of the processes of the vertebrae, the **spinous process (12)** is most distinct (exceptions are the first cervical vertebra and the caudal vertebrae). The **transverse processes (13)** are well developed on the cervical and lumbar vertebrae. On the thoracic vertebrae, they have a **costal fovea (14)** that bears an articular facet for the costal tubercle (see below). From the first to the sixth cervical vertebrae there are **transverse foramina (15)** at the base of the transverse processes, which altogether form the transverse canal that transmits the vertebral artery, vein and nerve. The **cranial articular processes (16)** and the

6 **caudal articular processes (17)** form synovial joints between the vertebrae. A **costal process (18)** is present on the 3ʳᵈ – 6ᵗʰ cervical vertebrae as the ventrocranial extremity of the transverse process, which is bifurcate in this region. In the lumbar vertebral column the ends of the transverse processes represent costal processes that are remnants of the ribs, and can develop to form lumbar 'ribs.' An **accessory process (19)** is lacking or poorly developed in the caudal lumbar part of the lumbar vertebral column. In the cranial lumbar region it is developed as an independent process. At the transition to the thoracic vertebral column, it passes onto the caudal contour of the transverse process and no longer stands independently. The **mamillary process (20)** of the lumbar vertebrae is expressed in the cranial articular process (mamiloarticular process) and changes its position at the transition to the thoracic vertebral column, passing onto the transverse process, actually to the cranial contour of the transverse process. **Hemal processes (21)** are developed from the

7 4ᵗʰ caudal vertebra and become gradually indistinct caudally. On the 4ᵗʰ to the 7ᵗʰ or 8ᵗʰ caudal vertebra, they may unite to form a **hemal arch (22)**.

The interarcuate spaces are dorsal and, in life, closed off by the interarcuate ligaments. The **lumbosacral space (23)** and the **sacrococcygeal (sacrocaudal) space (24)** are especially wide and of significance in performing epidural anesthesia. The atlanto-occipital space is suitable for tapping the subarachnoid space, which is filled with cerebrospinal fluid.

Special features are present on the following cervical vertebrae: The **first cervical vertebra (atlas, −25)** has a broad-surfaced **lateral process (26)**, also designated the wing of the atlas (*Ala atlantis*). The **alar notch (27)** calar foramen of other domestic mammals) is cranial at the attachment of the wing of the atlas to the lateral mass (see below) and is occupied by the ventral branch of the first cervical nerve. Contrary to the other spinal nerves, the first cervical nerve does not exit the vertebral canal by an intervertebral foramen but by the **lateral vertebral foramen (28)**. The vertebral foramen of the atlas is also different in that it is bounded dorsally by a **dorsal arch (29)**, ventrally by a **ventral arch (30)**. The two arches are joined laterally by bone designated the lateral mass (*Massa lateralis*). The atlas is the only vertebra to have a ventral arch (30) in the place of the body. This is due to the caudal shift of a great part of the embryonal primordium of its vertebral body to form the dens of the axis. The **second cervical vertebra, the axis (31)**, for this reason contains

in its **dens (32)** the displaced part of the body of the atlas. The last cervical vertebra differs from the other cervical vertebra by its large spinous process, its caudal costal foveae for the first ribs and by the absence of the transverse foramen.

Lumbar vertebra

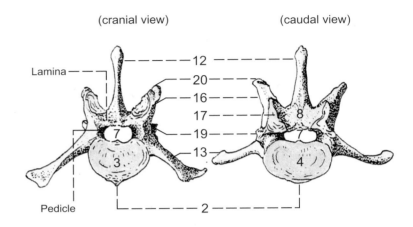

(cranial view)   (caudal view)

II. The **sacrum** is formed by the fusion of the three sacral vertebrae. Laterally, it bears the **sacral wing (33)**, whose **auricular surface (34)** forms a synovial joint with the auricular surface of the ilium. The **median sacral crest (35)** is formed by an incomplete fusion of the spinous processes. The lateral ends of the fused lateral (transverse) processes form the **lateral sacral crest (36)**. The **intermediate sacral crest (37)** results from the sequential arrangement of the fused mamilloarticular processes. The **promontory (38)** forms the cranioventral contour of the sacral bone and takes part in the limiting terminal line of the pelvic inlet. From the vertebral canal, the sacral nerves enter intervertebral foramina and leave the vertebral column after dividing into dorsal and ventral branches that emerge from the **dorsal (39)** and **ventral sacral foramina (40)**, respectively, that proceed from each intervertebral foramen.

b) Of the 13 **RIBS (COSTAE)**, the first through the ninth are **sternal ribs (41)**, connected to the sternum by synovial articulation. Ribs 10 – 12 are the freely moveable, 'breathing' **asternal ribs (42)**. By the overlapping of the cartilaginous parts of the asternal ribs, a costal arch is formed on both sides of the body. The last rib does not regularly participate in the formation of the arch. It usually terminates freely in the musculature of the abdominal wall as a 'floating' rib **(43)**. Ribs, sternum and thoracic vertebral column form the thorax, the inlet of which is bounded by the first pair of ribs and the outlet by the costal arches. The dorsal part of the rib is osseous (**Os costae, −44**). Its **head (45)** bears cranial and caudal **articular facets (46)**. The two articular facets are separated by a rough crest that, in most ribs, is indirectly in contact with the intervertebral disc by means of the intercapital ligament (see illustration, p. 11). An indistinct **neck of the rib (47)** connects the head to the **body of the rib (48)**. The proximodorsally located **costal tubercle (49)** bears an **articular surface (50)** for articulation with the costal fovea of the transverse process. The **angle of the rib (51)** is only indistinctly recognizable. The **costal cartilage (52)** begins at the costochondral junction and, slightly distal to this, there is a distinct bend, the **knee of the rib (53)** that in other domestic mammals is in the area of the costochondral junction.

c) The **STERNUM** consists of the **manubrium (54)**, the **body of the sternum (55)** with its six **sternebrae (56)**, and the **xiphoid process (57)**, which is bony cranially, cartilaginous caudally. The first pair of ribs articulates with the manubrium, the second at the synchondrosis that joins the manubrium to the body of the sternum, the third through the seventh at the following sternal synchondroses, and the eighth and ninth jointly at the synchondrosis joining the body to the xiphoid process.

Vertebral column and bones of thorax

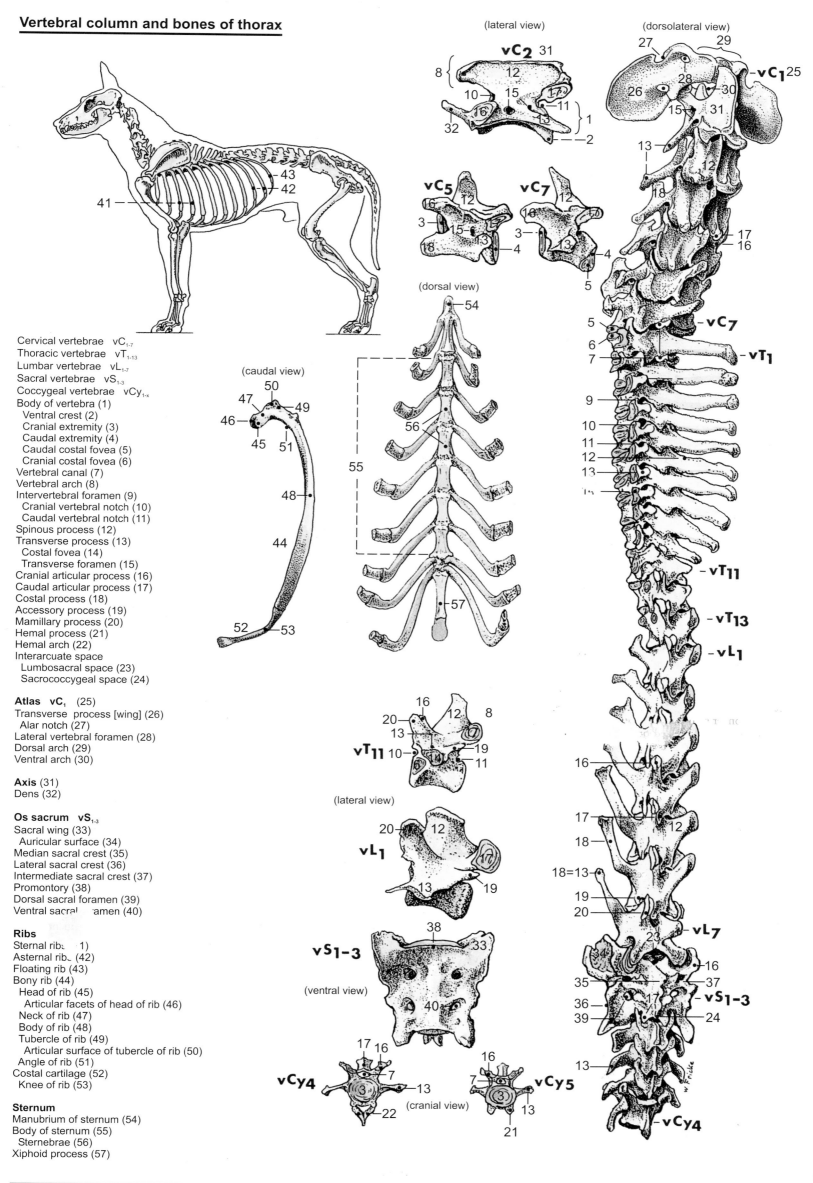

(lateral view)
vC₂ 31
(dorsolateral view)
vC₁ 25

vC₅ vC₇
vC₇

(dorsal view)

(caudal view)

vT₁₁

vL₁

vS₁₋₃
(ventral view)

vCy₄ vCy₅
(cranial view)

vC₇
vT₁
vT₁₁
vT₁₃
vL₁
vL₇
vS₁₋₃
vCy₄

Cervical vertebrae   vC₁₋₇
Thoracic vertebrae   vT₁₋₁₃
Lumbar vertebrae   vL₁₋₇
Sacral vertebrae   vS₁₋₃
Coccygeal vertebrae   vCy₁₋ₓ
Body of vertebra (1)
 Ventral crest (2)
 Cranial extremity (3)
 Caudal extremity (4)
 Caudal costal fovea (5)
 Cranial costal fovea (6)
Vertebral canal (7)
Vertebral arch (8)
Intervertebral foramen (9)
 Cranial vertebral notch (10)
 Caudal vertebral notch (11)
Spinous process (12)
Transverse process (13)
 Costal fovea (14)
 Transverse foramen (15)
Cranial articular process (16)
Caudal articular process (17)
Costal process (18)
Accessory process (19)
Mamillary process (20)
Hemal process (21)
Hemal arch (22)
Interarcuate space
 Lumbosacral space (23)
 Sacrococcygeal space (24)

Atlas vC₁   (25)
Transverse process [wing] (26)
Alar notch (27)
Lateral vertebral foramen (28)
Dorsal arch (29)
Ventral arch (30)

Axis (31)
Dens (32)

Os sacrum vS₁₋₃
Sacral wing (33)
 Auricular surface (34)
Median sacral crest (35)
Lateral sacral crest (36)
Intermediate sacral crest (37)
Promontory (38)
Dorsal sacral foramen (39)
Ventral sacral foramen (40)

Ribs
Sternal ribs (41)
Asternal ribs (42)
Floating rib (43)
Bony rib (44)
 Head of rib (45)
  Articular facets of head of rib (46)
 Neck of rib (47)
 Body of rib (48)
 Tubercle of rib (49)
  Articular surface of tubercle of rib (50)
 Angle of rib (51)
Costal cartilage (52)
 Knee of rib (53)

Sternum
Manubrium of sternum (54)
Body of sternum (55)
 Sternebrae (56)
Xiphoid process (57)

5. ARTICULATIONS OF THE VERTEBRAL COLUMN AND OF THE THORAX; ATLANTO-OCCIPITAL AND ATLANTO-AXIAL JOINTS

a) JOINTS (ARTICULATIONS)

NAME	PARTICIPATING BONES	FORM/ COMPOSITION	FUNCTION	REMARKS
I. Atlanto-occipital joint	Occipital condyles and cranial articular foveae of the atlas	Elliptical joint, simple joint	Hinge joint, dorsal and ventral flexion	Right and left joint cavities communicate ventrally.
II. Atlanto-axial joint	Fovea of the dens and caudal articular fossa of the atlas, dens and ventral articular surface of the dens	Trochoid joint, simple joint	Axial rotation of the head on the neck, head 'shaking'	The atlanto-axial joint communicates with the atlanto-occipital joint.
III. Joints of the articular processes	Articular processes of adjacent vertebrae	Plane joints	Sliding joints	Considerable mobility in the cervical region, decreasing in the thoracic and lumbar regions.
IV. Joint of the head of the rib (costovertebral joint)	Articular surface of the head of the rib and caudal costal fovea of the more cranial vertebra and cranial costal fovea of the more caudal vertebra with which the rib head articulates	Spheroid joint, composite joint	Hinge joint that, together with the vertebrae, makes possible the variation in thoracic volume in respiration	The convex rib-head joint surface is formed by two articular facets. The articular depression is formed by the costal foveae of the two vertebral bodies and the intervening fibrocartilage of the intervertebral symphysis. The last two to three ribs articulate only with the cranial costal fovea of the same-numbered (the more caudal) vertebra.
V. Joint of the rib tubercle (costotransverse joint)	Articular surface of the costal tubercle and the costal fovea of the trans-verse process of the same numbered (the more caudal) vertebra	Plane joint, simple joint	Hinge joint	On the last ribs, the costotransverse joint approaches and then fuses with the costovertebral joint.
VI. Sternocostal joint	Cartilaginous ends of the first to the eighth ribs and the sternum	Condylar joint, simple joint	Hinge joint	The first rib articulates with the manu-brium of the sternum. The ninth (last sternal) rib is not connected to the sternum by a synovial joint but by fibrous tissue.
VII. Costochondral synchondrosis	Costal bone and costal cartilage	Synchondrosis	Nearly rigid and immoveable	Postnatally a true joint may develop from a synchondrosis.
VIII. Sternal synchondroses	Manubrium of the sternum, sternebrae of the body of the sternum, xiphoid process	Synchondrosis	Increasingly rigid and immoveable	Of the sternal synchondroses, the manubriosternal and xiphosternal synchondroses are specially named.
IX. Intervertebral symphysis (joints between the bodies of adjacent vertebrae)	Bodies of adjacent vertebrae, starting with the axis and including the caudal vertebrae	Intervertebral disc without a space	Slight mobility	The discs in the intervertebral region of the sacrum ossify in the second year of life.
X. Sacroiliac joint	See joints of the pelvic limb.			

b) LIGAMENTS OF THE VERTEBRAL COLUMN

Three ligaments extend over longer areas of the vertebral column. Short liga-ments bridge over the space between individual vertebrae.

The **ventral longitudinal ligament** is attached ventrally to the bodies of the vertebrae and to the intervertebral discs. It extends from the second cervical vertebra to the sacrum.

The **dorsal longitudinal ligament** lies on the floor of the vertebral canal and attaches at the dorsal border of the intervertebral disc. It extends from the axis to the first caudal vertebrae.

The **nuchal ligament** (see p. 29) in the dog consists only of the paired elastic **funiculus nuchae**. It bridges over the cervical vertebral column from the cau-dal end of the spinous process of the axis and extends to the spinous process of the first thoracic vertebra. Here it is continued by the **supraspinous liga-ment** with loss of elasticity and attaches to the spinous process of all the ver-tebrae up to the third sacral vertebra.

The **ligamenta flava** extend as short elastic ligaments from vertebral arch to vertebral arch and thus close the interarcuate spaces dorsally.

Interspinous ligaments are lacking. The **M. interspinalis** lies between the spi-nous processes of adjacent vertebrae.

c) LIGAMENTS OF THE ATLANTO-OCCIPITAL AND ATLANTO-AXIAL JOINTS, AND OF THE THORAX

At the **atlanto-occipital joint**, the **dorsal atlanto-occipital membrane** rein-forces the joint capsule and bridges over the atlanto-occipital space (access to the cerebellomedullar cistern for withdrawal of cerebrospinal fluid for diag-nostic purposes). The **ventral atlanto-occipital membrane** is a ventral rein-forcement of the joint capsule. The **lateral ligament** is a lateral reinforcement of the joint capsule.

On the **atlanto-axial** joint the dens is held to the floor of the vertebral canal and to the occipital bone by the **apical ligament of the dens**, the **transverse atlantal ligament** and the **alar ligaments**. The transverse atlantal ligament is underlain by a synovial bursa and is attached to either side of the atlas. In the case of rupture of these ligaments or fracture of the dens following car acci-dents or strangulation, damage to the spinal cord may occur with paralysis and death as consequences. The elastic **dorsal atlanto-axial membrane** extends from the cranial projection of the spine of the axis to the dorsal arch of the atlas.

The **joints between the articular processes** of the vertebrae lack ligaments. The joint capsule is either tightly attached or more loose according to the degree of movement and influences the direction of the movement, which depends on the position of the articular surfaces.

At the **joint of the rib-head**, the **intra-articular ligament of the head of the rib** connects the costal heads of both sides and lies over the intervertebral disc. It is also called the **intercapital ligament**. It is lacking at the first and the last two pairs of ribs. The **radiate ligament of the head of the rib** is present as a strengthening of the joint capsule.

At the **costotransverse joints**, the joint capsule is reinforced by a **costotrans-verse ligament**.

Joints of the vertebral column and the thorax

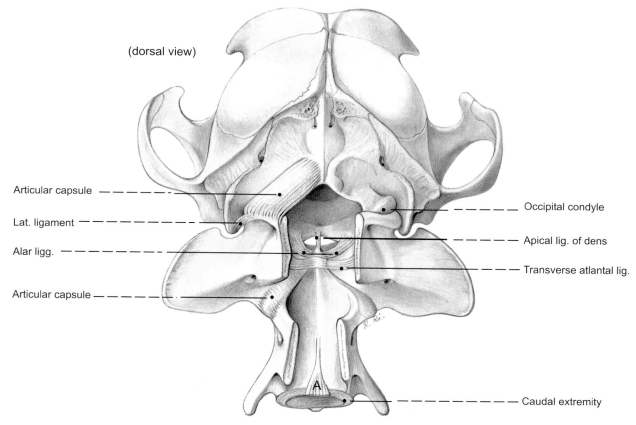

(dorsal view)

Articular capsule

Lat. ligament

Alar ligg.

Articular capsule

Occipital condyle

Apical lig. of dens

Transverse atlantal lig.

A

Caudal extremity

Atlanto-occipital and atlanto-axial joints

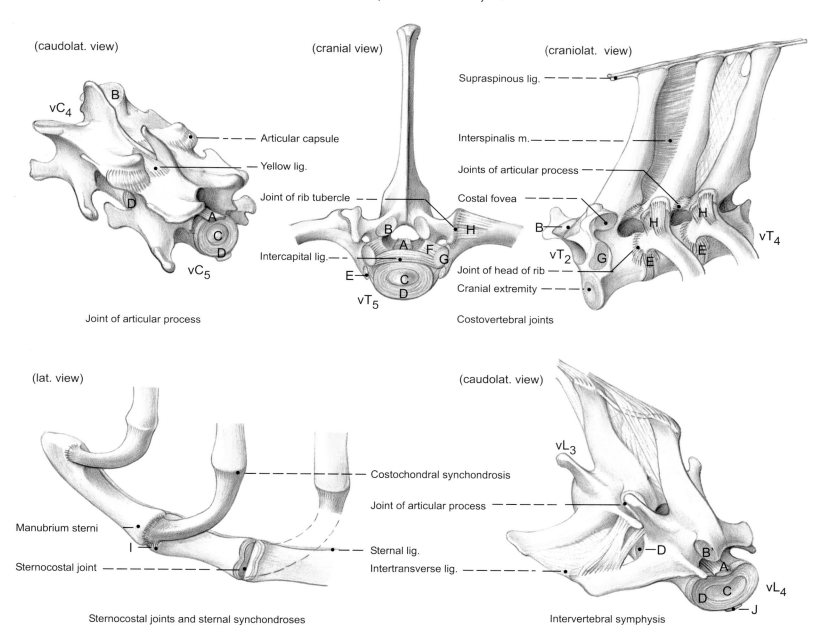

(caudolat. view)

vC₄

B

D

A

C

D

vC₅

Articular capsule

Yellow lig.

Joint of articular process

(cranial view)

Joint of rib tubercle

Intercapital lig.

B

A

F

G

H

E

C

D

vT₅

Costovertebral joints

(craniolat. view)

Supraspinous lig.

Interspinalis m.

Joints of articular process

Costal fovea

Joint of head of rib

Cranial extremity

B

vT₂

H

H

G

E

E

vT₄

(lat. view)

Manubrium sterni

Sternocostal joint

I

Costochondral synchondrosis

Joint of articular process

Sternal lig.

Intertransverse lig.

Sternocostal joints and sternal synchondroses

(caudolat. view)

vL₃

D

B'

A

D

C

J

vL₄

Intervertebral symphysis

(see pp. 9, 89, 91)

Legend :

A Dorsal longitudinal lig.
B Cran. articular process
B' Caud. articular process

Intervertebral disc:
C Nucleus pulposus
D Anulus fibrosus

E Radiate lig. of head of rib
F Intra-articular lig. of head of rib
G Cran. costal fovea

H Costotransverse lig.
I Radiate sternocostal lig.
J Ventral longitudinal lig.

11

CHAPTER 2: NECK AND CHEST REGION (CERVICAL AND THORACIC REGION)

1. CUTANEOUS MUSCLES AND CUTANEOUS NERVES OF THE NECK AND THORACIC WALL

To demonstrate the cutaneous muscles a longitudinal incision is made through the skin on the left side of the body. The incision should extend from the base of the ear to the midlevel of the scapula up to the ventral end of the last rib. In doing this, the cutaneous muscles must be preserved. At the ends of the incision at the base of the ear and at the level of the last rib, a transverse section is made through the skin, which is then reflected to the dorsal and ventral midlines. The external jugular and omobrachial veins, which are superficially located, are examined first in order to avoid unintended damage to the vessels and the smearing of the dissection site with the coagulated blood.

a) The **CUTANEOUS MUSCLES** end in the skin with the finest tendinous fibers and thus bring about movement of the skin, for example, to ward off insects.

The **cutaneus trunci muscle (4)** converges in its fiber course to the axillary fossa and to the ventromedian linea alba and is penetrated by fine cutaneous nerves. Its motor innervation is by the **lateral thoracic nerve (5)**, the branches of which can be seen through the ventral half of this thin muscle.

The **platysma (2)** can be seen extending from its origin on the dorsal midline to the border between head and neck where it is continued by the cutaneus faciei muscle.

The **nerve supply of the cervical platysma (3)** originates from the caudal auricular nerve of the seventh cranial nerve (facial nerve). It crosses deep to the muscle in a dorsal paramedian course. The nerve can be identified by spreading the coarse fiber bundles of the muscle.

The **superficial sphincter colli muscle (1)** is ventral on the neck with transverse fibers that are closely attached to the skin.

To demonstrate the cervical cutaneous nerves, cut the dorsal linear origin of the platysma and reflect the muscle cranially to the cranial transverse section of the skin. To demonstrate the thoracic cutaneous nerves, cut the cutaneus trunci muscle along the caudal transverse section of the skin at the level of the last rib as well as at the caudal border of the triceps brachii muscle and reflect it ventrally toward the linea alba. In the ventral thoracic and abdominal regions in all cases the aponeurosis of the external abdominal oblique muscle (34) should be preserved.

b) The **CUTANEOUS NERVES** supply the skin and are predominantly sensory (they also contain autonomic fibers); they are the parts of the spinal nerves that are visible subcutaneously. The spinal nerves (*e.g.*, nC4) divide at their exit from the intervertebral foramen into a **dorsal branch (d)** and a **ventral branch (v)** that further divide into a **medial branch (dm** or, respectively, **vm)** and a **lateral branch (dl** or, respectively, **vl)**. Except for the dorsal cervical region, the deeply located medial branches contain predominantly motor fibers, the lateral branches mainly sensory fibers for the supply of the skin. Of the eight cervical nerves, only nC1 passes through the lateral vertebral foramen of the atlas. The second through the seventh cervical nerves leave the vertebral canal cranial to the vertebra of the same number, and the eighth cervical nerve caudal to the seventh cervical vertebra. The first cervical nerve does not reach the skin of the neck with its dorsomedial branch (nC 1dm). The major occipital nerve (nC 2dm) runs deep to the superficial cervicoauricularis muscle to the occipital region. The following nC 3 dm to nC 6dm are often double. The last two, nC 7dm and nC 8dm are small and do not usually reach the skin but end in the thick muscular layer. The innervation of the dorsal cutaneous cervical region by dm-branches is different from the arrangement in other regions of the body in which the skin is supplied by lateral branches, and the musculature by medial. The difference is clear when one compares sites of emergence of the cutaneous nerves in the dorsal cervical and dorsal thoracic regions.

I. The **dorsal cutaneous branches of the cervical nerves** reach the dorsal midline in the company of cutaneous blood vessels and are formed by dm-branches.

II. The **dorsal cutaneous branches of the thoracic nerves** appear a handsbreadth dorsal and paramedian; that is, they are more lateral and are regularly formed by dl-branches. They are accompanied by cutaneous blood vessels. The thirteen thoracic nerves leave the vertebral canal caudal to the vertebra of the same number and divide into a dorsal and a ventral branch. The ventral branch passes as an intercostal nerve ventrally between the ribs and gives off a vl (prox. or lateral cutaneous)-branch about the middle of the length of the intercostal space and a vl (dist. or ventral cutaneous)-branch at the ventral end of the intercostal space.

III. The **ventral cutaneous branches of the cervical nerves** are in a ventrolateral row and are formed by vl-branches (nC 2vl to nC 5vl). The nC 2v through nC 5v communicate with each other and form a cervical plexus in the depth of the musculature. The ventral cutaneous nerve of C2 runs with its **great auricular nerve (11)** to the base of the ear and with its **transverse cervical nerve (12)** to the ventral cervical region and the caudal part of the mandibular space. The ventral branches of C6 to T2 join to form the brachial plexus with their main parts (see p. 19), and it is from this plexus that the plexus nerves of the thoracic limb originate.

IV. The **lateral cutaneous branches of the thoracic nerves** are formed by the proximal vl-branches (lateral cutaneous branches of the intercostal nerves) mentioned above.

V. The **ventral cutaneous branches of the thoracic nerves** are formed by the distal vl branches (ventral cutaneous branches of the intercostal nerves). These nerves are very small.

2. DORSAL EXTRINSIC LIMB MUSCLES

Knowledge of the bones of the shoulder girdle is required for the dissection (see p. 17). In the course of the dissection, the cleidocervical and trapezius muscles are cut along the course of the dorsal branch of the accessory nerve (cranial nerve XI) and reflected to either side. Following this, the division of the accessory nerve into a long dorsal and a short ventral branch can be demonstrated.

The origin of the muscles or, respectively, their attachment to the skull and the cervical and thoracic parts of the vertebral column, the ribs and sternum (collectively, the trunk) as well as to the thoracic limb is decisive for their designation as **trunk-limb muscles**. Because they insert on part of the shoulder girdle, it is also justified to designate them synonymously as muscles of the shoulder girdle. Of these muscles, the serratus ventralis provides the main synsarcotic junction between the trunk and the limb, its area of rotation being found in the middle of the serrate surface of the scapula.

The **trapezius muscle** originates with both its parts (according to Donat *et al.*, 1967, three parts) at the dorsal midline above the spinous processes of the cervical and thoracic vertebrae. Its **thoracic part (7)** ends in a cranioventral direction on the dorsal third of the spine of the scapula. The **cervical part (6)** inserts after a caudoventral course on the dorsal two-thirds of the spine of the scapula. Despite the different directions of their fiber course, both parts act as protractors of the limb. This is because the thoracic part inserts dorsal to and the cervical part ventral to the area of rotation of the synsarcotic trunk-limb junction. The **cleidocervical muscle (15)** according to the nomenclature proposal of Donat et al., 1967, is considered as a third part (clavicular part) of the trapezius muscle. It courses between the **clavicular intersection (16)** and the dorsal midline of the neck. The **dorsal branch of the accessory nerve (13)**, which innervates

this muscle, appears between the cleidocervical muscle and the cervical part of the trapezius muscle at the apex of a muscularly bounded triangle, and can be followed further where the transection of the trapezius muscle (see the dissection instructions) begins.

The **omotransversarius muscle (14)** runs as its name suggests between the acromion and shoulder (*omos*) and the transverse process (wing) of the atlas. **Innervation:** nC 4vm. Deep to its dorsomedial surface is the superficial cervical lymph node, which should be preserved.

The **latissimus dorsi muscle (8)** arises from the broad **thoracolumbar fascia (9)** and ends chiefly on the teres major tuberosity by common tendon with the teres major. It has attachments to the brachial fascia as well as to the major and minor tubercular crests of the humerus, by which a broad axillary arch is formed. The **thoracodorsal nerve** and vessels (see p. 19) enter the medial aspect of the muscle.

The **rhomboideus muscle (10)** is covered by the trapezius muscle and consists of the M. rhomboideus capitis (nC vm), M. rhomboideus cervicis (nC vm) and M. rhomboideus thoracis (nT vm). They originate at the nuchal crest and at the dorsal midline and end on the scapular cartilage. **Function:** To fix, elevate, and retract the thoracic limb; when the neck is lowered, to elevate the neck.

Cervical and pectoral regions

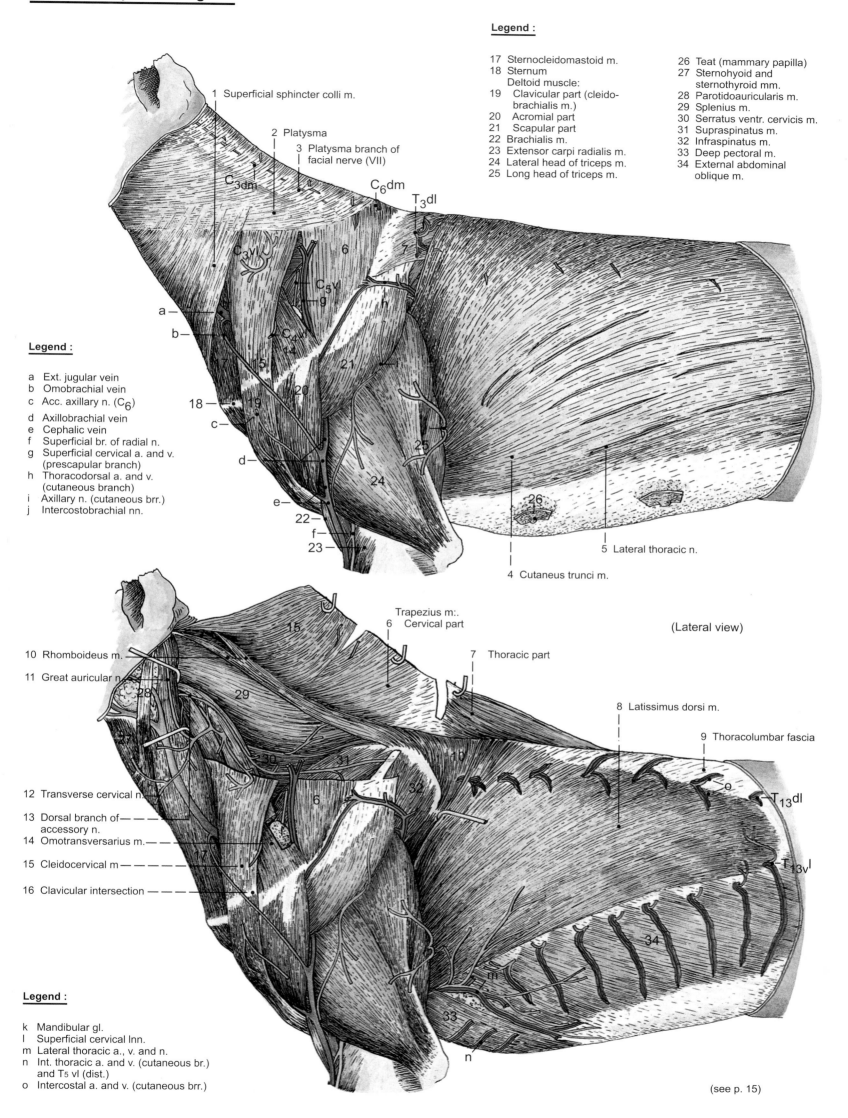

1 Superficial sphincter colli m.
2 Platysma
3 Platysma branch of facial nerve (VII)

C₃dm C₆dm T₃dl

Legend :

17 Sternocleidomastoid m.
18 Sternum
    Deltoid muscle:
19   Clavicular part (cleido-brachialis m.)
20   Acromial part
21   Scapular part
22 Brachialis m.
23 Extensor carpi radialis m.
24 Lateral head of triceps m.
25 Long head of triceps m.
26 Teat (mammary papilla)
27 Sternohyoid and sternothyroid mm.
28 Parotidoauricularis m.
29 Splenius m.
30 Serratus ventr. cervicis m.
31 Supraspinatus m.
32 Infraspinatus m.
33 Deep pectoral m.
34 External abdominal oblique m.

Legend :

a Ext. jugular vein
b Omobrachial vein
c Acc. axillary n. (C₆)
d Axillobrachial vein
e Cephalic vein
f Superficial br. of radial n.
g Superficial cervical a. and v. (prescapular branch)
h Thoracodorsal a. and v. (cutaneous branch)
i Axillary n. (cutaneous brr.)
j Intercostobrachial nn.

4 Cutaneus trunci m.
5 Lateral thoracic n.

Trapezius m:.
6 Cervical part
7 Thoracic part

(Lateral view)

10 Rhomboideus m.
11 Great auricular n.

8 Latissimus dorsi m.
9 Thoracolumbar fascia

T₁₃dl
T₁₃vl

12 Transverse cervical n.
13 Dorsal branch of accessory n.
14 Omotransversarius m.
15 Cleidocervical m
16 Clavicular intersection

Legend :

k Mandibular gl.
l Superficial cervical lnn.
m Lateral thoracic a., v. and n.
n Int. thoracic a. and v. (cutaneous br.) and T₅ vl (dist.)
o Intercostal a. and v. (cutaneous brr.)

(see p. 15)

3. VENTRAL EXTRINSIC LIMB MUSCLES

> In the course of the dissection, the superficial and deep pectoral muscles are transected a fingerbreadth lateral to the ventral midline. In this way, their innervation by cranial and caudal pectoral nerves can be observed.

The function of the **trunk-limb muscles** consists in the movement of the head, vertebral column and thoracic limb, and in the suspension of the trunk by the thoracic limbs. The more ventral muscles act more in the suspension of the trunk and therefore are rich in tendinous intersections; whereas, the more dorsal muscles are more functional in limb movement and the suspension of the thoracic limb is an accessory function.

With the clavicular part of the deltoid muscle (cleidobrachialis), the **superficial pectoral muscles** form the lateral pectoral groove. In the dog, the cephalic vein occupies only the most medial part of the groove as, at this level, it does not pass in the main part of the groove, but medially upon the superficial pectoral, deep to the cleidobrachialis. The broad **transverse pectoral muscle (14)** takes linear origin from the manubrium and cranial part of the body of the sternum. The more superficial **descending pectoral muscle (15)** arises only from the manubrium. The two parts of the superficial pectoral end on the crest of the major tubercle of the humerus.

The **principal portion of the deep pectoral muscle (17)** forms the base for the narrow, laterally located **accessory portion (16)**. The deep pectoral muscle has its origin from the manubrium and body of the sternum and terminates at the major and minor tubercles. The accessory portion inserts on the brachial fascia. The nerves that supply the deep pectoral can be seen on its cut surface.

The **serratus ventralis muscle (31)** is subdivided into the cervical serratus ventralis muscle (nCvm) and the thoracic serratus ventralis muscle (**long thoracic nerve —30**). The two fuse with each other in the area of the thoracic inlet. They originate from the transverse processes of the cervical vertebrae or, respectively, the ribs and insert jointly on the facies serrata of the scapula.

The **sternocleidomastoid muscle** (ventral branch of the accessory nerve) consists of three individual muscles: The **cleidomastoid (5)** and **sternomastoid (3) muscles** fuse cranially; the sternomastoid muscle and **sterno-occipital muscle (4)** fuse caudally. The lateral surface of the sternocleidomastoid muscle forms the jugular furrow for the external jugular vein. The innervation by the ventral branch of the accessory nerve is to the deep face of the sternomastoid and sterno-occipital muscles caudal to the mandibular gland. Here, the ventral branch (see p. 13) lies between the sternomastoid and sterno-occipital muscles, which form a continuous muscle and can only be separated artificially. The **accessory nerve** divides into the previously identified **dorsal ramus**, which communicates with nC 2, and into the short **ventral ramus** whose three branches end after a short course in the individual muscles that together comprise the sternocleidomastoideus.

The **deltoid muscle** has scapular, acromial, and clavicular parts; the **clavicular part** is also designated the **cleidobrachialis muscle (13)** because it extends from the clavicular intersection to the humerus, the bone of the brachium. The **scapular and acromial parts of the deltoid muscle** are supplied by the **axillary nerve**, a branch of the brachial plexus. The cleidobrachialis muscle is innervated by the **accessory axillary or brachiocephalic nerve (nC 6 – 12)**, the most cranial branch of the brachial plexus. It enters the deep surface of the cleidobrachialis two fingerbreadths distal to the clavicular intersection. The term **brachiocephalicus muscle** is a collective term for a continuous muscle that, in domestic mammals, is formed by parts of the deltoid and sternocleidomastoideus muscles, and by the cleidocervicalis. Its three parts have an attachment to the clavicular intersection and are the **cleidobrachialis, cleidomastoideus, and cleidocervicalis**. The cleidobrachialis extends from the humerus to the clavicular intersection. The **clavicular intersection** is a thin layer of connective tissue that crosses the brachiocephalicus muscle cranial to the shoulder; at its medial end, it contains a small cartilage and often a small bone that is visible radiographically. The intersection attaches the fibers of the cleidobrachialis on its distal side; the fibers of the cleidocervicalis and cleidomastoideus on its proximal side, and is a complete partition between the attaching muscle fibers. The cleidomastoideus arises from the clavicular intersection and joins the sternomastoideus (see above) to insert on the mastoid process of the temporal bone. The cleidocervicalis arises from the clavicular intersection superficial to the cleidomastoid. From the intersection, the cleidocervicalis extends craniodorsally to the median fibrous seam of the neck that attaches right and left muscles dorsally. The term **cleidocephalicus muscle** is applied to the cleidomastoid and cleidocervical muscles together and the brachiocephalicus may therefore be described as consisting of the cleidobrachialis and cleidocephalicus.

The **sternohyoid muscle (nC 1vm – 7)** and the **sternothyroid muscle (nC 1vm – 2)** do not belong to the trunk-limb musculature, but to the long hyoid muscles. The right and left sternohyoid muscles contact each other at the ventral midline of the neck. The sternothyroideus muscle is adjacent laterally.

4. NERVES, VESSELS, AND VISCERAL ORGANS OF THE NECK

> The jugular furrow and external jugular vein have been dissected. To demonstrate structures of the ventral neck, the sternohyoid muscles are separated in the midline and transected jointly with the sternothyroideus muscles.

a) Like the subclavian and internal jugular veins, the **EXTERNAL JUGULAR VEIN (8)** originates from the brachiocephalic vein at the level of the thoracic inlet. In caudal-cranial sequence, it gives off the cephalic, superficial cervical and omobrachial veins. It then divides at the caudal border of the mandibular gland into a dorsal branch, the **maxillary vein (19)**, and a ventral branch, the **linguofacial vein (18)**. At its union with the external jugular vein, the **cephalic vein (11)** lies in the medial part of the lateral pectoral groove and joins the external jugular just cranial to the thoracic inlet. The **superficial cervical vein (10)** is satellite to the extrathoracic part of the same-named artery; it joins the external jugular near the root of the neck, usually just opposite the cephalic vein. The **omobrachial vein (9)** courses superficially upon the deltoid and cleidocervical muscles; it extends between the **axillobrachial vein** and the external jugular. The **axillobrachial vein** passes dorsally from the cephalic along the lateral border of the cleidobrachialis muscle, then deep to the deltoid muscle to join the caudal circumflex humeral vein (see p. 21).

b) Of the **NEUROVASCULAR STRUCTURES OF THE VENTRAL NECK**, the **internal jugular vein (22)** runs along the dorsolateral border of the trachea and gives off branches for the brain, thyroid gland, larynx and pharynx. The left and right common carotid arteries originate at the level of the thoracic inlet from the arterial brachiocephalic trunk (see p. 49). The **common carotid artery (24)** courses cranially on the dorsolateral border of the trachea and dispatches branches to the thyroid gland, larynx and pharynx. The **vagosympathetic trunk (23)** is a large nerve that lies dorsal to the common carotid artery. It conducts sympathetic fibers from the thoracolumbar sympathetic trunk to the head (see p. 49). Parasympathetic constituents of the vagus nerve (tenth cranial nerve) reach from the head predominantly to the body cavities. After its separation from the sympathetic trunk, the vagus nerve gives off the recurrent laryngeal nerve (see p. 49) within the thoracic cavity and after this contains parasympathetic and sensory nerve fibers, and perhaps skeletal motor fibers for the esophagus. The **recurrent laryngeal nerve (26)** with its skeletal motor, autonomic and sensory fibers turns and passes cranially in the neck. It lies within the connective tissue laterally on the trachea that, like the esophagus, receives branches from it. The recurrent laryngeal nerve is easily found as it passes dorsal to the thyroid gland; its terminal part is the caudal laryngeal nerve that supplies parts of the larynx.

c) Of the **LYMPHATIC SYSTEM**, only the lymphatic trunks and the lymph nodes are considered here. The tracheal (jugular) lymphatic trunk is the large paired lymphatic trunk of the neck. It begins as the efferent drainage of the medial retropharyngeal lymph node, receives afferent vessels from the superficial and deep cervical lymph nodes and empties at the venous angle formed by the confluence of external and internal jugular veins. At its termination, the **left tracheal lymphatic trunk (28)** joins the **thoracic duct (29)**, which conducts the lymph from the body cavities. The **medial retropharyngeal lymph node (1)** lies at the cranial attachment of the sternothyroid muscle. It receives its lymph from the head. The **superficial cervical lymph node (27)** lies deep to the omotransversarius muscle, between it and the serratus ventralis. Its afferent vessels pass from the superficial cervical area, and also from the trunk, head, and thoracic limb. The deep cervical lymph nodes lie close to the trachea and consist of an inconstant cranial, middle and caudal group. Their afferents are from their immediate surroundings in the neck.

d) The **CERVICAL VISCERAL STRUCTURES** are the esophagus, trachea, thyroid and parathyroid glands. The cervical part of the **esophagus (25)** lies dorsal to the trachea in the middle of the neck and dorsolateral (to the left) at the thoracic inlet. Its reddish color is due to its external coat of striated muscle. This striated muscle of the visceral type is innervated by the vagus nerve. The **trachea (6)** consists of C-shaped incomplete cartilaginous rings that are closed off by a membranous part that contains transverse bundles of trachealis (smooth) muscle. The incomplete cartilaginous rings and their complementary membranous parts are connected to each other by anular ligaments. The tracheal lumen is kept open by the incomplete cartilaginous rings that are braced by fibroelastic tissue. The tension thus created makes possible the changes in tracheal length with respiration and swallowing and is responsible for the typical round cross-section of the trachea, which can be narrowed by contraction of the trachealis muscle. The **thyroid gland (21)** lies at the cranial end of the trachea with left and right lobes that sometimes may be connected by a slight ventral isthmus. The bilateral pairs of **parathyroid glands (20)** lie on the thyroid gland as pale, rounded glands with a diameter of about three millimeters. They lie on the lateral and medial surfaces of the thyroid or in the thyroid parenchyma.

Cervical and pectoral regions

(ventral view)

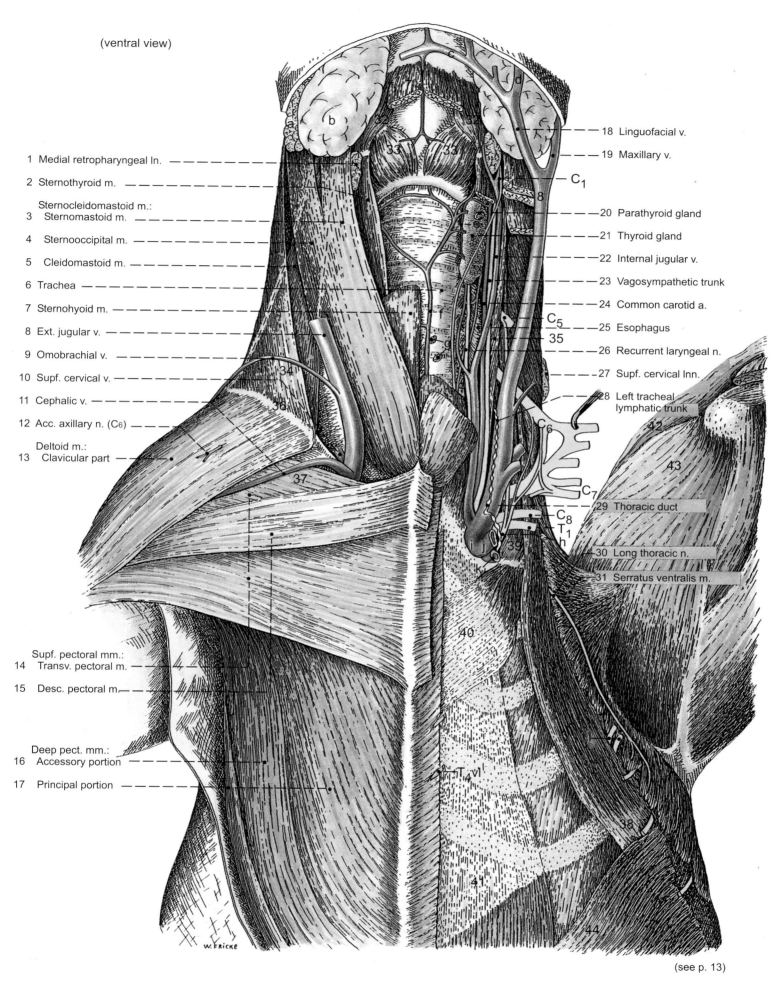

1 Medial retropharyngeal ln.
2 Sternothyroid m.

Sternocleidomastoid m.:
3   Sternomastoid m.
4   Sternooccipital m.
5   Cleidomastoid m.
6 Trachea
7 Sternohyoid m.
8 Ext. jugular v.
9 Omobrachial v.
10 Supf. cervical v.
11 Cephalic v.
12 Acc. axillary n. (C$_6$)

Deltoid m.:
13   Clavicular part

Supf. pectoral mm.:
14   Transv. pectoral m.
15   Desc. pectoral m.

Deep pect. mm.:
16   Accessory portion
17   Principal portion

18 Linguofacial v.
19 Maxillary v.
20 Parathyroid gland
21 Thyroid gland
22 Internal jugular v.
23 Vagosympathetic trunk
24 Common carotid a.
25 Esophagus
26 Recurrent laryngeal n.
27 Supf. cervical lnn.
28 Left tracheal lymphatic trunk
29 Thoracic duct
30 Long thoracic n.
31 Serratus ventralis m.

(see p. 13)

Legend :

32 Thyrohyoid m.
33 Cricothyroid m.
34 Cleidocervical m.
35 Longus capitis m.
36 Clavicular intersection
37 Lat. pectoral groove
38 Scalenus dors. m.

39 Scalenus med. m.
40 Rectus thoracis m.
41 Rectus abdominis m.
42 Supraspinatus m.
43 Subscapular m.
44 Ext. abdom. oblique m.

a   Parotid gland
b   Mandibular gland
c   Hyoid arch
d   Facial v.
e   Cran. thyroid a.
f   Caud. thyroid v.

g   Deep cervical lnn.
h   Phrenic n.
i   Brachiocephalic v.
j   Subclavian v.
k   Axillary a. and v.
l   Intercostobrachial nn.

15

CHAPTER 3: THORACIC LIMB

I. THE SKELETON OF THE THORACIC LIMB

The **pectoral (shoulder) girdle** consists of scapula, coracoid bone and clavicle, which are completely developed as individual bones in many vertebrates below the mammals (e.g., birds). In the domestic mammals there is a considerable reduction of the coracoid to a coracoid process of the scapula and of the clavicle to the clavicular intersection, a connective tissue strip within the brachiocephalicus muscle (see p. 14). There often remains as well a small bony remnant of the clavicle, which may be observed radiographically at the medial end of the clavicular intersection. It appears as a lamina of bone and cartilage ca. 10 x 5 mm.

a) The **SCAPULA** is the main constituent of the shoulder girdle. The **costal surface (1)** of the scapula is subdivided into a dorsally situated **facies serrata (2)**, the area of insertion of the serratus ventralis muscle, and a ventrally located **subscapular fossa (3)**, the area of attachment of the subscapularis muscle. The **lateral surface (4)** is subdivided by the **spine of the scapula (5)** into a **supraspinous fossa (6**, –origin of the supraspinatus muscle) and an **infraspinous fossa (7**, –origin of the infraspinatus muscle). At the ventral end of the spine of the scapula is the **acromion (8)** with a distal **hamate process (9)**. The **caudal margin (10)** of the scapula is nearly straight; the **cranial margin (11)** has a **scapular notch (12)** distally , and the **dorsal margin (13)** bears a narrow **scapular cartilage (14)**. Of its three angles (**caudal (15)**, **cranial (16)** and **ventral (17)** angles), the ventral one has a shallow oval **glenoid cavity (18)**. Caudodistal to the slight neck of the **scapula (19)** is the **infraglenoid tubercle (20)** and craniodistally from the neck, the **supraglenoid tubercle (21)** with the craniomedial **coracoid process (22)**.

b) The **HUMERUS** bears the **head of the humerus (23)** as an articular prominence for the shoulder joint. The head is separated distinctly from the **neck of the humerus (24)** only caudally. The **crest of the greater tubercle (26)** passes distally from the cranial margin of the **greater tubercle (25)**, and the **line of the triceps muscle (27)** passes proximocaudally from the deltoid tuberosity; it passes caudal to the greater tubercle. The **intertubercular groove (28)** seats the tendon of origin of the biceps brachii muscle and forms the deep furrow that defines the **lesser tubercle (29)** medially. From the lesser tubercle, the **crest of the lesser tubercle (30)** extends distally where it passes over into the lateral supracondylar crest. The **body of the humerus (31)** bears the **deltoid tuberosity (32)** laterally at the junction of its proximal and middle thirds. The deltoid tuberosity serves for the insertion of the deltoid muscle. From the deltoid tuberosity, the **humeral crest (33)** continues distally to the medial epicondyle. The crest bounds cranially the spirally coursing **groove of the brachialis muscle (34)**, which is occupied by the brachialis muscle. The **humeral condyle (35)** consists of a large **medial trochlea (36)** for articulation with the ulna and the small lateral **capitulum humeri**, which articulates with the radius. The humeral condyle bears an epicondyle on either side. From the **lateral epicondyle (38**, bearing roughnesses for the origin of the lateral collateral ligament and lateral digital extensor, and a caudal facet for the origin of the ulnaris lateralis muscle), the distinct lateral **supracondylar crest (38')** extends proximally. The **medial epicondyle (39)** is the process for attachment of the medial collateral ligament and, caudally, the digital and carpal flexors. The deep, caudal **olecranon fossa (40)** and the shallow **radial fossa (41)** communicate by the **supratrochlear foramen (42)**, which is closed off in life by membrane.

c) The **BONES OF THE ANTEBRACHIUM** are the radius and ulna.

I. On the **radius**, the **head of the radius (43)** has a caudomedial condylar **articular circumference (44)** for the proximal articulation with the ulna at its radial notch. The **neck of the radius (45)** is indistinct and bears caudomedially a small prominence, the **radial tuberosity (46)**, for the termination of the radial insertion of the biceps brachii muscle. The **body of the radius (47)** is continued distally by the **trochlea of the radius (48)**, which articulates distal-

ly with the carpal bones, and laterally, by means of the **ulnar notch (49)**, forms the distal articulation with the articular circumference of the ulna. The distal radius ends medially with the **medial styloid process (50)**.

II. The **ulna** projects beyond the head of the radius with its **olecranon (51)**, which is enlarged proximally to form the **tuber olecrani (52)**. The **semilunar trochlear notch (54)** begins at the pointed **anconeal process (53)** from which it curves distally, medially and laterally, to reach the **medial coronoid process (55)** or, respectively, **lateral coronoid process (56)**. The **radial notch (57)** lies at the transition to the **body of the ulna (58)**. The **head of the ulna (59)** forms the distal (!) end of the bone. It possesses the **articular circumference (60)** medially and ends distally with the **lateral styloid process (61)**. The **interosseous space of the antebrachium (62)** is especially wide in the distal third of the antebrachium.

d) The **CARPAL BONES** are laid down in the embryo in three rows and are reduced postnatally to two rows. The medial **radial carpal bone (63)** contains the intermediate carpal bone of the proximal row as well as the central carpal bone of the middle row and is also called the intermedioradial carpal bone. The **ulnar carpal bone (64)**, which is distal to the ulna, and the laterally projecting **accessory carpal bone (65)** complete the proximal row. **Carpal bones I – IV (66)** form the distal row and articulate with the metacarpal bones.

Synonyms for the carpal bones:

Radial carpal bone	Os scaphoideum	⎫
Intermediate carpal bone	Os lunatum	⎬ Intermedioradial
Ulnar carpal bone	Os triquetrum	
Accessory carpal bone	Os pisiformis	
Carpal bone I	Os trapezium	
Carpal bone II	Os trapezoideum	
Carpal bone III	Os capitatum	
Carpal bone IV	Os hamatum	

e) The **METACARPAL BONES I – V** have a **basis (67)** with an articular surface proximally, a long **body (68)** and finally a distal (!) **head (69)**. Metacarpal I may be absent or divided into two bones in which case the proximal part is fused with the first carpal bone.

f) The **BONES OF THE DIGIT** are the proximal, middle and distal phalanges. On digit I, the thumb (*pollex*), the middle phalanx is usually absent. The **proximal phalanx (70)** and the **middle phalanx (71)** have a **basis (72)** proximally, a **body (73)** and a distal **head (74)**. The indistinct **flexor tuberosity (75)** is proximopalmar on the middle phalanx; it serves for the termination of the superficial flexor tendon. The **distal phalanx** or **unguicular bone (76)** has an **articular surface (77)** proximodorsally, an indistinct **extensor process (78)** for the insertion of the extensor tendon and proximopalmarly an indistinct **flexor tubercle (79)** for the attachment of the deep flexor tendon. The sharp-edged **unguicular crest (80)** overlies the **unguicular sulcus (81)** and the basis of the **unguicular process (82)**, which bears the claw.

g) The **SESAMOID BONES** of the manus are the **sesamoid bone of the abductor digiti I muscle (83)**, which articulates with a small mediopalmar facet of the radial carpal bone, and **proximal sesamoid bones (84)**, which are palmar at the metacarpophalangeal joints. On the palmar side of the distal interphalangeal joint there is a **distal sesamoid (85)**. Dorsally on the proximal interphalangeal joint there is a **dorsal sesamoid (86)** that is always cartilaginous (sesamoid cartilage), and the sesamoid that is dorsal at the metacarpophalangeal joint is occasionally cartilaginous.

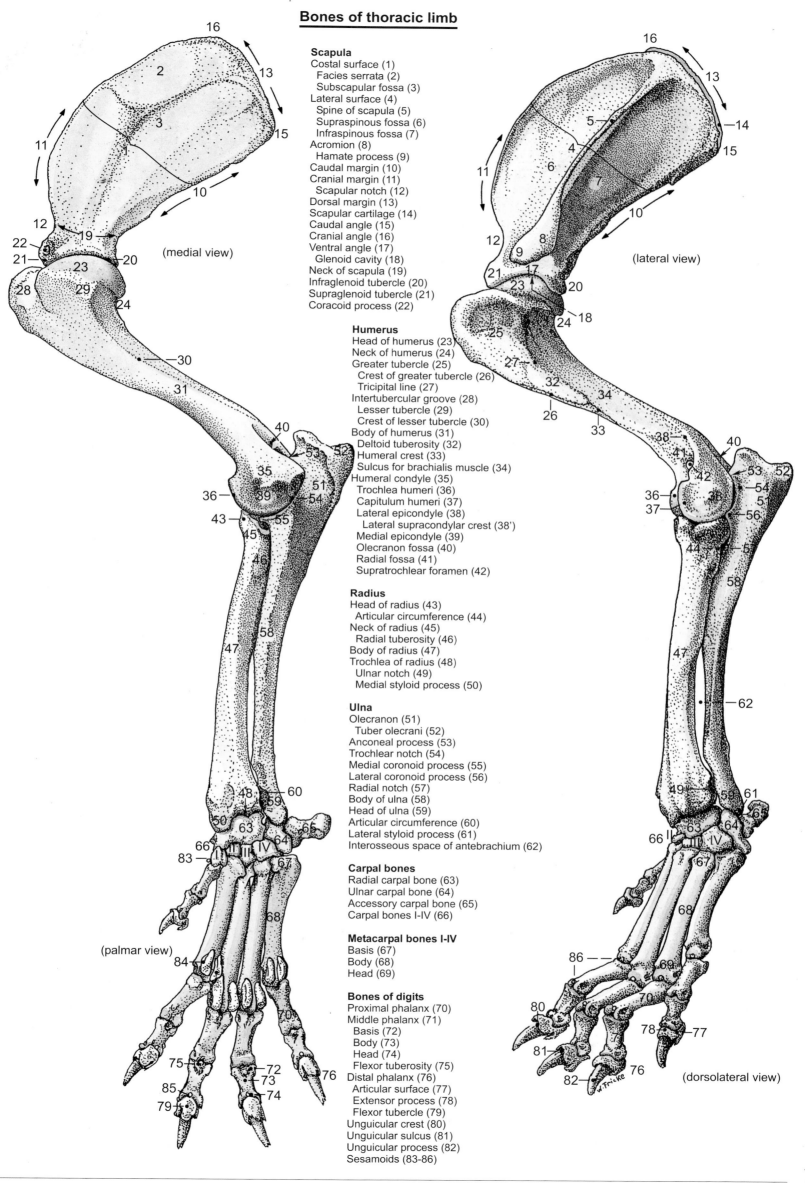

Bones of thoracic limb

Scapula
Costal surface (1)
  Facies serrata (2)
  Subscapular fossa (3)
Lateral surface (4)
  Spine of scapula (5)
  Supraspinous fossa (6)
  Infraspinous fossa (7)
  Acromion (8)
  Hamate process (9)
Caudal margin (10)
Cranial margin (11)
  Scapular notch (12)
Dorsal margin (13)
Scapular cartilage (14)
Caudal angle (15)
Cranial angle (16)
Ventral angle (17)
Glenoid cavity (18)
Neck of scapula (19)
Infraglenoid tubercle (20)
Supraglenoid tubercle (21)
Coracoid process (22)

Humerus
Head of humerus (23)
Neck of humerus (24)
Greater tubercle (25)
  Crest of greater tubercle (26)
  Tricipital line (27)
Intertubercular groove (28)
  Lesser tubercle (29)
  Crest of lesser tubercle (30)
Body of humerus (31)
Deltoid tuberosity (32)
Humeral crest (33)
Sulcus for brachialis muscle (34)
Humeral condyle (35)
  Trochlea humeri (36)
  Capitulum humeri (37)
  Lateral epicondyle (38)
    Lateral supracondylar crest (38')
  Medial epicondyle (39)
Olecranon fossa (40)
Radial fossa (41)
Supratrochlear foramen (42)

Radius
Head of radius (43)
  Articular circumference (44)
Neck of radius (45)
  Radial tuberosity (46)
Body of radius (47)
Trochlea of radius (48)
  Ulnar notch (49)
  Medial styloid process (50)

Ulna
Olecranon (51)
  Tuber olecrani (52)
Anconeal process (53)
Trochlear notch (54)
Medial coronoid process (55)
Lateral coronoid process (56)
Radial notch (57)
Body of ulna (58)
Head of ulna (59)
  Articular circumference (60)
  Lateral styloid process (61)
Interosseous space of antebrachium (62)

Carpal bones
Radial carpal bone (63)
Ulnar carpal bone (64)
Accessory carpal bone (65)
Carpal bones I-IV (66)

Metacarpal bones I-IV
Basis (67)
Body (68)
Head (69)

Bones of digits
Proximal phalanx (70)
Middle phalanx (71)
  Basis (72)
  Body (73)
  Head (74)
  Flexor tuberosity (75)
Distal phalanx (76)
  Articular surface (77)
  Extensor process (78)
  Flexor tubercle (79)
  Unguicular crest (80)
  Unguicular sulcus (81)
  Unguicular process (82)
Sesamoids (83-86)

(medial view)

(lateral view)

(palmar view)

(dorsolateral view)

2. MEDIAL VEINS OF THE THORACIC LIMB; MEDIAL SHOULDER AND ARM MUSCLES AND THEIR NERVE SUPPLY

For its further dissection, the thoracic limb is separated from the trunk. To do this, the cleidocephalicus muscle (see p. 14) is cut proximal to the clavicular intersection, and the other trunk-limb muscles are severed a few fingerbreadths proximal to their insertion on the thoracic limb. The external jugular vein is transected cranially from the origin of the omobrachial vein, and the subclavian vein from the brachiocephalic vein shortly after the latter's division into subclavian and external jugular. The axillary artery is cut just lateral to the first rib. The segmental nerve roots (nCv 6 to nTv 2) are sectioned a short distance before their confluence to form the brachial plexus, in which case the three roots of the phrenic nerve (nCv 5 through 7) should be cut near their origin from plexus nerves nCv 6 – 7, and preserved in their course to the thoracic inlet. With the thoracic limb removed, the skin of the limb is reflected to the level of the metacarpophalangeal joints. In doing this, observe the carpal pad at the carpus, the metacarpal pad at metacarpophalangeal joint level and the digital pads at the level of the distal interphalangeal joints. The distal end of the limb must be kept wrapped and moistened to avoid its drying out. In reflecting the skin, especially on the flexor aspect of the elbow joint and on the cranial contour of the antebrachium, preserve for later dissection the superficial veins and the cutaneous nerves that accompany them. Medially at the elbow joint, the pronator teres muscle (42) is cut in order to demonstrate the veins.

a) The **VEINS** are identified on the basis of their area of drainage. The sequence of branches serves only as an auxiliary criterion because it varies considerably in the venous system. In the arterial and nervous systems, the variations are less.

The very short subclavian vein is continued at the level of the first rib by the **axillary vein (21)**, which releases first the (often doubly developed) **external thoracic vein (22)** to the pectoral muscles. A further venous branch, the **lateral thoracic vein (4)**, is given off and passes with the same-named artery and nerve. It runs along the lateral border of the deep pectoral muscle (see p. 13) or, respectively, of the latissimus dorsi muscle. At its origin, it contacts the **axillary lymph node (21)** and, at the level of the second intercostal space, the **accessory axillary lymph node (3)**. From the axillary vein then the **subscapular vein (5)** courses to the same-named muscle and the **thoracodorsal vein (2)** to the medial aspect of the latissimus dorsi muscle. The subscapular vein releases the **caudal circumflex humeral vein (18)**, which passes deeply, coursing in an arciform manner laterally upon the caudal aspect of the humeral joint capsule, and anastomosing laterally with the **cranial circumflex humeral vein (23)** (see p. 25). The latter is a very slight vein that originates from the axillary vein and courses to the hilus area of the biceps brachii muscle. After branching off the axillobrachial vein (see p. 25), which can also originate from the caudal circumflex humeral vein, the axillary vein is continued by the **brachial vein (6)**. On the flexor aspect of the elbow joint, the latter gives off the **superficial brachial vein (10)**, the continuation of which, the **median cubital vein (27)**, originates from the cephalic vein. The brachial vein passes deep to the pronator teres, gives off the **common interosseous vein (12)** and is continued by the **median vein (13)**.

1   b) The **SPINAL NERVES** nCv 6 to nTv 2 form the roots of the brachial plexus in which the ventral branches of these several spinal nerves intermesh with an exchange of fibers. The major nerves of the thoracic limb originate as branches of the brachial plexus. In the following identification of nerves and muscles, the nerves serve as guiding structures in determining the homologies of the muscles and, on the other hand, the nerves are identified on the basis of their area of supply.

The **axillary nerve** (nC 7 and 8, −17) sends a branch to the teres major muscle (1), the muscle arising proximally at the caudal margin of the scapula and terminating, with the latissimus dorsi, on the humerus. The axillary nerve innervates additionally the caudal part of the subscapular muscle as well as the shoulder joint. At the caudal border of the subscapular muscle, the nerve passes deeply, runs laterally ventral to the long head of triceps and appears finally on the lateral surface of the shoulder (see p. 21). The **accessory axillary nerve** (brachiocephalic nerve, nC 6 and 7, −15) is the most cranial branch of the brachial plexus (its origin as a branch of the brachial plexus is disputed by some authors). It extends to the clavicular part of the deltoid, providing the motor supply to that muscle, and penetrates the muscle with its sensory cutaneous branch. The **subscapular nerve** (nC 6 and 7, −16) enters the subscapular muscle (16) with two branches. The subscapular muscle originates in the subscapular fossa and ends on the lesser tubercle of the humerus. The **suprascapular nerve** (nC 6 and 7, −14) passes laterally, deeply between the subscapular and supraspinatus muscles. It crosses the cranial aspect of the neck of the scapula and appears on the lateral surface of the scapula deep to the supraspinatus and infraspinatus muscles (see p. 21). The **musculocutaneous nerve** (nC 6 – nT 1, −25) lies upon the cranial face of the brachial artery. Its proximal muscular branch supplies the coracobrachialis and biceps brachii muscles and, a fingerbreadth proximal to the elbow joint, the musculocutaneous nerve communicates with the median nerve. It then proceeds craniomedially deep to the biceps brachii and ends in a distal muscular branch for the brachialis (there may be an additional branch to the biceps brachii muscle) and the **medial cutaneous antebrachial nerve (11)**. The latter nerve passes craniodistally between the biceps and brachialis muscles, arriving subcutaneously and descending the craniomedial forearm. The short, fusiform **coracobrachialis muscle (20)** originates on the coracoid process and terminates at the level of the proximal third of the humerus caudal to the lesser tubercle. The tendon of origin of the long **biceps brachii muscle (26)** arises from the supraglenoid tubercle of the scapula and, enveloped by a cranial extension of the synovial joint capsule, passes in the intertubercular groove where it is held in place by the transverse humeral ligament. Its tendon of insertion (see text-illustration) splits Y-like distal to the flexor aspect of the

2

elbow joint and inserts on the proximal radius (radial tuberosity) and ulna. The **brachialis muscle** (see text-illustration) runs with its insertion tendon between the branching tendons of the biceps brachii, reaching the proximal medial margin of the ulna and the radius. The brachialis originates caudal to the head of the humerus, winds spirally in the groove of the brachialis muscle from caudal to laterocranially around the humerus, then distomedially, and ends on the proximal ulna. The **radial nerve** (nC 7 – nT 2, −19) passes deeply distal to the strong insertion tendon of the teres major muscle, entering between the medial and long heads of the triceps brachii muscle, which it innervates. Before it enters the triceps, it gives off a small branch to the **tensor fasciae antebrachii muscle (7)**. The latter muscle originates from the insertion tendon of the latissimus dorsi muscle and terminates on the olecranon and the medial antebrachial fascia. The **ulnar nerve** (nC 8 – nT 2, −8) and **median nerve** (nC 8 – nT 2, −24) originate jointly from the brachial plexus and separate from each other in the distal arm region, the ulnar inclining caudally. Throughout their course in the proximal arm, the two nerves lie together caudal to the brachial artery and in association with the brachial vein. The smaller median nerve is the more cranial. At the distal third of the humerus, the ulnar nerve dispatches the **caudal cutaneous antebrachial nerve (9)**, which passes on the extensor aspect of the elbow joint and distally on the caudal forearm. The **cranial and caudal pectoral nerves**, the **long thoracic nerve**, the **thoracodorsal nerve** and the **lateral thoracic nerve** are also accounted as nerves of the brachial plexus.

3

4

Biceps brachii, brachialis coracobrachialis mm.

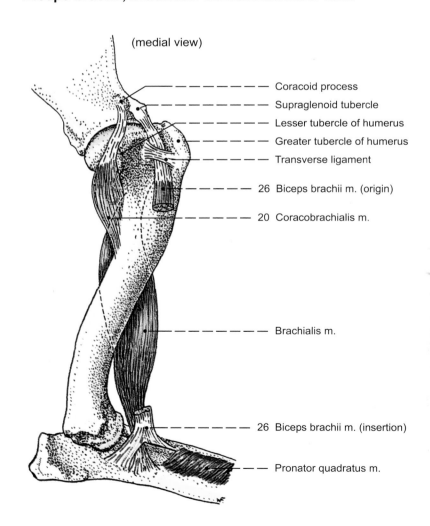

(medial view)

- Coracoid process
- Supraglenoid tubercle
- Lesser tubercle of humerus
- Greater tubercle of humerus
- Transverse ligament
- 26 Biceps brachii m. (origin)
- 20 Coracobrachialis m.
- Brachialis m.
- 26 Biceps brachii m. (insertion)
- Pronator quadratus m.

18

Thoracic limb

(caudomedial view)

1 Teres major m.
2 Thoracodorsal a., v. and n.
3 Accessory axillary ln.
4 Lateral thoracic a., v. and n.
5 Subscapular a. and v.
6 Brachial a. and v.
7 Tensor fasciae antebrachii m.

8 Ulnar nerve
9 Caud. cutaneous antebrachial n.
10 Superficial brachial vein
11 Medial cutaneous antebrachial n.
12 Common interosseous vein
13 Median vein and artery

14 Suprascapular a., v. and n.
15 Accessory axillary n.
16 Subscapular n. and m.
17 Axillary nerve
18 Caudal circumflex humeral vein
19 Radial nerve
20 Coracobrachialis m.
21 Axillary v. and ln.
22 Ext. thoracic a. and v. and cran. pectoral n.
23 Cranial circumflex humeral a. and v.
24 Median nerve
25 Musculocutaneous n.
26 Biceps brachii m.
27 Median cubital vein

(see pp. 23, 25)

3. LATERAL VEINS OF THE THORACIC LIMB; LATERAL SHOULDER AND ARM MUSCLES AND THEIR NERVE SUPPLY

> To demonstate the anastomoses between the medial deep and the lateral superficial venous systems as well as the muscular branches of the axillary nerve, the scapular and acromial parts of the deltoid muscle are severed at their origin from the scapula (see text-illustration). To demonstrate the muscular branches of the radial nerve, the lateral head of the triceps brachii muscle is cut in its middle and the stumps reflected.

a) The **LATERAL SUPERFICIAL CUTANEOUS VEINS** course in the scapular and arm region unaccompanied by same-named arteries. From the external jugular, the **cephalic vein (19)** passes briefly laterally in the lateral pectoral groove, then deeply between the cleidobrachialis and superficial pectoral muscles to reach the lateral border of the cleidobrachialis. Here it joins the **axillobrachial vein (7)**. Before the axillobrachial vein passes deep to the scapular part of the deltoid muscle, it receives the **omobrachial vein (6)**. At the flexor aspect of the elbow joint, the cephalic vein gives off the **median cubital vein (20)**, the continuation of which, as the superficial brachial vein, reaches the medially situated brachial vein. The cephalic vein in its course upon the cranial contour of the antebrachium is accompanied by both branches of the superficial ramus of the radial nerve and by the distal continuation (cranial superficial antebrachial artery) of the weak superficial antebrachial artery. Three fingerbreadths proximal to the carpus, the cephalic vein passes onto the medial side of the limb, then caudopalmarly to reach the palmar surface of the manus. Distal to this point, its straight direct-distal course upon the cranial aspect of the limb is continued by the **accessory cephalic vein (21)**, which dispatches the dorsal common digital veins on the dorsum of the manus.

b) The **NERVES** that supply the **LATERAL MUSCLES** of the shoulder and brachium originate medially at the shoulder from the brachial plexus, where their initial portions were previously identified (see p. 19).

The **axillary nerve** gives off muscular branches to the medial aspect of the scapular and acromial parts of the deltoid muscle and to the fusiform teres minor muscle. After this, the axillary nerve terminates with its **cranial lateral cutaneous brachial nerve (10)** and its **cranial cutaneous antebrachial nerve (11)**. These nerves appear subcutaneously at the caudal border of the deltoid muscle in the company of the axillobrachial vein. The **deltoid muscle** originates from the scapular spine with its **scapular part (3)** and from the acromion with its **acromial part (4)**. Both parts end on a common tendon that inserts on the deltoid tuberosity of the humerus. The **clavicular part of the deltoid (5, cleidobrachial muscle)**, runs between the clavicular intersection and the distal end of the humeral crest. It is supplied by the accessory axillary nerve (brachiocephalic nerve, –nC 6). The teres minor muscle (see text-illustration) originates at the infraglenoid tubercle and the caudal margin of the scapula and terminates at the teres minor tuberosity. The **suprascapular nerve (2)**, previously identified, innervates the supraspinatus muscle. It crosses the neck of the scapula cranially, and turns caudally on the lateral surface of the scapula at the base of the acromion, finally entering the deep face of the infraspinatus muscle. The **supraspinatus muscle (1)** originates in the supraspinous fossa and inserts cranially on the greater tubercle of the humerus. The **infraspinatus muscle (9)** lies deep to the scapular part of the deltoid muscle. Its origin is the infraspinatus fossa and spine and cartilage of the scapula. It ends on the infraspinatus facet of the humerus, a little distal to the greater tubercle. Where its tendon crosses over the cartilage-covered caudal part of the greater tubercle, it is underlain by a subtendinous bursa. The insertion tendons of the infraspinatus and subscapularis have the function of lateral or, respectively, medial contractile ligaments at the shoulder joint, which lacks proper collateral ligaments. Deep within the fibrous joint capsule there are lateral and medial fibrous reinforcements that are designated glenohumeral ligaments (see p. 26). The **radial nerve (15)**, passing deep to the lateral head of the triceps, supplies with its proximal muscular branches the heads of the triceps brachii muscle and the anconeus muscle. The continuing radial nerve passes distally upon the brachialis muscle and divides into a **deep branch (17)** for the digital and carpal joint extensors (and the ulnaris lateralis) and a **superficial branch (16)** that accompanies the cephalic vein on either side with lateral and medial branches. These branches continue on the distal limb alongside the accessory cephalic vein. Their dorsal common digital nerves supply the dorsum of the manus. The triceps brachii muscle (see also the small illustration) originates with its **long head (12)** on the caudal margin of the scapula, with its **accessory head (14)** caudally on the humerus, with its **lateral head (13)** from the line of triceps and, with its **medial head (8)**, proximomedially from the humerus. Deep to their common termination at the olecranon, a subtendinous bursa is present laterally. Proximal to the olecranon there is an inconstant subcutaneous olecranon bursa. The **anconeus (18)** originates at the margins of the olecranon fossa and ends with a fleshy attachment laterally on the olecranon.

Muscles of scapula

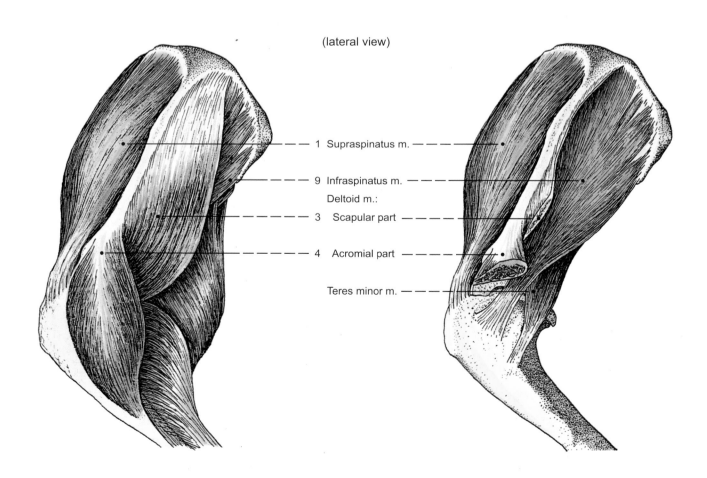

(lateral view)

1 Supraspinatus m.

9 Infraspinatus m.

Deltoid m.:

3 Scapular part

4 Acromial part

Teres minor m.

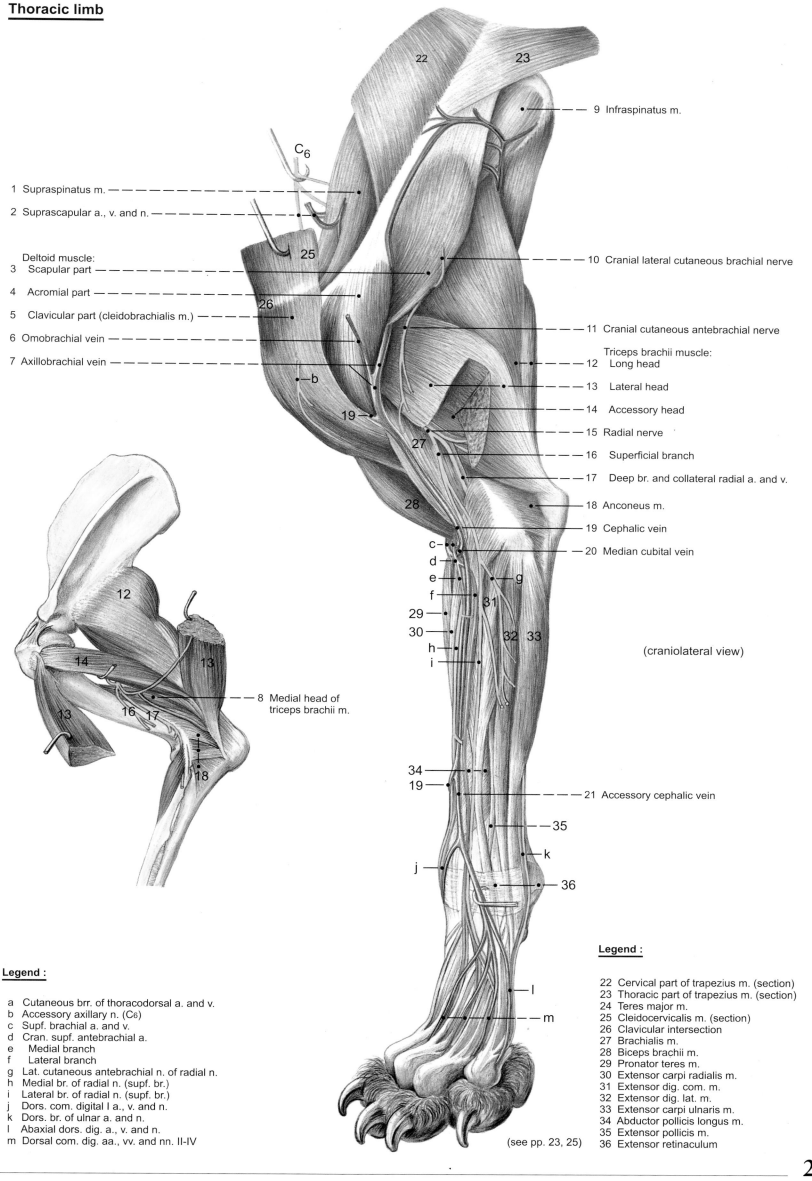

1 Supraspinatus m. — — — — — —

2 Suprascapular a., v. and n. — — — — — — —

C6

Deltoid muscle:
3   Scapular part — — — — — — — —

4   Acromial part — — — — — — —

5   Clavicular part (cleidobrachialis m.) — — — —

6 Omobrachial vein — — — — — — —

7 Axillobrachial vein — — — — — — —

8 Medial head of triceps brachii m.

9 Infraspinatus m.

10 Cranial lateral cutaneous brachial nerve

11 Cranial cutaneous antebrachial nerve

Triceps brachii muscle:
12   Long head

13   Lateral head

14   Accessory head

15   Radial nerve

16   Superficial branch

17   Deep br. and collateral radial a. and v.

18 Anconeus m.

19 Cephalic vein

20 Median cubital vein

21 Accessory cephalic vein

(craniolateral view)

(see pp. 23, 25)

4. ANTEBRACHIAL (FOREARM) MUSCLES AND THEIR NERVE SUPPLY

To clearly differentiate between the individual carpal and digital flexor muscles, the termination of their tendinous insertions has to be identified. To do this, the carpal canal, passage for the two digital flexor tendons and associated structures on the palmar carpus, must be opened. First, the superficial lamina of the flexor retinaculum extending between the accessory carpal bone and the medial styloid process is cut. The superficial flexor tendon is lifted up from the carpal canal. Then the deep lamina of the flexor retinaculum, which lies between the flexor tendons, is cut. After lifing up the deep flexor tendon, the palmar carpal ligament, which forms the deep boundary of the canal, can be seen. To see the insertions of the extensor and flexor tendons, the skin of the second digit will be completely reflected. The manica flexoria of the superficial flexor tendon is incised laterally and the passage of the deep flexor tendon through the manica can then be more easily observed.

1 **a)** The **CAUDOMEDIAL FOREARM MUSCLES** are the two digital flexors, the two flexors of the carpal joint and the two pronators of the radioulnar joints.

The **origin of all of these muscles** except one (pronator quadratus) is from the medial epicondyle of the humerus; additional to its origin from the medial epicondyle, the deep digital flexor has radial and ulnar heads. The pronator quadratus muscle is composed of horizontal fibers that occupy the antebrachial interosseous space. Two of the muscles have, in addition to their origin from the medial epicondyle, an origin from the ulna (flexor carpi ulnaris muscle) and an origin from the ulna and radius (deep digital flexor muscle). Thus, the flexor carpi ulnaris has two heads of origin, the deep digital flexor, three.

The **insertion of the two digital flexors** is on the digital bones; of the two carpal joint flexors, at the carpus or proximal metacarpus; of the two pronators on the radius and ulna (these are things to consider in identifying the different muscles).

I. Of the two **digital flexor muscles**, the **superficial digital flexor (10)** is continued at the distal third of the antebrachium by its tendon, which divides in the proximal metacarpus into four branches, each inserting on a digit (II – V). Proximal to their termination on the flexor tuberosity of the middle phalanx the tendon is modified to form a tunnel or sleeve-like **manica flexoria (20)** for the corresponding tendon-branch of the deep digital flexor. The **deep digital flexor muscle** has a strong **humeral head (8)** and weak **ulnar (7)** and **radial (6) heads** that join in the distal third of the antebrachium to form the deep flexor tendon. The deep flexor tendon then divides at the distal carpus and proximal metacarpus into five tendons of insertion (I – V), four of which pass through the sleeve of the corresponding manica flexoria and end on the flexor tubercle of the distal phalanx of digits II – V. The branch of the deep flexor to the distal phalanx of digit I is unaccompanied by a tendon of the superficial flexor.

2 **II.** Of the two carpal joint flexors, the two heads of the **flexor carpi ulnaris muscle (15)** remain separate up to their insertion on the accessory carpal bone. The ulnar head is mainly tendinous, the humeral head predominantly fleshy. The **flexor carpi radialis muscle (2)** has a divided terminal tendon and inserts on the proximopalmar aspect of metacarpal bones II and III.

III. Of the two **pronator muscles** of the radioulnar joints, the **pronator teres muscle** (see text-illustration) inserts craniomedially on the proximal radius. The **pronator quadratus muscle (4)** occupies the antebrachial interosseous space palmarly, and extends between the radius and ulna.

The **nerve supply** is by the **median (5) and ulnar nerves (9)**, in which case the more medially located muscles (pronator teres, pronator quadratus and flexor carpi radialis muscles as well as the radial head of the deep digital flexor muscle) are supplied alone by the median nerve. The median nerve also supplies the superficial digital flexor, the most caudal of the medial muscles. The more caudally located muscles (flexor carpi ulnaris muscle and ulnar head of the deep digital flexor muscle) are supplied only by the ulnar nerve. The humeral head of the deep digital flexor muscle, consisting of three bellies and found in the middle of both areas of supply is innervated by both the ulnar and median nerves. The **ulnar nerve** divides in the proximal antebrachial third into the palmar branch and the dorsal branch. The **dorsal branch of the ulnar nerve (14)** runs distally along the caudolateral border of the ulnaris lateralis muscle (extensor carpi ulnaris muscle), crosses the accessory carpal bone laterally, and ends as abaxial dorsal digital nerve V on the dorsum of the manus. The **palmar branch of the ulnar nerve (17)** courses deeply, within the carpal canal medial to the accessory carpal bone and between the accessorometacarpal ligaments (ligaments that extend from the accessory carpal bone to metacarpal bones IV and V; see illustration on p. 27), to reach the lateral palmar surface of the manus.

b) The **CRANIOLATERAL FOREARM MUSCLES** are the digital extensors, two muscles of the pollex (digit I, homologous to the thumb of human beings), two carpal extensors and two supinators of the radioulnar joints (see text-illustration).

The **origin** of the craniolateral forearm muscles is predominantly from the lateral supracondylar crest (brachioradialis, extensor carpi radialis, common digital extensor), the lateral epicondyle of the humerus and the lateral collateral ligament of the elbow joint (supinator, lateral digital extensor, extensor carpi ulnaris or ulnaris lateralis). The long abductor of digit I (*m. abductor pollicis longus*) and the extensor of digit I (*m. extensor pollicis*) arise from the cranial surface of the ulna and radius and the interosseous ligament that joins the two bones.

The **insertion** of these muscles is brought into play in distinguishing the different muscles of the craniolateral group. Of the four muscle groups, each consisting of two individual muscles, the digital extensors insert distally on

the extensor process of the distal phalanx, the pollex muscles between the metacarpus and the distal phalanx of digit I, the carpal extensors directly distally to the carpus and the metacarpus, and the supinators on the radius.

I. Of the two **digital extensors**, the **common digital extensor muscle (13)** ends on digits II – V and the **lateral digital extensor muscle (16)** on digits III – V.

II. Of the two **pollex (digit I) muscles**, the **long abductor of digit I (11)** inserts proximally on the first metacarpal bone, and the **extensor of digit I (12)** ends with two very weak tendons on the first and second digits.

III. Of the two **extensors of the carpal joint** (both are named 'extensors'; only the extensor carpi radialis functions as an extensor of the joint), the **extensor carpi radialis muscle (3)** ends by dividing into two tendons that insert proximally on metacarpal bones II and III. The **extensor carpi ulnaris (ulnaris lateralis, –18)**, which acts chiefly as an abductor of the paw and partial flexor of the carpus ends on the proximal lateral prominence of metacarpal V and with a transverse branch that attaches to the accessory carpal bone.

IV. Of the two supinators (see text-illustration), the **supinator muscle** lies deep to the origins of the digital extensors and terminates proximocranially on the radius. The **brachioradialis muscle** passes superficially on the flexor aspect of the elbow joint and inserts on the craniomedial margin of the radius at the junction of its middle and distal thirds.

The **nerve supply** of these muscles is by the **radial nerve**, which, by its **deep branch (1)**, supplies all of the craniolateral forearm muscles. The superficial branch (see p. 21) lies on both sides of the cephalic vein with its medial and lateral branches, and gives off the lateral cutaneous antebrachial nerve as the several branches that extend caudally from the lateral branch onto the craniolateral antebrachium. In the company of the accessory cephalic vein, both the medial and lateral branches continue distally onto the dorsum of the manus and branch here into the **dorsal common digital nerves (19)**, each of which ends by dividing proximal to the metacarpophalangeal joints into dorsal proper digital nerves that extend toward the ends of neighboring digits.

Antebrachial muscles

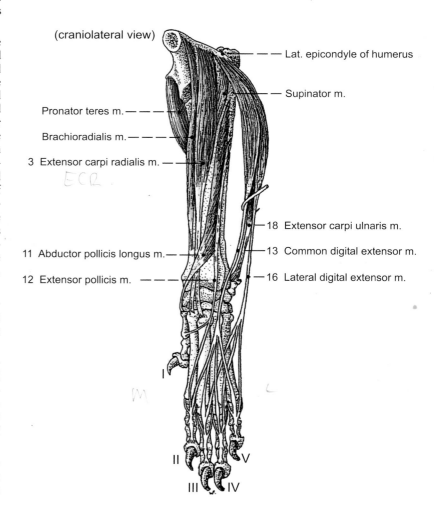

(craniolateral view)

- Lat. epicondyle of humerus
- Supinator m.

Pronator teres m.

Brachioradialis m.

3 Extensor carpi radialis m.

11 Abductor pollicis longus m.

12 Extensor pollicis m.

18 Extensor carpi ulnaris m.

13 Common digital extensor m.

16 Lateral digital extensor m.

I

II V

III IV

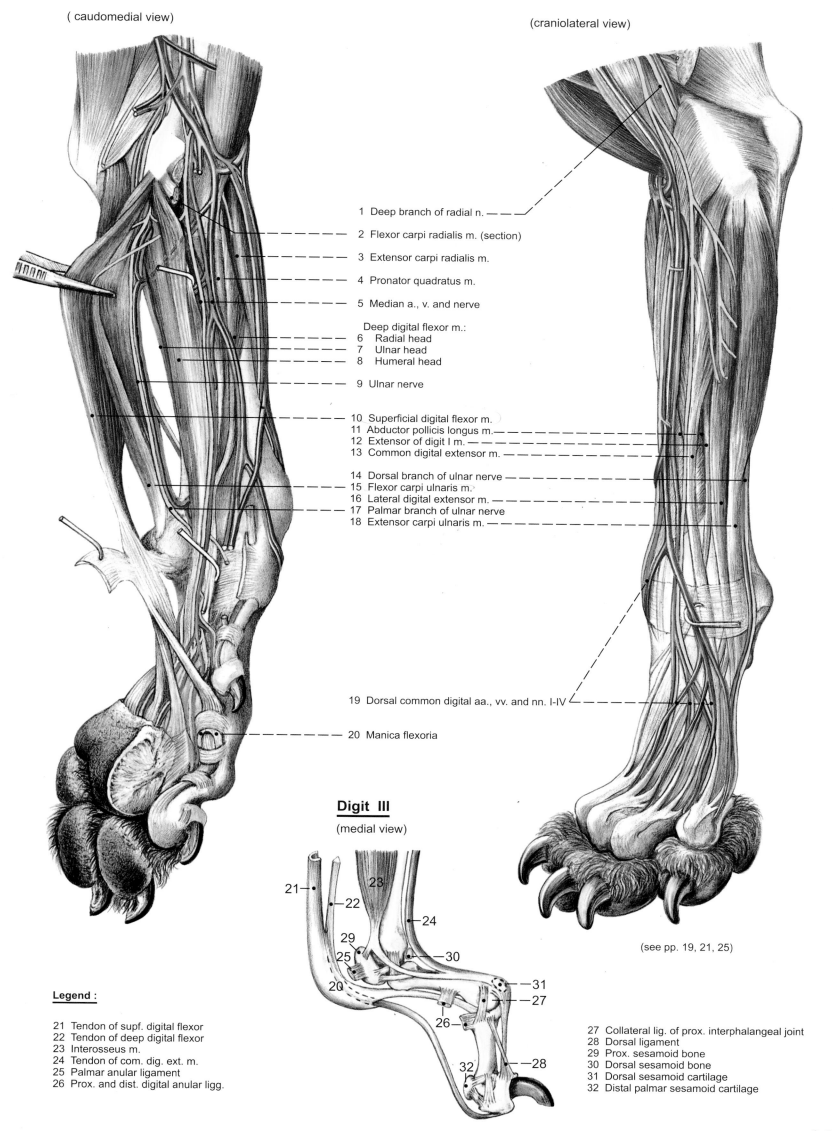

(caudomedial view)

(craniolateral view)

1 Deep branch of radial n.
2 Flexor carpi radialis m. (section)
3 Extensor carpi radialis m.
4 Pronator quadratus m.
5 Median a., v. and nerve

Deep digital flexor m.:
6   Radial head
7   Ulnar head
8   Humeral head
9 Ulnar nerve

10 Superficial digital flexor m.
11 Abductor pollicis longus m.
12 Extensor of digit I m.
13 Common digital extensor m.
14 Dorsal branch of ulnar nerve
15 Flexor carpi ulnaris m.
16 Lateral digital extensor m.
17 Palmar branch of ulnar nerve
18 Extensor carpi ulnaris m.

19 Dorsal common digital aa., vv. and nn. I-IV

20 Manica flexoria

Digit III

(medial view)

(see pp. 19, 21, 25)

Legend :

21 Tendon of supf. digital flexor
22 Tendon of deep digital flexor
23 Interosseus m.
24 Tendon of com. dig. ext. m.
25 Palmar anular ligament
26 Prox. and dist. digital anular ligg.

27 Collateral lig. of prox. interphalangeal joint
28 Dorsal ligament
29 Prox. sesamoid bone
30 Dorsal sesamoid bone
31 Dorsal sesamoid cartilage
32 Distal palmar sesamoid cartilage

23

5. VESSELS AND NERVES OF THE THORACIC LIMB

a) SHOULDER, BRACHIUM (ARM) AND ANTEBRACHIUM (FORE-ARM) are supplied by blood vessels and nerves that run mainly medially and cranially on the limb. At the joints they are generally found on the protected, flexor, aspect of the joint. The blood supply of the thoracic limb is by a single artery, the axillary artery. The venous drainage is by several veins: the medially situated axillary vein, the craniolaterally located cephalic and the axillobrachial and omobrachial veins.

The **axillary artery and vein (15)** lie at the bend of the shoulder joint, superficial to the axillary nerve. At the level of the first rib, they continue the long subclavian artery or, respectively, the very short subclavian vein and give off the external thoracic and lateral thoracic vessels before ending by dividing into the subscapular artery and vein and the brachial artery and vein. The cranial circumflex humeral vessels usually arise at the terminal division of the axillary vessels or from the brachial artery and vein. With the cranial pectoral nerve, the **external thoracic artery and vein (16)** enter the superficial pectoral muscle. The **lateral thoracic artery and vein (3)** pass with the same-named nerve on the lateral border of the deep pectoral muscle; they supply the axillary lymph node and the inconstant accessory axillary lymph node and the thoracic mammae. Branches of the lateral thoracic vessels, joined by caudal pectoral nerves, pass to the deep face of the deep pectoral muscle. The **subscapular artery and vein (1)** course at the caudal border of the subscapular muscle. The subscapular artery gives off caudally the **thoracodorsal artery (2)**; whereas, the **thoracodorsal vein (2)** usually arises from the axillary vein. With the same-named nerve, both vessels enter the medial aspect of the latissimus dorsi muscle. Additional branches of the subscapular artery and vein are the **caudal circumflex humeral artery and vein (4)**, which run deeply, passing laterally caudal to the shoulder joint, ventral to the long head of triceps, and anastomose with the weak cranial circumflex humeral vessels. The **cranial circumflex humeral artery and vein (17)** pass cranially from the axillary or brachial vessels and enter the biceps brachii muscle at its hilus. The **brachial artery and vein (5)**, which proceed as end-branches of the axillary vessels, give off the deep brachial, bicipital, collateral ulnar, superficial brachial and transverse cubital arteries and veins. After passing deep to the pronator teres muscle, the brachial vessels end at the level of the proximal interosseous space by dividing into common interosseous and median vessels. About the middle of the brachium, accompanied by the radial nerve, the **deep brachial artery and vein (6)** pass deeply between the medial and long heads of the triceps, which they supply. In the distal brachium, the **bicipital artery and vein (18)** pass cranially to supply the biceps brachii muscle. The **collateral ulnar artery and vein (7)** accompany the ulnar nerve to the extensor aspect of the elbow joint and anastomose distally with the recurrent ulnar vessels that proceed from the ulnar artery and vein. The **superficial brachial artery (8)** originates in the distal third of the brachium; the same-named vein closer to the level of the elbow joint. The artery and vein pass first superficially and transversely across the flexor aspect of the elbow joint. The superficial brachial artery passes over distally into the superficial antebrachial artery, whose branches initially join the cephalic vein and, continuing, pass onto the dorsum of the manus, with the accessory cephalic vein. On the flexor aspect of the elbow joint, the very short **superficial brachial vein (8)** is continued by the median cubital vein. The arrangement of the veins here is like the letter 'H.' The superficial brachial and median cubital veins form the bar of the H. The longitudinal branches of the 'H' are formed medially by the brachial vein, laterally by the cephalic vein. The **transverse cubital artery and vein (9)** pass deep to the terminal part of the biceps brachii muscle at the level of the flexor aspect of the elbow joint. The **common interosseous artery and vein (10)** give off the **ulnar artery and vein (11)**, which pass distally with the ulnar nerve. The common interosseous vessels end by dividing into cranial and caudal interosseous vessels. The caudal interosseous vessels run distally deep to the pronator quadratus muscle. The cranial interosseous vessels emerge cranially from the proximal interosseous space and supply the craniolateral forearm muscles. The **median artery and vein (12)** arise as end-branches of the brachial vessels. In the proximal third of the antebrachium, they give off caudally the **deep antebrachial vessels (13)** for the caudomedial forearm muscles and, a fingerbreadth distal, the small **radial artery and vein (14)** that pass along the medial margin of the radius. After this, the median artery (the satellite veins become very small) passes in the carpal canal and reaches the palmar surface of the deep digital flexor tendon.

b) The **VESSEL AND NERVE SUPPLY OF THE MANUS** is by deep and superficial arteries, veins and nerves. On the dorsal and palmar surfaces of the manus, the deeply located vessels and nerves are designated *metacarpal* arteries, veins, and nerves; dorsal or palmar according to the surface of the manus supplied. The superficially located vessels and nerves are designated *common digital* arteries, veins, and nerves; again, dorsal or palmar according to the surface of the manus. The common digital vessels and nerves divide distally into proper digital vessels and nerves.

I. On the **dorsum of the manus**, the dorsal common digital arteries I – IV proceed from the two branches of the superficial antebrachial artery. Dorsal common digital veins I – IV are from the accessory cephalic vein. Dorsal common digital nerves I – IV are from the medial and lateral branches (rami) of the superficial ramus of the radial nerve. The dorsal branch of the ulnar nerve ends on the dorsum of the manus as the dorsal abaxial digital nerve of digit V. The deeply located dorsal metacarpal arteries and veins I – IV originate from the respective arterial and venous *rete carpi dorsale*. The venous carpal rete (carpal network) is formed by dorsal carpal branches of the accessory cephalic and radial veins. The arterial carpal rete is formed by dorsal carpal branches of the caudal interosseous, ulnar and radial arteries.

II. On the **palmar surface of the manus**, the palmar common digital arteries and veins I – IV arise from the respective arterial and venous superficial palmar arches. The arterial superficial palmar arch is formed in the proximal metacarpus. The medial arm of the arch is from the median and radial arteries; its lateral arm proceeds from the union of the ulnar artery and palmar carpal branch of the caudal interosseous artery. The venous superficial palmar arch lies farther distally, at the proximal margin of the metacarpal pad. It is formed by a confluence of the cephalic and radial veins medially, by the ulnar and caudal interosseous veins laterally. The palmar metacarpal arteries and veins I – IV originate in the proximal metacarpus from the respective arterial and venous deep palmar arches. The arterial arch is formed medially by the radial artery and laterally by a confluence of the ulnar and caudal interosseous arteries. The venous arch is formed by the cephalic and radial veins medially and laterally by a confluence of the ulnar and caudal interosseous veins. The palmar common digital nerves I – III arise from the median nerve, palmar common digital nerve IV from the superficial branch of the palmar branch of the ulnar nerve. Palmar metacarpal nerves I – IV originate from the deep branch of the palmar branch of the ulnar nerve.

c) The **LYMPH DRAINAGE** of the thoracic limb (see pp. 15 and 19) is by superficially and deeply located lymph vessels. The superficial lymph vessels predominantly accompany the superficial lateral cutaneous veins and pass to the **superficial cervical lymph nodes** from which the lymph drains to the venous angle at the junction of internal and external jugular veins. The deep lymph vessels accompany the deep blood vessels and pass to the axillary and accessory axillary lymph nodes, which also drain the lymph from the thoracic wall and the three cranial mammae. The disc-shaped **axillary lymph node**, about 2 cm in diameter, can be palpated in the caudal angle between the lateral thoracic and axillary vessels. The **accessory axillary lymph node** is located one intercostal space farther caudal on the course of the lateral thoracic artery and vein. The lymph passes from the axillary and accessory axillary lymph nodes to the venous angle also.

Legend (see figure on opposite page)

19 Circumflex scapular a. and v.	33 Axillobrachial v.	52 Cranial cutaneous antebrachial n.
20 Brachiocephalic v.	34 Median n.	53 Suprascapular n.
21 Subclavian v.	35 Recurrent ulnar a. and v.	54 Accessory axillary (brachiocephalic) n. (C6)
22 Collateral radial a. and v.	36 Cranial interosseous a. and v.	55 External jugular v.
23 Ulnar n.	37 Caudal interosseous a. and v.	56 Cephalic v.
24 Caudal cutaneous antebrachial n.	38 Interosseous branch	57 Median cubital v.
25 Palmar branch	39 Dorsal branch of the ulnar a. and n.	58 Accessory cephalic v.
26 Deep branch	40 Deep palmar arch	59 Omobrachial v.
27 Superficial branch	41 Musculocutaneous n.	60 Palmar metacarpal aa., vv. and nn. I – IV
28 Palmar abaxial a. and n. of digit V	42 Medial cutaneous antebrachial n.	61 Dorsal abaxial n. of digit I (dorsal view)
29 Superficial palmar arch	43 Radial n.	Palmar abaxial n. of digit I (palmar view)
30 Dorsal common digital aa., vv. and nn. (dorsal view)	44 Superficial ramus	62 Dorsal carpal branch of the radial a. and v.
Palmar common digital aa., vv. and nn. (palmar view)	45 Lateral branch (ramus)	63 Dorsal carpal branch of the caudal interosseous a.
31 Dorsal proper digital aa., vv. and nn. (dorsal view)	46 Medial branch (ramus)	64 Dorsal carpal branch of the accessory cephalic v.
Palmar proper digital aa., vv. and nn. (palmar view)	47 Deep branch	65 Dorsal carpal branch of the ulnar a.
32 Phrenic nerve	48 Cranial superficial antebrachial a.	66 Rete carpi dorsale
	49 Lateral branch (ramus)	67 Dorsal metacarpal aa. and vv. I – IV
	50 Medial branch (ramus)	68 Abaxial dorsal digital a., v. and n. of digit V
	51 Axillary n.	

Arteries, Veins, Nerves of thoracic limb

(Basset Artésien - Normand)

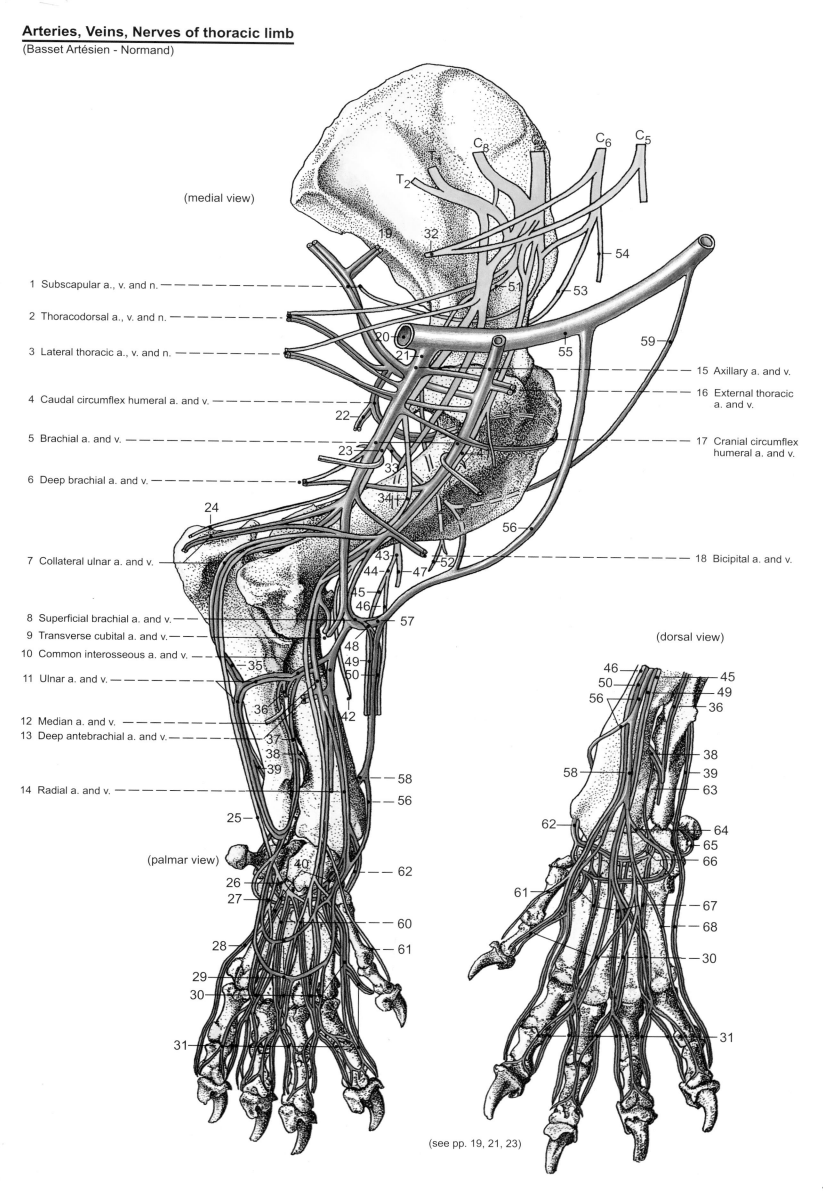

(medial view)

T$_1$
T$_2$
C$_8$
C$_6$
C$_5$

19   32   54

51   53

1 Subscapular a., v. and n.

2 Thoracodorsal a., v. and n.

3 Lateral thoracic a., v. and n.

20   55   59

21

4 Caudal circumflex humeral a. and v.

22

5 Brachial a. and v.

23

6 Deep brachial a. and v.

33

34

24

7 Collateral ulnar a. and v.

43
44   47   52
45
46

8 Superficial brachial a. and v.

57

9 Transverse cubital a. and v.

48

10 Common interosseous a. and v.

49
50

35

11 Ulnar a. and v.

36

12 Median a. and v.

42

13 Deep antebrachial a. and v.

37
38
39

14 Radial a. and v.

58
56

25

(palmar view)

40

26

27

28

29

30

31

15 Axillary a. and v.

16 External thoracic a. and v.

17 Cranial circumflex humeral a. and v.

18 Bicipital a. and v.

(dorsal view)

46   45
50   49
56   36

38
39

58   63

62   64
65
66

61   67
68
30

31

62   60   61

(see pp. 19, 21, 23)

25

6. SYNOVIAL STRUCTURES OF THE THORACIC LIMB

a) JOINTS OF THE THORACIC LIMB

	NAME	BONES INVOLVED	FORM/ COMPOSITION	FUNCTION	COMMENTS
1	I. Shoulder (humeral) joint	Glenoid cavity of the scapula, head of the humerus	Spheroid joint/ Simple joint	Movement in all directions, chiefly a hinge joint (ginglymus).	A capsular synovial sheath invests the tendon of origin of the biceps brachii muscle, which is kept in position by the transverse retinaculum that bridges the intertubercular groove.
2	II. Elbow (cubital) joint a) Humero-ulnar joint	Humeral condyle, trochlear notch of the ulna	Compound joint/ Ginglymus	Snapping hinge joint	Craniolateral recess deep to the common digital extensor muscle; 2. Craniomedial recess deep to the biceps brachii muscle; 3. Caudal recess between the lateral epidondyle and the olecranon.
	b) Humero-radial joint	Humeral condyle, head of the radius	Ginglymus		
3	c) Proximal radio-ulnar joint	Articular circumference of the radius, radial notch of the ulna	Trochoid joint	Rotation of the radius on its long axis	
3	III. Distal radioulnar joint	Ulnar notch of the radius, radial circumference of the ulna	Trochoid joint/ Simple joint	Rotation of the radius on its long axis	The joint cavity communicates with the carpal joint. For treatment of growth disturbances, the radioulnar ligament may be cut.
	Joints of the Manus				
4	IV. Carpal joint a) Antebrachiocarpal joint	Trochlea of the radius, ulna, radial carpal bone, ulnar carpal bone	Ellipsoid joint, compound joint	Predominantly a hinge joint with slight abduction/ adduction movement	The joint cavity consists of two parts that communicate with each other. Proximal part: a) and e), which communicate with the radioulnar joint. Distal part: b) and c). The carpal joint has dorsal fascial reinforcement, the extensor retinaculum, which retains the extensor tendons in position. On the palmar aspect, the flexor retinaculum bridges the carpal canal. The lateral and medial collateral ligaments are relatively short ligaments since they bridge only the antebrachiocarpal joint.
	b) Middle carpal joint	Proximal and distal rows of the carpal bones	Condylar joint/ Compound joint		
	c) Carpometacarpal joint	Carpal bones I – IV and MC I – V	Plane joint/ Compound joint		
	d) Intercarpal joints	Joints between the carpal bones of a row (perpendicular joints)	Plane joint/ Compound joint		
	e) Joints of the accessory carpal bone	Accessory carpal bone, ulnar carpal bone, ulna	Plane joint/ Compound joint	Amphiarthrosis (little movement)	
	V. Metacarpophalangeal joints	Proximal phalanges; proximal sesamoid bones; dorsal sesamoid bones; metacarpal bones	Compound joint	Mainly a hinge joint with slight abduction and adduction as well as axial rotation	Metacarpophalangeal and interphalangeal joints have each in their joint capsules a dorsal and a palmar outpouching. The joint capsule attaches at the margin of the articular surfaces of the participating sesamoids. At the metacarpophalangeal joint there are proximal sesamoids palmarly and a single dorsal sesamoid.
	VI. Proximal interphalangeal joints of the manus	Proximal and middle phalanges	Saddle joint/ Simple joint		Dorsal sesamoid is present.
	VII. Distal interphalangeal joints of the manus	Middle phalanges and distal phalanges	Saddle joint/ Simple joint		Distal sesamoid is present.

The **shoulder joint** lacks typical ligaments external to the joint capsule. Their function is taken over by contractile tension-bands, the tendons of the infraspinatus and subscapular muscles. The lateral and medial glenohumeral ligaments are 'internal' capsular reinforcements.

At the **elbow joint** the collateral ligaments bifurcate, forming radial and ulnar attachments. The anular ligament of the radius grips around the head of the radius and extends from the medial coronoid process of the ulna to the lateral collateral ligament.

b) SYNOVIAL BURSAE

The **subtendinous bursa of the infraspinatus muscle** is located between its terminal tendon and the cartilage-covered lateral surface of the greater tubercle.

The **subtendinous bursa of the subscapularis muscle** lies between the insertional tendon of its muscle and the shoulder joint capsule.

The **subtendinous bursa of the triceps brachii muscle** is expanded between the olecranon and the insertion of the triceps brachii muscle.

5 The **subcutaneous olecranon bursa** is an acquired synovial bursa.

The **bicipitoradial bursa** lies between the tendon of the biceps and the radius and is frequently fused with the subtendinous bursa of the brachialis muscle.

The **subtendinous bursa of the brachialis muscle** is located between the endtendon of the brachialis and the radius.

c) SYNOVIAL SHEATHS

Synovial sheaths protect the tendon of origin of the coracobrachial muscle (*Vagina synovialis m. coracobrachialis*), and of the biceps brachii muscle in the intertubercular groove (*Vagina synovialis intertubercularis*). The latter is an extension of the shoulder joint capsule with which it communicates. The end-tendons of the carpal joint extensors are protected by a synovial sheath (long abductor of digit I) or by synovial sheaths and bursae (extensor carpi radialis). The ulnaris lateralis end-tendon and its caudal extension to the accessory carpal are protected by a synovial bursa. The radial carpal flexor end-tendon is protected by a synovial sheath; the ulnar carpal flexor by a bursa. The digital extensors are protected by synovial sheaths at the carpus, the digital flexors on the digits. The deep flexor usually has a synovial sheath at the carpus.

Joints, synovial bursae and sheaths

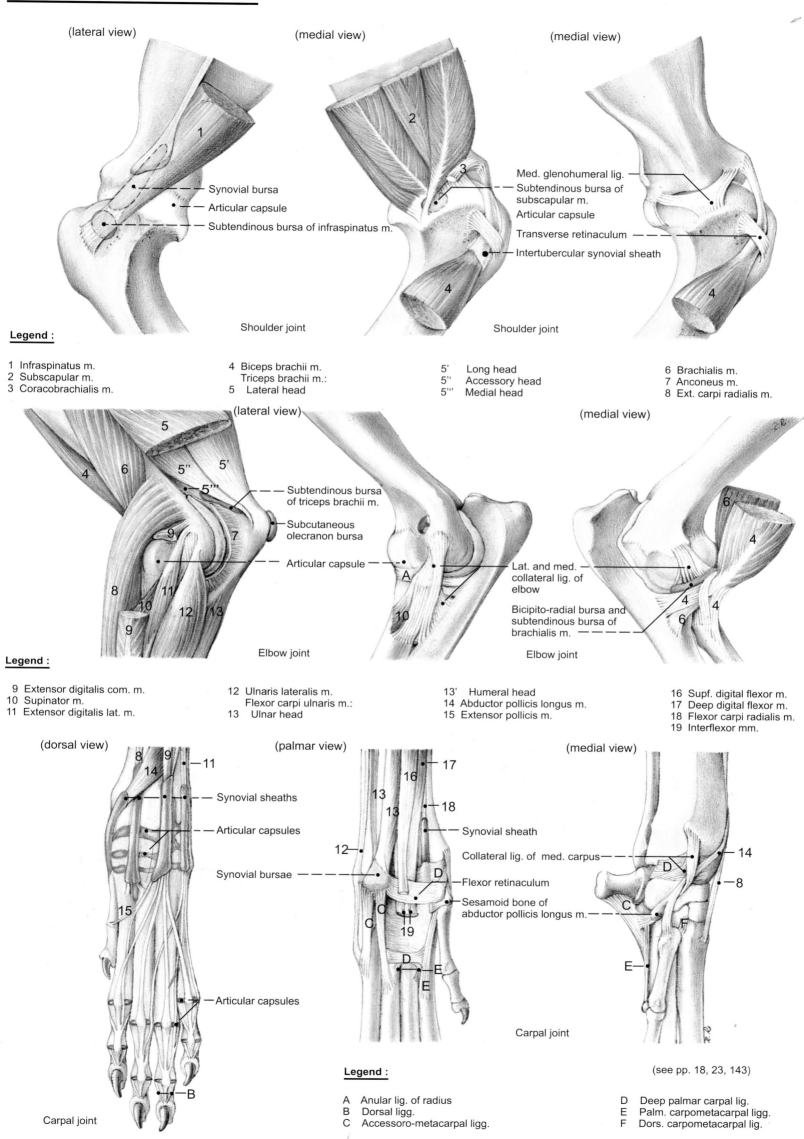

(lateral view)

(medial view)

(medial view)

Synovial bursa
Articular capsule
Subtendinous bursa of infraspinatus m.

2

3

4

Med. glenohumeral lig.
Subtendinous bursa of subscapular m.
Articular capsule
Transverse retinaculum
Intertubercular synovial sheath

4

Shoulder joint

Shoulder joint

Legend :

1 Infraspinatus m.
2 Subscapular m.
3 Coracobrachialis m.

4 Biceps brachii m.
Triceps brachii m.:
5 Lateral head

5' Long head
5'' Accessory head
5''' Medial head

6 Brachialis m.
7 Anconeus m.
8 Ext. carpi radialis m.

(lateral view)

(medial view)

5

4 6

5'' 5'

5'''

9 7

8

11

10

12 13

9

Subtendinous bursa of triceps brachii m.
Subcutaneous olecranon bursa
Articular capsule

A

10

Lat. and med. collateral lig. of elbow
Bicipito-radial bursa and subtendinous bursa of brachialis m.

6

4

4

6

Elbow joint

Elbow joint

Legend :

9 Extensor digitalis com. m.
10 Supinator m.
11 Extensor digitalis lat. m.

12 Ulnaris lateralis m.
Flexor carpi ulnaris m.:
13 Ulnar head

13' Humeral head
14 Abductor pollicis longus m.
15 Extensor pollicis m.

16 Supf. digital flexor m.
17 Deep digital flexor m.
18 Flexor carpi radialis m.
19 Interflexor mm.

(dorsal view)

(palmar view)

(medial view)

8 9
14
11

Synovial sheaths
Articular capsules
Synovial bursae

15

Articular capsules

B

Carpal joint

16 17

13

13

12

18

Synovial sheath

D

C

C

19

D

E

E

Flexor retinaculum
Sesamoid bone of abductor pollicis longus m.

Collateral lig. of med. carpus
14
8
D
C
F
E

Carpal joint

(see pp. 18, 23, 143)

Legend :

A Anular lig. of radius
B Dorsal ligg.
C Accessoro-metacarpal ligg.

D Deep palmar carpal lig.
E Palm. carpometacarpal ligg.
F Dors. carpometacarpal lig.

CHAPTER 4: THORACIC AND ABDOMINAL WALL

1. MUSCLES OF THE VERTEBRAL COLUMN, NUCHAL LIGAMENT, AND LUMBAR CUTANEOUS NERVES

To demonstrate the muscles of the vertebral column, the skin is removed from the lateral body wall, the dorsum, and the sacral region as far as the caudal end of the sacrum. Then one removes the remnants of the extrinsic muscles of the thoracic limb. The m. serratus dorsalis cranialis (33) is detached from its rib insertions and reflected dorsally. The thoracolumbar fascia (22, see also text-illustration p. 30) is incised longitudinally along a line parallel to and 2 cm from the dorsal midline. In the lumbosacral area, the underlying lumbodorsal tendon (39) is incised longitudinally at the same level as the fascia, and a transverse incision is made at the caudal end of the parent cut. Then the tendon is detached from the underlying musculature. The lumbodorsal tendon divides at the lateral border of the m. longissimus lumborum. The deep lamina is directed between the mm. iliocostalis and longissimus lumborum as an intermuscular septum (see text-illustration p. 30) and the superficial lamina runs over the m. iliocostalis. In the neck, the m. splenius and m. semispinalis are transected after being exposed. The sequence to be followed in the dissection of the muscles corresponds to the numeration in the table below.

a) The **MUSCLES OF THE VERTEBRAL COLUMN** are subdivided into a dorsal and a ventral group, and a specific epaxial group that moves the head. All the dorsal vertebral muscles (Nos. I to X) function in the extension and lateral movement or inclination of the vertebral column. The **innervation of all dorsal vertebral muscles** and the **dorsal muscles that act on the atlanto-occipital and atlanto-axial joints** ('head movers', — Nos. XIV to XVII) is by the dorsal rami of the spinal nerves.

The ventral vertebral muscles (Nos. XI to XIII) flex the vertebral column and incline it laterally. The **innervation of all ventral vertebral muscles** is by ventral rami of the segmental spinal nerves. The muscles situated ventral to the lumbar part of the vertebral column, namely the mm. quadratus lumborum, psoas major and psoas minor, belong to the sublumbar or inner loin muscles and are dealt with on p. 60.

MUSCLES OF THE VERTEBRAL COLUMN

Dorsal muscles of the vertebral column		Ventral muscles of the vertebral column	Dorsal muscles moving the head
I. m. splenius	VI. mm. multifidi	XI. mm. scaleni	XIV. m. rectus capitis dors. major
II m. iliocostalis	VII. m. sacrococcygeus (-caud.) dors. med.	XII. m. longus capitis	XV. m. rectus capitis dors. minor
III. m. longissimus	VIII. m. sacrococcygeus (-caud.) dors. lat.	XIII. m. longus colli	XVI. m. obliquus capitis caud.
IV. m. semispinalis capitis	IX. mm. interspinales		XVII m. obliquus capitis cran.
V. m. spinalis et semispinalis cervicis et thoracis	X. mm. intertransversarii		

I. The **m. splenius (1)**, previously transected in its middle, extends from the spinous processes of the first three thoracic vertebrae to the nuchal crest of the skull. II. The **m. iliocostalis** arises from the wing of the ilium and inserts onto the lumbar transverse process **(m. iliocostalis lumborum, —24)**, the angles of the ribs, and the transverse processes of the last two cervical vertebrae **(m. iliocostalis thoracis, —17)**. III. Also extending caudally to the wing of the ilium, the **m. longissimus** is divided along its length into the **mm. longissimus lumborum (23), thoracis (16), cervicis (12)** and **capitis (2)**. Corresponding to their region, these muscles insert onto lumbar transverse processes, tubercles of the ribs, cervical transverse processes and the mastoid process of the cranium respectively. IV. The **m. semispinalis capitis** lies in the neck region dorsal to the m. longissimus and consists of a dorsal **m. biventer cervicis (4)**, characterized by tendinous intersections directed transversely, and a ventral **m. complexus (3)**. Both muscles extend from the cervico-thoracic boundary to the cranium. V. The **m. spinalis et semispinalis thoracis et cervicis (15)** lies medial and adjacent to the m. longissimus and courses between the second cervical and eleventh thoracic vertebrae. VI. The multipennate **mm. multifidi** extend from the axis to the sacrum. In the caudal half of the neck, the m. **multifidus cervicis (10)** lies deep to the m. complexus and is traversed by dorsal branches of cervical nerves on its ventrolateral aspect. The m. multifidus thoracis is situated deeply, and the **m. multifidus lumborum (26)** lies deep to the thoracolumbar fascia, adjacent to lumbar vertebrae and their spinous processes. VII. At the level of the seventh lumbar vertebra the **m. sacrococcygeus (-caud.) dorsalis medialis (27)** continues the oblique pennate m. multifidus by means of an approximating fiber-flow directed caudally. VIII. The **m. sacrococcygeus (-caud.) dorsalis lateralis (25)** begins acutely at the fourth lumbar vertebra and, as the caudomedial continuation of the m. longissimus, proceeds to the tail by a strong terminal tendon. IX. The **mm. interspinales** lie deeply between the spinous processes. X. The **mm. intertransversarii (8)** are superficial in the neck; whereas, in the thoracolumbar region they are situated deeply along the vertebral column. The mm. intertransversarii cervicis are located ventral to the line of insertion of the m. longissimus cervicis. XI. The **mm. scaleni** extend from the fourth or fifth cervical vertebra to the eighth rib **(m. scalenus dorsalis, —14)** and the first rib **(m. scalenus ventralis, m. scalenus medius, —13)**. XII. The **m. longus capitis (9)** lying adjacent and ventromedial to the mm. scaleni is situated ventrolateral to the cervical vertebrae. Arising from the sixth cervical vertebra it inserts on the muscular tubercle of the occipital bone. XIII. The **m. longus colli** (see text-illustration), which appears plaited, is situated ventromedially on the cervical and thoracic parts of the vertebral column. Arising on the first cervical vertebra it extends to the sixth thoracic. XIV. The **m. rectus capitis dorsalis major (6)** continues cranially from the spinous process of the axis. Between the spinous process of the axis and the occipital bone it overlies the deeper **m. rectus capitis dorsalis minor (XV.)**. XVI. The **m. obliquus capitis caudalis (7)** extends from the lateral surface of the spinous process of the axis to the dorsal surface of the wing of the atlas. XVII. The **m. obliquus capitis cranialis (5)** runs from the wing of the atlas to the occipital bone.

b) The **NUCHAL LIGAMENT (11)**, which is paired, lies dorsomedian above the spinous processes of the cervical vertebrae and connects the spi-

nous processes of the second cervical and first thoracic vertebrae. Caudally it passes over into the supraspinous ligament. The yellow color of the nuchal ligament indicates a predominance of elastic fibers.

c) The **LUMBAR CUTANEOUS NERVES** form a dorsal, a lateral and a ventral series of cutaneous nerves by means of their serial passage through the strata of skeletal muscles.

I. The series of **dorsal lumbar cutaneous nerves** is formed from nL1 to 4 dl (dorsal clunial nn.) and becomes subcutaneous approximately 8 cm from the dorsal midline. As a rule the nL5 to 7 dl do not reach the cutaneous field of innervation.

II. The series of **lateral lumbar cutaneous nerves** arises from branches of the cranial iliohypogastric (nL1 vl), caudal iliohypogastric (nL2 vl), ilioinguinal (nL2 and 3 vl) and lateral cutaneous femoral (nL3 and 4 vl) nn. These nerves pass through the abdominal muscles on a line directed caudodorsally from the ventral end of the last rib to the tuber coxae. The **cranial iliohypogastric n. (18, —with accompanying blood vessels)**, and the **caudal iliohypogastric n. (19)** pierce the m. obliquus externus abdominis. The **ilioinguinal n. (20, —sometimes absent)** and the **lateral cutaneous femoral n. (21, —with accompanying blood vessels)** become subcutaneous over the dorsal border of the m. obliquus externus abdominis.

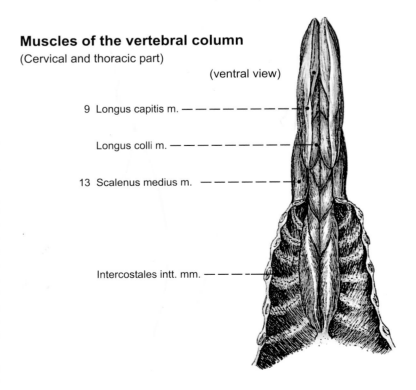

Muscles of the vertebral column
(Cervical and thoracic part)

(ventral view)

9 Longus capitis m. —————

Longus colli m. —————

13 Scalenus medius m. —————

Intercostales intt. mm. —————

Cervical and thoracic muscles

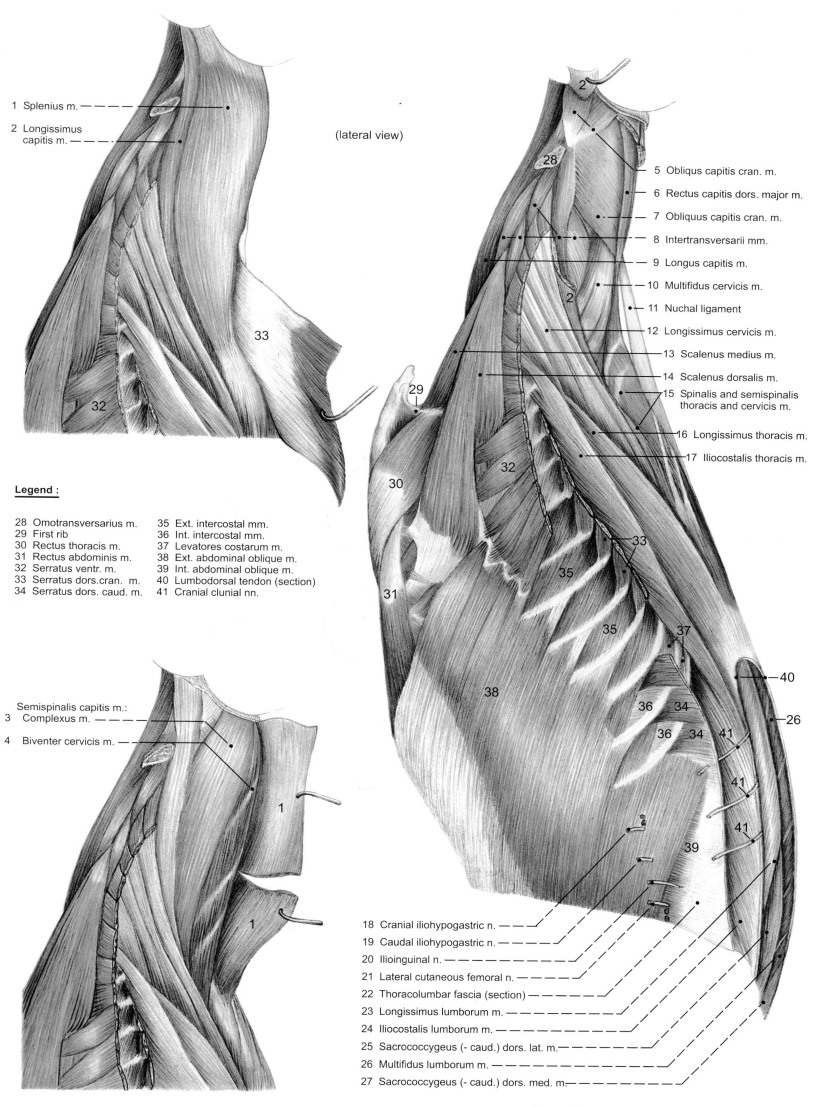

1 Splenius m.

2 Longissimus capitis m.

(lateral view)

2

28

5 Obliqus capitis cran. m.

6 Rectus capitis dors. major m.

7 Obliquus capitis cran. m.

8 Intertransversarii mm.

9 Longus capitis m.

10 Multifidus cervicis m.

11 Nuchal ligament

12 Longissimus cervicis m.

13 Scalenus medius m.

14 Scalenus dorsalis m.

15 Spinalis and semispinalis thoracis and cervicis m.

16 Longissimus thoracis m.

17 Iliocostalis thoracis m.

33

32

29

30

32

35

31

35

38

37

36 34

36 34 41

41

41

39

40

26

Legend :

28 Omotransversarius m.
29 First rib
30 Rectus thoracis m.
31 Rectus abdominis m.
32 Serratus ventr. m.
33 Serratus dors.cran. m.
34 Serratus dors. caud. m.

35 Ext. intercostal mm.
36 Int. intercostal mm.
37 Levatores costarum m.
38 Ext. abdominal oblique m.
39 Int. abdominal oblique m.
40 Lumbodorsal tendon (section)
41 Cranial clunial nn.

Semispinalis capitis m.:
3 Complexus m.
4 Biventer cervicis m.

1

1

18 Cranial iliohypogastric n.
19 Caudal iliohypogastric n.
20 Ilioinguinal n.
21 Lateral cutaneous femoral n.
22 Thoracolumbar fascia (section)
23 Longissimus lumborum m.
24 Iliocostalis lumborum m.
25 Sacrococcygeus (- caud.) dors. lat. m.
26 Multifidus lumborum m.
27 Sacrococcygeus (- caud.) dors. med. m.

(see p. 31)

2. RESPIRATORY MUSCLES

The thoracic cavity is opened after displaying the external respiratory muscles. To facilitate this, the right thoracic limb and its extrinsic muscles are removed and the following structures are severed or transected on both sides of the body: The mm. obliquus externus abdominis and scalenus dorsalis at their tendinous margins, and the first to ninth ribs of the right side and the second to ninth of the left inclusive. Dorsally the ribs in question are transected along the lateral border of the m. iliocostalis and ventrally along that of the m. rectus abdominis. In this way the line of insertion of the diaphragm remains intact. This runs from the ninth costal cartilage, across the eleventh costochondral articulation and caudodorsally to the middle of the thirteenth rib, and represents the boundary between the thoracic and pleural cavities on the one side and the abdominal and peritoneal cavities on the other. With the thoracic cavity opened, the five layers of the thoracic wall can be studied; namely, skin, external fascia of the trunk, a musculoskeletal layer, internal fascia of the trunk, and pleura. To expose the m. intercostalis internus, the m. intercostalis externus is removed from the tenth intercostal space.

The **respiratory muscles** lie upon the thorax and are known therefore as muscles of the thorax. From the functional viewpoint they are divided into an expiratory and an inspiratory group.

The main respiratory muscle, the diaphragm, and the other obligatory respiratory muscles, are supported functionally by auxiliary respiratory muscles, which have been discussed in connection with other muscle groups, for example the muscles of the vertebral column. The mm. scalenus and serratus ventralis are auxiliary inspiratory muscles and the m. iliocostalis and abdominal muscles are auxiliary expiratory muscles, although some authors consider the mm. scalenus to be obligatory. Keeping in mind their positional relationship to the thorax, the obligatory respiratory muscles are also divided into external, middle and internal respiratory muscles.

The **innervation of the diaphragm** is provided by the phrenic n. of its respective side and that of the remaining respiratory muscles by intercostal nn.

RESPIRATORY MUSCLES

Expiratory Muscles		Inspiratory Muscles
I. m. serratus dorsalis caudalis	external respiratory muscles	IV. m. serratus dorsalis cranialis V. m. rectus thoracis
II. mm. intercostales interni incl. mm. subcostales and retractor costae	middle respiratory muscles	VI. mm. intercostales externi incl. mm. levatores costarum
III. m. transversus thoracis	internal respiratory muscles	VII. Diaphragm

a) The **EXPIRATORY MUSCLES** run to the caudal borders of the ribs, their fibers being directed cranioventrally. They draw the ribs caudomedially and in so doing narrow the thorax.

I. The **m. serratus dorsalis caudalis (2)** takes origin from the thoracolumbar fascia (see text-illustration) and its fibers course cranioventrally to insert on the caudal borders of the last three ribs.

II. The **mm. intercostales interni (5)** lie dorsal to the costochondral articulations and deep to the mm. intercostales externi. They also appear deep to the m. rectus abdominis in the spaces between the costal cartilages. The **mm. subcostales** and the **m. retractor costae (34)** belong to the system of internal intercostal muscles. As a longer muscle portion, each of the mm. subcostales passes over the medial surface of a rib to insert onto the next or the next but one. The m. retractor costae extends from the transverse processes of the first three lumbar vertebrae to the caudal border of the last rib.

III. The **m. transversus thoracis (13)**, situated cranial to the diaphragm, is the cranial continuation of the **m. transversus abdominis**. It arises on the internal surface of the sternum and inserts in a crenate manner onto the medial surface of each **genu costae** (bend of the costal cartilage).

b) The **INSPIRATORY MUSCLES** run to the cranial borders of the ribs, the fiber bundles being directed caudoventrally. They draw the ribs craniolaterally and widen the thorax.

IV. The **m. serratus dorsalis cranialis (3)** takes origin from the supraspinous ligament dorsal to the first eight thoracic spinous processes and terminates by seven to nine fleshy insertions onto the cranial borders of ribs three to ten.

V. At the level of the fourth costal cartilage, the **m. rectus thoracis (6)** continues the m. rectus abdominis cranially. It runs obliquely over the aponeurotic origin of the latter as far as the first rib.

VI. The **mm. intercostales externi (4)** are situated mainly between the osseous ribs, and extend ventrally as far as the costochondral articulations at the approximate level of the lateral border of the m. rectus abdominis. Only sparse muscle bundles lie further ventrally. As the vertebral portions of the mm. intercostals externi, the **mm. levatores costarum (1)** can also be classified with the system of external intercostal muscles. Each of the mm. levatores costarum runs in approximately the same direction from the transverse process of one thoracic vertebra over the angle of the rib to the cranial border of the subsequent caudal rib. The mm. levatores are largely covered by the mm. iliocostalis and serratus dorsalis caudalis.

VII. The **diaphragm** is a musculotendinous septum between the thoracic and abdominal cavities. Its tendinous cupola situated ventrally projects a considerable way into the thoracic cavity. The diaphragm functions as the main respiratory muscle, the contraction of which flattens the cupola laterally. The crown of the cupola is fixed at the caval foramen and during respiration, its position remains largely constant.

The diaphragm is divided into a peripheral muscular portion and a centrally placed tendinous portion, the central tendon. The muscular portion consists of a **sternal part (15)** inserting onto the sternum, a **costal part (13)** inserting onto ribs nine to thirteen inclusive, and a **lumbar part**, the crura of which insert onto the third and fourth lumbar vertebrae. The free medial border of the weak **left crus (8)** and that of the stronger **right crus (7)** bound the **aortic hiatus (9)**. This affords passage to the aorta, thoracic duct and right azygos v. The free dorsolateral borders of the crura form the lumbocostal arches, which are crossed dorsally by the sympathetic trunk and the ramifying greater splanchnic n. The slit-like **esophageal hiatus (10)** provides a transit for the esophagus and the accompanying dorsal and ventral vagal trunks. It lies in the muscular part of the diaphragm bordering the central tendon. The **central tendon (14)** is V-shaped and exhibits the **foramen venae cavae (11)** to the right, in the region of the cupola. The foramen gives passage to the caudal vena cava.

Innervation is by the **phrenic n. (12)**, which arises by three roots from the fifth to seventh cervical nerves. The nerve passes over the pericardium and heart at the level of the coronary groove. The right phrenic n. accompanies the caudal vena cava, both lying within the *plica venae cavae* that extends between the heart and the diaphragm. The left phrenic n. reaches the diaphragm in a short fold of the mediastinal pleura of the left pleural sac.

Thoracolumbar fascia

(transverse section)

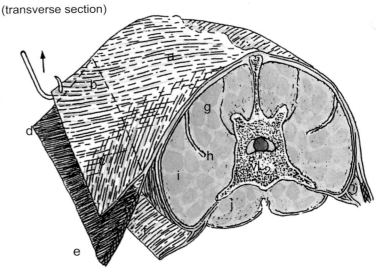

a	Thoracolumbar fascia	g	Longissimus lumborum m.
b	Latissimus dorsi m.	h	Intermuscular septum
c	Ext. abdom. oblique m.	i	Iliocostalis lumborum m.
d	Serratus dors. caud.	j	Quadratus lumborum and
e	Int. abdom. oblique m.		psoas minor mm.
f	Transversus abdominis m.		

Thoracic muscles

(left lateral view)

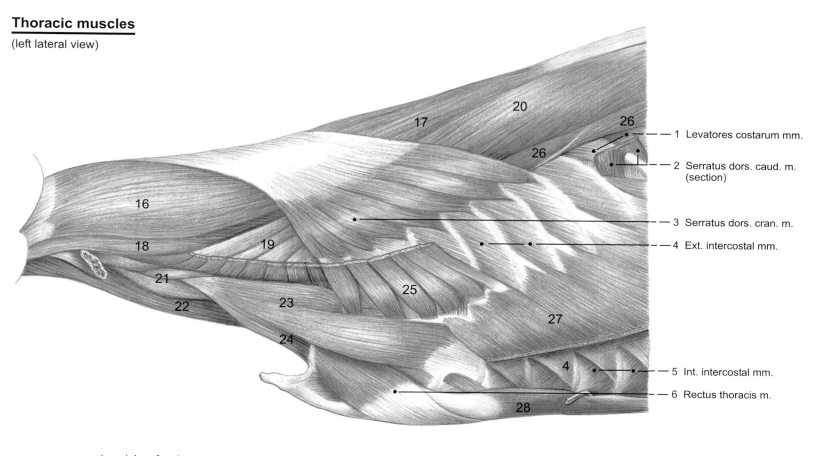

1 Levatores costarum mm.
2 Serratus dors. caud. m. (section)
3 Serratus dors. cran. m.
4 Ext. intercostal mm.
5 Int. intercostal mm.
6 Rectus thoracis m.

(cranial surface)

Diaphragma

(caudal surface)

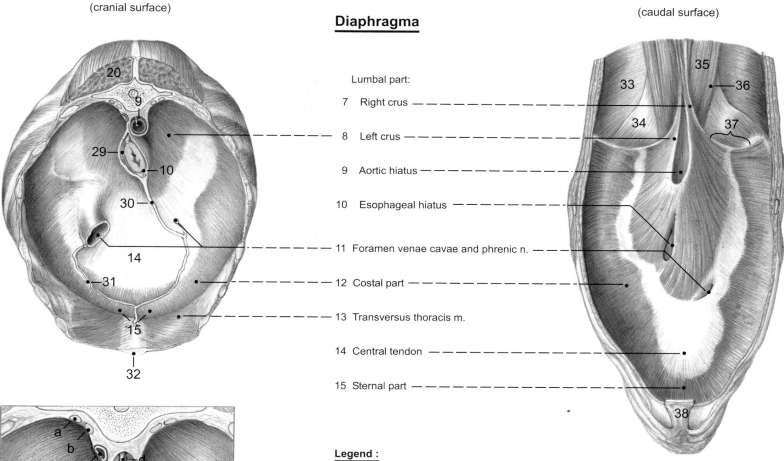

Lumbal part:

7 Right crus
8 Left crus
9 Aortic hiatus
10 Esophageal hiatus
11 Foramen venae cavae and phrenic n.
12 Costal part
13 Transversus thoracis m.
14 Central tendon
15 Sternal part

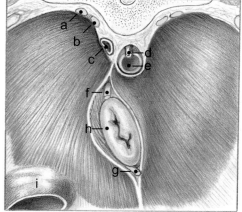

Legend :

a Sympathetic trunk
b Greater splanchnic n.
c Right azygos v.
d Thoracic duct
e Aorta
f Dorsal vagal trunk
g Ventral vagal trunk
h Esophagus
i Caudal vena cava

Legend :

16 Splenius m.
17 Spinalis and semispinalis thoracis m.
18 Longissimus capitis m.
19 Longissimus cervicis m.
20 Longissimus thoracis m.
21 Intertransverse m.
22 Longus capitis m.
23 Scalenus dorsalis m.
24 Scalenus medialis m.
25 Serratus ventralis m.
26 Iliocostalis thoracis m.
27 Ext. abdom. oblique m.

28 Rectus abdominis m.
29 Serosal cavity of mediastinum
30 Mediastinum
31 Plica venae cavae
32 Sternum
33 Transversus abdominis m.
34 Retractor costae m.
35 Psoas minor m.
36 Quadratus lumborum m.
37 Lumbocostal arch
38 Xiphoid process

3. BODY WALL, PREPUCE AND MAMMARY GLANDS (MAMMAE)

The remaining skin of the abdomen is removed from both sides of the body, keeping intact the mammae or the penis as the case may be. In the bitch, the mammae of the left side are preserved by incising the skin abound the base of each teat. Beginning laterally, the mammae of the right side are removed after cutting through the right m. supramammarius and the suspensory ligament of the mammae. In the male one removes the hairy outer skin adjacent to the penis and its cranial continuation, the external lamina of the prepuce, while keeping intact the m. preputialis cranialis and the suspensory ligament of the penis. The preputial laminae will be cut as shown in the accompanying figure.

a) The **PREPUCE (PREPUTIUM)** covers the glans penis. The caudal part, which passes over into the haired skin in the region of the body of the penis, is attached to the ventral body wall. The cranial part reaches nearly to the umbilicus and ends freely, ring-like, passing over at the preputial orifice into the internal lamina that lines the preputial cavity. The prepuce consists of a haired **external lamina (7)**, which is continuous at the **preputial ostium (1)** with the hairless cutaneous mucous membrane of the **internal lamina (8)**. At the **preputial fundus (10)**, at the level of the greatest circumference of the bulbus glandis, the internal lamina is reflected onto the glans penis as the **penile lamina (9)**, which clothes the glans. In the fundus region, the internal lamina and the penile lamina exhibit numerous lymph nodules. With erection of the penis, the penis lengthens, emerging from the prepuce. The internal lamina is drawn cranially onto the lengthened penis, and the fundus and preputial cavity are then no longer present.

b) The **MAMMAE** lie on both sides of the median intermammary groove and as a rule consist of five mammary gland complexes per side; namely, a cranial and caudal thoracic mammary gland complex, a cranial and caudal abdominal mammary gland complex, and an inguinal mammary gland complex. The mammae of the male are characterized by insignificant mammary papillae or teats. A mammary gland complex consists of the **body of the mamma** with about eight to twenty mammary glands (usually about 12 glands are developed) and a teat (*Papilla mammae*).

Before birth, from the tip of each teat-anlage, at first several solid epidermal buds sprout deeply into the subcutaneous tissue, a process which takes place in the male sex without recognizable differences. At the time of birth, the epithelial buds contain a lumen.

A sex-specific difference becomes distinct only with **sexual maturity** and the first estrus. Especially under the effect of estrogen, the epithelial sprouts divide and form a partial lumen. Moreover, estrogen brings about the deposition of fat within the mammary gland. This is transitory and later the fat tissue is replaced by the further development of the epithelial sprouts into well developed glands. In the non-lactating bitch the glandular and adipose tissue are so slightly developed that the bodies of the glands exhibit no swelling and can scarcely be separated from one another.

With pregnancy, sprouting, ramification and lumen-formation increase. This is induced by an elevated blood-estrogen level. In the second half of pregnancy alveoli develop at the ends of these mammary gland canals; this is brought about especially by the effect of progesterone.

During the lactation period, about thirty days in length, the alveoli guarantee the secretion of milk. Thus, from an individual epidermal sprout a large gland with alveoli, lactiferous ducts, lactiferous sinus and papillary duct develops. From the alveoli the milk reaches the **lactiferous sinus (4)** first by smaller and then by larger **lactiferous ducts (3)**. The sinus is without subdivision by a transverse fold as is typical for larger animals. Its predominant part is in the papilla (*Pars papillaris*) and extends only with its initial part, that receives the lactiferous ducts, into the body of the gland (*Pars glandularis*). The lactiferous sinus reaches the surface of the body as a more narrow **papillary duct (5)**. The duct is located in the distal third of the teat and, usually independent of neighboring glands, opens by a **papillary ostium (6)** on the end of the **teat (Papilla mammae, —2)**. Erectile blood vessels of the teat with typical thick-walled (muscular) veins are less developed in the bitch. Smooth muscle cell bundles surround the individual papillary ducts circularly as sphincters.

After the lactation period a large part of the duct system, and especially the glandular alveoli, undergoes involution.

The **fascial and muscular suspensory apparatus** as well as the vascular and nerve supply of the mammae and prepuce are alike in many ways and, for that reason, are studied together.

I. The **suspensory ligament of the mammae** or, respectively, **of the penis (20)** as the continuation of the deep fascia of the trunk splits off at the level of the linea alba and passes around the mammary complex or into the prepuce and around the penis as the fascia penis. The **cranial supramammary muscle (female)** or **cranial preputial muscle (18, —male)** arises from the linea alba at the level of the xiphoid cartilage and extends onto the basis of the abdominal mammae or, respectively, into the prepuce. The caudal muscles of the same name are inapparent.

With respect to the **blood and lymph vascular and nerve supply**, there is a cranial field of supply for the two thoracic mammae and the cranial abdominal mamma as well as a caudal supply field for the caudal abdominal and inguinal mammae, or, respectively, for the prepuce, the skin in the region of the penis, and the scrotum. Anastomoses occur between the two fields of supply at the level of the umbilicus.

II. For the cranial thoracic mammae, the **blood vessels** of the cranial supply field arise from the **lateral thoracic artery and vein (13)** and from the **internal thoracic artery and vein**. Perforating branches of the latter vessels emerge near the linea alba to supply the two thoracic mammae and end with the **cranial superficial epigastric artery and vein (17)**. The cranial superficial epigastric vessels perforate the thoracic wall at the level of the costal arch and, after supplying the cranial abdominal mammae, anastomose with the like-named caudal vessels at the level of the umbilicus. The blood vessels of the caudal supply field arise from the **external pudendal artery and vein (26)**, which, after traversing the inguinal rings and canal, divide at the level of the inguinal teat into the **ventral labial** or, respectively, **ventral scrotal artery and vein (27)** and the **caudal superficial epigastric artery and vein (23)**. These vessels give off mammary or, respectively, preputial branches. The cranial and caudal superficial epigastric vessels are the main vessels and also take over the supply of the teats. Additional contributing vessels are the intercostal arteries and veins, the cranial abdominal vessels and the deep circumflex iliac vessels. Individual vessel-branches (predominantly veins) can cross the midline (*Linea alba*) and take part in the supply of the contralateral mammae.

III. The **lymph vessels** of the cranial supply field run to the axillary (11) and accessory axillary (12) lymph nodes. The lymph vessels of the caudal supply field drain both caudal mammae and the prepuce, the external skin covering the penis and the scrotum. They run to the **superficial inguinal lymph nodes** situated at the base of the inguinal mamma where the external pudendal artery and vein divide into ventral labial or scrotal branches and the caudal superficial epigastric artery and vein.

IV. The **sensory nerve supply** is derived from the **intercostal nerves** cranially and the **cranial and caudal iliohypogastric nerves** caudally. These approach the mammae by means of **lateral cutaneous branches (15 and 21** of the lateral series of thoracic and lumbar cutaneous nerves) and by **ventral cutaneous branches (14 and 22)** near the linea alba. Caudal to the 10th intercostal nerve, no ventral cutaneous branch is dispatched by the thoracic or cranial lumbar spinal nerves, the ventral skin being supplied by the ventral extension of the lateral cutaneous branch and, the inguinal mamma caudally, by the **genitofemoral nerve (24)**, which traverses the inguinal canal in the company of the external pudendal artery and vein.

c) Before commencing the dissection, details should be provided on the **RELATIONSHIP OF THE FASCIAE** (see also pp. 36 and 146).

I. The superficial and deep fasciae of the trunk are classified as the **external fasciae of the trunk**. The **superficial trunk fascia** is closely united to the skin and ensheathes the cutaneous muscles of the abdomen by means of two laminae. The **deep trunk fascia (19)** is intimately united to the surface of the external abdominal muscle. Dorsally, in the lumbar region, it is known as the **thoracolumbar fascia** (see p. 30), which courses over the muscles of the vertebral column between spinous and transverse processes. In the midline ventrally, the deep fascia fuses with the linea alba, and there the suspensory ligament of the mammae separates off from it. In the inguinal region the external fascia of the trunk (comprising the superficial and deep fasciae of the trunk) continues as the **external spermatic fascia**. This envelops the vaginal tunic of the peritoneum externally, and at the inguinal groove passes onto the thigh as the **fascia lata (28)**.

II. By and large, the **internal fascia of the trunk** is adherent to the serosa and is known by different terms depending on its location. In the thoracic cavity it is known as the **endothoracic fascia**, in the abdominal cavity as **transversalis fascia**, on the ventral surface of the sublumbar muscles as the **iliac fascia**, and within the pelvic cavity as the **pelvic fascia**. The internal fascia of the trunk, or more particularly the transversalis fascia, continues as the **internal spermatic fascia** that invests the vaginal tunic of the peritoneum.

Mammary region and Preputial region

Mammary gland

Prepuce

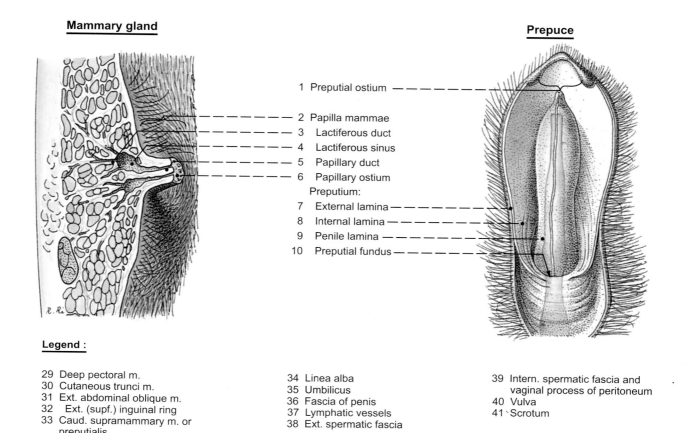

1 Preputial ostium
2 Papilla mammae
3 Lactiferous duct
4 Lactiferous sinus
5 Papillary duct
6 Papillary ostium
Preputium:
7 External lamina
8 Internal lamina
9 Penile lamina
10 Preputial fundus

Legend :

29 Deep pectoral m.
30 Cutaneous trunci m.
31 Ext. abdominal oblique m.
32 Ext. (supf.) inguinal ring
33 Caud. supramammary m. or preputialis

34 Linea alba
35 Umbilicus
36 Fascia of penis
37 Lymphatic vessels
38 Ext. spermatic fascia

39 Intern. spermatic fascia and vaginal process of peritoneum
40 Vulva
41 Scrotum

(ventral surface)

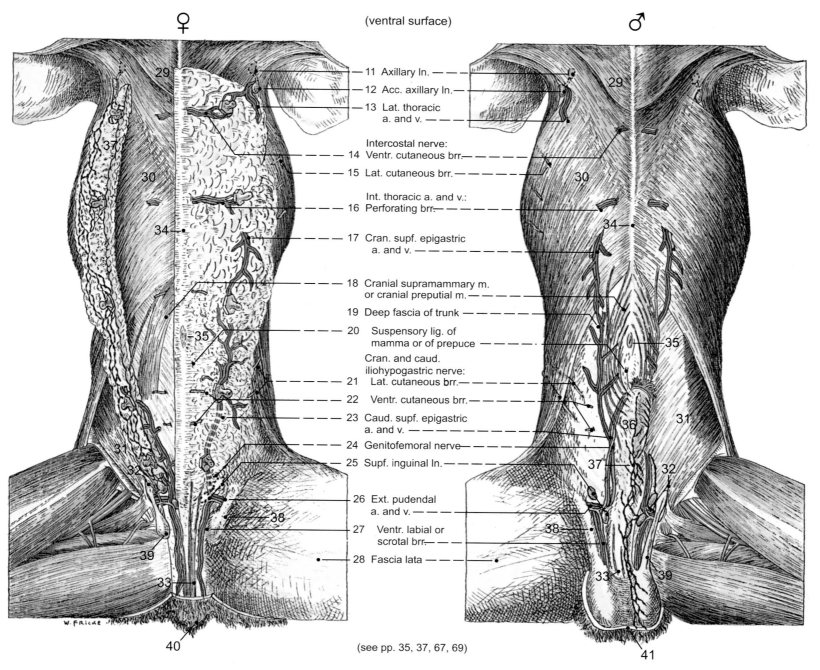

11 Axillary ln.
12 Acc. axillary ln.
13 Lat. thoracic a. and v.
Intercostal nerve:
14 Ventr. cutaneous brr.
15 Lat. cutaneous brr.
Int. thoracic a. and v.:
16 Perforating brr.
17 Cran. supf. epigastric a. and v.
18 Cranial supramammary m. or cranial preputial m.
19 Deep fascia of trunk
20 Suspensory lig. of mamma or of prepuce
Cran. and caud. iliohypogastric nerve:
21 Lat. cutaneous brr.
22 Ventr. cutaneous brr.
23 Caud. supf. epigastric a. and v.
24 Genitofemoral nerve
25 Supf. inguinal ln.
26 Ext. pudendal a. and v.
27 Ventr. labial or scrotal brr.
28 Fascia lata

(see pp. 35, 37, 67, 69)

4. ABDOMINAL MUSLES, RECTUS SHEATH, PREPUBIC TENDON

To expose the abdominal muscles and the sheath of the m. rectus abdominis, the m. obliquus externus abdominis and the overlying deep fascia of the trunk on the left side are transected 2 cm ventral and parallel to the origin of the external oblique muscle from the ribs and thoracolumbar fascia (see text-illustration on p. 30). The ventral muscle remnant is reflected ventrally as far as the lateral border of the m. rectus abdominis. Then the m. obliquus internus abdominis is transected 2 cm dorsal and parallel to the border between the muscle and its aponeurosis, and also reflected.

a) Taking into consideration their sites of origin, the ABDOMINAL MUSCLES are subdivided into parts; namely, the costal part taking origin from the ribs, the sternal part from the sternum, the lumbar part from the **thoracolumbar fascia** (see text-illustration p. 30), and the inguinal part from the **inguinal ligament (7)**. With the exception of the m. rectus abdominis, each inserts at the linea alba in the ventral midline by means of an aponeurosis or abdominal tendon. The m. obliquus internus abdominis also inserts along the costal arch by means of a costal tendon and the m. obliquus externus abdominis terminates by a pelvic tendon or lateral crus at the pecten ossis pubis. Lateral to their midventral insertions the aponeuroses of the abdominal muscles form the **sheath of the m. rectus abdominis** (rectus sheath, — see also p. 36), the layers passing external to the rectus abdominis forming the external lamina of the sheath, the layers passing internal to the rectus forming the internal lamina. Ventral and paramedian, the aponeuroses of the external lamina of the sheath form a meshlike zone that is anchored to the **tendinous intersections (2)** of the m. rectus abdominis. Midventrally, the **linea alba (10)** arises as a consecutive series of crossing, interweaving, tendon fibers. It begins at the mesosternum as a ventromedian 'anchoring raphe' for the aponeuroses of the abdominal muscles. At its widest, it encircles the **umbilical ring (11)** by means of two umbilical crura and terminates by tapering abruptly at the cranial end of the pelvic symphysis.

I. The **m. obliquus externus abdominis (8)** arises as costal and lumbar parts that pass over into an abdominal and a pelvic tendon. Known respectively as the **abdominal tendon** or **medial crus (8')** and the **pelvic tendon** or **lateral crus (8")**, they bound the **external (superficial) inguinal ring** (see p. 37). The aponeurosis of the muscle contributes entirely to the external lamina of the rectus sheath and inserts caudally with the abdominal and pelvic tendon at the pelvis, joining the prepubic tendon. Deep fibers of the abdominal tendon of the contralateral external abdominal oblique muscle also end on the prepubic tendon as **fibrae reflexae (13)**.

Rectus sheath
(cranial abdominal region)

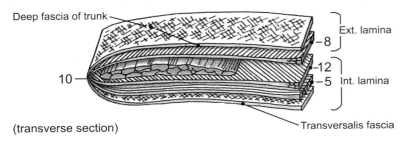

(transverse section)

II. The **m. obliquus internus abdominis (12)** has lumbar and inguinal parts. Its aponeurosis participates in the sheath of the m. rectus abdominis in three ways: 1) A cranial 2 cm-wide section of aponeurosis subscribes to the internal lamina only. 2) A subsequent 2-4 cm-wide section participates in forming both external and internal laminae in the umbilical region. 3) Caudally the aponeurosis only passes to the external surface of the m. rectus abdominis.

Rectus sheath
(middle abdominal region)

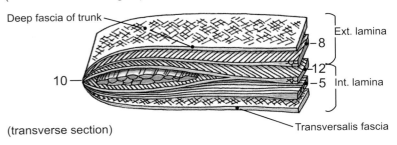

(transverse section)

III. The **m. transversus abdominis (5)** contributes to the sheath in a manner similar to the m. obliquus internus abdominis. However, its contribution to both laminae occurs approximately one to two vertebral lengths more caudally. On the lateral surface of the muscle, ventromedial branches of thoracic and lumbar nn. (cranial and caudal iliohypogastric and ilioinguinal nn.) run ventrally, parallel to the muscle fibers.

Rectus sheath
(caudal abdominal region)

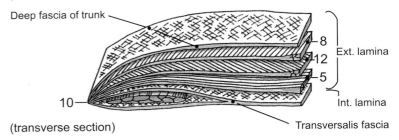

(transverse section)

IV. The **m. rectus abdominis (1)** arises from the first rib and the first four sternebrae and could therefore be said to have a costal and a sternal part. It ends at the pecten ossis pubis. Caudal to the sternal ribs it is enclosed in its sheath formed from the aponeuroses of the remaining three abdominal muscles and the internal and external fasciae of the trunk. The external trunk fascia contributes entirely to the external lamina and internal trunk fascia to the internal lamina of the rectus sheath except caudally where it is double-layered.

Innervation of the four abdominal muscles is by intercostal nn., by the **cranial (3) and caudal (4) iliohypogastric nn.**, and by the **ilioinguinal n. (6)**. By means of their vm branches, all such nerves course across the lateral surface of the m. transversus abdominis. The vl branches of the nerves run on the external abdominal oblique muscle to the mammae (see p. 33).

To demonstrate the prepubic tendon, in the accompanying figure on the right side the abdominal wall over the urinary bladder (and the prostate in males) was fenestrated. The external and internal oblique abdominal muscles, including the transversalis fascia and parietal peritoneum, are cut at the lateral border of the rectus abdominis muscle and the latter is lifted caudally after being sectioned transversely at the level of the tuber coxae. In the caudal region of the left side, the abdominal tendon of the external abdominal oblique muscle is removed. The prepubic tendon is split parallel to the muscle fibers by a section between the pelvic tendon of the external abdominal oblique muscle and the medial and lateral tendons of origin of the pectineus (and long adductor) muscle. This section also cuts through the iliopubic cartilage.

b) The **PREPUBIC TENDON (9)** is represented by a stout tendinous mass extending ventrally from the brim of the pelvis. It consists mainly of the tendons of insertion of the right and left rectus abdominis muscles, and of the lateral and medial tendons of origin of the (ipsilateral) **pectineus muscle (and long adductor, —15)** (see under IV.) as well as the cranially bordering **pelvic tendon of the external abdominal oblique muscle** (lateral crus), which is specially fixed by the fibrocartilaginous **iliopubic cartilage (14)**. The externally palpable iliopubic cartilage reinforces the caudal angle of the external (superficial) inguinal ring that connects the abdominal and pelvic tendons of the external abdominal oblique muscle. The cartilage also serves as a medial,

superficial origin for the pectineus muscle. An additional, strong, fleshy origin of the pectineus muscle is present as a medial, deep origin from the **iliopubic eminence** (see p. 37). The lateral tendon of origin comes from the psoas minor tubercle. The medial tendon of origin of the ipsilateral pectineus (long adductor) muscle does not cross the medial tendon of origin of the contralateral muscle of the same name. Thus, the dog lacks a bilateral attachment of the pectineus muscle, which for the large domestic animals is of paramount significance in safeguarding the connection of both pelvic halves at the pelvic symphysis.

Abdominal muscles and Inguinal region

(caudoventral view)

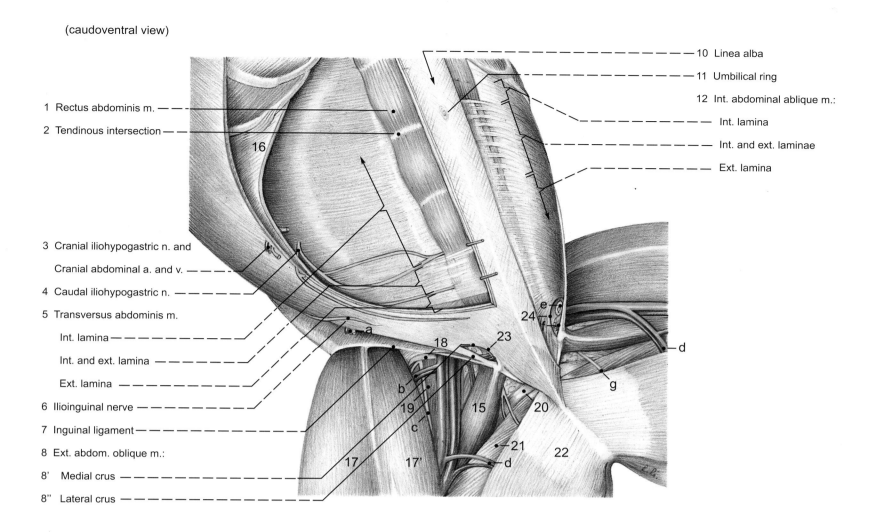

1 Rectus abdominis m.
2 Tendinous intersection
16
3 Cranial iliohypogastric n. and
  Cranial abdominal a. and v.
4 Caudal iliohypogastric n.
5 Transversus abdominis m.
   Int. lamina
   Int. and ext. lamina
   Ext. lamina
6 Ilioinguinal nerve
7 Inguinal ligament
8 Ext. abdom. oblique m.:
8' Medial crus
8" Lateral crus

10 Linea alba
11 Umbilical ring
12 Int. abdominal ablique m.:
   Int. lamina
   Int. and ext. laminae
   Ext. lamina

Legend :

Int. abdom. oblique m.:
16 Costal tendon
Sartorius m.:
17 Cranial part
17' Caudal part
18 Ext. iliac fascia
19 Iliopsoas m.

20 Adductor brevis m.
21 Adductor magnus m.
22 Gracilis m.
23 Ext. inguinal ring (supf.)
24 Int. inguinal ring (deep)
25 Transversalis fascia of trunk and
   Peritoneum

a Lat. cutaneous femoral n. and
   deep circumflex iliac a. and v.
b Lat. circumflex femoral a. and v.
c Saphenous n.
d Prox. caud. femoral a. and v.
e Vaginal process of peritoneum and
   ext.cremaster m.

f Genitofemoral n. and
   ext. pudendal a. and v.
g Obturator nerve
h Femoral a., v. and n.
i Urinary bladder
j Prostate

(caudoventral view)

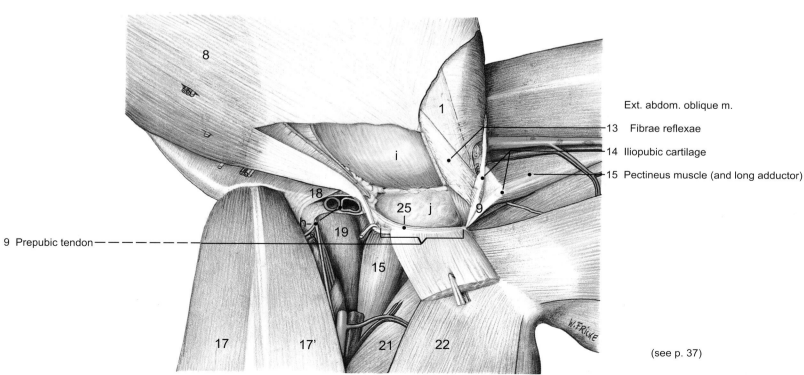

Ext. abdom. oblique m.
13 Fibrae reflexae
14 Iliopubic cartilage
15 Pectineus muscle (and long adductor)

9 Prepubic tendon

(see p. 37)

35

5. INGUINAL REGION, INGUINAL SPACE (INGUINAL CANAL), NEUROMUSCULAR AND VASCULAR LACUNAE

In the inguinal region three conduits are exposed, namely the inguinal space (canal), the lacuna neuromusculorum and the lacuna vasorum. Initially, the right inguinal mamma is reflected medially, and following this, one is able to study the participation of the five layers of the abdominal wall in the formation of the inguinal space. This begins at the internal or deep inguinal ring and ends at the external or superficial inguinal ring. Observe the continuation of the external fascia of the trunk as the tubelike external spermatic fascia. Externally, this envelops the vaginal process and its covering of internal spermatic fascia. Then on the right side, the external trunk fascia, the three expansive abdominal muscles, the transversalis fascia and the peritoneum are transected and reflected. This incision is made along the long axis of the external inguinal ring as far as the costal arch. In so doing, each individual abdominal layer is studied.

1 a) The **INGUINAL SPACE (INGUINAL CANAL)** extends from the internal to the external inguinal ring. The caudal angles of both rings lie one above the other, whereas the cranial angle of the internal ring lies approximately 2 cm craniolateral to that of the external ring. This results in a corresponding lengthening of the inguinal space.

I. The **skin** does not participate in the formation of the inguinal space and merges with the integument of the scrotum (male) or of the labia of the vulva (female).

II. The **external fascia of the trunk (5)** turns at the external inguinal ring to envelop the **vaginal process of the peritoneum (24)** with its tubular content and is then known as the **external spermatic fascia (21)**. The vaginal process is designated the **vaginal tunic in the male (24)**, and contains the spermatic cord; whereas, in the bitch, it houses the round ligament of the uterus and its enveloping body of fat. In contrast to most other female mammals, the bitch possesses a vaginal process of peritoneum and an accompanying external spermatic fascia in most of the cases. The **external pudendal a. and v. (20)**, the **genitofemoral n.** and the m. cremaster (externus) pass through the space on the outside of the vaginal process and then enter the tubular external spermatic fascia. Within a few millimeters the two blood vessels and nerve pierce the fascia and the vessels branch into the **caudal superficial epigastric a. and v.** (see p. 14A – 9) and the **ventral scrotal or ventral labial rami** (see p. 33) in the vicinity of the superficial inguinal lymph node.

III. By a cleavage in its aponeurosis, the **m. obliquus externus adominis** forms the **lateral crus (16)** and **medial crus (15)** of the **external (superficial) inguinal ring (17)**.

The free caudal border of the **m. obliquus internus abdominis (14)** contributes to the formation of the **internal (deep) inguinal ring (18)** together with the lateral border of the **m. rectus abdominis (19)** and the internal surface of the inguinal ligament.

The **m. cremaster (externus, —22)** is distinct in the male; whereas it seems weaker in the bitch. In rodents the **m. cremaster (externus, —22)** is divided into a primary part derived from the m. transversus abdominis and a secondary part from the m. obliquus internus abdominis. To a large degree in domestic mammals, the united m. cremaster (externus) has lost its direct connection with the two abdominal muscles. The resulting independent muscle takes origin from the inguinal ligament and passes through the inguinal space outside the vaginal process.

The **m. transversus abdominis (6)** does not contribute to the formation of the inguinal space since its free caudal border is at the level of the tuber coxae.

IV. **The internal fascia of the trunk (7, —transversalis fascia)** is adherent to the peritoneum. It protrudes through the inguinal space as the tubular **internal spermatic fascia (23)** and envelops the vaginal tunic.

V. The **peritoneum (8)** evaginates as a tubular vaginal process, penetrates the inguinal space and is adherent to the enveloping internal spermatic fascia. The **vaginal ring (9)** in the caudolateral part of the abdominal cavity is the site of evagination and remains as the entrance into the vaginal process; it does not belong to the inguinal space.

b) The **NEUROMUSCULAR LACUNA** (see also text-illustration) is passage for the m. iliopsoas and the femoral n. contained within it. At the level of the lacuna and the transition from lateral to dorsal body wall, the **transversalis**

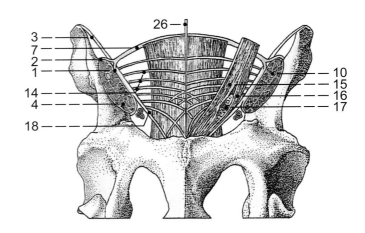

fascia (7) extends over the **m. iliopsoas (4)** and is designated here as the **iliac fascia**. The inguinal ligament is woven into this fascial covering and subdivides the iliac fascia into an **internal iliac fascia (1)** on the abdominal cavity side and an **external iliac fascia (2, —iliac lamina)** on the femoral side. The two layers of fascia end on the ilium. Occasionally absent, the very weak **inguinal ligament (3)** arises at the tuber coxae. In the region of the lacuna neuromusculorum it is interwoven with the iliac fascia to provide a connective tissue reinforcement for the origin of the m. obliquus internus abdominis. At the level of the inguinal space more ventrally, the ligament unites with the lateral crus of the m. obliquus externus abdominis; both radiate into the prepubic tendon and end on the pecten ossis pubis. With the m. iliopsoas, the **femoral n. (10)** and its branch, the **saphenous n. (11)**, pass through the lacuna neuromusculorum. This is bounded by the inguinal ligament ventrally and the ilium dorsally. Subsequently, the saphenous n. attains the **femoral trigone (12)**, whose boundaries are formed by the inguinal ligament, the m. pectineus, and the caudal part of the m. sartorius. The femoral trigone forms the borders of the **femoral space (13, —femoral canal)**, which is bounded deeply by the m. iliopsoas and covered superficially by the medial femoral fascia. Besides the saphenous n. the space houses the femoral a. and v.

c) The **VASCULAR LACUNA** (see also text-illustration) is the passage for the femoral vessels. It is bounded by the lacuna neuromusculorum dorsolaterally, by the body of the ilium dorsomedially, and by the inguinal ligament ventrally. The medial section of the lacuna vasorum that is not occupied by blood vessels is known as the **femoral ring**. Due to its covering of peritoneum **2** and transversalis fascia, the femoral ring is a self-contained access to the femoral space (femoral canal) and is the site of femoral hernia.

PARTICIPATION OF LAYERS OF THE ABDOMINAL WALL IN FORMING THE INGUINAL SPACE (INGUINAL CANAL) AND RECTUS SHEATH

Abdomen	Ring	Process	Rectus Sheath
I. Skin	—	Skin of scrotum	—
II. External trunk fascia	—	Ext. spermatic fascia	Ext. lamina
III. M. obl. ext. abdom.	Ext. inguinal ring	} Ing. space (canal)	Ext. lamina
III. M. obl. int. abdom.	Int. inguinal ring		Ext. lam.; ext. and int. lam.; int.
	– – – – – – – – – – – – – –	M. cremaster (ext.)	—
III M. transv. abdom.	—		Ext. lam.; ext. and int. lam.; int.
IV. Internal trunk fascia	—	Int. spermatic fascia	Lam. int.
V. Peritoneum	Vaginal ring	Vaginal process (female) Vaginal tunic (male)	—

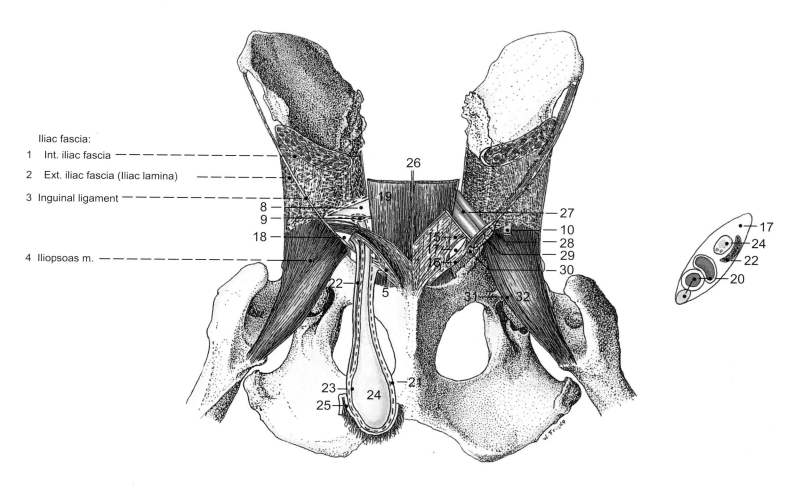

Iliac fascia:

1 Int. iliac fascia

2 Ext. iliac fascia (Iliac lamina)

3 Inguinal ligament

4 Iliopsoas m.

(caudoventral view)

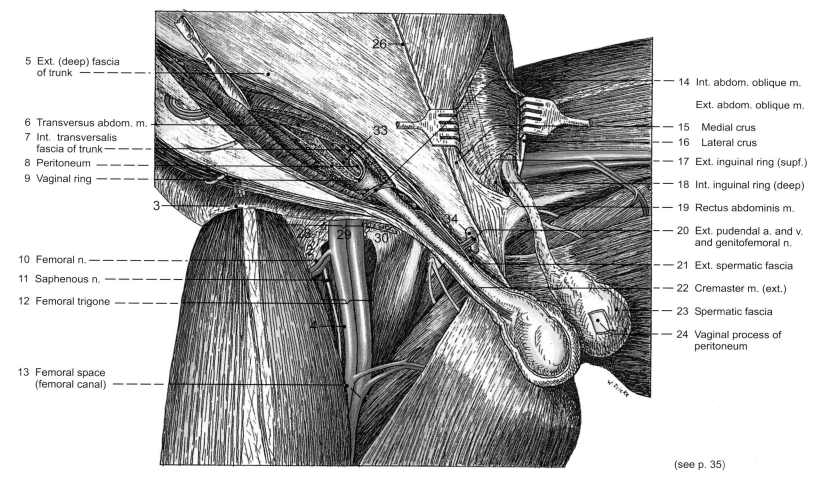

5 Ext. (deep) fascia
of trunk

6 Transversus abdom. m.

7 Int. transversalis
fascia of trunk

8 Peritoneum

9 Vaginal ring

3

10 Femoral n.

11 Saphenous n.

12 Femoral trigone

13 Femoral space
(femoral canal)

14 Int. abdom. oblique m.

Ext. abdom. oblique m.

15 Medial crus

16 Lateral crus

17 Ext. inguinal ring (supf.)

18 Int. inguinal ring (deep)

19 Rectus abdominis m.

20 Ext. pudendal a. and v.
and genitofemoral n.

21 Ext. spermatic fascia

22 Cremaster m. (ext.)

23 Spermatic fascia

24 Vaginal process of
peritoneum

(see p. 35)

Legend :

25 Skin of scrotum	28 Lacuna musculorum	Iliopsoas m.:	33 Testicular a. and v. and
26 Linea alba	29 Lacuna vasorum	31 Iliacus m.	Deferent duct
27 Ext. iliac a. and v.	30 Femoral ring	32 Psoas minor m.	34 Supf. inguinal ln.

CHAPTER 5: THORACIC CAVITY

1. LUNGS, TRACHEAL BIFURCATION AND BRONCHI

1 In the **lung field**, the triangular field that projects the lung onto the lateral thoracic wall of its respective side, this main respiratory organ is externally accessible for auscultation and percussion. In a dog in the normal standing attitude, the **cranial border of the triangle** is at the level of the 5th rib. With the thoracic limb drawn forward, the lung field can be increased about the width of two ribs. The **dorsal border of the triangle** is the lateral border of the iliocostalis muscle, and the **caudoventral (basal) border** ascends from the costochondral junction of the sixth rib to the middle of the eighth rib to the vertebral end of the 11th rib.

The external **form of the lungs** is inconstant as the lungs necessarily follow the varying dimensions of the thoracic cavity in the movements of respiration. Together, the two lungs resemble a cone (each lung forming a 'half-cone') with a cranially situated **apex of the lung (Apex pulmonis)** that projects slightly beyond the thoracic inlet, and a large **base (Basis pulmonis)** that abuts the diaphragm.

The **lung surface** is covered by pulmonary (visceral) pleura (see p. 42). After embalming the cadaver, as a reflection of the plasticity of the lung parenchyma, the **costal surface** *in situ* shows distinct costal impressions. The **medial surface** (see text-illustration) extends dorsally with its **vertebral part** up to the vertebral column; ventrally, in its **mediastinal part**, the following can be identified: the **aortic impression (12)**, **esophageal impression (13)** as well as the **sulcus for the caudal vena cava (14)**, and continuing ventrally from the caval sulcus, the **cardiac impression**. The **diaphragmatic surface (16)** lies smoothly upon the diaphragm.

2 a) The **LUNGS** (see text-illustration) of the dog are distinctly asymmetrical because the right lung with its four lobes is considerably larger than the left lung with only two lobes.

Externally the pulmonary lobes in the dog are subdivided or set off by **interlobar fissures** that are very deep and in part reach to the subdivision of the bronchi.

I. The **right lung (Pulmo dexter)** is divided by **cranial (2)** and **caudal (3)** interlobar fissures into **cranial (5)**, **middle (4)**, and **caudal (1) lobes,** and the small **accessory lobe** (see text-illustration, −17) that extends from the medial surface into the mediastinal recess (see p. 42). The accessory lobe cannot be seen in lateral view. It partly passes over the caudal vena cava, forming the *sulcus venae cavae caudalis*. On the ventral border of the lung, the cranial interlobar fissure passes over into the **right cardiac notch (6)**. The caudal interlobar fissure separates the middle lobe from the caudal lobe, which, medially, is fused with the accessory lobe.

II. The **left lung (Pulmo sinister)** has a **cranial lobe (7)** that is subdivided into a **cranial part (8)** and **caudal part (9)**. The cranial part overlaps laterally the cranial portion of the caudal part or the latter overlaps laterally the caudal portion of the cranial part. The intralobar fissure that separates cranial and caudal parts opens at the ventral border of the lung into the shallow **left cardiac notch (10)**. The **caudal lobe (11)** is undivided and with its diaphragmatic surface lies upon the diaphragm.

Bronchial tree and pulmonary vessels (dorsal view)

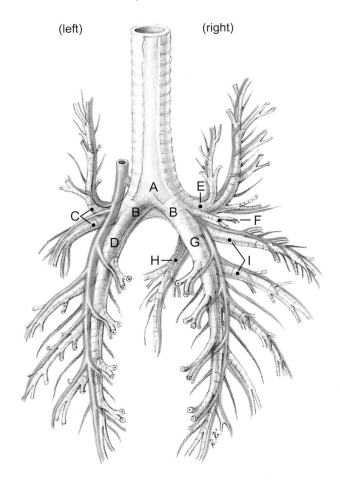

(left) (right)

b) The **BIFURCATION OF THE TRACHEA** (see text-illustration, above −A) and its division into the **principal bronchi (B)** determines the subdivision into right and left lung. The subdivision of the principal bronchi into **lobar bronchi**, which cannot be discerned externally, is more significant in defining the lobes of the lung than the visible fissures, which are partly between the lobes, partly within a lobe.

The tracheal bifurcation is ventral to the esophagus, and is about halfway between the thoracic inlet and the diaphragm. For the ventilation of each lobe of the lung the principal bronchi divide into two **lobar bronchi** for the **left lung (cranial lobar bronchus −C and caudal lobar bronchus −D)**, and in the **right lung** into four lobar bronchi **(cranial lobar bronchus −E, middle −F, caudal −G and accessory −H)**.

The lobar bronchi give off **segmental bronchi (I)**, which are designated according to their position as dorsal, ventral, lateral, and medial segmental bronchi. The segments can be defined, for example, by anatomical corrosion casts. In the dog, the branches of the pulmonary artery accompany the segmental bronchus (bronchoarterial type of supply) in the caudal lobe. They run in the center of the segments and the branches of the pulmonary veins mark the periphery of the segments. In the cranial and middle lobes the segmental bronchi are not only accompanied by arterial branches but also by venous ones (bronchovascular type of supply). Because the pulmonary segment is ventilated by only one segmental bronchus, in case of bronchial occlusion, on a radiograph the segment is visible as a wedge-like shadow with a central wedge-shaped tip and a peripheral base. There, where the bronchial cartilages disappear, the smaller branches of the segmental bronchi continue as bronchioles, which are smaller than 1 mm in diameter. The terminal parts of the air conducting system, the terminal bronchioles, continue as the gas-exchange system, to which belong the respiratory bronchioles (diameter smaller than 0.5 mm), the alveolar ducts and alveolar sacs, and finally the alveolus.

Right and left lung (medial aspect)

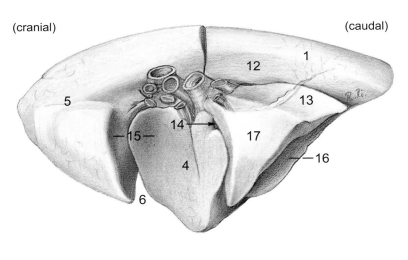

(cranial) (caudal)

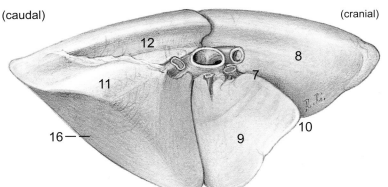

(caudal) (cranial)

Thoracic cavity and lungs

(right lung)

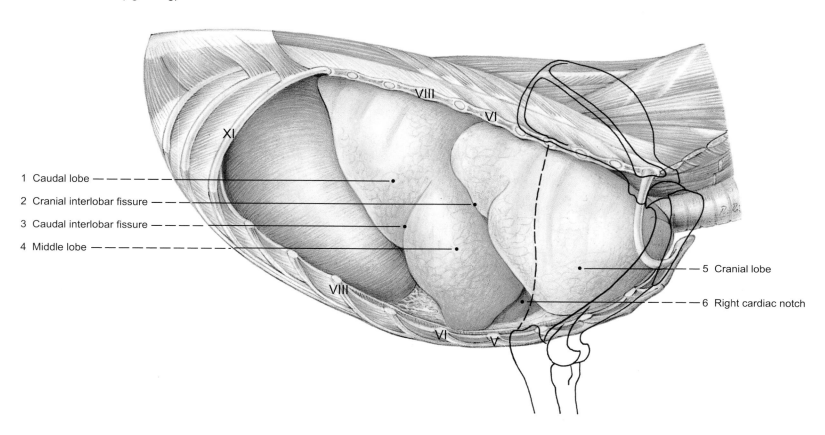

1 Caudal lobe
2 Cranial interlobar fissure
3 Caudal interlobar fissure
4 Middle lobe

5 Cranial lobe
6 Right cardiac notch

(left lung)

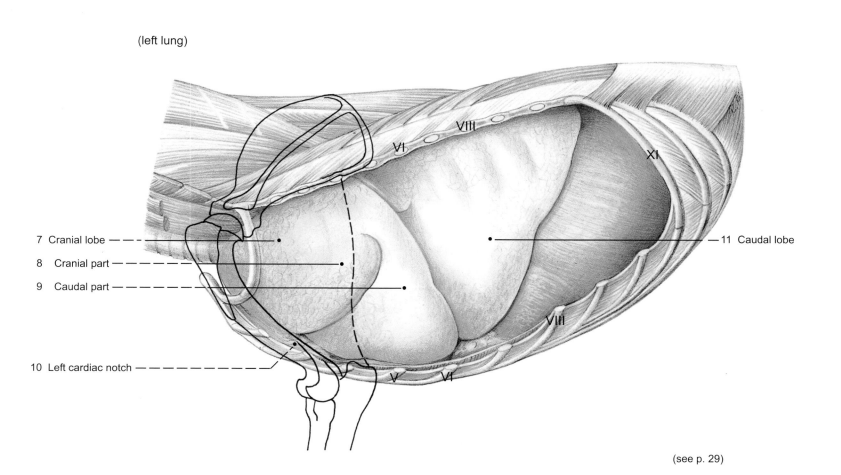

7 Cranial lobe
8 Cranial part
9 Caudal part
10 Left cardiac notch

11 Caudal lobe

(see p. 29)

2. BLOOD VESSELS, NERVES, AND LYMPHATIC SYSTEM OF THE LUNGS; AORTIC ARCH, LYMPH NODES OF THE THORACIC CAVITY, THYMUS

1 a) The **BLOOD SUPPLY OF THE LUNGS** is furnished by the pulmonary circulation (pulmonary arteries and veins) and the broncho-esophageal artery and vein.

In contrast to the systemic circulation with its higher blood pressures, the pulmonary circulation is called the low pressure system. This is due to the lower blood pressures in its vessels, which facilitate the functional supply of the lungs. From the right ventricle of the heart, the venous blood reaches the hilus of the right and left lungs by way of the arterial **pulmonary trunk (10)** and its principal branches, the right and left pulmonary arteries. The blood, oxygenated in the pulmonary capillaries is returned to the left atrium of the heart by 5 – 8 **pulmonary veins (14)**.

The paired broncho-esophageal arteries originate from the aorta or an originating intercostal artery at the level of the 5th – 7th ribs. They enter the hilus of the right or, respectively, left lung and provide the nutritive supply of the bronchial tree and its immediate environs. In the border region between the air-conducting and gas exchange systems in some species, anastomoses of broncho-esophageal and pulmonary capillaries have been observed. The mixing of functional and nutritive blood in the dog is disputed. The broncho-esophageal vein usually opens into the right vena azygos.

2 b) The **NERVE SUPPLY OF THE LUNGS** is provided by the plexus of autonomic fibers from the sympathetic and parasympathetic nervous systems. There are also visceral sensory fibers with the autonomic nerves. These enter the root of the lung without, however, supplying the pulmonary parenchyma with pain conducting fibers.

c) The **LYMPHATIC SYSTEM OF THE LUNGS** (see text-illustration) comprises the **pulmonary lymph nodes (E)**, which belong to the bronchial lymph center and lie within the pulmonary parenchyma, and the **tracheobronchial lymph nodes: right (D), middle (C), and left (13, B)**. The latter are found at the cranial border of the right principal bronchus, dorsal at the tracheal bifurcation, and caudodorsal at the left principal bronchus. Their tributaries pass from the lung and the heart. Their efferent lymphatic vessels go directly, or indirectly after traversing the cranial mediastinal lymph nodes, to the large lymphatic trunks that end in the venous angle between the internal and external jugular veins.

3 d) The aortic arch first gives off the **brachiocephalic trunk (7)**, which gives off the **left common carotid artery (1)** and **right common carotid artery**, and the **right subclavian artery**. The **left subclavian artery (9)** leaves the convexity of the aortic arch a fingerbreadth distal. Right and left subclavian arteries each give off four arteries: The **vertebral artery (3)** crosses the **costocervical trunk (2)** medially and, with the same-named nerve and vein, reaches the *Canalis transversarius* of the cervical vertebral column. The

internal thoracic artery (5, –see also p. 49) passes caudoventrally, then deep to the transverse thoracic muscle. Its branches perforate the thoracic wall and send **mammary branches** to the thoracic mammary gland complexuses. At the level of the xiphosternum, it gives off an artery to the diaphragm before dividing into the **cranial epigastric and cranial superficial epigastric arteries**. The latter vessels run caudally on the internal surface of the rectus abdominis muscle or, respectively, on the superficial aspect of the external lamina of the rectus sheath and anastomose with the same-named caudal vessels. The **superficial cervical artery** dispatches the deltoid branch to the lateral pectoral sulcus and ramifies in the lateral cervical region in relation to the superficial cervical lymph nodes. The **broncho-esophageal arteries** proceed directly from the **descending aorta (12)** or from intercostal arteries V – VII. The **intercostal arteries (11)** pass with the same-named veins and nerves directly caudal to the ribs and connect the aorta with the internal thoracic artery.

4 e) The **LYMPH NODES OF THE THORACIC CAVITY** comprise the **cranial mediastinal lymph nodes (6, A**; middle and caudal mediastinal lymph nodes are absent in the dog; see also the text-illustration). The cranial mediastinal nodes are located in the precardial mediastinum, especially attached to the great vessels or the viscera. The **cranial sternal lymph nodes (4**; caudal sternal lymph nodes are absent in the dog) are at the cranial border of the transverse thoracic muscle. **Intercostal lymph nodes** are inconstant. When present, they are proximal at the 5th or 6th intercostal space. Their tributary areas are in the direct neighborhood of the particular lymph node. Efferent lymphatic vessels of the cranial mediastinal lymph nodes pass to the venous angle. Efferents from the cranial sternal and intercostal lymph nodes pass to the cranial mediastinal lymph nodes or directly to the venous angle.

5 f) The **THYMUS (8)** produces T-lymphocytes. Corresponding to its origin from the third and fourth pharyngeal pouches, the thymus is regarded as a lymph-epithelial organ which, on the cut surface, shows an arrangment into medulla and cortex. Outpocketings of the arbor-like, branching, medulla are covered by cortex and surrounded by a connective tissue capsule, thus presenting a pseudo-lobation.

The thymus is fully developed in the perinatal phase. Its involution commences at the age of 4 – 6 months. In this process the parenchyma is more and more replaced by fat tissue. However, there remain always tiny active thymic islands, even in old age.

The thymus of the newborn extends from the heart to a few millimeters cranial to the thoracic inlet. The paired organ is fused medially and is located in the mediastinal space.

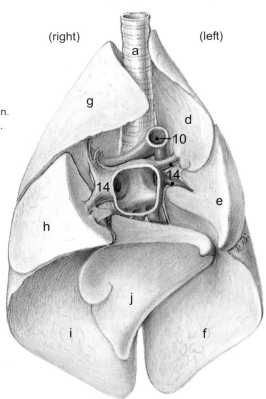

Lungs and bronchial lc. (dorsal view)

(left)   (right)

Lungs (ventral view)

(right)   (left)

Legend :

A   Cran. mediastinal ln.
B   Left tracheobronchial ln.
C   Middle tracheobronchial ln.
D   Right tracheobronchial ln.
E   Pulmonary lnn.

a   Trachea
b   Bifurcation of trachea
    Left lung:
c   Cran. lobe
d   Cran. part
e   Caud. part
f   Caud. lobe
    Right lung:
g   Cran. lobe
h   Middle lobe
i   Caud. lobe
j   Acc. lobe

Thoracic cavity (left side)

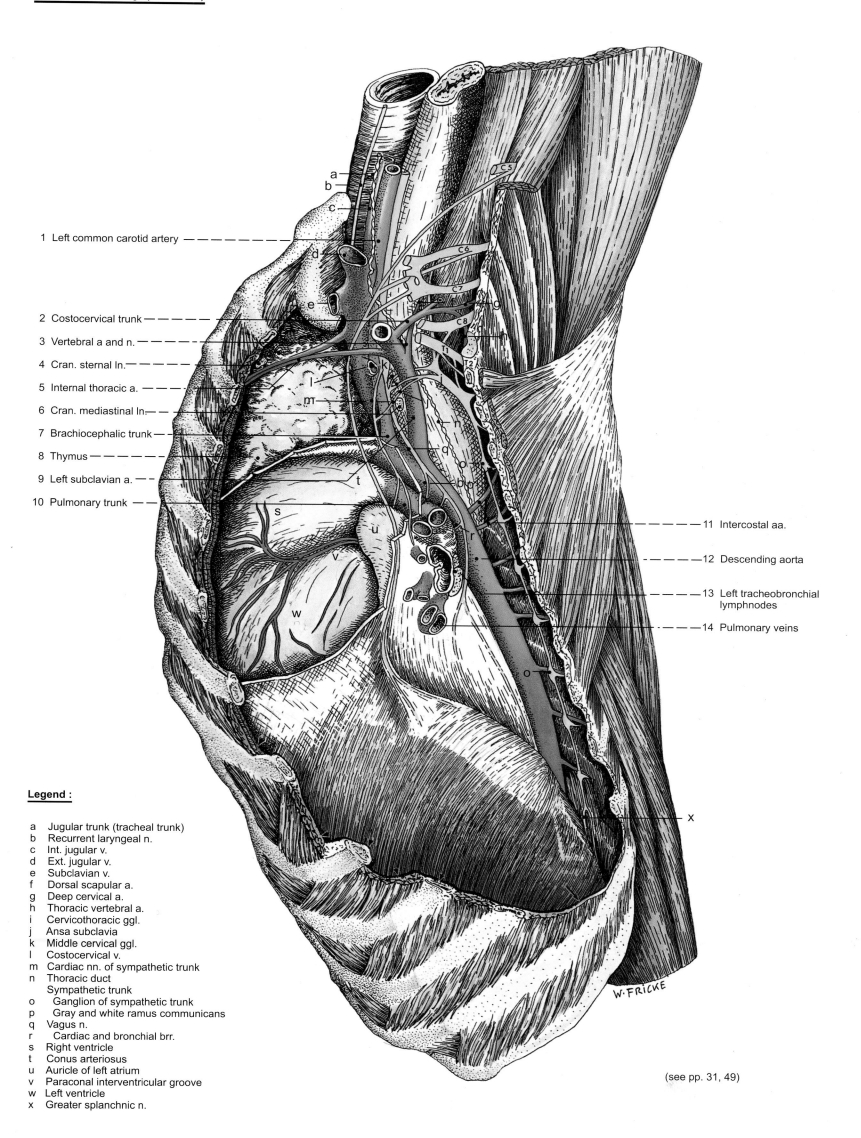

1 Left common carotid artery

2 Costocervical trunk

3 Vertebral a and n.

4 Cran. sternal ln.

5 Internal thoracic a.

6 Cran. mediastinal ln.

7 Brachiocephalic trunk

8 Thymus

9 Left subclavian a.

10 Pulmonary trunk

11 Intercostal aa.

12 Descending aorta

13 Left tracheobronchial lymphnodes

14 Pulmonary veins

Legend :

a Jugular trunk (tracheal trunk)
b Recurrent laryngeal n.
c Int. jugular v.
d Ext. jugular v.
e Subclavian v.
f Dorsal scapular a.
g Deep cervical a.
h Thoracic vertebral a.
i Cervicothoracic ggl.
j Ansa subclavia
k Middle cervical ggl.
l Costocervical v.
m Cardiac nn. of sympathetic trunk
n Thoracic duct
   Sympathetic trunk
o Ganglion of sympathetic trunk
p Gray and white ramus communicans
q Vagus n.
r Cardiac and bronchial brr.
s Right ventricle
t Conus arteriosus
u Auricle of left atrium
v Paraconal interventricular groove
w Left ventricle
x Greater splanchnic n.

W·FRICKE

(see pp. 31, 49)

41

3. THORACIC CAVITY, PLEURA, AND VEINS OF THE THORACIC CAVITY

a) The **THORACIC CAVITY (CAVUM THORACIS**; see also text-illustration) is cranial to the diaphragm. It is enclosed by the thorax comprising the thoracic vertebrae, ribs and sternum. Caudal to the diaphragm, the thorax encloses the intrathoracic part of the abdominal cavity. The thoracic cavity is lined with serous membrane, the **pleura**, which also covers the organs within the thoracic cavity. The pleural lining of the thoracic wall is referred to as **parietal pleura**, the parts of which, depending on their location, are designated **costal pleura (F)**, **diaphragmatic pleura (H)** and **mediastinal pleura (G)**. The **visceral pleura** covers the lung and is therefore named **pulmonary pleura (D)**. The mediastinal pleura of each side together with an intermediate fibrous layer form the **mediastinum (8)**, corresponding to the mesentery of the abdominal cavity, q.v. The mediastinum may be regarded as the mesentery of the esophagus. It inserts onto the vertebral bodies dorsally, the sternum ventrally and the diaphragm caudally. There the line of insertion is pushed farther to the left of the midline. The following structures pass through the mediastinum in a craniocaudal direction: **right azygos vein (10)**, **thoracic duct (12)**, **descending aorta (C)**, **dorsal vagal trunk (13)**, **esophagus (19)**, **ventral vagal trunk (18)** and **trachea (9)** with tracheal bifurcation. The **pulmonary ligament (17)** extends from the caudal lobe of the lung to the mediastinum, and thus connects the pulmonary pleura with the mediastinal pleura.

Within the thoracic cavity the pleura forms two **pleural cavities (B)**, which pass through the thoracic inlet into the neck region as **pleural cupulae (A)**. That of the left extends about the width of two ribs cranial to the thoracic inlet; the right cupula about one rib-width. The most caudal part of the pleural cavity is the **costodiaphragmatic recess (20)**, which lies immediately cranial to the line of insertion of the diaphragm. The pleural cavities are fluid-filled crevices of capillary dimension. Pulmonary and parietal pleura are adjacent to each other and are closely bound together by cohesive forces, so that the lung must follow the thoracic wall. As a result, inspiration develops by enlargement of the thorax. In addition, due to the asymmetrical caudal insertion of the mediastinum, the left pleural cavity has a **costomediastinal recess (P)**. In contrast, the right pleural cavity has a left **mediastinodiaphragmatic recess (O)**. The caudal vena cava traverses the right pleural cavity in a proper plica venae cavae, a folded part of the mediastinum. The latter produces a further niche, the **mediastinal recess (15)**, for the accessory lobe of the right lung. An additional cavity, the **serous cavity of the mediastinum (16)** is situated within the mediastinum to the right of the esophagus and caudal to the bifurcation of the trachea. This is the result of a 'pinching off' of a part of the peritoneal cavity during ontogenesis. The serous cavity of the mediastinum and accompanying tension in the pulmonary ligament can be seen by raising the caudal lobe of the right lung. The serous cavity of the mediastinum is opened by an incision directed ventroparallel to the line of insertion of the pulmonary ligament. One is able to probe its extent with the index finger from the diaphragm to the root of the lung. The **pericardial cavity (J)**, containing the heart, is situated in the mediastinum ventral to the esophagus and the bifurcation of the trachea. With the pericardium opened, one recognizes the **serous pericardium** and its **parietal lamina (K)**. At the base of the heart this becomes the **visceral lamina (epicardium —L)**, which invests the heart surface. The **fibrous pericardium (M)** is the outer enveloping connective tissue foundation of the pericardium. It is continuous with the **phrenicopericardiac ligament (N)** and the **endothoracic fascia (E)**, which is the connective tissue base of the parietal pleura. The portion of the **mediastinal pleura** covering the pericardium laterally is termed the **pericardiac pleura (I)**.

b) VEINS OF THE THORACIC CAVITY

Near the heart, the **cranial vena cava (7)** gives off the **right azygos vein (10)** and at the thoracic inlet in sequence the **costocervical vein (5)** and **internal thoracic vein (6)**, before it divides into **left and right brachiocephalic veins (4)**. The brachiocephalic vein gives off the subclavian, **external jugular (1)** and **internal jugular (2)** veins. The **caudal vena cava (11)** has its own pleural covering, the **plica venae cavae**, which is split off from the mediastinum.

Thoracic cavity

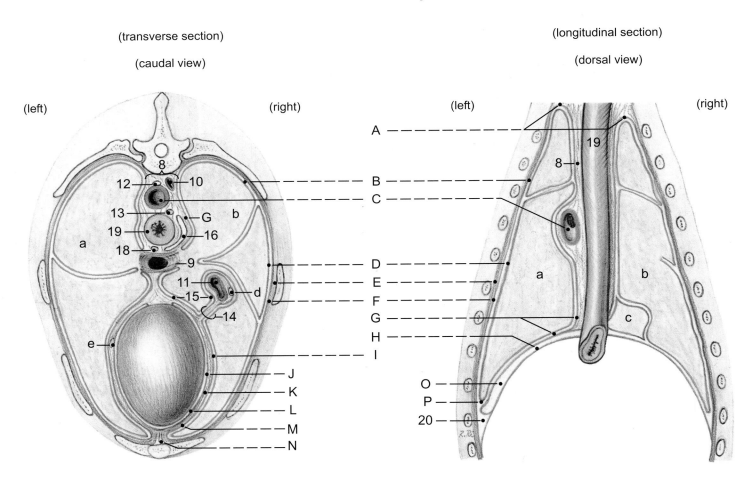

(transverse section)

(caudal view)

(longitudinal section)

(dorsal view)

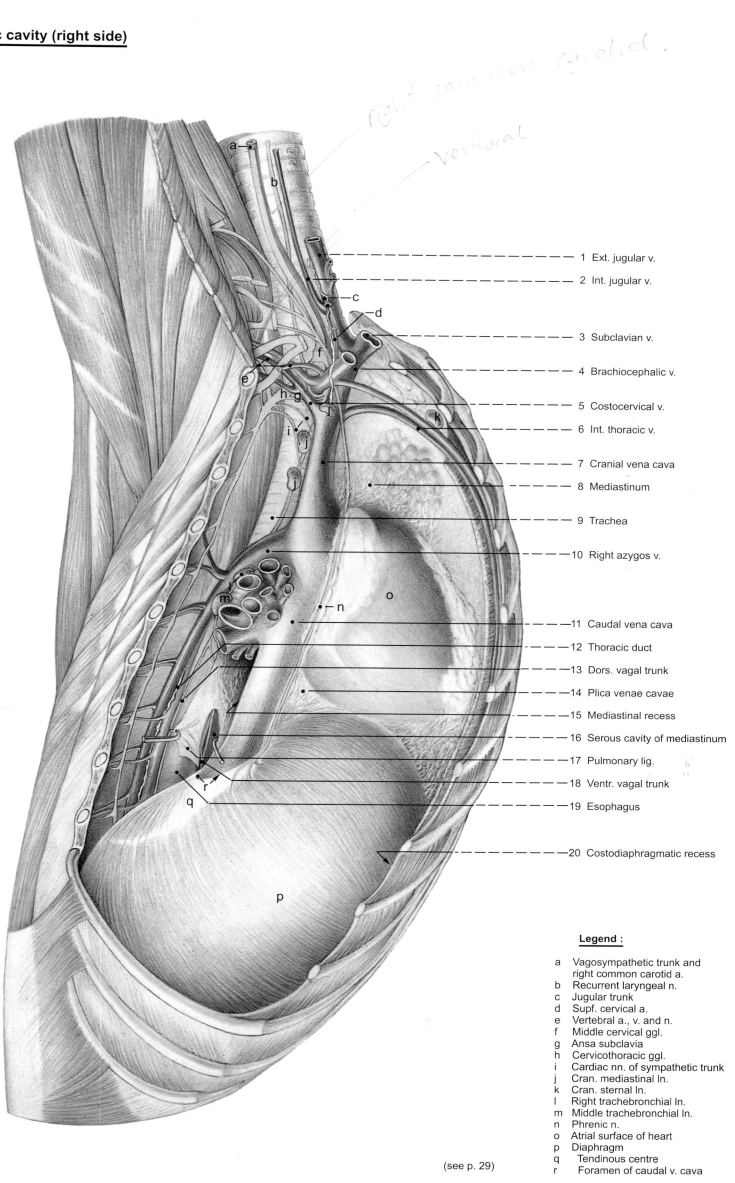

right common carotid.

vertebral

1 Ext. jugular v.
2 Int. jugular v.
3 Subclavian v.
4 Brachiocephalic v.
5 Costocervical v.
6 Int. thoracic v.
7 Cranial vena cava
8 Mediastinum
9 Trachea
10 Right azygos v.
11 Caudal vena cava
12 Thoracic duct
13 Dors. vagal trunk
14 Plica venae cavae
15 Mediastinal recess
16 Serous cavity of mediastinum
17 Pulmonary lig.
18 Ventr. vagal trunk
19 Esophagus
20 Costodiaphragmatic recess

Legend :

a   Vagosympathetic trunk and
    right common carotid a.
b   Recurrent laryngeal n.
c   Jugular trunk
d   Supf. cervical a.
e   Vertebral a., v. and n.
f   Middle cervical ggl.
g   Ansa subclavia
h   Cervicothoracic ggl.
i   Cardiac nn. of sympathetic trunk
j   Cran. mediastinal ln.
k   Cran. sternal ln.
l   Right trachebronchial ln.
m   Middle trachebronchial ln.
n   Phrenic n.
o   Atrial surface of heart
p   Diaphragm
q   Tendinous centre
r   Foramen of caudal v. cava

(see p. 29)

4. HEART, SURFACE OF THE HEART, HEART WALL AND RELATIONSHIPS IN THE INTERIOR OF THE HEART

On the isolated heart, the pericardium is opened by a circular section at the level of the coronary sulcus. The aorta should be cut close enough to the heart so that the aortic valve is visible. The pulmonary trunk should be cut in small steps until the pulmonary trunk valve is visible. After this dissection, the surface of the heart should be examined. To study the internal relationships of the heart the right atrium is opened by scissors. Begin the section at the tip of the right auricle, follow the ventral border of the auricle and, at the coronary groove, continue it farther through the atrial wall to the interatrial septum. The left atrium is opened in a like manner. The ventricles are opened by different sections. The right ventricle is opened by a longitudinal section that starts at the pulmonary trunk valve, runs parallel to the interventricular septum and ends halfway to the apex of the heart. From this point a cross-section is made through the total right ventricle, but without damaging the papillary muscles. To open the left ventricle, a longitudinal section is conducted alongside the left ventricular border, thus bisecting the parietal cusp of the bicuspid valve.

1; 2 The heart combines the functions of a pressure and suction pump to maintain the circulation of the blood. It is situated in the mediastinal space and forms a caudally open angle of 45-50 degrees with its longitudinal axis. The apex of the heart extends to the ventral insertion of the diaphragm. The heart lies between the 3rd and 7th ribs, 4/7 on the left, and 3/7 to the right of the midline.

3 a) The **HEART SURFACE** is characterized by a **base**, at which the great vessels connect to the organ, and an **apex (7)** with its muscle arranged like a vortex. The apices of the **auricles (2, −right auricle; 4, −left auricle)** of the right and left atria respectively denote the **auricular surface (8)**. The surface opposite, where the auricles are absent, is designated **atrial surface (12)**. Externally, the left or arterial side of the heart is differentiated from the right or venous side by its greater extent, the left ventricle alone forming the apex. Apart from this it has a thicker, more compact ventricular wall. The **right (3) and left (5) ventricular margins** lie between the two heart surfaces in the region of the respective ventricles of the heart. Between the apices of the two

4 auricles is the curved outflow tract of the right ventricle, the **conus arteriosus (9)**, that propels blood from the right ventricle to the pulmonary trunk. At the level of the line of reflection of the pericardium, the **ligamentum arteriosum (1)** travels between aorta and pulmonary trunk; it is the remnant of the embryonic ductus arteriosus. The **paraconal interventricular groove (6)** lies beside the conus arteriosus and represents the boundary between the ventricles externally. It contains the paraconal interventricular branch or 'long limb' of the left coronary artery and its satellite vein. The indistinct **subsinuosal interventricular groove (11)** lies opposite. It runs ventrally from the origin of the coronary sinus (at the area of discharge of the great and middle cardiac veins) toward the heart's apex. The **coronary groove (10)**, which contains the 'circular limbs' of the coronary arteries, is the externally recognizable boundary between the atria and the ventricles.

b) The **HEART WALL** consists of the very thin endocardium, the strong
5 myocardium and the very thin epicardium. The **endocardium (k)** lines the internal surface and continues as the inner lining of the large blood vessels
6 that lead to the heart or carry blood from the heart. The **myocardium (j)** is subdivided into a 'work' (contracting) myocardium and a 'stimulus-conducting' myocardium. The contracting myocardium far outweighs the conducting myocardium. Its thickness is adapted to local pressure differences. It consists of striated cardiac muscle cells that are attached end-to-end, forming an acute-angled network. The cardiac muscle cells are arranged in three layers (external, middle and internal) which mix with each other in the form of a whorl at the tip of the heart. In the area of the conus arteriosus there are circularly arranged muscle cell bundles. The musculature of the atria and the ventricles is not a continuum but, coming from the corresponding direction (the atrial musculature from dorsal; the ventricular muscle from ventral), insert on the heart skeleton (see p. 46). The myocardial cells of the internal conducting system have only very few myofibrils and, as a result of their specialization for conducting impulses, have lost their ability to contract. The
7 **epicardium (i)** is a serosal layer on the heart that corresponds to the visceral lamina of the serous pericardium.

c) The **INTERNAL RELATIONSHIPS OF THE HEART** are described according to the direction of blood flow. Within the **right atrium (A)** is a smooth walled region, the **sinus venarum cavarum** or **sinus venosus) (a)**, into which the cranial and caudal caval veins open. This is separated indistinctly from the atrial region proper with its furrowed, reticulate internal relief. The heart veins open ventral to the opening of the caudal vena cava into the **coronary sinus (b)** (great cardiac v. and the middle cardiac v.), which represents a tubular outpouching of the right atrium. The right **cardiac vv. (d)** and the *vv. cordis minimae* are located in the right atrium, between the **mm. pectinati (c)**, which project into the atrial lumen in a comb-like manner. A fewer number of vv. cordis minimae appear in the left atrium and the left and right ventricles. At the entrance to the **right ventricle (B)**, the three cusps of the **tricus-**
8 **pid valve (e)** are anchored to the anulus fibrosus of the cardiac skeleton. From the **parietal cusp (e'₁)**, chordae tendineae extend chiefly to the great **papillary muscle (m. papillaris magnus, −e"₁)**, from the **septal cusp (e'₂)**

mainly to the unremarkable **small papillary muscles (mm. papillares parvi, −e"₂)**, and from the indistinct **angular cusp (e'₃)** situated in the angle between the other two cusps, mainly to the **subarterial papillary muscle (e"₃)** lying ventral to the arterial pulmonary trunk. The **pulmonary trunk valve (f)** is
9 characterized by having three cusps that, corresponding to their positions relative to right and left sides of the heart, are designated **right (f₁)**, **left (f₂)** and **intermediate (f₃) semilunar valvules**.

In the atrial region between the two halves of the heart, is the **interatrial septum (g)**. If the septum is held against a light source, the translucent **fossa ovalis (h)** can be discerned. Since the epicardium and myocardium are lacking here, the fossa ovalis consists only of a duplicature of the endocardium. Blood flows into the two ventricles through a right and a left **atrioventricular ostium (1)** respectively. The two ventricles are separated completely from one another by a thick **interventricular septum (m)**. In both ventricles, tendon-like **septomarginal trabeculae (n)**, conduction musculature, extend from the septum to the marginal region, particularly to the papillary muscles. **Trabeculae carneae (o)**, particularly distinct in the region of the apex of both ventricles, project into the ventricular lumen as fleshy trabeculae. The **chordae tendineae (p)** are tendinous filaments that connect each cusp of the atrioventricular valves with each of two papillary muscles.

Five to eight ostia of the **pulmonary vv. (q)** are present in the **left atrium (C)**. At its entrance, the **left ventricle (D)** has the **bicuspid valve (r)**, whose **parietal cusp (r'₁)** is connected by chordae tendineae chiefly to the **subauricular papillary muscle (r"₁)** and with its **septal cusp (r'₂)** mainly to the subatrial **papillary muscle (r"₂)**. The route of expulsion of the blood to the **aortic valve (s)** lies between the septal cusp and the ventricular septum. The crescent-shaped valvules of the aortic valve are denoted according to their positions with reference to right and left sides of the heart and the ventricular septum. They are designated the **right (s₁)**, the **left (s₂)** and the **septal (s₃) semilunar valvules**.

Legend (see figures on opposite page)

A	Right atrium			**C**	Left atrium
a	Sinus venarum cavarum [Sinus venosus]	g	Interatrial septum	q	Openings of the pulmonary veins
		h	Fossa ovalis		
b	Coronary sinus	i	Epicardium		
c	Pectinate muscles (Musculi pectinati)	j	Myocardium		
d	Right cardiac veins	k	Endocardium		

B	Right ventricle			**D**	Left ventricle
e	Tricuspid valve (Right atrioventricular valve)	l	Atrioventricular ostium	r	Bicuspid (mitral) valve (Left atrioventricular valve)
e'₁	Parietal cusp			r'₁	Parietal cusp
e'₂	Septal cusp	m	Interventricular septum	r'₂	Septal cusp
e'₃	Angular cusp				
e"₁	Large papillary muscle	n	Septomarginal trabeculae	r"₁	Subauricular papillary muscle
e"₂	Small papillary muscles			r"₂	Subatrial papillary muscle
e"₃	Subarterial papillary muscle	o	Trabeculae carneae		
f	Pulmonary trunk valve	p	Chordae tendineae	s	Aortic valve
f₁	Right semilunar valvule			s₁	Right semilunar valvule
f₂	Left semilunar valvule			s₂	Left semilunar valvule
f₃	Intermediate semilunar valvule			s₃	Septal semilunar valvule

Right ventricle

(Auricular surface)

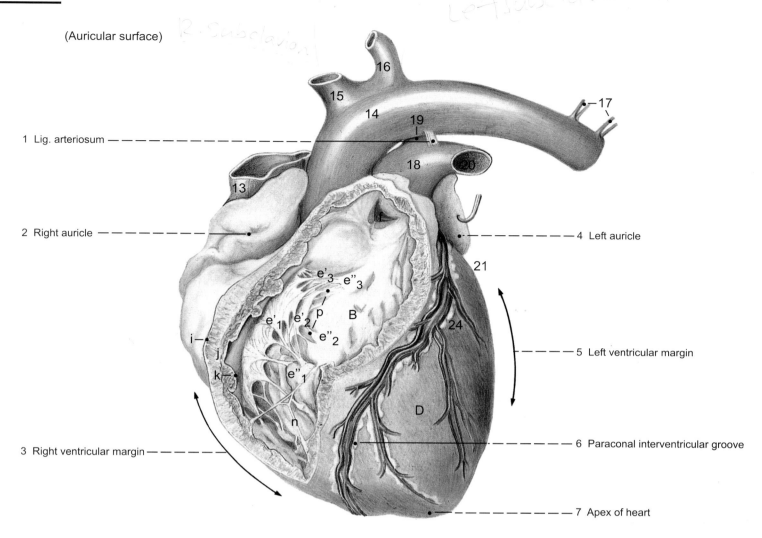

1 Lig. arteriosum

2 Right auricle

3 Right ventricular margin

4 Left auricle

5 Left ventricular margin

6 Paraconal interventricular groove

7 Apex of heart

Legend :

13 Cran. vena cava
14 Aorta
15 Brachiocephalic trunk
16 Left subclavian a.
17 Intercostal aa.

18 Pulmonary trunk
19 Right pulmonary a.
20 Left pulmonary a.
21 Great cardiac v.
22 Right coronary a.

23 Left coronary a.
24 Paraconal interventricular br.
25 Circumflex branch
26 Subsinuosal interventricular br.
27 Middle cardiac v.

28 Caud. vena cava
29 Pulmonary vv.

Base of heart

Left atrium and left ventricle

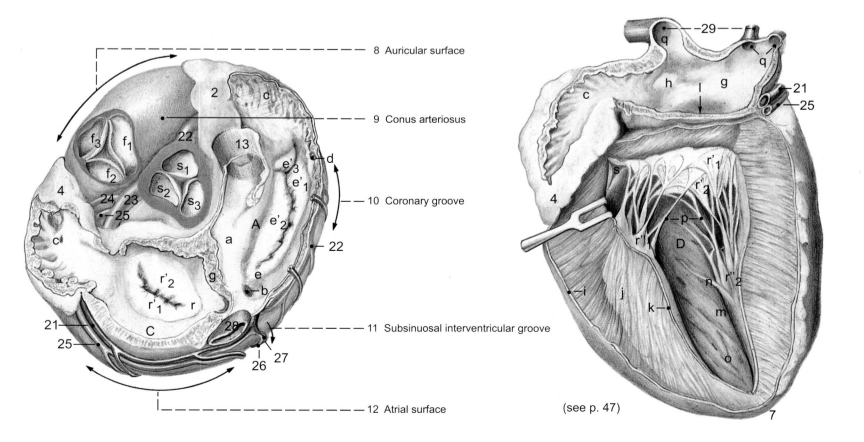

8 Auricular surface

9 Conus arteriosus

10 Coronary groove

11 Subsinuosal interventricular groove

12 Atrial surface

(see p. 47)

5. HEART, CORONARY VESSELS, HEART VALVES, CARDIAC CONDUCTION SYSTEM

a) The **HEART VESSELS** are the coronary arteries and the cardiac veins. The arteries are termed coronary arteries because their main branches run in the coronary groove. They lie beneath the epicardium and are surrounded by adipose tissue. Left and right coronary arteries originate from the first part of the aorta, opposite the left and right semilunar cusps. The coronary arteries can show variations with respect to their course and the area of the heart supplied, and may, in the diagnosis of blood vascular disturbances, contribute to disorders.

I. The **two coronary arteries (Aa. coronariae)** convey about 10% of the stroke-volume of blood to the heart muscle. The **left coronary artery (5,** –see also p. 45) leaves the first part of the aorta and, crossing ventral to the left auricle, divides into two principal branches: The first principal branch, the **paraconal interventricular branch (7)**, courses in the same named longitudinal groove, where it releases a proximal and distal collateral vessel to the left ventricular wall. The second principal branch, the **circumflex branch (6)**, after passing ventral to the left auricle runs in the coronary sulcus between left ventricle and atrium to the subsinuosal interventricular groove where in most cases it continues as the **subsinuosal interventricular branch (8)**.

The **right coronary artery (2,** –see also page 45) originates from the aorta between the origin of the pulmonary trunk and the right auricle. With its **circumflex branch (3)**, after passing ventral to the right auricle, it runs in the right semicircumference of the coronary groove.

II. The **cardiac veins** are subdivided into one large, one middle-sized, small (right) and minimal veins. The **great cardiac vein (1,** –V. cordis magna; also called the *great coronary vein*) at first courses in the paraconal interventricular groove and, after this, in the coronary groove with the circumflex branch of the left coronary artery. It continues, without changing its direction, into the coronary sinus of the right atrium. The **middle cardiac vein (V. cordis media** –9) accompanies the subsinuosal interventricular ramus and empties into the coronary sinus. The small **right cardiac veins (Vv. cordis dextrae** –4) conduct blood from the right ventricular wall directly to the right atrium. The **minimal cardiac veins (Vv. cordis minimae)** drain the blood from the subendocardial tissue directly into the four internal chambers of the heart, especially into the atria.

b) The **VALVULAR APPARATUS** consists of the cardiac skeleton and the heart valves, which are formed as atrioventricular and semilunar valves. The **cardiac skeleton** is formed by **fibrous rings (Anuli fibrosi)**, which surround the openings between atrium and ventricle and the openings of the aorta and pulmonary trunk. In places the rings contain embedded cartilage. Between the atrioventricular openings and the aorta the heart skeleton is formed as a **right trigone cartilage** and as a **septal cartilage**. In addition to serving as the place of insertion for the myocardium, the heart skeleton functions as the attachment of the heart valves and, in the electrophysiological view, to separate the atrial musculature from the ventricular muscle so that atrial excitation does not pass diffusely into the ventricles. An opening is left only for the passage of the atrioventricular bundle of the cardiac conduction system.

Since the four heart valves are nearly in a single plane, one speaks of a 'valvular plane.' Externally, the valvular plane is marked by the circular coronary groove. The valvular plane changes its position during contraction of the heart. With ventricular systole (contraction) it is moved toward the apex of the heart and during diastole (relaxation) of the ventricular muscle it is returned to its original position. During systole blood is ejected, and by lowering the valvular plane, blood is at the same time sucked in from the atrium and the large veins near the heart (functions as a pressure and a suction pump).

The **atrioventricular valves (bicuspid valve** –15 and **tricuspid valve** –12), which close the atrioventricular ostia, are kept on a level with the valvular plane by the **chordae tendineae (13)** and the **papillary muscles (14)**, so that the cusps are not everted into the atrium with reversal of blood flow. Instead their free borders contact to complete valve closure. The papillary muscles do not serve to open the valves, which are opened passively by the blood-flow similar to the opening of a door by a gust of wind.

The **semilunar valves (Valva trunci pulmonalis** and **Valva aortae**, see also p. 45) consist of three individual cusps, each shaped like a pocket. They function strictly passively. The free border of each cusp, which projects into the lumen of the vessel, flutters with the physiological direction of the blood stream. With reversal of blood flow, the cusp is expanded by the inflow of blood; their free borders contact one another and close the valvular orifice.

c) The **CARDIAC STIMULUS-GENERATING AND STIMULUS-CONDUCTION SYSTEM** enables the heart to have an independent heart-action that, even with loss of consciousness, continues to function. This system consists of modified cardiac cells, the myocardium of the conducting system, which, gross-anatomically, is difficult to demonstrate. It is not a nervous tissue, but is regulated by the autonomic nervous system, which accelerates the stimulus generation (sympathetic nerves) or slows it down (parasympathetic nerves).

The **sinoatrial node (10)**, the normal pacemaker, is the superintending stimulus-generating center and is located in the region of the sinus venosus, between the mouth of the cranial vena cava and the right auricle. The rhythmic impulses formed here first reach the atrial myocardial cells and finally the **atrioventricular node (11)**, where conduction of the stimulus is retarded. The **atrioventricular bundle (16)**, the bundle of HIS, passes through an opening in the heart skeleton to reach the interventricular septum where it divides into two branches (**right bundle-branch** –17 and **left bundle-branch** –18). The two bundle-branches extend subendocardially in the corresponding ventricle toward the apex of the heart. Some fibers take an abbreviated course, passing by way of **septomarginal trabeculae (19)** to the ordinary myocardium and papillary muscles of the free wall, thus bypassing the heart's apex. Both branches divide into finer fibers (PURKINJE-fibers), which conduct impulses to the contractile myocardium and the papillary muscles of the ventricles.

d) The **CARDIAC NERVES** (see p. 49) of the autonomic nervous system modify the inherent rhythm of the heart. **Sympathetic fibers in the cardiac nerves** originate from the cervicothoracic ganglion (stellate ganglion) and the middle cervical ganglion. With the parasympathetic cardiac fibers of the vagus nerve (X) or of its recurrent laryngeal branch, they form the cardiac plexus. From the plexus, nerves pass to the heart, especially the blood vessels as well as the myocardial cells of the conducting system and the contractile myocardium. In addition, they form a subendocardial nerve plexus. Sympathetic and **parasympathetic fibers** are antagonistic with respect to their action on the heart. Sympathetic stimulation increases the frequency of heart contractions (positive chronotropic effect), shortens the conduction time for the spread of excitation (positive dromotropic effect) and increases the strength of heart contraction (positive inotropic effect). Parasympathetic stimulation has negative chrono-, dromo-, and inotropic action.

Efferent neurons of the sympathetic cardiac nerves are predominantly postganglionic; their synapses take place predominantly in the ganglia of the sympathetic trunk. Efferent parasympathetic neurons extending to the cardiac plexus and to the heart are presynaptic neurons. Their synapses take place in the small ganglia that are located predominantly subepicardially in the atrial walls.

Afferent fibers also pass with the sympathetic and parasympathetic fibers. Afferents passing with the sympathetic fibers are pain fibers, and those passing with the parasympathetic fibers lead from stretch receptors.

Endocrine (modified) myocardial cells are present in the wall of the atria. They secrete the natriuretic peptide hormone cardiodilatin, which serves to regulate blood pressure and blood volume.

Coronary arteries and veins of heart

(Auricular surface)

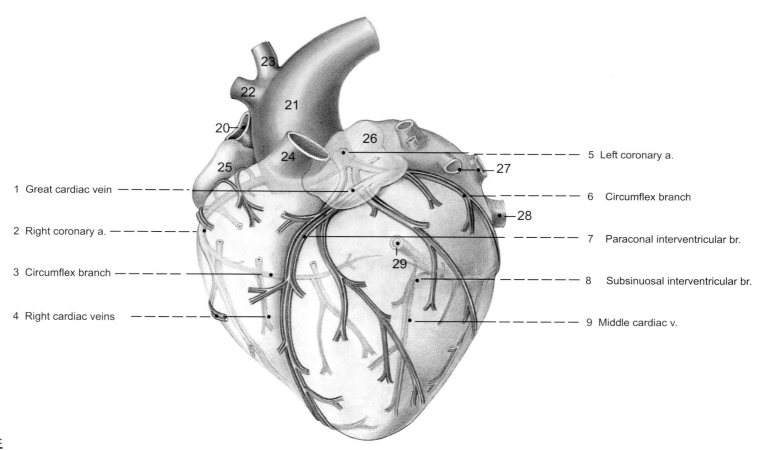

1 Great cardiac vein

2 Right coronary a.

3 Circumflex branch

4 Right cardiac veins

5 Left coronary a.

6 Circumflex branch

7 Paraconal interventricular br.

8 Subsinuosal interventricular br.

9 Middle cardiac v.

Legend :

20 Cran. vena cava
21 Aorta
22 Brachiocephalic trunk
23 Left subclavian a.

24 Pulmonary trunk
25 Auricle of right atrium
26 Auricle of left atrium
27 Pulmonary veins

28 Caudal vena cava
29 Coronary sinus
30 Right atrium
31 Right ventricle

32 Aortic valve
33 Left ventricle

Conducting system of heart

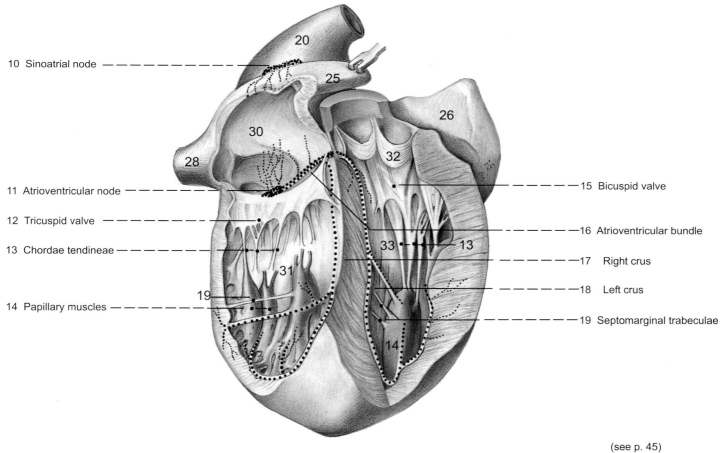

10 Sinoatrial node

11 Atrioventricular node

12 Tricuspid valve

13 Chordae tendineae

14 Papillary muscles

15 Bicuspid valve

16 Atrioventricular bundle

17 Right crus

18 Left crus

19 Septomarginal trabeculae

(see p. 45)

6. AUTONOMIC NERVOUS SYSTEM

1 The **autonomic (vegetative) nervous system** is composed of a **sympathetic part** (sympathetic nervous system) and a **parasympathetic part** (parasympathetic nervous system). The **intramural (intestinal) system** is considered a part of the autonomic nervous system and is observed in the gastrointestinal tract, *e.g.*, as submucosal, myenteric, and subserosal plexuses. The autonomic (vegetative) nervous system regulates the internal functions of the body autonomously; that is, without conscious control. For example, the smooth musculature of the glands, vessels and organ systems, by which metabolic activities, water and heat balance as well as other different body functions are carried out, is regulated and coordinated (*e.g.*, circulatory and respiratory systems) without conscious control. The autonomic nervous system regulates the autonomy of the stimulus-generating and conducting system within the heart. Contrary to the somatic nervous system, the autonomic nervous system is autonomous, not completely, but in a limited manner. It can fulfill its functions, which are partially essential for life, for example, during sleep, unconsciousness and general anesthesia. A limited autonomy exists also in relation to the vegetative centers of the brain (*e.g.*, of the diencephalon) and the humoral coordinating systems (*e.g.*, of the pituitary gland). As in the somatic nervous system with its sensory afferents and motor efferents, there are afferent fibers (visceral afferent neurons) associated with the autonomic nervous system; but today most regard the autonomic nervous system as an efferent system of fibers that pass from the brain and spinal cord to smooth muscle, heart muscle and gland. Visceral sensory (afferent) fibers conduct visceral pain and other modalities and regulate the graduation and modification of peripheral stimuli. The cell bodies of afferent visceral neurons of the sympathetic nervous system are located in the spinal ganglia, and their nerve fibers run within the dorsal root of the spinal nerves to the spinal cord. In the sympathetic part, it is only in the dorsal root that visceral afferent fibers are separate from the autonomic efferent nerve fibers. In the sympathetic part, the efferent pathway leaves the spinal cord by the ventral root of a spinal nerve, and consists of two neurons that synapse in sequence. The first neuron has its cell body in the spinal cord, its axon passing in the ventral root; the second neuron has its cell body in a peripheral ganglion, and its axon reaches the organ innervated.

The main parts of the autonomic system the sympathetic and parasympathetic, differ from each other in their topography and histochemically by their transmitter substances. As transmitter substance (neurotransmitter), in the parasympathetic part, acetylcholine is released at the ends of the pre- as well as the postsynaptic parasympathetic fibers. In the sympathetic part, acetylcholine is released by the presynaptic nerve fibers but predominantly norepinephrine by the postsynaptic fibers. Functionally, the sympathetic part and the parasympathetic part are predominantly antagonistic. The arrector pili muscles and the smooth muscle of the vessels of the skin are exclusively supplied by the sympathetic part. The sympathetic part is functionally activating, increasing the utilization of energy, the blood pressure and the heart rate, and other functions. The parasympathetic part furthers the recovery and maintenance of the body, building up energy reserves by activating the digestive system. The autonomic nervous system forms nerve plexuses. The plexuses contain ganglia of the same name and differ significantly from the plexuses of the somatic nervous system (brachial and lumbosacral plexus). The ganglia contain perikarya (nerve cell bodies) and here the synapse from the myelinated preganglionic to the unmyelinated postganglionic nerve fiber takes place.

The intramural (gastrointestinal) system consists of nerve fibers and nerve cells. A part of the nerve cells is responsible for the synapsing from the central to the peripheral neuron of the parasympathetic part. Other nerve cells belong to the short intramural reflex arcs that regulate the glandular activity and the motor activity of the intestines by neuropeptide transmitters.

a) The **sympathetic nervous system** with its paired sympathetic trunks extends from the head-neck border to the tail. Caudal to the thoracic inlet the sympathetic trunk is roughly segmented by its **ganglia (sympathetic trunk ganglia —10)** with their communicating branches. By longitudinal **interganglionic branches (11)** a chain of ganglia is formed that lies ventrolaterally on the vertebral bodies. For this reason, the ganglia are also called paravertebral ganglia. The original perikarya are within the lateral horn of the thoracolumbar part of the spinal cord. Their central myelinated nerve fibers leave the spinal nerve in the white communicating branches (rami) and, as efferent fibers, reach the ganglia of the sympathetic trunk. A part of these nerve fibers will synapse within the ganglia of the sympathetic trunk. From the ganglia, peripheral unmyelinated nerve fibers pass in the grey communicating branches (rami) to the somatic spinal nerves (details, see p. 60). Unmyelinated and myelinated nerve fibers are often found jointly in mixed communicating branches. The cervical sympathetic nerve trunk is different from the other parts of the trunk in that it lies at a distinct distance from the vertebral column united with the cervical part of the vagus nerve to form the vagosympathetic trunk. Also, at its three ganglia (cranial, middle and caudal cervical ganglia), it does not here receive contributions from the spinal cord. Thus a segmental subdivision is lacking.

The first three paravertebral ganglia of the thoracic sympathetic nerve trunk, together with the caudal cervical ganglion, form the **cervicothoracic (stellate) ganglion (5)**. From the latter the two branches of the **ansa subclavia (6)** are **2** released. After having embraced the left or, respective, right subclavian artery both branches reunite at the small **middle cervical ganglion (4)**. From here the sympathetic fibers within the vagosympathetic trunk conduct impulses that, by way of the cranial cervical ganglion (k), pass to the head (see p. 102). From the cervicothoracic ganglion the following groups of branches are given off: First, unmyelinated nerve branches pass to the thoracic viscera and are named according to the viscus innervated (*e.g.*, **cardiac nerves —7**). These branches receive also contributions from the ansa subclavia and the middle cervical ganglion. The sympathetic nerves of the thoracic organs mix with parasympathetic fibers from the vagus and, with these, form mixed plexuses for the thoracic viscera (cardiac, esophageal and pulmonary plexuses). Secondly, the **vertebral nerve (2)**, with the accompanying vertebral artery and vein, reaches the transverse canal of the cervical vertebral column and here gives off its sympathetic fibers to the cervical nerves. Thirdly, slender **grey communicating branches (3)** pass to the brachial plexus and to the first four intercostal nerves and furnish sympathetic fibers to them.

From the thoracic sympathetic nerve trunk, before its transition into the lumbar sympathetic trunk, at the level of the 10th to the 13th thoracic vertebra, the strong **major splanchnic nerve (13)** is given off. It runs over the lumbocostal arch of the diaphragm into the abdominal cavity to the solar (celiacomesenteric) plexus (see p. 60). After the major splanchnic nerve is given off, the thoracic sympathetic trunk becomes very thin and continues into the lumbar sympathetic nerve trunk, where it increases in thickness (see p. 61).

b) The **parasympathetic part (parasympathetic nervous system)** is composed of a cranial, cerebral, part and a caudal, sacral, part. Of the cranial nerves III, VII, IX and X, which carry parasympathetic fibers, the **vagus nerve (X —8)** passes to the body cavities. In the cervical region it is joined to the sympathetic trunk, forming the vagosympathetic trunk. At the level of the sympathetic middle cervical ganglion the vagus nerve separates from the sympathetic trunk and accompanies the trachea to the root of the lung where it gives off **cardiac and bronchial branches (9)** to the cardiac and pulmonary plexuses. Caudal to the root of the lung, the right and left vagus nerves divide each into a long dorsal and a short ventral branch which, dorsal and ventral to the esophagus, unite to form the **dorsal vagal and ventral vagal trunks (12)**. The vagal trunks accompany the esophagus through the esophageal hiatus into the abdominal cavity where they supply the abdominal viscera up to the transverse colon inclusively. Within the thoracic cavity the vagus nerve gives off the recurrent laryngeal nerve. The right recurrent laryngeal nerve loops **3** around the right subclavian artery near that artery's origin, and the **left recurrent laryngeal nerve (1)** loops medially around the aortic arch at the base of the heart. After this, the nerves of both sides return ventral to the common carotid artery and alongside the trachea to the larynx. Each recurrent laryngeal nerve gives off tracheal and esophageal branches and ends as the caudal laryngeal nerve of its side. After the origin of the recurrent laryngeal nerve with its motor and sensory branches the vagus nerve contains, beside visceral sensory fibers, exclusively parasympathetic fibers. The synapse of parasympathetic fibers, from the myelinated preganglionic fiber to the non-myelinated postganglionic fiber, takes place near the organ innervated, predominantly in the intramural ganglia (for the parasympathetic pathways from the sacral spinal cord, see pp. 60 and 70).

Legend (see opposite illustrations):

a	Ciliary ganglion	n	Celiac ganglion
b	Pterygopalatine ganglion	o	Minor splanchnic nerve
c	Lacrimal gland	p	Adrenal branch
d	Mandibular ganglion and sublingual ganglion	q	Cran. mesenteric ganglion
e	Sublingual gland	r	Abdominal aortic plexus
f	Mandibular gland	s	Lumbar splanchnic nn.
g	Otic ganglion	t	Caud. mesenteric ganglion
h	Zygomatic gland	u	Hypogastric n.
i	Parotid gland	v	Sacral splanchnic nn.
j	Distal (nodose) ganglion	w	Pelvic nn.
k	Cran. cervical ganglion	x	Pelvic plexus
l	Vagosympathetic trunk	y	Esophageal hiatus
m	White ramus communicans (white communicating branch)		

Cervical and thoracic arteries, veins and nerves

(Left surface)

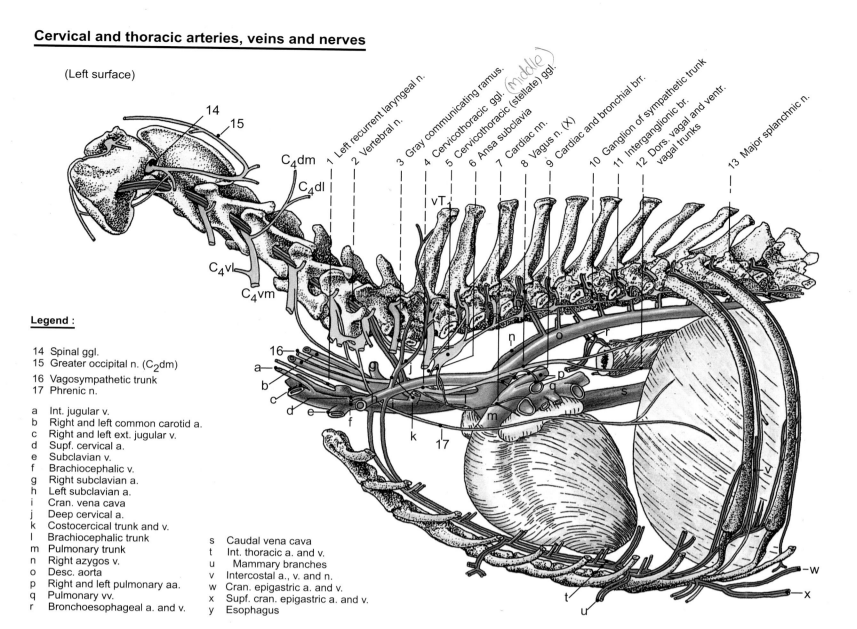

1 Left recurrent laryngeal n.
2 Vertebral n.
3 Gray communicating ramus.
4 Cervicothoracic ggl.
5 Cervicothoracic (stellate) ggl.
6 Ansa subclavia
7 Cardiac nn.
8 Vagus n. (X)
9 Cardiac and bronchial brr.
10 Ganglion of sympathetic trunk
11 Interganglionic br.
12 Dors. vagal and ventr. vagal trunks
13 Major splanchnic n.

C4dm
C4dl
C4vl
C4vm

vT1

Legend :

14 Spinal ggl.
15 Greater occipital n. (C2dm)
16 Vagosympathetic trunk
17 Phrenic n.

a Int. jugular v.
b Right and left common carotid a.
c Right and left ext. jugular v.
d Supf. cervical a.
e Subclavian v.
f Brachiocephalic v.
g Right subclavian a.
h Left subclavian a.
i Cran. vena cava
j Deep cervical a.
k Costocervical trunk and v.
l Brachiocephalic trunk
m Pulmonary trunk
n Right azygos v.
o Desc. aorta
p Right and left pulmonary aa.
q Pulmonary vv.
r Bronchoesophageal a. and v.

s Caudal vena cava
t Int. thoracic a. and v.
u   Mammary branches
v Intercostal a., v. and n.
w Cran. epigastric a. and v.
x Supf. cran. epigastric a. and v.
y Esophagus

Autonomic nervous system

(see pp. 41, 61)

Sympathetic part:
 ——— Preganglionic nerve fiber
 - - - Postganglionic nerve fiber

Parasympathetic part:
 ——— Preganglionic nerve fiber
 - - - Postganglionic nerve fiber

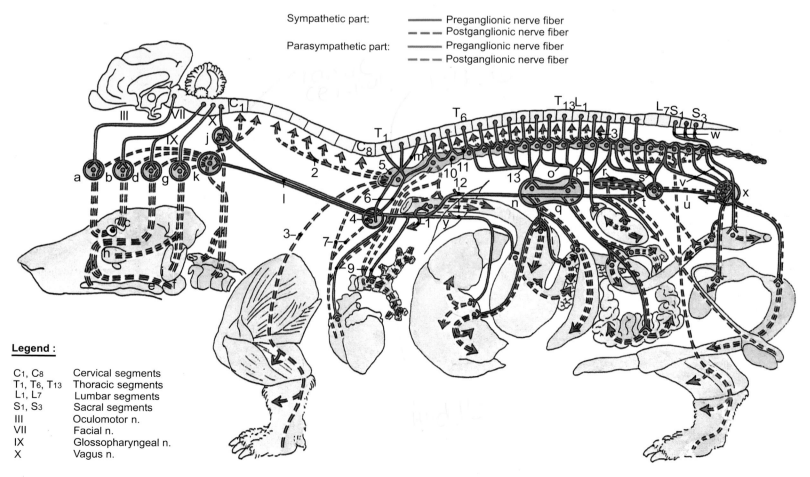

Legend :

C1, C8   Cervical segments
T1, T6, T13   Thoracic segments
L1, L7   Lumbar segments
S1, S3   Sacral segments
III   Oculomotor n.
VII   Facial n.
IX   Glossopharyngeal n.
X   Vagus n.

49

CHAPTER 6: ABDOMINAL CAVITY
1. TOPOGRAPHY OF THE ABDOMINAL ORGANS AND RELATIONSHIPS OF THE PERITONEUM

Avoiding damage to abdominal organs, the abdominal cavity is opened by a paramedian section from the diaphragm to the pecten ossis pubis and by a transverse section at the level of the last rib. After this, the position of those abdominal organs that are not covered by the greater omentum should be studied. Then, beginning caudally, the greater omentum is lifted up and pulled cranially over the stomach. Most abdominal organs can now be viewed in their normal position.

a) The **ABDOMEN** is subdivided by natural borders into **abdominal regions** which can be projected onto the abdominal wall and which are made up of those organs lying underneath. The **cranial abdominal region** extends from the diaphragm to a transverse plane that connects the most caudal points of both costal arches. The **middle abdominal region** lies between this cranial transverse plane and a caudal transverse plane that connects right and left tubera coxarum. The **caudal abdominal region** extends from this caudal transverse plane to the terminal line of the pelvic inlet. The terminal line starts at the sacral promontory dorsally and extends by way of the arcuate line laterally to the pecten ossis pubis ventrally. These regions are additionally subdivided into subregions.

I. In the **cranial abdominal region** are the **liver (1)**, which covers the gall bladder (see p. 59), the first part of the **duodenum**, the main part of the **pancreas (5)** and the **spleen**. If the stomach is not very full, the entire **stomach (2)** will also be in the cranial abdomen.

Projected onto the **xiphoid region** – separated by the pre-umbilical fat body of the **falciform ligament (10)** – are the quadrate lobe and portions of the left and right medial lobes of the liver and also the greater curvature of the stomach and the gall bladder which, covered by the liver, lies to the right of the median plane at the level of the 7th intercostal space.

In the **left hypochondriac region**, the left medial lobe of the liver (region of the 6th – 8th intercostal space), the left lateral lobe of the liver (region of the 10th intercostal space), and the **spleen (11)** at the level of the 11th and 12th intercostal space are in contact with the body wall.

In the **right hypochondriac region** the right medial lobe of the liver (region of the 6th – 8th intercostal space), the right lateral lobe of the liver (region of the 8th – 9th intercostal space) and the caudate process of the liver, which invests the cranial pole of the right kidney, the **descending duodenum (–3,** –region of the 11th – 12th intercostal space) and the right lobe of the pancreas project onto the thoracic wall.

II. In the **middle abdominal region**, the intestinal mass, except its commencement and termination, caudal portions of the **spleen (11)** and in the female, the **ovary (7)**, including uterine tube and **uterine horns (8)** are in contact with the abdominal wall.

In the **umbilical region** the **jejunal loops (6)** contact the ventral abdominal wall.

In the **left lateral abdominal region**, the left kidney, dorsally, and following caudally, the left ovary and portions of the descending colon, jejunum and cecum, and the ascending colon, are projected onto the abdominal wall.

In the **right lateral abdominal region** are the caudal pole of the right kidney, the right ovary, the descending duodenum and portions of the jejunum as well as the cecum and ascending colon.

III. In the **caudal abdominal region**, there are the **urinary bladder (9)**, the initial portion of the rectum and, in the bitch, the body of the uterus; in the male dog, the ends of the deferent ducts.

In the **pubic region** the urinary bladder is found, and in older male dogs the prostate gland is present.

Jejunal loops and portions of the uterus project onto the **left inguinal and right inguinal regions.**

b) Before undertaking to distinguish the abdominal cavity from the peritoneal cavity and the retroperitoneal space, the **PERITONEUM** will be considered.

The **peritoneum** is a serous membrane that consists of a superficial mesothelium, a connective tissue layer, the lamina propria serosae, and a tela subserosa of loose connective tissue as a 'gliding' layer. As **parietal peritoneum**, it lines the peritoneal cavity and, as **visceral peritoneum**, it covers the surface of the abdominal viscera. The latter organs are suspended by a duplication of the serosa designated in the case of the intestine as mesentery, of the stomach as dorsal and ventral mesogastrium or omentum, and, in relation to organs other than the stomach and intestine, as various peritoneal ligaments, mesovarium in the case of the ovary, etc. The tela subserosa may contain fat tissue. At normal nutritional conditions only a little fat is present in association with the parietal and visceral peritoneum. The mesenteries contain predominantly greater amounts of fat tissue in the subserous layer. In the **mesogastrium** (see p. 53), strands of subserous fat surround lace-like arranged blood and lymph vessels. Between these strands, in the reticular meshes, the subserous fat tissue is scarce or absent. Because of this structure parts of the **ventral mesogastrium** are designated **lesser omentum** and the elongate **dorsal mesogastrium**

is designated **greater omentum**. Where the abdominal organs develop in the ventral mesogastrium (liver) or in the dorsal mesogastrium (pancreas, spleen) the reticular structure is lacking on the surface of the organ and there is only a small amount of subserous fat.

The **extent to which the abdominal organs are covered by the peritoneum** depends on their position. *According to one point of view*, chiefly used by the continental European countries, abdominal organs are **intraperitoneal** (within the peritoneal cavity), **retroperitoneal** (outside the peritoneal cavity but invested in part by peritoneum), or **extraperitoneal** (entirely external to the peritoneum and having no part covered by peritoneum). In this view, however, organs like the intestine that are invested by peritoneum except at the narrow line of attachment of the mesentery are regarded as intraperitoneal; that is, as lying within the peritoneal cavity. In this view, an organ like the liver is also regarded as intraperitoneal as it is invested by peritoneum except at the narrow line of attachment of the ligaments of the liver. *In another view*, employed in many countries of the western hemisphere, no abdominal organ is regarded as intraperitoneal—located within the peritoneal cavity. In this view, all organs are excluded from the peritoneal cavity by their serous covering. In this view, all abdominal organs are extraperitoneal (outside the peritoneal cavity) and only a little serous fluid is located intraperitoneally. *In both points of view*, the term *retroperitoneal* describes organs of the abdominal cavity that are covered by the peritoneum only on a part of their surface. Retroperitoneal organs have a substantial part of their surface uncovered by the peritoneum. The kidneys are an example. Most countries of the western hemisphere also account as retroperitoneal organs that are entirely caudal to the peritoneal cavity; *e.g.*, the caudal vagina and vestibule, the pelvic urethra, etc. In the continental European countries, the term *extraperitoneal* is limited to those organs that are sufficiently far removed from the peritoneum that no part is covered by the peritoneum; *e.g.*, the caudal rectum. In the first point of view, organs that follow the longitudinal axis of the body as, for example, the rectum, change from an intraperitoneal position to an extraperitoneal one. In the second point of view, the rectum, and all other abdominal organs, are always entirely extraperitoneal.

c) The **ABDOMINAL CAVITY** comprises that space between the diaphragm and pelvic inlet, which becomes free after the removal of all abdominal organs, including the peritoneum.

d) The **PERITONEAL CAVITY** is that space which is enclosed by the parietal peritoneum and contains, in the one point of view, the intraperitoneally located organs with their mesenteries, omenta, peritoneal ligaments, etc. (gastrointestinal tract, liver, spleen, pancreas, ovary, uterine tube and uterus of the bitch). In the other point of view, discussed above, the peritoneal cavity contains only a small amount of serous fluid.

e) In the dog, the greater omentum reaches from its attachment at the greater curvature of the stomach caudally nearly to the pelvic inlet. In doing so, it lies between the abdominal organs and the ventral abdominal wall. Accordingly, many **ABDOMINAL ORGANS** are not ordinarily in contact with the ventral abdominal wall.

Abdominal organs that are not covered by the **greater omentum (4)** but covered by the visceral peritoneum are in direct contact with the abdominal wall. Cranially, these are portions of the **liver** including the **gall bladder** (see p. 59) and, caudally, parts of the **stomach**. To the left, the **spleen** lies superficially on the intestinal mass. Caudally the **urinary bladder** projects freely into the hypogastrium. On the right side, the **descending duodenum** is uncovered by the greater omentum from the level of the umbilicus to the liver.

Those abdominal organs that are **covered by the greater omentum** become visible after removal of the greater omentum. The **velar part of the greater omentum** (Velum omentale –12) is spread out between the hilus of the spleen and the descending mesocolon, and **coils of the small intestine (jejunum)** with the **pancreas** can be seen. Exceptions are only for the transitional area between duodenum and jejunum and for the initial portions of the colon, which after displacement also are visible. In the bitch, the **ovary**, surrounded by the ovarian bursa, and the **uterine horns** can be seen; in the male dog, the terminal part of the deferent duct.

f) The **RETROPERITONEAL SPACE** (see also the discussion of this space in 'b)' above) is located at the dorsolateral abdominal wall between the parietal peritoneum and the sublumbar muscles and contains the kidneys including the adrenal glands as well as numerous vessels, nerves and lymph vessels, including the aorta and caudal vena cava. It can be observed after the part of the peritoneum that covers each kidney, together with the kidneys, is removed from underlying structures.

Abdominal cavity and digestive apparatus

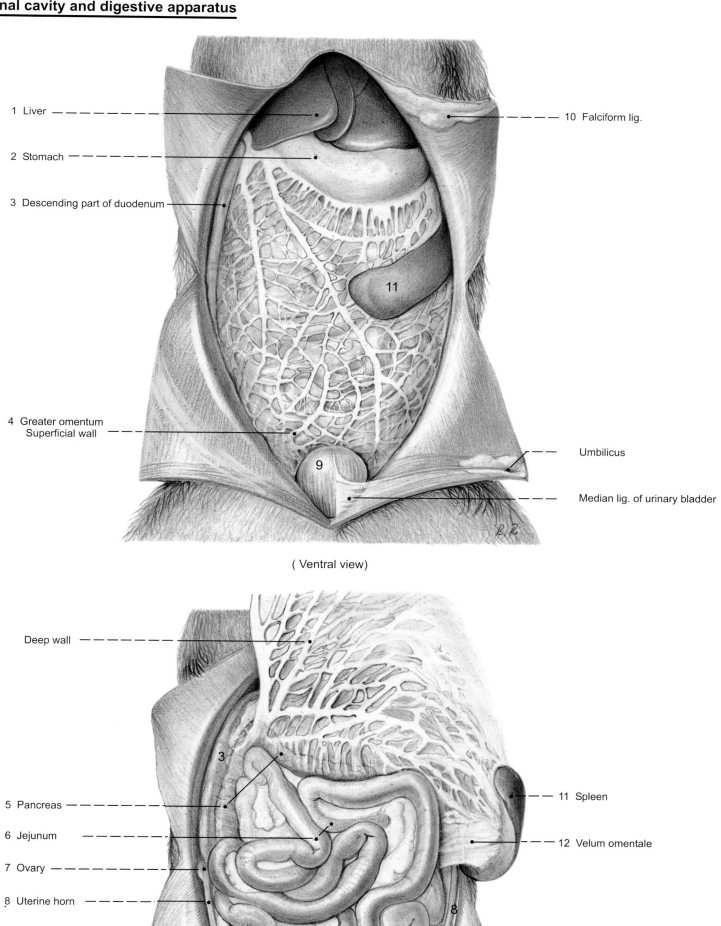

1 Liver — — — — — — — — — — — — — — — 10 Falciform lig.

2 Stomach — — — — — — — — — —

3 Descending part of duodenum — — —

4 Greater omentum
  Superficial wall — —

Umbilicus

9

Median lig. of urinary bladder

11

(Ventral view)

Deep wall — — — — — — — —

3

5 Pancreas — — — — — — — — —

6 Jejunum — — — — — — — —

7 Ovary — — — — — — — —

8 Uterine horn — — — — — —

11 Spleen

12 Velum omentale

8

6

9 Urinary bladder — — — — — — —

(see pp. 53, 55, 57, 59)

2. PERITONEAL CAVITY, LYMPH NODES OF STOMACH AND INTESTINE, CISTERNA CHYLI AND SPLEEN

a) The **PERITONEAL CAVITY** ends caudally within the pelvic cavity with three excavations (pouches) of the **parietal peritoneum (15)**, which are situated one above the other. The dorsally located **rectogenital pouch (3)** extends most caudal and is dorsally bounded by the rectum and ventrally by the uterus or deferent ducts. Between the genital organs and the urinary bladder is the **vesicogenital pouch (5)**. The ventrally located **pubovesical pouch (2)** is found between the urinary bladder and the pubic bone. This pouch has only a short caudal extension and is subdivided by the **median ligament of the urinary bladder (1)**. The vaginal process is an extension of the peritoneum external to the abdominal cavity; it is like the finger of a glove, commencing at the **vaginal ring (7)** and traversing the inguinal rings and canal (inguinal space). In addition, cranially, the serosal mediastinal cavity (43) separates during ontogenesis owing to the development of the diaphragm. It extends cranially within the mediastinum to the base of the heart.

b) The **PERITONEUM** that joins the parietal peritoneum of the abdominal wall to the visceral peritoneum that invests the stomach and intestine (see also pp. 156, 157) is designated the greater omentum and lesser omentum (26, 27, 28; 20, 21, 22; —see also the text-illustration) of the stomach and the common dorsal mesentery of the intestine.

I. The **dorsal mesogastrium (17,** greater omentum, omentum majus or epiplöon**)** to a great extent covers the intestinal tract ventrally and laterally. The **greater omentum (26)** is composed of superficial and deep laminae. Each lamina consists of a double lamella of serosa. The greater omentum starts as a **deep leaf or visceral wall (Paries profundus, −28)** jointly with the transverse mesocolon at the dorsal abdominal wall, lies ventrolateral to the intestinal mass and reflects at the pelvic inlet as the **superficial leaf or parietal wall (Paries superficialis, −27)**. The latter wall is in contact with the ventral abdominal wall (Paries) and extends to the greater curvature of the stomach. Here both serosal lamellae separate and cover the surface of the stomach as **visceral peritoneum (4)**. At the lesser curvature of the stomach the lamellae meet each other again. Here the ventral mesogastrium (lesser omentum) begins. The superficial and deep walls of the greater omentum, with the visceral surface of the stomach and a small part of the visceral surface of the liver, form the wall of the omental bursa, which reaches caudally to the pelvic inlet with its caudal extension, the **caudal omental recess (50)**. The left lobe of the pancreas develops between the two lamellae of the deep wall; and between the lamellae of the superficial wall, the spleen develops. The **epiploic (omental) foramen (16)** lies caudal to the liver, ventral to the caudal vena cava and dorsal to the portal vein. It is the opening to the **vestibule of the omental bursa (19)**, which, with the caudal omental recess, forms the total omental bursa. The vestibule of the omental bursa lies between the dorsal abdominal wall and the lesser omentum and, at the lesser curvature of the stomach, has access to the caudal recess of the omental bursa (*Aditus ad recessum caudalem*). Particular named parts of the greater omentum are the **gastrosplenic or gastrolienal ligament (24)** and the **velar part of the greater omentum (Velum omentale, see p. 51)**. The omental velum lies left in the body and runs between the deep wall of the greater omentum and the descending mesocolon. It is the only part of the greater omentum that does not join in the formation and bordering of the cavity of the omental recess.

II. The **ventral mesogastrium** begins at the lesser curvature of the stomach and ends at the diaphragm and the ventral abdominal wall between the diaphragm and the umbilicus. The liver develops in the ventral mesogastrium. By the development of the liver, the lesser omentum is subdivided into a proximal (visceral) and a distal (parietal) part. The proximal part is the **lesser omentum (20)**, which consists of the **hepatogastric ligament (21)** and the **hepatoduodenal ligament (22)**. The distal part of the ventral mesogastrium is the **falciform ligament (23)**, which runs between the liver and the diaphragm and ventral abdominal wall. In the fetus, in its free border, the falciform ligament contains the umbilical vein. After birth, the umbilical vein and much of the falciform ligament undergo complete involution leaving only a fatty, caudal, remnant at the umbilicus and a short fold ventral to the caudal vena cava at the diaphragmatic face of the liver. The other hepatic ligaments (triangular and coronary ligaments, see p. 58) are secondarily developed peritoneal folds without significant vessels.

III. The **common dorsal mesentery (10)** extends from the beginning of the duodenum to the rectum and, for the individual parts of the intestine, is specifically designated as mesoduodenum, mesojejunum, mesoileum, mesocecum, mesocolon and mesorectum. The elongation of the intestine with simultaneous rotation during ontogenesis brings about a dorsal twisting of the cranially located mesentery at the origin of the cranial mesenteric artery. This forms the **root of the mesentery (13)**. The **mesocolon (9)** of the descending colon and the **mesorectum (6)**, which follow caudally from the area of the root, are linearly fixed at the dorsal abdominal and pelvic wall. A ventral mesentery does not develop caudal to the cranial part of the duodenum.

c) The **LYMPH NODES** of the gastrointestinal tract lie predominantly in the mesenteries and omenta of those parts of the viscera which form part of the afferent area of the corresponding lymph nodes. The **hepatic (portal) lymph nodes (18)** are cranial to the pancreas, on both sides of the portal vein. The **jejunal lymph nodes (12)** lie in the proximal third of the mesojejunum in series, one after the other. The solitary lymph nodes may have a length up to 20 cm. The **lienal (splenic) lymph nodes** are grouped around the ramification of the splenic artery and vein. A **gastric lymph node** is inconstant. When present it is found near the pylorus at the lesser curvature of the stomach. The **colic lymph nodes (14)** lie near the attachment of the ascending mesocolon and the transvese mesocolon of the intestine. The **caudal mesenteric lymph nodes (8)** are at the terminal branching of the caudal mesenteric artery. The efferent vessels draining the above-mentioned lymph nodes predominantly unite to form the visceral trunk, which opens at the level of the kidneys into the cisterna chyli.

d) The **CISTERNA CHYLI** (see p. 61) is dorsally situated upon the abdominal aorta at the level of the kidneys, between the crura of the diaphragm. As main tributaries of the cisterna chyli, the **lumbar trunk** drains the lymph from the pelvis including the total limb area, and the **visceral trunk** drains the lymph from the internal organs. From the cistern, the lymph passes in the **thoracic duct**, which, passing through the aortic hiatus, continues cranially alongside the aorta to reach the previously mentioned venous angle at the thoracic inlet (see p. 41).

e) The position of the **spleen** (Lien, −11; see text-illustration) depends on the degree of filling of the stomach. Spleen and stomach are loosely connected by the gastrosplenic ligament. If the stomach is almost completely empty the ventral extremity of the spleen lies caudal to the left costal arch and may reach beyond the midline to the right side of the body. At the **splenic hilus (Hilus lienis, −25)** both serosal lamellae of the superficial wall of the greater omentum are fixed. The more superficial lamella invests the spleen as its peritoneal cover. On the cut surface of the spleen the red and white splenic pulp can barely be distinguished with the unaided eye or they may remain undetected. Red and white pulp have principally different functions. The **red splenic pulp** has its main function in the circulatory system of the blood. In this pulp the blood flows partly outside the blood vessels (open circulation of the spleen) and partially inside the wide-lumen thin-walled blood sinuses (closed circulation of the spleen). In the red pulp the aged erythrocytes are broken down and the blood is stored (storage spleen). The numerous smooth muscle cells of the splenic capsule and of the radiating splenic trabeculae may squeeze out the blood as if from a sponge. Because the blood from the splenic vein reaches the portal vein, the spleen functions as a regulator of the blood pressure, especially of the portal circulation (see p. 57). The splenic artery (*A. lienalis*), which originates from the celiac artery, releases several branches to the elongate splenic hilus. The **white splenic pulp** (splenic nodules and **periarterial lymph sheath, PALS**) is chiefly functional in the immune defense mechanisms of the body and has functions similar to the lymph nodes (formation of lymphocytes and humoral defense substances; filter for the blood; recirculation of lymphocytes). The lymphocytes are in the blood only a short time. After they leave the blood stream they pass to lymphatic organs like the spleen. **Splenic vessels;** see p. 57; **splenic nerves** from the vagus and sympathetic nerves, see p. 49.

(lateral view)

Pancreas 28

15 19 21

Intestine

28

27

Omental bursa
(caudal recess)

Spleen

23

Diaphragm

Liver

Stomach

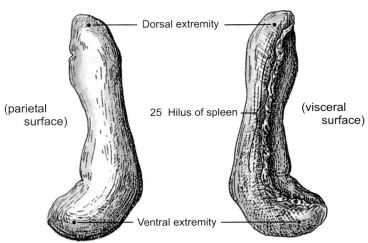

Dorsal extremity

(parietal surface)

25 Hilus of spleen

(visceral surface)

Ventral extremity

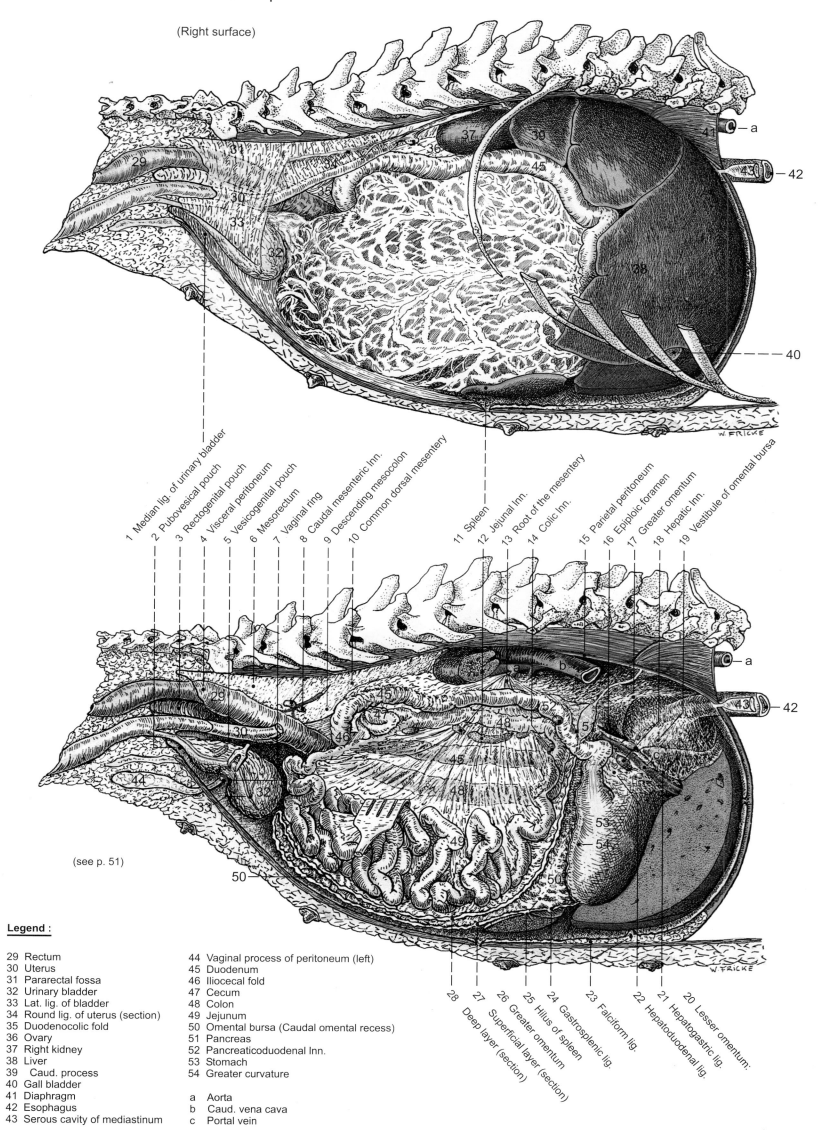

(Right surface)

(see p. 51)

1 Median lig. of urinary bladder
2 Pubovesical pouch
3 Rectogenital pouch
4 Visceral peritoneum
5 Vesicogenital pouch
6 Mesorectum
7 Vaginal ring
8 Caudal mesenteric Inn.
9 Descending mesocolon
10 Common dorsal mesentery
11 Spleen
12 Jejunal Inn.
13 Root of the mesentery
14 Colic Inn.
15 Parietal peritoneum
16 Epiploic foramen
17 Greater omentum
18 Hepatic Inn.
19 Vestibule of omental bursa

28 Deep layer (section)
27 Superficial layer (section)
26 Greater omentum
25 Hilus of spleen
24 Gastrosplenic lig.
23 Falciform lig.
22 Hepatoduodenal lig.
21 Hepatogastric lig.
20 Lesser omentum

Legend :

29 Rectum	44 Vaginal process of peritoneum (left)
30 Uterus	45 Duodenum
31 Pararectal fossa	46 Iliocecal fold
32 Urinary bladder	47 Cecum
33 Lat. lig. of bladder	48 Colon
34 Round lig. of uterus (section)	49 Jejunum
35 Duodenocolic fold	50 Omental bursa (Caudal omental recess)
36 Ovary	51 Pancreas
37 Right kidney	52 Pancreaticoduodenal Inn.
38 Liver	53 Stomach
39 Caud. process	54 Greater curvature
40 Gall bladder	
41 Diaphragm	a Aorta
42 Esophagus	b Caud. vena cava
43 Serous cavity of mediastinum	c Portal vein

53

3. STOMACH AND SMALL INTESTINE, PANCREAS

a) The **ESOPHAGUS** with its **thoracic part** lies in the mediastinum and courses through the esophageal hiatus of the diaphragm into the abdominal cavity. The very short **abdominal part (25)** enters the stomach immediately. Both the thoracic and abdominal part have an outer serosal membrane and differ by this from the cervical part, which is surrounded by an adventitia.

1
2
b) The **STOMACH (VENTRICULUS, GASTER, —7)** is the continuation of the esophagus. The **function of the stomach** consists of a transitory storage of food and of the regulation of its further transport in small portions into the small intestine. The hydrochloric acid of the stomach has a disinfecting action and functions to activate the pepsinogen formed by the gastric glands, which, as pepsin, initiates digestion. The stomach is glandular throughout and of unilocular, simple type in comparison with the stomach of othe domestic mammals. Like the wall of the intestine, the stomach wall consists of a
3 mucous membrane (*Tunica mucosa* with a *Lamina epithelialis, propria* and *muscularis mucosae*), submucosa (*Tela submucosa*) as a gliding layer, muscu-
4 lar tunic and an external serosal tunic. The position and shape of the stomach vary considerably depending on its fullness. The stomach that is nearly empty lies with its longitudinal axis roughly transverse to the longitudinal axis of the body. The fundus of the stomach contacts the diaphragm. The stomach is separated by the liver from the ventral abdominal wall and is almost entirely located in the intrathoracic part of the abdominal cavity. With filling of the stomach, the pylorus projects far into the middle abdominal region to the level of the third lumbar vertebra. The stomach is then found with its broad surface at the lateral and ventral abdominal wall.

5 The **cardiac part** with its **cardiac ostium (27)** and the surrounding **cardiac sphincter muscle**, is related on the left to the **cardiac notch (26)** and the **greater curvature of the stomach (30)** and the **blind-sac-like fundus (28)**. To the right the cardiac part is related to the **lesser curvature (15)** and passes over without a distinct boundary to the **body of the stomach (29)**. The **gastric groove (14)** is on the internal surface of the body of the stomach in the region of the lesser curvature, where the **angular notch (16)** marks the border to the pyloric part. The groove is flanked on both sides by longitudinal muscle bundles that are able to close the gastric groove to form a tube. The pyloric part consists of the thin-walled and wide-lumened **pyloric antrum (22)**, which at an internal transverse fold continues cone-like into the tapering **pyloric canal (17)**. The pylorus, which follows the pyloric canal, has increasing sphincter-like circular muscular bundles and communicates with the duodenum at its **pyloric ostium (18)**. On its internal surface, the stomach
6 wall is protected by a mucus layer that prevents self-digestion. The **gastric mucous membrane** is thrown up into centimeter-thick gastric folds that are erased with increasing fullness of the stomach. Superficial gastric areas (*Areae gastricae*) are mound-like projections with a diameter of a few millimeters, and are separated at the sides by gutter-like depressions. On the gastric areas, gastric pits can just be seen with the naked eye. Here the united secretory ducts of several gastric glands open. The gastric mucous membrane has in its cardiac part the narrow, ring-like cardiac gland zone, at the fundus and body the zone of proper gastric glands, and in the pyloric part the pyloric gland region, which in the area of the lesser curvature may extend onto the body of the stomach. The **muscular** tunic contains besides the external longitudinal layer, which continues onto the esophagus and the duodenum, and the internal circular layer, which is thickened to form the **cardiac sphincter muscle (27)** and the **pyloric sphincter muscle (18)**, also obliquely coursing fibers (*Fibrae obliquae*). The latter are especially distinct in the fundus and are also distinct in the body of the stomach. The **serous tunic** continues at the greater curvature into the dorsal and at the lesser curvature of the stomach into the ventral mesogastrium.

7 I. The **blood supply** (see p. 57) of the stomach is provided by the vascular arcades that course at the greater and lesser curvatures and give off numerous coiled branches that straighten with increasing fullness of the stomach. The arterial arch at the lesser curvature joins the left and right gastric arteries. The arterial arch at the greater curvature of the stomach is formed by the left and right gastroepiploic arteries. In addition, the splenic artery furnishes short gastric branches to the dorsal left part of the greater curvature. The **gastric veins** join the portal vein (see p. 57).

II. The **lymph drainage** is to the gastric lymph node, which is inconstant. When present, it lies toward the pyloric extremity of the lesser curvature. Lymph drainage is also furnished by the splenic, pancreaticoduodenal and hepatic lymph nodes.

III. The **nerve supply** of the stomach is by the gastric plexus of the autonomic nervous system. The parasympathetic constituents reach the stomach by way of the dorsal and ventral vagal trunks in company with the esophagus, and

pass to the gastric plexus. They supply the gastric glands and the musculature of the stomach. Synapse with the second, postganglionic, neurons takes place in the wall of the stomach in the myenteric and submucosal plexuses.

8 c) The **PANCREAS** (see also p. 57) consists of two parts with very different functions, the predominant exocrine portion and the small endocrine part. The surface of the organ is lobular and partially nodular. The color depends on the blood content and is pale to deep red. The pancreas is roughly hookshaped with a total length of about 25 cm in a medium-sized dog of 15 kg. The **body of the pancreas (2)** is adjacent to the cranial part of the duodenum, and its associated **left lobe (8)** is directed left toward the spleen. The left lobe is also called the splenic lobe or transverse branch. The **right lobe of the pancreas (4)** or duodenal lobe is on the right side within the descending mesoduodenum. The exocrine portion of the pancreas originates embryologically from two organ-primordia and, in agreement with this, usually two excretory ducts are present. The **pancreatic duct (21)** merges either in common with or directly beside the **ductus choledochus (common bile duct, —19)** on the **major duodenal papilla (20)** in the area of the body of the pancreas. The **accessory pancreatic duct (24)** terminates a few cm farther caudally on the **minor duodenal papilla (23)** at the cranial part of the right pancreatic lobe. Both ducts communicate within the pancreas and, in the case of the obliteration of the terminal part of the pancreatic duct, which rarely occurs, only the opening of the accessory pancreatic duct on the minor duodenal papilla remains. At the opening of the pancreatic excretory ducts, their circular smooth muscle is reinforced to form a sphincter by which a reflux of (activated) pancreatic juice and a self-digestion of the organ is prevented. Within the pancreas, lipid-, carbohydrate-, and protein-splitting enzymes are formed. These are in part formed as inactive precursors that become activated in the intestine by an enterokinase. The pin-point-sized **pancreatic islets (LANGERHANS islets)** reach a maximum diameter of only 0.5 mm and form altogether the endocrine portion, which represents more or less 1–2% of the pancreas. The pancreatic islets have a dense capillary network, and their hormones (mainly insulin and glucagon) are drained by the blood vascular system.

I. The **blood supply** is from the celiac artery (pancreatic branches of the splenic artery and cranial pancreaticoduodenal artery) and also from pancreatic branches of the caudal pancreaticoduodenal artery of the cranial mesenteric artery. Venous drainage is to the portal vein.

II. **Lymph drainage** is to the pancreaticoduodenal lymph nodes, which are located at the beginning duodenum. Besides these, lymph reaches the hepatic and jejunal lymph nodes.

III. The **parasympathetic nerve supply** is secretory to the exocrine pancreas and is supported by hormones of the wall of the intestine. Sympathetic nerves act to inhibit secretion.

9 d) The digestion and absorption of nutrients take place within the **SMALL INTESTINE** (see also p. 57). Associated with this function, the internal intestinal surface is considerably increased by circular folds, intestinal villi, crypts of the mucous membrane and microvilli of its enterocytes. The small intestine consists of duodenum, jejunum and ileum and extends from the pylorus to the opening of the ileum into the large intestine. It is about three and one-half times the length of the body.

I. The **duodenum** is shaped like a hook and surrounds the pancreas. It begins with the **cranial part (1)**, which ascends to the right and dorsal as far as the porta of the liver and after this continues at the cranial duodenal flexure as
10 the descending part. The **descending part (3)** bears at its beginning internally the major duodenal papilla (see above). Three fingerbreadths farther caudal the minor duodenal papilla is located. The descending part continues at the caudal flexure as the **transverse part (6)**. The latter lies caudal to the cranial mesenteric artery and, after a transverse course to the left across the midline, continues as the **ascending part (5)**. At the **duodenojejunal flexure (10)** the ascending part is continued as jejunum. The boundary is at the cranial indistinct border of the **duodenocolic fold (11)** where the mesentery becomes longer.

II. The **jejunum (9)** is by far the longest portion of the small intestine and is suspended by a long mesojejunum that permits a wide distribution of the jejunal loops between the stomach and the pelvic inlet.

III. The short **ileum (13)** begins at the indistinct free end of the **ileocecal fold (12)**. The site of termination of the arterial and venous **antimesenteric ileal branch** indicates more distinctly the border with the jejunum. The ileum ends with a fairly straight course at the ileal ostium and surrounding ileal sphincter muscle at the junction with the ascending colon (see p. 56).

Stomach, Intestine and Pancreas

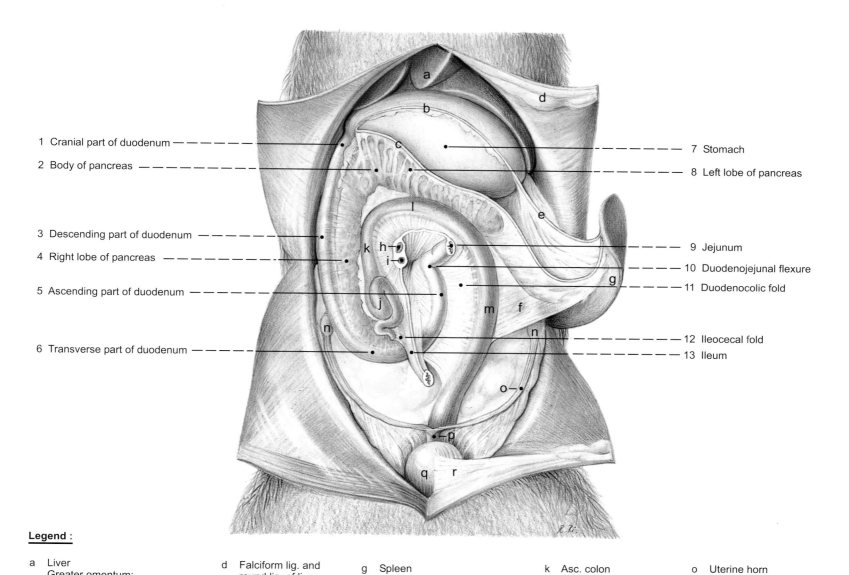

1 Cranial part of duodenum

2 Body of pancreas

3 Descending part of duodenum

4 Right lobe of pancreas

5 Ascending part of duodenum

6 Transverse part of duodenum

7 Stomach

8 Left lobe of pancreas

9 Jejunum

10 Duodenojejunal flexure

11 Duodenocolic fold

12 Ileocecal fold

13 Ileum

Legend :

a Liver	d Falciform lig. and	g Spleen	k Asc. colon	o Uterine horn
Greater omentum:	round lig. of liver	h Com. mesenteric v.	l Transv. colon	p Body of uterus
b Superficial wall (section)	e Gastrosplenic lig.	i Cran. mesenteric a.	m Desc. colon	q Urinary bladder
c Deep wall (section)	f Velum omentale	j Cecum	n Ovary	r Median lig. of bladder

Stomach

(sectioned visceral surface)

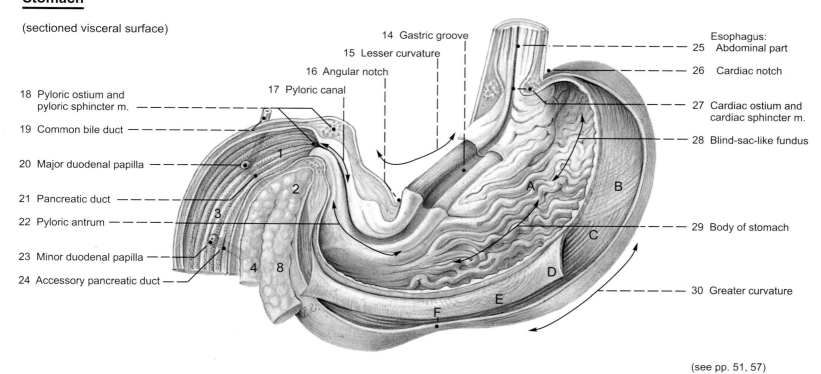

14 Gastric groove

15 Lesser curvature

16 Angular notch

17 Pyloric canal

18 Pyloric ostium and pyloric sphincter m.

19 Common bile duct

20 Major duodenal papilla

21 Pancreatic duct

22 Pyloric antrum

23 Minor duodenal papilla

24 Accessory pancreatic duct

Esophagus:
25 Abdominal part

26 Cardiac notch

27 Cardiac ostium and cardiac sphincter m.

28 Blind-sac-like fundus

29 Body of stomach

30 Greater curvature

(see pp. 51, 57)

Legend :

A Mucous membrane and gastric folds	Muscular tunic: B Ext. oblique fibers	C Longitudinal layer D Circular layer	E Int. oblique fibers F Serous layer

55

4. LARGE INTESTINE, BLOOD VESSELS OF STOMACH AND INTESTINE

1   **a)** It is in the **LARGE INTESTINE** that the reabsorption of water, and dissolved electrolytes together with the digestive juices, takes place. On the lumenal surface of the large intestine, villi are absent and the crypts of the large intestine are particularly deep. The mucosa bears longitudinal folds that disappear in cases of intestinal impaction and a two- to threefold increase in intestinal diameter. The canine large intestine is short and simply formed in comparison to this part of the gut in other domestic animals. The large intestine is composed of cecum, colon, rectum and anal canal.

I. The **cecum** is coiled like a corkscrew (H, see also text-illustration below left) and consists of an apex, and a body that abuts on the ascending colon. The cecum lies on the right side within the concavity of the C-shaped duodenum. The cecum can be considered as a diverticulum of the colon. Both parts of the large intestine are in communication at the **cecocolic ostium**, which is found beside the **ileal ostium** that also opens into the ascending colon.

2   II. The **colon** is shaped like a hook and commences on the right side from the cecocolic ostium with the short **ascending colon (I – J)**, which ascends to the level of the cranial mesenteric artery. At the right colic flexure, cranial to the cranial mesenteric artery, the **transverse colon (J – K)** continues its course, which again opens into the **descending colon (K – L)** at the left colic flexure on the left side.

III. The **rectum (L – M)** commences at the pelvic inlet, about at the T-shaped termination of the caudal mesenteric artery into the left colic artery and cranial rectal artery. Just cranial to its continuation as anal canal it is dilated as the **rectal ampulla**.

3   IV. The **anal canal** (see text-illustration, below, right) consists of three zones, each lying caudal to the other: the **columnar zone** commences at the anorectal line where the simple columnar epithelium of the intestinal mucosa, which contains intestinal glands, terminates. The columnar zone is characterized by columnar folds of the anal mucosa. The mucous membrane is lined by a stratified squamous epithelium and contains solitary lymph nodules and anal glands. The columns of mucous membrane cover longitudinally running blood vessels and form by this an erectile body that supports closure of the anus. The **intermediate zone** (also called anocutaneous line) that follows can be seen as a 1 mm wide indistinct circular fold at the transition to the modified external cutis. The terminal **cutaneous zone** is about 4 cm wide and has

4   at its beginning a few hairs, which increase in number caudally. Hepatoid circumanal glands are also present. Laterally between the anal canal and the

5   external anal sphincter muscle are the **paranal sinuses** that open laterally between the intermediate and the cutaneous zone.

Anal closure is chiefly brought about by internal and external anal sphincter muscles. The **internal anal sphincter muscle** is an enlargement of the circular muscle layer of the muscular tunic of the rectum. The cross-striated **external anal sphincter muscle** closes the anus and in doing so compresses the paranal sinus, thus emptying it.

b) The **ARTERIES OF STOMACH AND INTESTINE** originate from the celiac, cranial and caudal mesenteric arteries, which are ventral branches of the abdominal aorta.

The **celiac artery (22)** divides into three main branches: The **left gastric artery (17)** gives off an esophageal branch and supplies the left part of the lesser curvature of the stomach. The **splenic artery (21, –A. lienalis)** releases pancreatic branches, lienal or **splenic branches (18)** and **short gastric arteries (Aa. gastricae breves, –16)** and the **left gastroepiploic artery (20)** for the left-ventral part of the greater curvature of the stomach. The **hepatic artery (5)** passes to the *Porta hepatis* and, after release of the **right gastric artery (4)** for the pylorus-sided part of the lesser curvature of the stomach and the **hepatic branches (1)** for the liver, continues as the **gastroduodenal artery (3)**. The latter bifurcates into the **right gastroepiploic artery (7)** for the right-ventral part of the greater curvature and the **cranial pancreaticoduodenal artery (6)**. The right gastroepiploic artery anastomoses at the greater curvature with the same-named left artery, the right gastric artery anastomoses at the lesser curvature with the same-named left artery and the cranial pancreaticoduodenal artery anastomoses on the duodenum with the same named caudal vessel that is a branch of the cranial mesenteric artery.

The **cranial mesenteric artery (23)** releases the **ileocolic artery (27)**, the often double **caudal pancreaticoduodenal artey (11)**, 12 – 15 **jejunal arteries (29)**, and ends as the **ileal artery (14)**. The ileocolic artery branches into the **middle colic artery (24)** for the transverse colon, the **right colic artery (9)** and the **colic branch (Ramus colicus –10)** for the ascending colon and divides into the **cecal artery (12)** and the **mesenteric ileal branch (13)**. The cecal artery is continued onto the ileum as the **antimesenteric ileal branch (15)**. The mesenteric ileal branch anastomoses with the ileal artery that forms a common stem with the last jejunal artery.

The **caudal mesenteric artery (30)** gives off the **cranial rectal artery (31)** to the rectum and the **left colic artery (28)**, which anastomoses on the descending colon with the middle colic artery.

c) The **PORTAL VEIN (–2**, see also p. 59**)** is formed by three main   **6** branches*, the veins of which behave principally like the same-named arteries that they accompany. These are 1. The **gastroduodenal vein (3)**, which at the level of the stomach opens into the portal vein from the right side, and 2. the **splenic vein (19)**, which passes from the left and opens into the portal vein about 4 cm caudal to the gastroduodenal vein. By reason of its receiving the left gastric vein, the splenic vein is also designated the gastrosplenic vein *(V. gastrolienalis)*. 3. The strongest contribution to the portal vein is by the **common mesenteric vein (8)**, which is formed by the confluence of the **cranial mesenteric vein (26)** and **caudal mesenteric vein (25)**.

Lymphatic system of the intestinal canal (see p. 52)

Nerve supply of the intestine (see p. 60)

Cecum and Ileum

(ventral view)

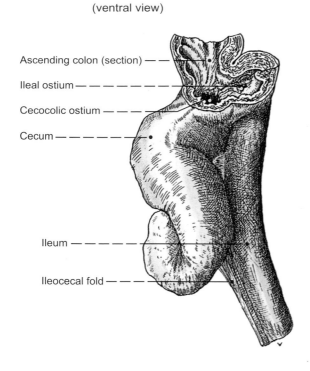

Ascending colon (section)

Ileal ostium

Cecocolic ostium

Cecum

Ileum

Ileocecal fold

Rectum and anal canal

(dorsal view)

Rectum

Rectal ampulla

Ext. anal sphinter m.

Int. anal sphincter m.

Paranal sinus

Anal canal:

Columnar zone

Intermediate zone

Cutaneous zone

56

*) In another point of view, the portal vein begins at the confluence of the cranial and caudal mesenteric veins and receives the gastroduodenal and splenic veins as tributaries. In this view, no 'common mesenteric vein' is formed.

Intestine

(Ventral view)

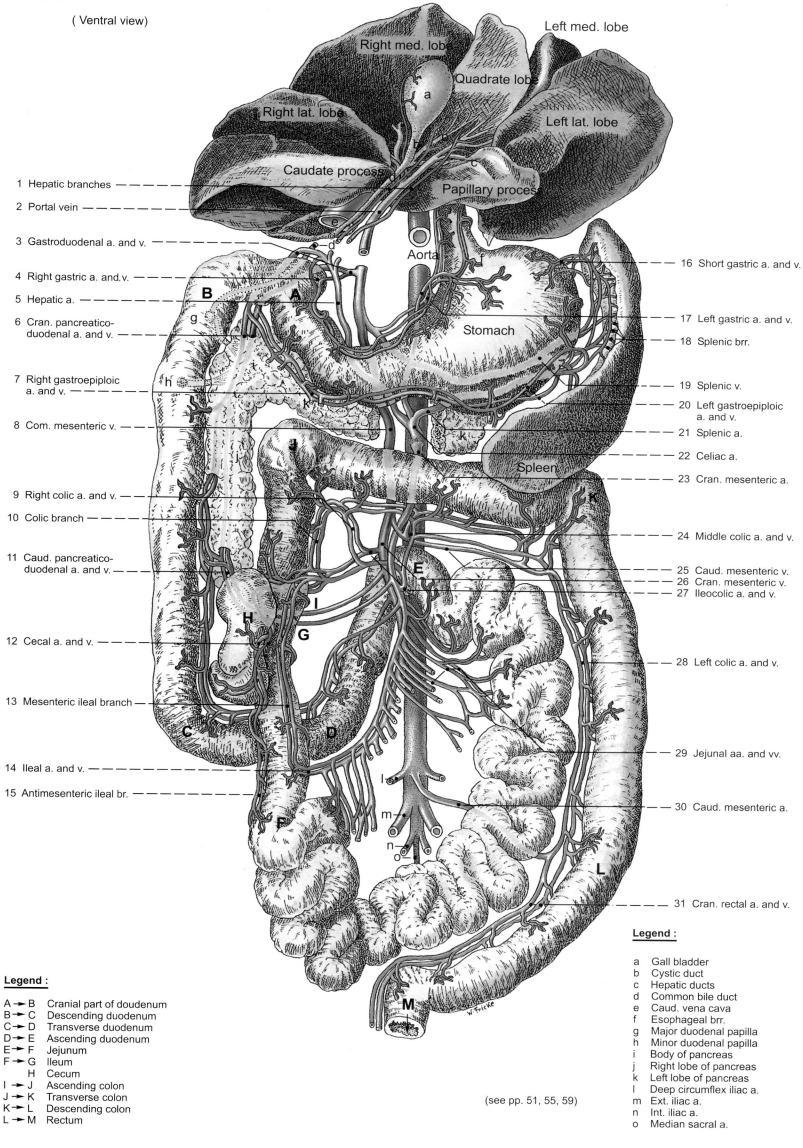

Right med. lobe   Left med. lobe

Quadrate lobe

Right lat. lobe   Left lat. lobe

a

Caudate process

Papillary process

1 Hepatic branches
2 Portal vein
3 Gastroduodenal a. and v.
4 Right gastric a. and v.
5 Hepatic a.
6 Cran. pancreatico-duodenal a. and v.
7 Right gastroepiploic a. and v.
8 Com. mesenteric v.
9 Right colic a. and v.
10 Colic branch
11 Caud. pancreatico-duodenal a. and v.
12 Cecal a. and v.
13 Mesenteric ileal branch
14 Ileal a. and v.
15 Antimesenteric ileal br.

Aorta

Stomach

Spleen

16 Short gastric a. and v.
17 Left gastric a. and v.
18 Splenic brr.
19 Splenic v.
20 Left gastroepiploic a. and v.
21 Splenic a.
22 Celiac a.
23 Cran. mesenteric a.
24 Middle colic a. and v.
25 Caud. mesenteric v.
26 Cran. mesenteric v.
27 Ileocolic a. and v.
28 Left colic a. and v.
29 Jejunal aa. and vv.
30 Caud. mesenteric a.
31 Cran. rectal a. and v.

Legend :

A → B	Cranial part of doudenum
B → C	Descending duodenum
C → D	Transverse duodenum
D → E	Ascending duodenum
E → F	Jejunum
F → G	Ileum
H	Cecum
I → J	Ascending colon
J → K	Transverse colon
K → L	Descending colon
L → M	Rectum

Legend :

a	Gall bladder
b	Cystic duct
c	Hepatic ducts
d	Common bile duct
e	Caud. vena cava
f	Esophageal brr.
g	Major duodenal papilla
h	Minor duodenal papilla
i	Body of pancreas
j	Right lobe of pancreas
k	Left lobe of pancreas
l	Deep circumflex iliac a.
m	Ext. iliac a.
n	Int. iliac a.
o	Median sacral a.

(see pp. 51, 55, 59)

LIVER AND GALL BLADDER

1   **a)** The functions of the **LIVER (HEPAR s. JECUR)** are manifold and correlate with the remarkable size of the organ, which is about 3.3 % of the body weight. Besides metabolic functions in the metabolism of carbohydrate, protein and fat, the liver has significant functions in inactivating hormones and detoxifying foreign substances as well as therapeutic agents (for particulars, see clinical-functional anatomy and textbooks of biochemistry). Prenatally, this largest of the internal organs has an even greater share of the total body weight; because in the fetus there is in addition the important function of blood cell formation.

The **position of the liver** is predominantly intrathoracic. The right lateral lobe of the liver and the caudate process of the caudate lobe abut on the right kidney at the level of the last rib. The lateral border of the liver courses roughly parallel to the costal arch. Only the ventral portion of the liver is extrathoracic, resting on the falciform ligament with its abundant fat tissue.

The **surface of the liver** with its smooth convex **diaphragmatic surface** is in contact with the diaphragm and matches the form of the diaphragmatic cupola. Its concave **visceral surface** is directed to the abdominal organs. Stomach, duodenum, colon and the right kidney bring about impressions on the plastic, firm-elastic surface of the organ. Of the borders of the liver, the dorsal border is blunt and bears the **esophageal impression (16)**; whereas, the other margins of the healthy organ are sharp.

I. The **lobes of the liver** of the dog are well demarcated by deep interlobar fissures **(13)**. The resulting distinct lobation is supposed to correlate with the clearly expressed dynamics of the vertebral column.

The **lobation of the liver** follows according to the comparative anatomical point of view. From that point of view, the liver is subdivided by two lines that extend from its dorsal to its ventral border. The left line runs beweeen the dorsally located esophagus and the ventrally situated round ligament of the liver, which, in the mature dog, is usually absent. The right line connects the caudal vena cava, which is dorsal and the ventrally located gall bladder. Between the two lines, the **quadrate lobe (11)** is ventral to the *Porta hepatis* and the **caudate lobe** is dorsal. The caudate lobe consists of the large **caudate process (7)**, which is connected to the right kidney by the hepatorenal ligament, and the small, left-projecting **papillary process (15)**, which is ventral to the lesser omentum. Lateral to the connecting lines are right and left lobes, which are separated by intralobar fissures into a **right medial lobe (2)** and a **right lateral lobe (6)** and a **left medial (12)** and **left lateral lobe (14)**.

The **lobulation of the liver** is not so distinct as in the pig; nevertheless it is easily recognized on the hepatic surface. The hepatic lobules have a diameter of 1 – 1.5 mm and a height of 1.5 – 2 mm. The afferent blood vessels, branches of the portal vein and hepatic artery, surround the periphery of the lobules and mark the corner points of a hexagonal, classical hepatic lobule. The central vein is central within the liver lobule. It represents the first part of the hepatic venous system (hepatic veins), which drains blood from the liver (on other principles of classification, for example, portal venous lobules, see textbooks of histology).

II. The **ligaments of the liver** (see also p. 59, below) fix the organ predominantly to the diaphragm. The **right and left triangular ligaments** fix the right and left lateral lobes. The **coronary ligament** that continues medially from them fixes the right and left medial lobes. The **hepatorenal ligament (9)** runs between the caudate process and the right kidney. The **falciform ligament (10)** is the distal portion of the ventral mesogastrium. In the fetus the umbilical vein of the liver runs in the free border of the falciform ligament from the umbilicus to the liver. In the mature dog, the umbilical vein is lost, the **round ligament of the liver** does not persist, and the falciform ligament is present only as a short fold ventral to the caudal vena cava as it departs the liver cranially and a much larger fat-filled fold caudally at the level of the umbilicus. The *Area nuda* of the liver is a zone of adhesion where the liver is joined to the diaphragm by connective tissue; this area is free of peritoneum and lies to the right and left of the caudal vena cava as it passes through the liver. The lesser omentum is subdivided into the hepatoduodenal and hepatogastric ligaments, which originate from the named origins and converge to the porta of the liver (*Porta hepatis*; see p. 53). The ductus choledochus runs in the free border of the hepatoduodenal ligament and, beside it, are the portal vein and hepatic artery.

III. The following structures pass to and from the liver at the **porta (Porta hepatis)**: portal vein (functional blood vessel), the hepatic artery (nutrient blood vessel), hepatic ducts, vagal and sympathetic branches as well as lymph vessels that pass to the hepatic (portal) lymph nodes.

2   The **blood supply** (see opposite page, lower figures) of the liver is from two sources: With respect to size, the **portal vein (18)** with its branches is the main supply, providing venous blood rich in nutrients. The small calibered

hepatic artery **(17)** with its branches conveys oxygenated blood to the liver. After entering the liver, the portal vein divides into right and left branches that supply the liver chiefly. The hepatic artery divides similar to the portal vein; both send their blood within the hepatic lobule through the hepatic capillaries, which as liver sinusoids are especially permeable. The venous blood from the liver sinusoids reaches the center of the liver lobule and the central vein and after this by way of collecting veins into the **hepatic veins,** which, at the dorsal border of the liver, open into the embedded **caudal vena cava (19)**.

The principle of the portal venous circulation can be explained following the description of the blood supply of the liver: Within the portal circulation the blood flows in the venous branch through successive capillary beds. Initially it flows through the first capillary bed in the intestinal wall and is collected finally in the tributaries of the portal vein. After this it flows through the second capillary bed in the liver lobules. The portal vein of the liver collects blood from organs of the gastrointestinal tract and the spleen. This blood has been carried to these unpaired organs by way of unpaired arteries: celiac, cranial and caudal mesenteric arteries.

The **lymph drainage** of the liver is to the hepatic (portal) lymph nodes **(8)**, which are located near the porta.

The **sympathetic and parasympathetic nerve supply** is by the hepatic plexus, the constituents of which enter the liver at the porta in the company of the hepatic artery.

The **path of the bile** (see text-illustration) commences intralobularly in the liver with bile canaliculi, which, lacking their own walls, lie between the hepatic cells. Interlobularly the bile of the liver is first drained by way of smaller hepatic ducts and finally by several isolated **hepatic ducts (4)**. Outside the liver, at the opening of the last hepatic duct, the **cystic duct (3)** of the gall bladder is continued by the **ductus choledochus (5)**, which has a sphincter muscle *(M. sphincter ductus choledochus)*. The ductus choledochus opens on the major duodenal papilla.

Hepatic duct and gall bladder

(Visceral surface)

(right)   (left)

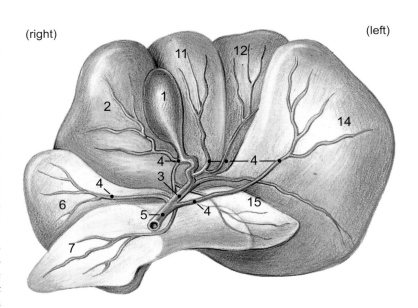

3   **b)** The **GALL BLADDER (1)** stores the bile insofar as it has not flowed directly into the duodenum. In the gall bladder, the golden colored bile is first dehydrated. This makes the bile thicker and changes its color to dark green. The gall bladder lies between the right medial lobe of the liver and the quadrate lobe. In the adult dog the **fundus of the gall bladder** extends to the diaphragm. The **body of the gall bladder** is continued by a constricted part, the **neck of the gall bladder.** The latter continues as the cystic duct. The bile may traverse the cystic duct in different directions: During digestion, into the duodenum; in intervals between digestion, from the liver for storage in the gall bladder.

Liver (Visceral surface)

(ventral)

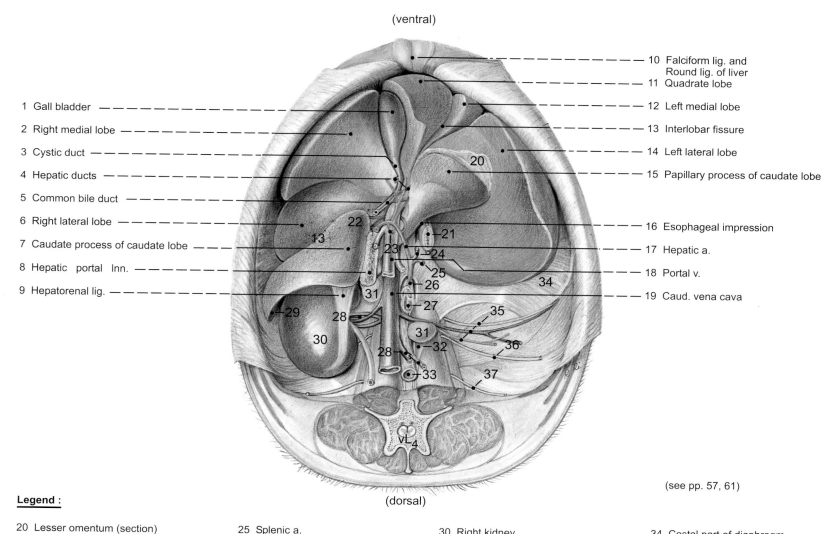

1 Gall bladder
2 Right medial lobe
3 Cystic duct
4 Hepatic ducts
5 Common bile duct
6 Right lateral lobe
7 Caudate process of caudate lobe
8 Hepatic portal lnn.
9 Hepatorenal lig.

10 Falciform lig. and Round lig. of liver
11 Quadrate lobe
12 Left medial lobe
13 Interlobar fissure
14 Left lateral lobe
15 Papillary process of caudate lobe
16 Esophageal impression
17 Hepatic a.
18 Portal v.
19 Caud. vena cava

(dorsal)

(see pp. 57, 61)

Legend :

20 Lesser omentum (section)
21 Esophagus and vagal trr.
22 Gastroduodenal a.
23 Right gastric a.
24 Left gastric a.

25 Splenic a.
26 Celiac a.
27 Cran . mesenteric a.
28 Renal a. and v.
29 Renal impression

30 Right kidney
31 Adrenal gland
32 Left crus of lumbar part of diaphragm
33 Aorta

34 Costal part of diaphragm
35 Cran. abdom. a. and v. and cran. iliohypogastric n.
36 Caud. iliohypogastric n.
37 Ilioinguinal n.

Visceral surface

(Portal v. and hepatic a.)

(right)

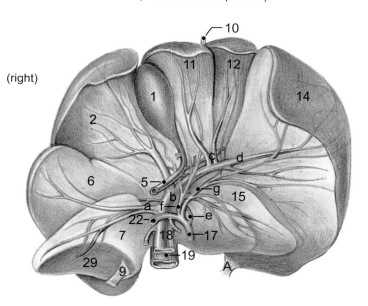

Diaphragmatic surface

(Hepatic vv.)

(left)   (right)

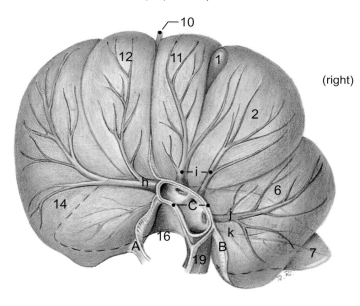

Legend :

A Left triangular lig.
B Right triangular lig.
C Coronary lig. of liver

Portal vein:
a Right br.
b Left br.
c Umbilical part
d Transverse part

Hepatic a.:
e Right lat. br.
f Right med. br.
g Left br.

Hepatic vv.:
h Left hepatic v.
i Middle hepatic v.
j Right hepatic v.
k Right acc. hepatic v.

59

6. AUTONOMIC NERVOUS SYSTEM, ABDOMINAL AORTA, CAUDAL VENA CAVA, SUBLUMBAR MUSCLES AND THE LUMBAR PLEXUS

The abdominal organs are shifted to the right side to demonstrate the left lumbar sympathetic nerve trunk and the abdominal aorta with its large originating intestinal arteries. For this dissection, first the kidney with its peritoneal cover is loosened from the underlying tissues to permit access to the retroperitoneal space, the aorta and the lumbar sympathetic trunk.

a) The **LUMBAR SYMPATHETIC TRUNK** lies in the lumbar region, medially, beside the psoas minor muscle. From the first three lumbar ganglia two to three thin nerves are released; these form the lumbar splanchnic nerves. In the sacral region, right and left sympathetic trunks, including the sacral ganglia, join to form an unpaired sacral sympathetic nerve trunk with the impar ganglion that is contained within it. The caudal continuation is the unpaired coccygeal sympathetic nerve trunk with its unpaired ganglia. In contrast to the first part of the lumbar sympathetic trunk, the last lumbar, sacral and coccygeal ganglia do not receive segmentally coursing white communicating rami; instead, the sympathetic nerves extend longitudinally within the lumbar sympathetic nerve trunk through the sacral- to the coccygeal sympathetic nerve trunk. Predominantly in the lumbar sympathetic trunk ganglia or only in the prevertebral ganglia that follow distally (see below) do synapses take place from myelinated preganglionic to unmyelinated postganglionic neurons. In comparison to the parasympathetic system, the synapse with the postganglionic neurons of the sympathetic system is brought about mainly near the central nervous system. After the synapse of the preganglionic neurons within the ganglia of the sympathetic nerve trunk, the unmyelinated postganglionic neurons again contact the segmental (somatic) spinal nerves as grey communicating branches and contribute sympathetic fibers to them. The grey and white communicating branches (*Rami communicantes grisei et albi*) can take their course close to the ganglion of the sympathetic nerve trunk either separately or in a common nerve trunk. The lesser number of myelinated preganglionic neurons, which pass through the ganglia of the sympathetic nerve trunk without synapse, run in the **lumbar splanchnic nerves (13)** and the sacral splanchnic nerves, and also through the **aortic plexus (9)** and the adrenal plexus (4), to the prevertebral plexus and the prevertebral ganglia within it. The prevertebral ganglia are the **celiac ganglion (1)** and the **cranial mesenteric ganglion (2)** (which with their associated plexuses collectively form the celiacomesenteric plexus) and the **caudal mesenteric ganglion (15)**. It is in these ganglia, which lie at the origin of the same-named artery, that the synapse onto the postganglionic unmyelinated neurons takes place. The postganglionic neurons form periarterial plexuses in the adventitia of the arteries and reach the internal organs with the ramifications of the arteries. The lumbar splanchnic nerves pass caudoventrally from the lumbar sympathetic nerve trunk to reach the caudal mesenteric ganglion. From the caudal mesenteric ganglion, sympathetic nerves pass as the **hypogastric nerves (25)** to reach the pelvic plexus within the pelvic cavity (see also p. 49).

b) The **PARASYMPATHETIC SYSTEM OF THE SACRAL SPINAL CORD** sends its nerves in retrograde fashion into the abdominal cavity up to the transverse colon. The parasympathetic supply of the organs situated cranial to the transverse colon is from the vagus nerve that, with its dorsal and ventral vagal trunks, enters the abdominal cavity, distributing branches to the diaphragmatic face of the stomach, to the liver and duodenum, and giving off branches to the celiacomesenteric (solar) plexus also.

c) The **ABDOMINAL AORTA (10)** releases the segmentally arranged paired lumbar arteries from its dorsal surface. These pass in company with the veins to the lumbar vertebral column and associated soft tissues. From the lateral wall of the aorta originate the common trunk of the caudal phrenic artery and cranial abdominal artery as well as the renal, ovarian or testicular, and deep circumflex iliac arteries. The same-named veins accompany all of these arteries. From the ventral wall of the aorta originate the unpaired celiac, cranial and caudal mesenteric arteries. In the initial portion of their course to the internal organs these arteries are unaccompanied by veins. The **celiac artery (1)** originates immediately caudal to the aortic hiatus at the level of the 13th thoracic vertebra. A little caudal to that the **cranial mesenteric artery (2)** follows at the level of the 1st lumbar vertebra. At the level of the 2nd lumbar vertebra the **cranial abdominal artery (5)** originates from the aorta jointly with the caudal phrenic artery (not labeled in the figure). The **renal artery (6)** follows immediately caudal, still at the level of the 2nd lumbar vertebra. The **ovarian artery (11)** or, respectively, testicular artery originates at

the level of the 3rd lumbar vertebra. The **caudal mesenteric artery (15)** leaves the aorta at the level of the 4th lumbar vertebra, and can be observed easily by putting tension on the mesentery of the large intestine at the level of the colon-rectum junction. The **deep circumflex iliac artery (17)** arises a short distance caudal to the caudal mesenteric artery at the level of the 4th lumbar vertebra, at a right angle to the aorta, cranial to the aorta's dividing into the **external iliac arteries (19)** and **internal iliac arteries (21)**, which is at the level of the 5th lumbar vertebra.

d) The **CAUDAL VENA CAVA (18)** lies to the right of the aorta and receives veins that are satellite to all the above-mentioned arteries; except that the celiac, cranial and caudal mesenteric arteries are, at their origin, unaccompanied by veins.

e) The **SUBLUMBAR MUSCLES** are located ventrolateral to the lumbar vertebral column and are supplied by ventral branches of the lumbar nerves. The **quadratus lumborum muscle (12)** originates at the last three thoracic vertebrae and the transverse processes of the lumbar vertebrae and courses to its region of insertion, which extends from the alar spine to the auricular surface of the iliac bone. The **psoas major muscle (22)** arises from the vertebral end of the last two ribs and from the lumbar vertebrae and, at the level of the pelvis, joins the iliacus muscle to form the iliopsoas muscle (see p. 37). The iliopsoas traverses the muscular lacuna to insert at the lesser trochanter of the femur (femoral bone). The **iliacus muscle (24)** takes origin from the sacropelvic surface of the ilium and from the lateral surface of the insertion tendon of the psoas minor muscle. The **psoas minor muscle (14)** arises from the last three thoracic and first four lumbar vertebrae where it lies ventral to the psoas major muscle. It terminates with a flat tendon at the psoas minor tubercle of the ilium.

f) The **LUMBAR PLEXUS** of the somatic nervous system (see also text-illustration) is formed from nLv 3 by ventral branches of the lumbar nerves and is connected with the sacral plexus to form the lumbosacral plexus. The nerve plexus lies within the sublumbar muscles and is seen only by removing the muscles (see p. 71). The **cranial iliohypogastric nerve (nLv1, −3)** and **caudal iliohypogastic nerve (nLv 2, −7)**, which as segmental nerves are not derived from the lumbar plexus, and the first plexus nerve (**ilioinguinal nerve −nLv2 and 3, −8**) emerge between the psoas minor and quadratus lumborum muscles. After a subperitoneal course, they penetrate the transverse abdominal muscle about 3 cm lateral to the quadratus lumborum and divide into a ventrolateral (vl) and ventromedial (vm) branch. The vl branches penetrate the abdominal muscles in an extended oblique course and supply the ventrolateral abdominal cutis (see p. 33). The vm branches supply the abdominal muscles and the peritoneum. They pass ventrally on the lateral surface of the transverse abdominal muscle to the rectus abdominis muscle and, near the linea alba, may reach the abdominal skin and the mammary gland. The **lateral cutaneous femoral nerve (nLv 3 and 4, −16)** emerges between the psoas major and minor muscles and with the deep circumflex iliac artery and vein, extends laterally through the transversus abdominis and internal abdominal oblique muscles. This branch supplies the skin in the area of the fold of the flank. The **genitofemoral nerve (nLv3 and 4, −20)** appears medial to the terminal tendon of the poas minor muscle. It accompanies the external iliac artery laterally and divides ventrally on this artery into a weak femoral and a strong genital branch. The femoral branch traverses the vascular lacuna to reach the femoral canal. The strong genital branch, after having traversed the inguinal canal, supplies the skin of the scrotum and prepuce or, respectively, the inguinal mammary gland complex. The **femoral nerve (nLv 4 − 5, −23)** passes within the iliopsoas muscle through the muscular lacuna and, before entering the quadriceps femoris muscle, gives off the long saphenous nerve. The **obturator nerve (nLv 4 − 6, −26)** passes lateral to the iliopsoas muscle, crosses the ilium medially and, after perforating the levator ani muscle, extends through the obturator foramen to reach the adductor muscles.

Lumbar plexus

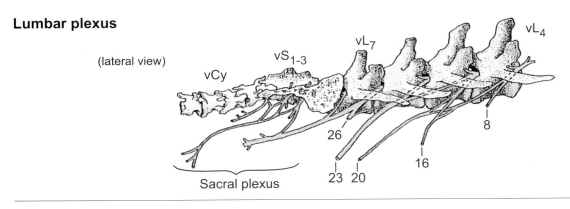

(lateral view)

vCy · vS~1-3~ · vL~7~ · vL~4~

26 · 23 · 20 · 16 · 8

Sacral plexus

(caudoventral view)

(right)   (left)

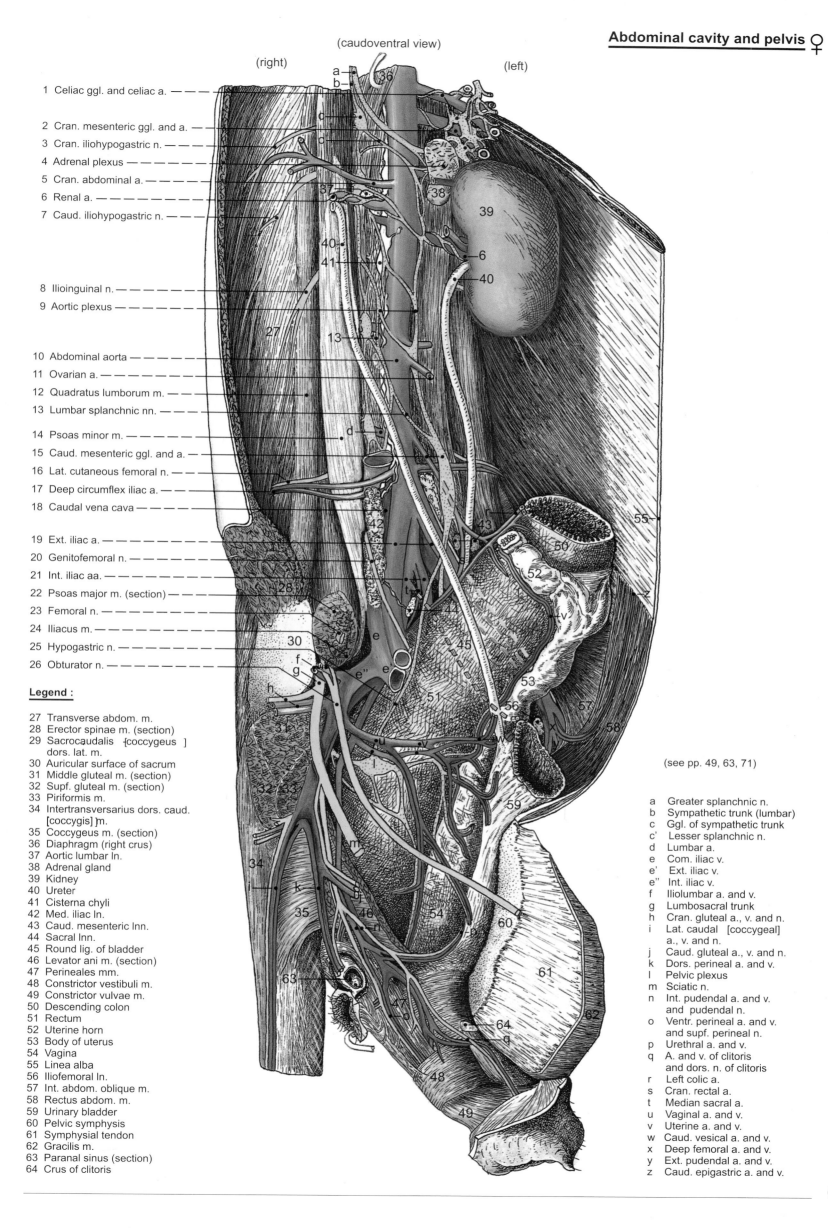

1 Celiac ggl. and celiac a.
2 Cran. mesenteric ggl. and a.
3 Cran. iliohypogastric n.
4 Adrenal plexus
5 Cran. abdominal a.
6 Renal a.
7 Caud. iliohypogastric n.

8 Ilioinguinal n.
9 Aortic plexus

10 Abdominal aorta
11 Ovarian a.
12 Quadratus lumborum m.
13 Lumbar splanchnic nn.
14 Psoas minor m.
15 Caud. mesenteric ggl. and a.
16 Lat. cutaneous femoral n.
17 Deep circumflex iliac a.
18 Caudal vena cava

19 Ext. iliac a.
20 Genitofemoral n.
21 Int. iliac aa.
22 Psoas major m. (section)
23 Femoral n.
24 Iliacus m.
25 Hypogastric n.
26 Obturator n.

Legend :

27 Transverse abdom. m.
28 Erector spinae m. (section)
29 Sacrocaudalis [coccygeus] dors. lat. m.
30 Auricular surface of sacrum
31 Middle gluteal m. (section)
32 Supf. gluteal m. (section)
33 Piriformis m.
34 Intertransversarius dors. caud. [coccygis] m.
35 Coccygeus m. (section)
36 Diaphragm (right crus)
37 Aortic lumbar ln.
38 Adrenal gland
39 Kidney
40 Ureter
41 Cisterna chyli
42 Med. iliac ln.
43 Caud. mesenteric lnn.
44 Sacral lnn.
45 Round lig. of bladder
46 Levator ani m. (section)
47 Perineales mm.
48 Constrictor vestibuli m.
49 Constrictor vulvae m.
50 Descending colon
51 Rectum
52 Uterine horn
53 Body of uterus
54 Vagina
55 Linea alba
56 Iliofemoral ln.
57 Int. abdom. oblique m.
58 Rectus abdom. m.
59 Urinary bladder
60 Pelvic symphysis
61 Symphysial tendon
62 Gracilis m.
63 Paranal sinus (section)
64 Crus of clitoris

(see pp. 49, 63, 71)

a Greater splanchnic n.
b Sympathetic trunk (lumbar)
c Ggl. of sympathetic trunk
c' Lesser splanchnic n.
d Lumbar a.
e Com. iliac v.
e' Ext. iliac v.
e" Int. iliac v.
f Iliolumbar a. and v.
g Lumbosacral trunk
h Cran. gluteal a., v. and n.
i Lat. caudal [coccygeal] a., v. and n.
j Caud. gluteal a., v. and n.
k Dors. perineal a. and v.
l Pelvic plexus
m Sciatic n.
n Int. pudendal a. and v. and pudendal n.
o Ventr. perineal a. and v. and supf. perineal n.
p Urethral a. and v.
q A. and v. of clitoris and dors. n. of clitoris
r Left colic a.
s Cran. rectal a.
t Median sacral a.
u Vaginal a. and v.
v Uterine a. and v.
w Caud. vesical a. and v.
x Deep femoral a. and v.
y Ext. pudendal a. and v.
z Caud. epigastric a. and v.

61

CHAPTER 7: URINARY AND GENITAL ORGANS, PELVIS

1. URINARY ORGANS

After double ligation between colon and rectum with preservation of the caudal mesenteric ganglion, the intestine is transected. The cranial part of the body, including the gastrointestinal canal with liver and pancreas is removed. For the study of the kidney, median, paramedian, sagittal and transverse sections are performed. The lymph nodes illustrated (**sacral, –8; medial iliac, –7** and **lumbar aortic lymph nodes, –6**) and the **adrenal glands (1)** will first be identified. They are described in more detail on p. 68.

Of the **urinary organs**, the kidneys, the ureter and the urinary bladder are described here and the urethra later, in common with the genital organs.

1 **a)** The **KIDNEYS** lie retroperitoneally within the **retroperitoneal space (4)**. The **left kidney** lies ventral to the first three lumbar vertebrae and the **right kidney** a half vertebral length more cranial. Classified according to comparative anatomical criteria, the canine kidney belongs to the smooth unipapillary type of kidney. Its **renal lobes (23)**, which in some marine mammals (*e.g.*, seals) are separated from each other and are attached to the renal branches of the ureter like grapes on a stalk, show a fusion of the cortical areas in the dog, which results in a smooth surface of the kidney. The **renal medulla (24)** retains a recognizable lobar arrangement. The pyramid-like medullary substance (**renal pyramid, –25**) of the renal lobe consists of a peripheral pyramidal base (or **external part, –27**) and a central renal papilla (or **internal part, –26**), which projects into the internal hollow space of the kidney (**renal sinus, –14**). In the median plane of the kidney the renal papillae are fused to form what may appear as a large, single, common renal papilla (**renal crest, –12**). On both sides of the median plane of the kidney, parts of the renal papillae that are not fused project as individual renal pyramids between the **pelvic recesses (19)** into the renal sinus. The kidneys are embedded in an external capsule of fat tissue, the **adipose capsule (2)**. The **fibrous capsule (13)** that follows internally is, after section, easily removed from the normal renal parenchyma, but this is not possible in certain pathological conditions. In the **renal cortex (18)**, which is about two centimeters thick, renal corpuscles can be seen as pinpoint circumscribed vascular spaces. A renal corpuscle consists of a coil of blood capillaries, the glomerulus, and a surrounding capsule, into which the primary urine – an ultrafiltrate of the blood plasma – passes. The renal corpuscle, with the proximal convoluted tubule that passes from it and the following nephron loop (HENLE's loop) and distal convoluted tubule form the nephron (see text-illustration). It is into the renal corpuscle of the nephron that the primary urine (about 150 liters daily) is filtered, and it is within its tubular system that the resorption of fluid, including glucose and electrolytes from the primary urine, takes place. In the opposite direction waste products, especially nitrogen containing end-products of protein metabolism, in particular, urea, and also certain drugs, are excreted. A connecting tubule joins the nephron to a collecting tubule. Several arched collecting tubules join like the branches of a tree to form a straight collecting tubule that unites with other collecting tubules to form a papillary duct. Within the collecting tubules, owing to an osmotic pressure difference, and under the influence of the antidiuretic hormone of the posterior hypophysis, a further resorption of water is realized from the filtrate. Thus is formed the secondary urine (about 1.5 liter daily). On the common renal papilla (renal crest) numerous papillary ducts discharge. They are predominantly single, with the result that an elongate sieve-like plate (*Area cribrosa* –21), is easily seen on viewing the **renal crest (22)**. At both ends of the area cribrosa there is an ca. 2 mm long slit-like opening, the **common papillary duct (20)**, which takes up several papillary ducts before its opening on the crest.

The **renal pelvis (11)** lies within the renal sinus. In the area of the renal hilus it is separated from the renal vessels that enter there, and the renal parenchyma, by fat tissue and at the perimeter of the common renal papilla (renal crest) its external adventitia is fused with the fine connective tissue that joins the tubules of the renal parenchyma. Its internal layer of epithelium is continued onto the renal crest and is continuous with the epithelium lining the papillary ducts that discharge there.

I. The blood vascular system of the kidney (see also text-illustration) has complicated topographical relations to the urine conducting, looplike renal tubules. The **renal artery (3)** divides into **interlobar arteries (15)**, which run between the lobes and are continued by the **arcuate arteries (16)**. The latter course arch-like at the interface between cortex and medulla. From the arcuate artery, **interlobular arteries (17)** pass in a peripheral direction. They supply predominantly the renal cortex and demarcate a lobule on either side. (Grossly, the renal lobules can scarcely be distinguished as subunits of the renal lobes.) The interlobular arteries give off the afferent glomerular arterioles, which at the vascular pole of each renal corpuscle are continued by a glomerulus. The efferent glomerular arteriole originates from the vascular pole of the glomerulus and is continued by a dense capillary net in the area of the renal tubules. The first capillary net (glomerulus) filters the primary urine and is found within the arterial limb of the blood vascular system. It is designated the glomerular capillary network. From the second capillary network (renal tubule net) the venous drainage of the kidney commences.

II. The **lymph** from the kidney drains into the lumbar aortic lymph nodes.

III. **Autonomic innervation** of the kidney is by sympathetic and parasympathetic nerve fibers that proceed chiefly from the abdominal aortic plexus.

2 **b)** The **URETER (5)** courses between the renal pelvis and the urinary bladder. It lies retroperitoneally, adjacent to the sublumbar muscles. Its caudal portion is located within a fold of peritoneum, crosses the deferent duct in the male dog and traverses the wall of the neck of the urinary bladder in a long oblique course.

Renal arteries and veins

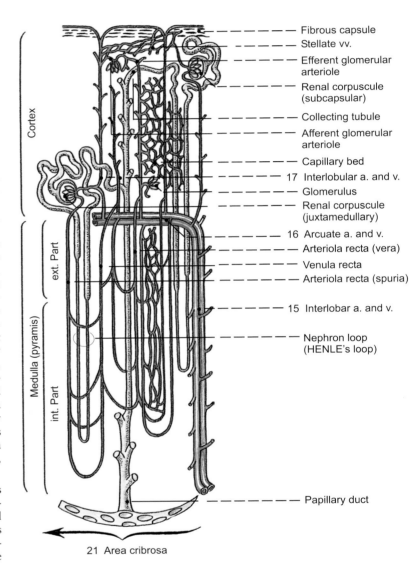

Fibrous capsule
Stellate vv.
Efferent glomerular arteriole
Renal corpuscle (subcapsular)
Collecting tubule
Afferent glomerular arteriole
Capillary bed
17 Interlobular a. and v.
Glomerulus
Renal corpuscle (juxtamedullary)
16 Arcuate a. and v.
Arteriola recta (vera)
Venula recta
Arteriola recta (spuria)
15 Interlobar a. and v.
Nephron loop (HENLE's loop)
Papillary duct

Cortex
ext. Part
Medulla (pyramis)
int. Part

21 Area cribrosa

c) The **URINARY BLADDER** (see also p. 64) lies clothed by the peritoneum. From it the **median ligament of the urinary bladder (10)** courses to the ventral midline and thus to the linea alba. During fetal development the urinary bladder leads to the embryonal urinary duct (urachus) and by that means to the umbilicus. The paired **lateral ligament of the urinary bladder (9)** extends to the dorsolateral body wall and contains the umbilical artery, which in many cases is obliterated to form the **round ligament of the bladder –9)** and in other cases supplies blood to the urinary bladder by cranial vesical arteries.

Abdominal cavity and urinary organs

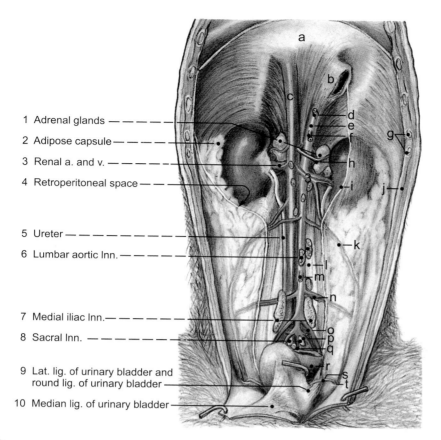

1 Adrenal glands
2 Adipose capsule
3 Renal a. and v.
4 Retroperitoneal space
5 Ureter
6 Lumbar aortic Inn.
7 Medial iliac Inn.
8 Sacral Inn.
9 Lat. lig. of urinary bladder and round lig. of urinary bladder
10 Median lig. of urinary bladder

Legend :

a Diaphragm
b Esophagus
c Caud. vena cava
d Celiac a.
e Aorta
f Cran. mesenteric a.
g Ribs
h Cran. abdominal v.
i Peritoneum (section)
j Abdominal mm.
k Testicular a. and v.
l Psoas minor m.
m Caud. mesenteric a.
n Deep circumflex iliac a. and v.
o Ext. iliac a.
p Int. iliac a.
q Median sacral a.
r Rectum
s Deferent duct
t Vaginal ring

(see p. 69)

Left kidney

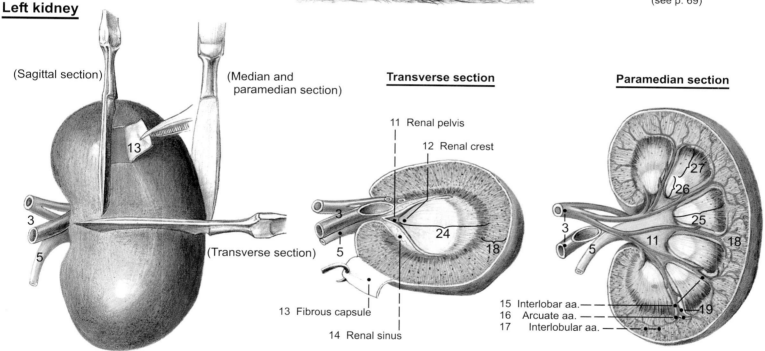

(Sagittal section)

(Median and paramedian section)

13

3

5

(Transverse section)

Transverse section

11 Renal pelvis
12 Renal crest

3
5
24
18

13 Fibrous capsule

14 Renal sinus

Paramedian section

27
26
3
25
11
5
18

15 Interlobar aa.
16 Arcuate aa.
17 Interlobular aa.
19

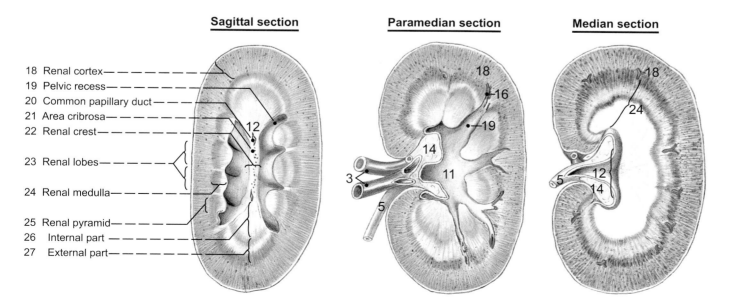

Sagittal section

18 Renal cortex
19 Pelvic recess
20 Common papillary duct
21 Area cribrosa
22 Renal crest
23 Renal lobes
24 Renal medulla
25 Renal pyramid
26 Internal part
27 External part

12

Paramedian section

18
16
19
14
3
11
5

Median section

18
24
12
5
14

2. URINARY BLADDER AND PERITONEAL RELATIONSHIPS OF THE GENITAL ORGANS

In the male dog on the right side of the body the scrotum (see clinical-functional anatomy) is cut, parallel to the raphe scroti with attention to the tunica dartos. The smooth musculature of the tunica dartos is also present in the scrotal septum, which separates the two vaginal tunics with their enclosed testes. The peritoneal vaginal tunic including the laterally adjacent (external) cremaster muscle and surrounding external spermatic fascia as well as the internal spermatic fascia is loosened from the scrotum and, by a longitudinal section, opened up to the vaginal ring. The bitch is treated similarly, insofar as a vaginal process is present.

a) The **URINARY BLADDER** (see also p. 62 and text-illustration) has a cranial **apex (Vertex)**, a central **body (Corpus vesicae)** and a caudal **neck (Cervix vesicae)**. Dorsally, at the neck of the bladder, the ureters, converging, traverse the wall obliquely. They lie just deep to the mucosa and create internally a moderate swelling, the **ureteral columns (Columnae uretericae)**, that can be traced caudally to the **opening of each ureter (Ostium ureteris)** into the bladder. **Ureteral folds** continue caudally from the openings, uniting at the transition of the urinary bladder to the **urethra**, the **internal urethral ostium**. It is here that the ureteral folds are continued as the median dorsal **urethral crest** that, in male dogs, extends to the **seminal colliculus** and, in the bitch, to the end of the urethra.

The **blood supply** of the urinary bladder is chiefly from the caudal vesical artery, which originates from the prostatic or, respectively, vaginal artery and runs from the pelvic cavity to the urinary bladder. The total venous drainage passes to the caudal vesical vein (see also p. 71).

The **lymph vessels** pass to the sacral lymph nodes.

The **autonomic innervation** is from the pelvic plexus. Within the wall of the urinary bladder intramural nerve plexuses containing ganglion cells regulate the contraction of the muscular wall.

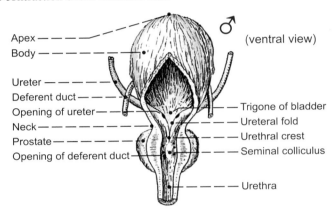

b) The **PERITONEAL FOLDS** of the internal genital organs of the female dog are subdivided into **mesovarium (proximal and distal)**, **mesosalpinx** and **mesometrium** and **gonadal ligaments**. Mesovarium, mesosalpinx and mesometrium collectively are named the **broad ligament of the uterus (Lig. latum uteri)**.

I. The **mesovarium (6)** conducts the ovarian artery and vein to the ovary. Near the ovary, the **mesosalpinx (9)** splits off laterally, the point of its origin defining a subdivision of the mesovarium into a long **proximal mesovarium (7)** and a short **distal mesovarium (8)** the epithelium (mesothelium) of which is continued onto the ovary as a surface epithelium (germinal epithelium). Between the two lamellae of the mesosalpinx there is lateral to the ovary the thin terminal portion, and medial to the ovary the thicker initial portion, of the uterine tube, which courses in an arc around the ovary. The short distal mesovarium with the suspended ovary and the long mesosalpinx form together the wall of the **ovarian bursa (10)**. The bursa exhibits at the free distal border of the mesosalpinx medially the **ostium of the ovarian bursa (11)** and laterally a fat-free place ('window') through which the ovary can be seen (see p. 67). Caudally, the mesovarium is continuous with the **mesometrium (4)**. Its attachment to the uterus, **parametrium (12)**, invests with its two lamellae the uterine artery and vein and continues as **perimetrium (13)** upon the uterine surface.

II. The **gonadal ligaments of the bitch** (see also p. 67) are the suspensory ligament of the ovary, the proper ligament of the ovary and the round ligament of the uterus. The **suspensory ligament of the ovary (1)** is the cranial gubernaculum that, lateral to the kidney, passes from the last rib at the attachment of the diaphragm to the ovary. The **caudal gubernaculum (Lig. inguinale ovarii)** follows caudally from the suspensory ligament. At the junction of the uterine tube with the horn of the uterus, it is subdivided into the **proper ligament of the ovary (2)**, which extends between the ovary and the termination of the uterine tube, and the **round ligament of the uterus (Lig. teres uteri, —3)** that follows the proper ligament. The round ligament is fixed laterally to the mesometrium and passes through the **vaginal ring (5)** up to the end of the **vaginal process of the peritoneum**. Even when the vaginal process is absent, which occurs in about 25% of the bitches on one or both sides of the body, the connective tissue portion of the round ligament of the uterus passes without peritoneal coverage through the inguinal space and may reach the pubic region.

As only a slight ovarian descensus has taken place, the ovaries are found near the location of their development, and the peritoneal folds that approach the ovary from cranial and caudal remain intact during ontogenesis and are not obliterated.

III. The **peritoneal folds of the internal genital organs of the male dog** are the mesorchium (proximal and distal), mesoductus deferens, mesofuniculus and mesepididymis. The **proximal mesorchium (15)** is found in the peritoneal cavity as the **vascular fold (Plica vasculosa)** containing the testicular vessels. It passes through the **vaginal ring (5)** into the vaginal process of the peritoneum. Here, in the **vaginal canal**, the proximal mesorchium is united with the **mesoductus deferens** (or fold of the deferent duct —Plica ductus deferentis, —24), both proceeding from that part of the mesorchium, the **mesofuniculus (23)**, that is continuous with the parietal vaginal tunic (the parietal vaginal tunic is designated *perifuniculus* in the figure). The **vaginal canal** and the **vaginal cavity** that follows caudally have (comparable to the peritoneal cavity) a **parietal vaginal tunic (Tunica vaginalis parietalis, —22 and 25**; designated *periorchium* and *perifuniculus* in the figure), from which the peritoneal lamellae containing the testicular vessels and nerves and the ductus deferens (*Mesorchium* and *Mesoductus*, respectively) fold off, and a **visceral vaginal tunic (Tunica vaginalis visceralis, —21**; designated *epiorchium* in the figure) that forms a thin serous covering upon the testis and epididymis.

The mesofuniculus is that part of the mesorchium that is between the origin of the mesorchium from the parietal vaginal tunic and the origin of the mesoductus from the medial side of the mesorchium (see p. 65).

The **spermatic cord (Funiculus spermaticus)** consists of seven structures: testicular artery, testicular vein, autonomic nerve plexus and testicular lymph vessels, deferent duct with deferent artery and vein, —a – g and their peritoneal coverings, the mesorchium and mesoductus. Close to the testicle, at the lateral origin of the short **mesepididymis (18)**, the long proximal mesorchium is continued by the **distal mesorchium (19)**. Between these two peritoneal folds, the **testicular bursa (or epididymal sinus, —20)** is found. The opening into the bursa is lateral.

IV. The **gonadal ligaments of the male dog** are subdivided into the cranial and caudal gubernaculum. The **cranial gubernaculum (suspensory ligament of the testis, —14)** is more or less completely reduced. Should it occur, it extends laterally from the proximal mesorchium and can be followed lateral to the kidney extending toward the diaphragm. The **caudal gubernaculum (Lig. inguinale testis)** is subdivided by the epididymis; that is to say, the **proper ligament of the testis (16)** courses between the testicle and the tail of the epididymis, and the **ligament of the tail of the epididymis (17)** is the band that, if distinct, extends with the scrotal ligament as a continuous cord from the tail to the dermis layer of the scrotal skin. The fundus of the vaginal tunic is attached to the internal scrotal surface by the extraperitoneal portion of the caudal gubernaculum and subcutaneous connective tissue. In the dog, the caudal end of the tail of the epididymis is uncovered by peritoneum and the connective tissue joining it to the dermis of the scrotal skin is usually poorly defined. The connective tissue here constitutes both the ligament of the tail of the epididymis and the **scrotal ligament**.

PERITONEAL RELATIONSHIPS OF THE GENITAL ORGANS

Peritoneal Folds of the Gonads			Ligaments of the gonads	
Bitch		**Male Dog**	**Bitch**	**Male Dog**
Proximal mesovarium		Proximal mesorchium (Plica vasculosa)	Suspensory ligament of the ovary (between ovary and diaphragm)	Suspensory ligament of the testis (extensively involuted)
Distal mesovarium	Ovarian bursa or Testicular bursa	Distal mesorchium	Proper ligament of the ovary (between the ovary and the termination of the uterine tube)	Proper ligament of the testis (between the testis and the tail of the epididymis)
Mesosalpinx (splits off laterally between the proximal and distal mesovarium)		Mesepididymis (splits off laterally between the proximal and distal mesorchium)	Round ligament of the uterus (between the termination of the uterine tube and the fundus of the vaginal process of the peritoneum)	Ligament of the tail of the epididymis (between the tail of the epididymis and the fundus of the vaginal tunic)
Mesometrium		Mesoductus deferens		

Urogenital ligaments

(right side)

Legend :

26 Ovary
27 Duodenum
28 Horn of uterus
29 Body of uterus
30 Vagina
31 Rectum
32 Rectogenital pouch
33 Vesicogenital pouch
34 Pubovesical pouch
35 Urethra
36 Lat. lig. of bladder and round lig. of bladder
37 Urinary bladder
38 Median lig. of bladder
39 Greater omentum
40 Uterine tube

♀

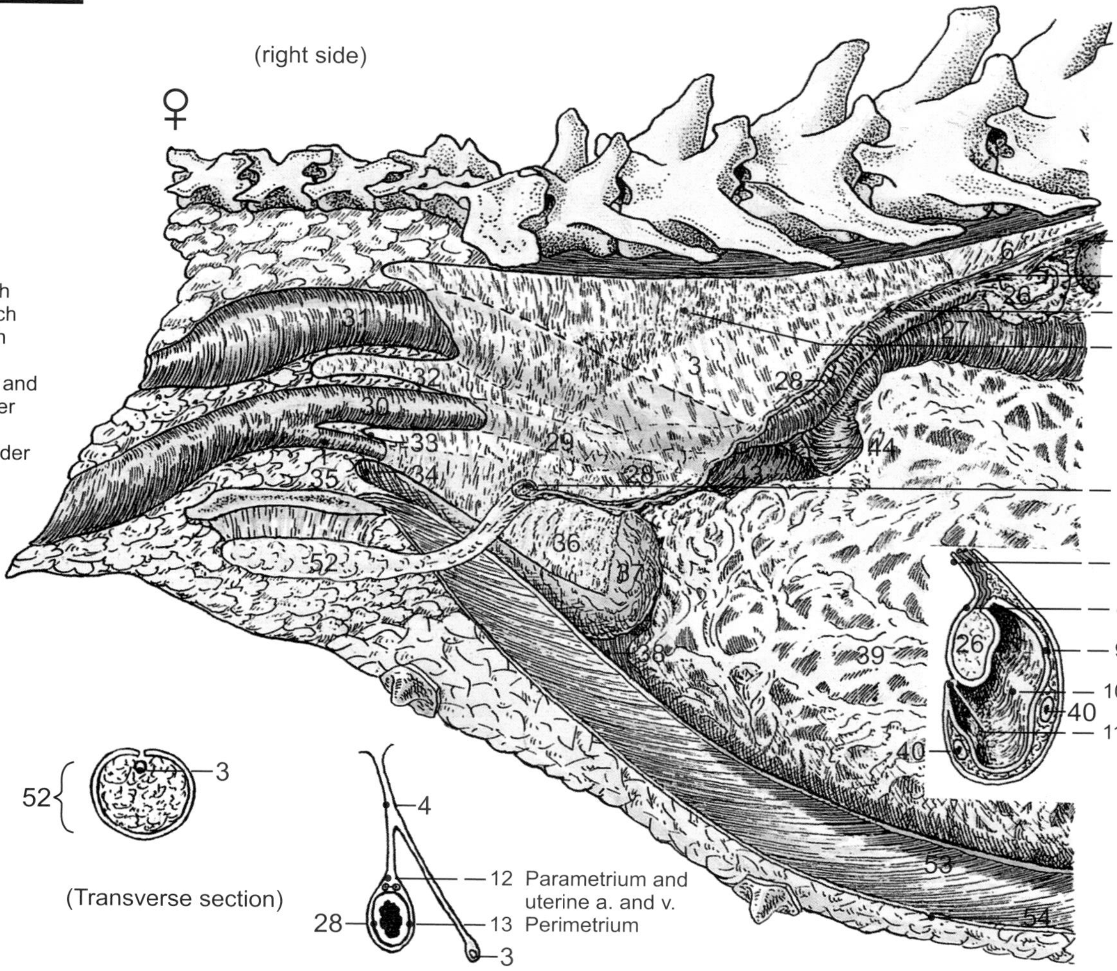

1 Suspensory lig. of ovary
2 Proper lig. of ovary
3 Round lig. of uterus
4 Mesometrium
5 Vaginal ring
6 Mesovarium:
7 Prox. mesovarium and ovarian a. and v.
8 Distal mesovarium
9 Mesosalpinx
10 Ovarian bursa
11 Ostium of ovarian bursa
12 Parametrium and uterine a. and v.
13 Perimetrium

(Transverse section)

41 Caudal vena cava
42 Aorta
43 Descending colon
44 Duodenocolic fold
45 Prostate
46 Retractor penis m.
47 Root of penis
48 Body of penis
49 Glans penis
50 Epididymis
51 Testis
52 Vaginal process of peritoneum
53 Ext. abdom. oblique m.
54 Linea alba

♂

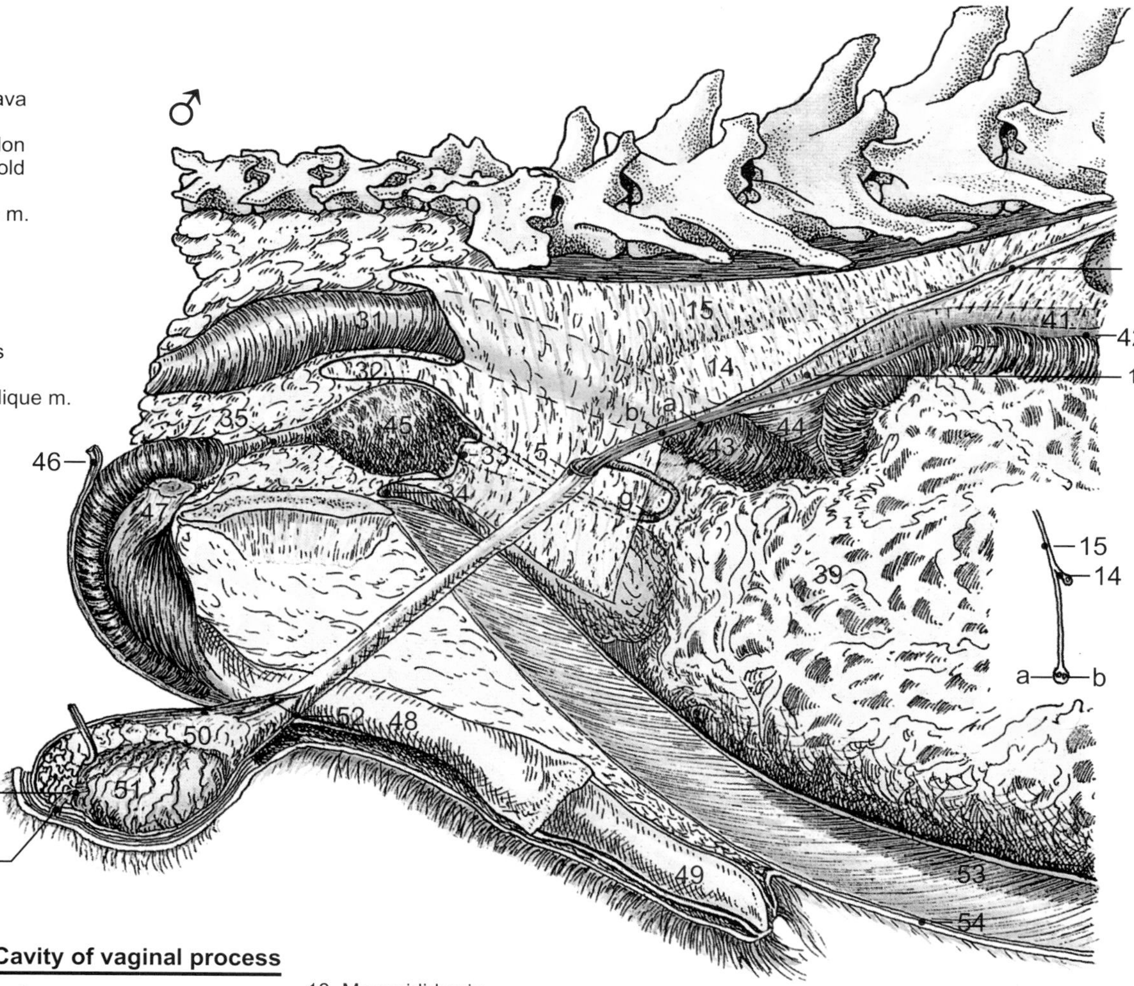

14 Suspensory lig. of testis
15 Prox. mesorchium
16 Proper lig. of testis
17 Lig. of tail of epididymis

(see pp.67,69,71)

Cavity of vaginal process

(Transverse section)

18 Mesepididymis
19 Distal mesorchium
20 Testicular bursa (Epididymal sinus)
21 Epiorchium
22 Periorchium

Vaginal canal

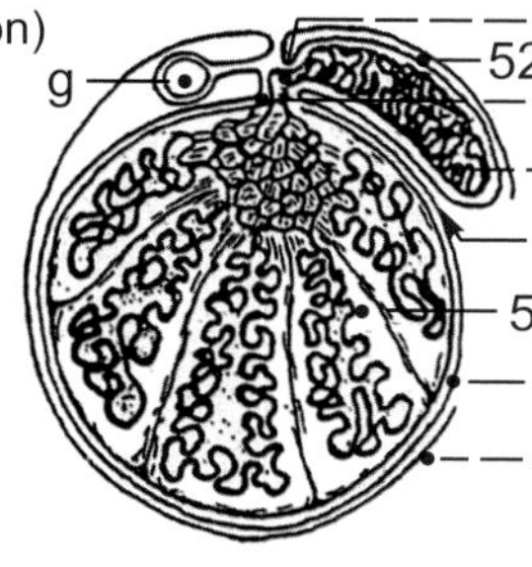

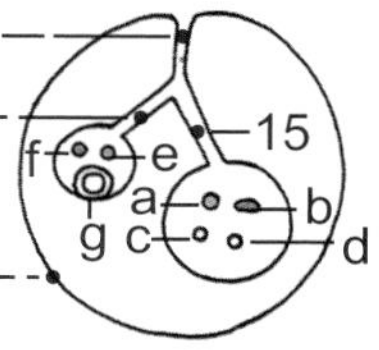

23 Mesofuniculus
24 Plica ductus defferentis
25 Perifuniculus

Legend :

a Testicular a.
b Testicular v.
c Lymphatic vessel
d Testicular nerve plexus
e A. of deferent duct
f V. of deferent duct
g Deferent duct

3. FEMALE GENITAL ORGANS

In the bitch, the ostium of the ovarian bursa is enlarged longitudinally and the ovary is everted through the opening. The ovary is then sectioned longitudinally into halves. The uterine tube is exposed in its entire length. Uterus, cervix, vagina, vaginal vestibule and vulva are opened on the dorsal midline in their total length so that their internal relations can be studied.

A **common basic structural plan is distinctly recognizable for both sexes even with respect to the genital organs** and becomes particularly clear during ontogenesis. In both genders, the genital organs may be subdivided into internal and external.

a) The **INTERNAL GENITAL ORGANS** are the gonads, the germ cell producing organs, and the uterine tube and uterus, the conducting organs, that convey the germ cell. During pregnancy, the uterus is the place for development of the fertilized germ cell. The vagina and vestibule of the vagina (usually designated only 'vestibule') are the copulatory organs that follow caudal to the uterus.

1   **I.** The **ovary (9)**, the female gonad, produces the germ cells and functions in addtion as an endocrine gland. The ovary is bilaterally flattened. Its size is dependent on the stage of the sexual cycle and is about 15 x 10 x 6 mm. The ovary is concealed within the **ovarian bursa (1)**, which is a space whose walls consist of the mesovarium and mesosalpinx (see also p. 65). It is accessible through a medial slit, the **ostium of the ovarian bursa (2)**. In lateral view, the ovary can be seen through a fat-free 'window' of the mesosalpinx (Fenestra bursae ovaricae). The ovaries lie suspended by the mesovarium, caudal to the kidneys, at the level of the 4th or 5th lumbar vertebra. Cortical and medullary parts can be distinguished.

The **cortex of the ovary** contains ovarian follicles with their contained oocytes and, depending on the phase of the sexual cycle, also corpora lutea. The corpora lutea are formed from the wall of the follicle following ovulation (see clinical-functional anatomy).

The **ovarian medulla** is also called the heterosexual part of the ovary owing to the fact that embryologically it is comparable to the anlage of the testis. The medullary cords of the embryonic ovary correspond to the embryonal testicular cords; but in the mammal, the cords are lost early in development. The medulla contains a dense network of blood and lymph vessels as well as autonomic nerves (chiefly sympathetic).

2   **II.** After ovulation, the **uterine tube (salpinx, —10)** transports the ovum to the uterus and, moreover, functions as the site of fertilization. It is 5 – 10 cm long and only a few mm thick. In the wall of the ovarian bursa, in the mesosalpinx with its abundant fat, the initial portion of the tube with its fimbriated infundibulum (14) can be recognized externally. It projects partially externally at the ostium of the ovarian bursa. The end-portion of the uterine tube, the isthmus, can also be recognized externally, but the middle portion of the tube is usually well concealed by fat. The **infundibulum (14)** with the centrally located **abdominal ostium of the uterine tube (15)** and the surrounding **tubal fimbriae** are located lateral to the ovary at the margin of the bursal ostium. The **ampulla of the uterine tube (13)** descends ventrally and in so doing extends cranially around the ovary, continuing in the mesosalpinx that forms the lateral wall of the ovarian bursa as the slightly undulating **isthmus of the uterine tube (16)**. The isthmus is continued by the **uterine part (15)** that pierces the wall at the tip of the uterine horn and opens into the uterine lumen on the **uterine papilla** with the **uterine ostium of the uterine tube (18)**.

3; 4   **III.** According to comparative anatomical classification, the canine **uterus (Metra)** is bicornuate. In the sexually mature, non-pregnant, medium-sized bitch, the **uterine horns (6)** are about 12 cm long and, after their union, are continued caudally into the **uterine body (7)**. The body of the uterus is only 2 – 3 cm long and is shorter than it may at first appear in external view. This is because the horns, fused externally, remain separated internally by a uterine velum for a distance of 1 cm. Besides horns and body, the **cervix uteri (8)**

5   is that part of the uterus that has the narrowest lumen and the firmest muscular coat, which facilitates its demarcation by palpation. The uterine cervix is about 1 cm long and projects with its **vaginal portion (20)** into the vagina. The vaginal portion of the cervix projects dorsal to the ventral vaginal fornix and is as a semi-cylinder integrated into the dorsal vagina wall that with a tapering longitudinal swelling is continued caudally into the vagina. The narrow **cervical canal (22)** is bounded by longitudinal mucosal folds and commences with the **internal uterine ostium (23)** and ends in the center of the vaginal portion with the **external uterine ostium (21)**. The wall of the uterus consists of three-layers altogether: endo-, myo-, and perimetrium.

IV. The **vagina (30)** is remarkably distensible and as a copulatory organ has **6** distinct longitudinal and indistinct transverse mucosal folds. It is compressed dorsoventrally by adjacent organs (dorsally, the rectum; ventrally, the feminine urethra) and has dorsal and ventral walls and a narrow transverse lumen. The length of the vagina is about 12 cm, extending cranially to the **vaginal fornix (19)**, which surrounds the vaginal portion of the cervix ventrally and laterally, and caudally to the **vaginal ostium (29)**. Ventrally, at the vaginal ostium, the external urethral ostium is found upon the urethral tubercle and laterally radiating semicircular mucosal folds perhaps signify the presence of a hymen. Like the uterus, the vaginal wall is also three-layered.

V. The **vestibule of the vagina (27)** extends from the vaginal ostium to the vulvar cleft (*Rima pudendi s. Rima vulvae*). The vestibule is at first horizontally positioned and, after this, continued caudally by a ventral arch-like portion that becomes more prominent with increasing age. The cutaneous aglandular mucous membrane appears smooth. Within the lateral wall are the **vestibular bulb (25)**, which is enveloped laterally by the striated **constrictor vestibuli muscle (24)**. Smooth muscle of the vestibular wall is sparse. The **accessory genital glands (minor vestibular glands)** secrete a viscous fluid and open, one after the other, in two longitudinal rows that are caudolateral to the **external urethral ostium (28)**.   **7**

b) The **EXTERNAL GENITAL ORGANS** are the female vulva (*Pudendum femininum*), the clitoris, and the feminine urethra.

I. The vulva consists of the **vulvar lips (Labia pudendi, —11)** and the **vulvar cleft (12)**. The vulvar lips form a rounded commissure dorsally, and a pointed ventral commissure. They correspond to the *labia minora* of the human being. The constrictor vulvae muscle forms the muscular basis of each labium.

II. The **clitoris** is the female homologue to the penis and, like the penis, may **8** be considered to consist of a **root, body** and **head,** with two types of erectile bodies. The unpaired **corpus spongiosum of the clitoris** forms alone the glans of the clitoris, which is located caudally in the vestibule. It may project slightly from the **clitoridal fossa (26)**. The two remaining parts of the unpaired erectile body lie external to the clitoris as the **vestibular bulb (25)** under the mucous membrane of the vestibule. The **body of the clitoris** is attached to the ischial arch by the crura of the clitoris. The two crura unite caudally to form the body of the clitoris that is principally fat-filled and, different from the corpus cavernosum penis, lacking an apical ossification. Cartilage may however occur in the tip of the clitoris.

The **blood supply** of the vulva, including the vestibule, is provided by branches of the internal pudendal artery and vein that also give off the vaginal artery and vein that, in turn, dispatch the **uterine artery and vein (5)**. The uterine vessels course in the mesometrium, form arcades, and anastomose at the tip of the uterine horn with the **uterine branch (4)** of the **ovarian artery and vein (3)**. The latter vascularize the ovary and also participate in the blood supply of the uterine tube. The venous uterine ramus is especially strong as it is the main drainage of the uterus.

The **lymph drainage** of the ovary, uterine tube, and cranial tip of the uterine horn is to the aortic lumbar lymph nodes (*Lnn. lumbales aortici*); of the other parts of the uterus and the vagina including the vulva to the medial iliac and sacral lymph nodes (see also p. 68).

The **autonomic nerve supply** of the ovary, including the uterine tube, is by the abdominal aortic plexus with ovarian, intermesenteric, and caudal mesenteric plexuses. Uterus and vagina are supplied by the pelvic plexus. The external genital organs are supplied with autonomic, motor, and sensory fibers by the pudendal nerve.

III. The **feminine urethra** measures only a few centimeters and is considerably shorter than the male urethra. It begins at the neck of the urinary bladder with the internal urethral ostium and ends ventrally at the vaginal ostium between vagina and vestibule with the external urethral ostium that opens on the mucosal urethral tubercle (*Tuberculum urethrale*). The urethra is located between the pelvic floor and the vagina. The initial part is similar to the neck of the urinary bladder and is structured by external longitudinal and internal circular smooth muscle cell bundles. The caudal part contains in its wall a venous erectile body and the striated urethralis muscle that assure the closure of the urethra (continence).

Female genital organs

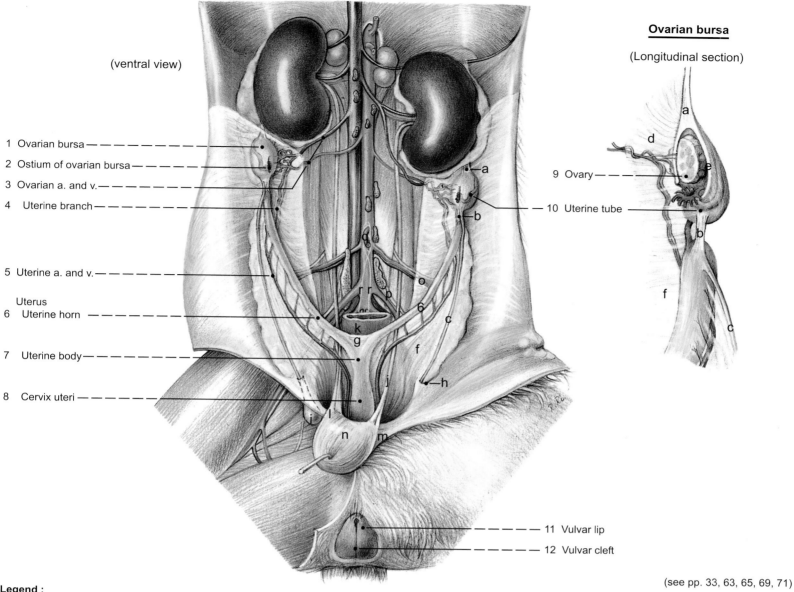

(ventral view)

1 Ovarian bursa
2 Ostium of ovarian bursa
3 Ovarian a. and v.
4 Uterine branch

5 Uterine a. and v.

Uterus
6 Uterine horn

7 Uterine body

8 Cervix uteri

Ovarian bursa

(Longitudinal section)

9 Ovary
10 Uterine tube

11 Vulvar lip
12 Vulvar cleft

(see pp. 33, 63, 65, 69, 71)

Legend :

a	Suspensory lig. of ovary	g	Intercornual lig.	m	Median lig. of bladder	r	Hypogastric nn.
b	Proper lig. of ovary	h	Vaginal ring	n	Urinary bladder	s	Perimetrium
c	Round lig. of ovary	i	Vaginal process of peritoneum	o	Deep circumflex iliac a. and v. and lat. cutaneous femoral n.	t	Myometrium
d	Mesovarium	j	Ureter	p	Genitofemoral n.	u	Endometrium
e	Mesosalpinx	k	Rectum			v	Fenestra bursae ovaricae
f	Mesometrium	l	Lat. lig. of urinary bladder	q	Caud. mesenteric a. and ggl.		

(dorsal view)

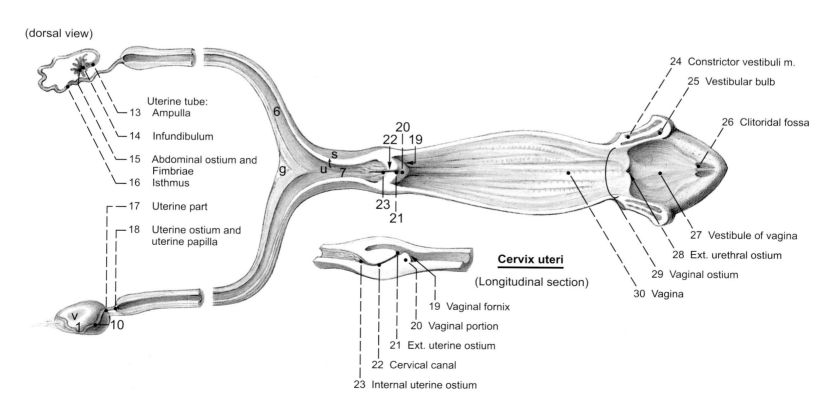

Uterine tube:
13 Ampulla
14 Infundibulum
15 Abdominal ostium and Fimbriae
16 Isthmus
17 Uterine part
18 Uterine ostium and uterine papilla

24 Constrictor vestibuli m.
25 Vestibular bulb
26 Clitoridal fossa

27 Vestibule of vagina
28 Ext. urethral ostium
29 Vaginal ostium
30 Vagina

Cervix uteri

(Longitudinal section)

19 Vaginal fornix
20 Vaginal portion
21 Ext. uterine ostium
22 Cervical canal
23 Internal uterine ostium

67

4. MALE GENITAL ORGANS, LYMPHATIC SYSTEM OF THE LUMBAR AND PELVIC REGIONS

In the male dog the testicle is cut into halves. The urinary bladder and the urethra are opened by a ventromedian section. The erectile bodies will be studied by making cross-sections of the penis at the level of the root, body and glans.

The genital organs of the male dog are, like those of the bitch, subdivided into internal and external genital organs. The accessory sex glands belong to the internal genital organs.

a) Following the descent of the testis into the scrotum, the **INTERNAL GENITAL ORGANS** are the testes, which are the germ cell forming organs (gonad: testis) and the organs that conduct the germ cell to the urethra (epididymis and deferent duct).

1 I. The **testicle (Testis or Orchis, −1)** lies in the scrotal cavity. It is invested by a firm tunica albuginea from which **connective tissue septa** radiate internally, joining together in the center of the testis to form the **mediastinum testis**. Between these septa, within the lobules of the testis, are the androgen producing interstitial or LEYDIG'S cells, and the convoluted seminiferous tubules *(Tubuli seminiferi convoluti)* that are continued by the straight seminiferous tubules *(Tubuli seminiferi recti)* into the rete testis, a tubular network within the mediastinum testis. The rete testis connects to 12 − 16 efferent ductules and by these to the epididymis (see clinical − functional anatomy).

2 II. The **epididymis** is divided into the thickened **head of the epididymis (16)**, which is the place where the efferent ductules unite to form the single epididymal duct, the slender **body of the epididymis (15)**, and the **tail of the epididymis (17)**, which is an enlargement at the caudal end of the body. The body and tail of the epididymis contain the strongly coiled epididymal duct, which has a length of several meters and, with a decrease in its coiling, is continued by the deferent duct at the medial aspect of the tail. The epididymis is the germ cell-conducting, germ cell-maturing, and for a limited period of time, a germ cell-storing organ.

3 III. The **deferent duct (ductus deferens, −8)** is the continuation of the epididymal duct. The first part of the deferent duct is in the **spermatic cord (26, −** see also p. 64), which is located within the **vaginal tunic (9)** of the peritoneum and extends to the **vaginal ring (4)**. The terminal portion of the deferent duct passes the vaginal ring and reaches the abdominal cavity. Just before its reaching the prostate, the duct has a very slight spindle-shaped enlargement **(ampulla of the ductus deferens, −5)** in the wall of which are accessory sex glands, the ampullary glands. The continuing narrow terminal part is surrounded by prostatic parenchyma and opens into the urethra on the **seminal**
4 **colliculus (24)**. Its opening is the *ejaculatory ostium*.

5 IV. The **prostate (23)** is the accessory sex gland, the ducts of which *(Ductuli prostatici)* open beside the seminal colliculus. The prostate has a **body (external part)** with two glandular lobes and a slight **disseminate part (internal part)**, the glandular lobules of which are located within the wall of the urethra and surrounded by the **urethralis muscle**. In other domestic mammals, there are in addition vesicular and bulbourethral glands.

b) The **EXTERNAL GENITAL ORGANS** are the penis and prepuce (see p. 33), the urethra, and the scrotum.

I. The penis consists of the **root of the penis**, the **body of the penis**, and the **glans penis** (designated here also as *Caput penis*) and is formed by two different types of cavernous body *(Corpora cavernosa)*. The one type is the **hard, paired erectile body (Corpus cavernosum penis or Corpus rigidum penis −18)***; the other part is the spongy, soft, **unpaired cavernous body of the urethra (Corpus spongiosum penis −19)**. On a cross-section through the penis, the tunica albuginea, trabeculae, and the cavernous tissue can be studied.

6 Erection of the penis is brought about by an increase in blood pressure within the vascular spaces of the cavernous tissue. This is the result of an increased inflow of blood that is supported by a dilatation of the penile arteries and a decrease in the drainage of the penile veins. At the **root of the penis**, each corpus cavernosum penis attaches to the ischial arch as a **crus penis (13)**. The corpus spongiosum penis, which is located between the crura, is well developed as the **bulb of the penis (12)** and is overlain by the bulbospongiosus muscle. In the area of the body of the penis both corpora cavernosa are fused at the median septum of the penis. They cover here roof-like the corpus spongiosum with its contained urethra. In the region of the glans penis, the paired
7 corpora cavernosa fuse to form the unpaired **os penis (22)**, which is hollowed out ventrally forming a deep groove. The unpaired corpus spongiosum penis, with the penile urethra that it envelops, lies in the ventromedian elongate groove of the penile bone. The **cavernous body of the glans (Corpus spongiosum glandis)** is derived from the corpus spongiosum penis. It consists of the prominent **bulb of the glans (21)**, which is at the level of the caudal third of the os penis, and cranial to the bulb, of the **long part of the glans (20)**.

II. The **masculine urethra (14)** commences at the **internal urethral ostium (25)** from the neck of the urinary bladder and ends at the **external urethral ostium (27)** at the tip of the glans of the penis. At the ejaculatory ostia, the path of the urine and that of the semen join. Caudal to the prostate, a cavernous body is present in the urethral wall. It is surrounded in circular fashion by the striated urethralis muscle. The pelvic part of the urethra passes over into the penile part in a caudally convex arch with a considerable increase in the girth of the erectile body.

The **blood supply** of the testicle, including the epididymis, is provided by the **testicular artery (7)**, which originates from the abdominal aorta about at the level of the third lumbar vertebra. It courses within the proximal mesorchium (vascular fold or *plica vasculosa*) and, within the spermatic cord, reaches the testicle before giving off its epididymal branches. The deferent duct, urethra and prostate are supplied by branches of the internal pudendal artery **(artery of the ductus deferens, −8**, and urethral and prostatic arteries). The penile artery of the internal pudendal artery gives off its artery of the bulb of the penis to the corpus spongiosum penis, including the corpus spongiosum glandis. Its deep artery of the penis passes to the corpus cavernosum penis, and its dorsal artery of the penis supplies parts of the corpus cavernosum penis, portions of the corpus spongiosum glandis and of the prepuce. The **testicular vein (7)** originates on the right side from the caudal vena cava, on the left from the left renal vein and forms the **pampiniform plexus (10)** dorsal to the head of the epididymis. The branches of the venous plexus enlace the testicular artery. The veins of the deferent duct, urethra and prostate drain − in the company of the same-named arteries (A. *ductus deferentis*, A. *urethralis* and A. *prostatica*) − the blood from the deferent duct, urethra and prostate to the internal pudendal vein. The penile veins accompany the same-named penile arteries. From the glans of the penis the blood is drained partially by the external pudendal vein by way of the inguinal space (inguinal rings and canal).

The **lymph drainage** of the testicle and epididymis, including the spermatic cord, is to the **medial iliac lymph nodes (2)** and the **lumbar aortic lymph nodes (1)**. From the prostate and the urethra the lymph reaches the **sacral (3) and medial iliac lymph nodes**. The **superficial inguinal or scrotal (6) lymph nodes** take up the lymph from the penis, prepuce and scrotum.

The **innervation** of the testicle and epididymis is by the testicular plexus and is within the spermatic cord. It has connections with the abdominal aortic and caudal mesenteric plexuses. The prostate and deferent plexuses supply the corresponding organs (prostate and deferent duct). They branch from the pelvic plexus and contain sympathetic, parasympathetic and sensory fibers. The pudendal nerve supplies the dorsal nerve of the penis, which conveys sensory, sympathetic and parasympathetic fibers.

c) The **LYMPH SYSTEM OF THE LUMBAR AND PELVIC REGIONS** is described in the following for both genders according to the natural direction of lymph flow in the caudocranial sequence.

The **sacral lymph nodes (2)** are located in the angle of origin between the right and left internal iliac arteries. The lymph flows from the nearby portions of the rectum and genital organs and from the sacrococcygeal vertebral column and their surroundings as well as the deep areas of the pelvic limbs. Efferent lymph vessels of the sacral nodes reach the medial iliac lymph nodes.

The **medial iliac lymph nodes (2)** lie at the aorta at the origin of the deep circumflex iliac artery (lateral iliac lymph nodes are absent in the dog). Afferent lymph vessels of the medial iliac lymph nodes proceed from the superficial inguinal lymph nodes and traverse the inguinal space. Moreover, they receive lymph from the abdominal and pelvic wall, the rectum, testicle, urinary bladder and the pelvic limb. The testicular lymph may bypass the medial iliac lymph nodes. For the most part the efferent vessels flow together into the lumbar trunk, which opens into the cisterna chyli. 8

The **lumbar aortic lymph nodes (1)** lie in an irregular manner along the abdominal aorta and receive the lesser part of the drainage of the medial iliac lymph nodes. Besides this, lymph from the caudal thoracic wall, abdominal wall, lumbar vertebral column and their surroundings and from the kidneys flows to the aortic lumbar nodes. Efferent vessels of these nodes open into the cisterna chyli.

*) In the formal nomenclature (Nomina Anatomica Veterinaria), the term corpus cavernosum penis is used.

Male genital organs

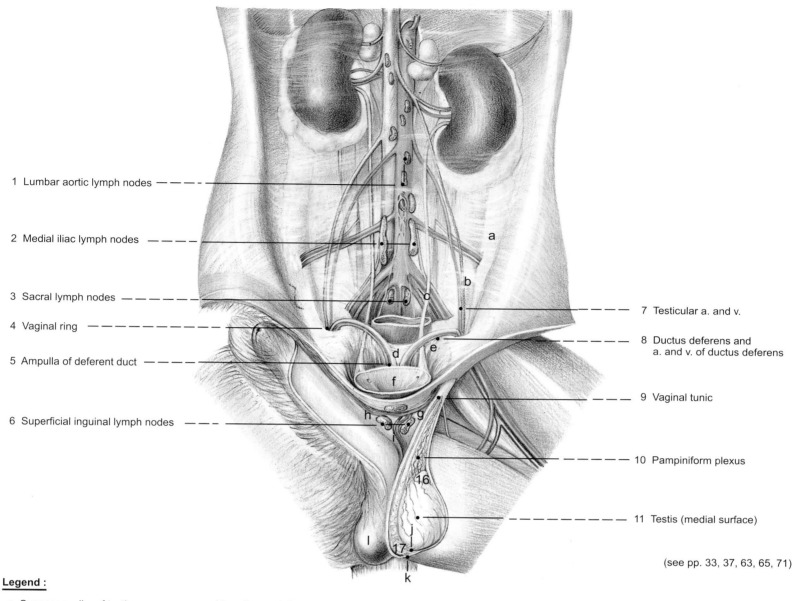

1 Lumbar aortic lymph nodes

2 Medial iliac lymph nodes

3 Sacral lymph nodes

4 Vaginal ring

5 Ampulla of deferent duct

6 Superficial inguinal lymph nodes

7 Testicular a. and v.

8 Ductus deferens and
   a. and v. of ductus deferens

9 Vaginal tunic

10 Pampiniform plexus

11 Testis (medial surface)

(see pp. 33, 37, 63, 65, 71)

Legend :

a Suspensory lig. of testis
b Prox. mesorchium
   [vascular fold]
c Ureter
d Plica genitalis

e Mesoductus deferens
   [deferential fold]
f Urinary bladder and
   Ureteral ostium
g Ext. pudendal a. and v.

h Caud. supf. epigastric a. and v.
i Ventral scrotal brr.
j Proper lig. of testis
k Lig. of tail of epididymis
l Scrotum

m Retractor penis m.
n Ischiocavernosus m.
o Urethralis m.
p Bulbospongiosus m.

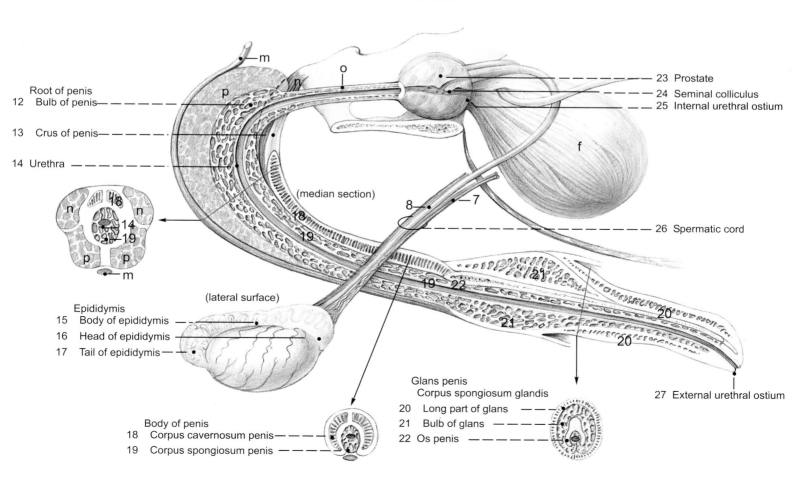

Root of penis
12 Bulb of penis

13 Crus of penis

14 Urethra

(median section)

(lateral surface)

Epididymis
15 Body of epididymis
16 Head of epididymis
17 Tail of epididymis

Body of penis
18 Corpus cavernosum penis
19 Corpus spongiosum penis

23 Prostate
24 Seminal colliculus
25 Internal urethral ostium

26 Spermatic cord

27 External urethral ostium

Glans penis
Corpus spongiosum glandis
20 Long part of glans
21 Bulb of glans
22 Os penis

69

5. ARTERIES, VEINS AND NERVES OF THE PELVIC CAVITY, ADRENAL GLANDS

The right pelvic limb together with the right portion of the bony pelvis is removed, preserving the arteries, veins, and nerves. The organs (rectum and urogenital organs) remain in the pelvic cavity. The pubic and ischiatic bones are cut with the saw a fingerbreadth to the right and parallel to the pelvic symphysis. The right ilium is separated from the sacrum at the sacroiliac joint. Then, the right crus of the penis (crus of the clitoris in the female) is cut from the ischial arch as well as the muscles, arteries, veins and nerves that course between thigh and pelvis.

a) The **TERMINAL DIVISION OF THE AORTA (21)** into the single median sacral artery and the paired external and internal iliac arteries is at the level of the last lumbar vertebra.

The unpaired **median sacral artery (18)** continues caudally from the aorta ventral to the sacrum and passes over caudally into the median coccygeal (caudal) artery.

The **external iliac artery (12)** is accompanied laterally by the genitofemoral nerve. Shortly before it traverses the vascular lacuna (*Lacuna vasorum*), the artery ends by dividing into **deep femoral (13)** and femoral arteries. Before its reaching the deep muscles of the medial thigh, the deep femoral artery dispatches the **pudendoepigastric trunk (14)** that divides into the **external pudendal artery (15)**, which traverses the inguinal space (canal), and the **caudal epigastric artery (27)**, which courses on the internal surface of the rectus abdominis muscle and anastomoses at the level of the umbilicus with the same-named cranial artery. The latter artery originates from the internal thoracic artery. On the external surface of the rectus abdominis muscle, at the level of the umbilicus, there is a superficial anastomosis between the superficial cranial epigastric artery and the superficial caudal epigastric artery. The cranial artery is a branch of the internal thoracic artery and the caudal artery passes from the external pudendal artery. It is not uncommon for the caudal epigastric and external pudendal arteries to arise independently from the deep femoral artery and, in that case, no pudendoepigastric trunk is formed.

At its origin, the **internal iliac artery (17)** gives off the umbilical artery that runs in the lateral ligament of the urinary bladder, and is either completely obliterated to form the **round ligament of the bladder** or as a cranial vesical artery supplies the cranial part of the urinary bladder. After a short course, the internal iliac artery ends by dividing into the **caudal gluteal artery (6)** and **internal pudendal artery (9)**. The caudal gluteal gives off the **iliolumbar (1)**, **cranial gluteal (3)**, **lateral coccygeal (caudal) (7)** and the **dorsal perineal artery (8)**, which as parietal arteries supply the pelvic wall. Before it enters the ischiorectal fossa, the internal pudendal artery gives off a visceral vessel for pelvic cavity organs; that is, the vaginal (female) or prostatic (male) artery with the middle rectal artery passing from its caudal branch and the uterine (female) or deferent artery (male), including the caudal vesical artery, passing from its cranial branch. The **vaginal artery (11)** and the corresponding **prostatic artery (11)** run ventrally, almost perpendicularly, to their area of supply, to the vagina or the prostate. The middle **rectal artery (10)** supplies the ventrolateral aspect of the ampulla of the rectum. The **uterine artery (24)** courses near the insertion of the mesometrium and anastomoses with the **uterine branch (23)** of the **ovarian artery (22)**. The ovarian artery is a direct branch of the aorta at the level of the 3rd lumbar vertebra. The **artery of the ductus deferens (24)** accompanies the deferent duct to the epididymis. When there is complete obliteration of the umbilical artery, the **caudal vesical artery (26)** supplies the entire urinary bladder.

BLOOD VESSELS OF THE PELVIC CAVITY

Aorta	Caudal vena cava
Median sacral a.	Median sacral v.
Median coccygeal (caudal) a.	Median coccygeal (caudal) v.
External iliac a.	Common iliac v.
Deep femoral a.	External iliac v.
Pudendoepigastric trunk	Deep femoral v.
Internal iliac a.	Pudendoepigastric v.
Umbilical a.	Internal iliac v.
Caudal gluteal a.	Iliolumbar v.
Iliolumbar a.	Vaginal or prostatic v.
Cranial gluteal a.	Uterine v. or v. of the ductus
Lateral coccygeal (caudal) a.	deferens
Dorsal perineal a.	Caudal vesical v.
Internal pudendal a.	Middle rectal v.
Vaginal or prostatic a.	Cranial gluteal v.
Uterine a. or a. of the ductus	Lateral coccygeal (caudal) v.
deferens	Caudal gluteal v.
Caudal vesical a.	Dorsal perineal v.
Middle rectal a.	Internal pudendal v.

b) The **terminal division of the caudal vena cava (20)** is at the level of the last lumbar vertebra where the very slight **median sacral vein (18)** continues the caudal course of the caudal vena cava. At this level, the caudal vena cava divides into the large right and left **common iliac veins (19)** that branch at the pelvic inlet into external and internal iliac veins. The **internal iliac vein (17)**, compared to the same-named artery, is very long and releases the visceral venous trunk (vaginal vein, female; prostatic vein, male) that accompanies the same-named artery that is a branch of the internal pudendal artery. After giving off the **iliolumbar vein (1)**, **cranial gluteal vein (3)** and **lateral coccygeal (caudal) vein (7)**, the long internal iliac vein is continued at the origin of the **last parietal vein (caudal gluteal vein, —6)**, at the level of the third caudal vertebra, by the **internal pudendal vein (9)**. The caudal gluteal vein gives off the **dorsal perineal vein (8)**.

c) The **SACRAL PLEXUS** of the lumbosacral plexus is formed by the ventral branches of the last two lumbar nerves and the sacral nerves. It can be subdivided into a stronger cranial part (lumbosacral trunk) and a weaker caudal part.

I. The **lumbosacral trunk (16)** originates from nLv 6 and nLv 7 as well as nSv 1 and gives off the **cranial gluteal nerve (3)** and **caudal gluteal nerve (6)**, which are accompanied by the same named blood vessels and supply the gluteal muscles and the skin overlying them. The lumbosacral plexus is then continued by the **ischiadic nerve (4)**, which crosses the greater ischiadic notch laterally to reach the thigh.

II. The **caudal part of the sacral plexus** gives off the **pudendal nerve** (nSv 1 – nSv 3, —9), which enters the ischiorectal fossa, accompanied by the internal pudendal artery and vein (see p. 73). The **caudal cutaneous femoral nerve (5)** originates mostly –with considerable individual variation in its origin – from nSv 2 and nSv 3. At its origin, it gives off muscular branches for the coccygeus and levator ani muscles (some authors regard these branches as independent branches of the sacral plexus), courses ventrolaterally along the sacrotuberous ligament, passes the ischiadic tuber and ends in the skin of the caudolateral thigh. Branches, as caudal clunial nerves, supply the gluteal region.

The caudal clunial nerves (see p. 73) consist also of cutaneous branches of the caudal gluteal nerve, which, together with the same-named blood vessels, enter the tela subcutanea proximally at the caudal border of the superficial gluteal muscle.

The middle clunial nerves (see p. 73) are formed by weak dorsal branches of the sacral nerves and by a cutaneous branch of the cranial gluteal nerve, which with the same-named blood vessels reaches the skin proximally at the cranial border of the superficial gluteal muscle. The cranial clunial nerves (see p. 29) are formed by dorsal branches of the lumbar cutaneous nerves and supply the skin of the lumbar region.

d) The **parasympathetic nervous system of the sacral spinal cord** is composed of the **pelvic nerves (2)**, which extend perpendicularly upon the lateral wall of the rectum at the level of the vaginal fornix or of the prostate and meet the horizontally running hypogastric nerve to form the pelvic plexus. The pelvic plexus consists of sympathetic and parasympathetic and visceral sensory fibers and contains within it small pelvic ganglia. From the plexus, which is delicate, nerves course in the company of blood vessels to the different organs of the pelvic cavity as rectal, vesical, prostatic, deferential, and uterovaginal plexuses.

e) The **ADRENAL GLANDS** (see p. 63) are endocrine glands that lie craniomedial to the kidney. Their cortical part has a yellowish tinge owing to the content of stored lipid substances utilized in the synthesis of steroid hormones. The yellow color is visible on the sectioned surface of the gland. The brownish to gray part of the sectioned gland, the medulla, produces the hormones epinephrine and norepinephrine (see textbooks of biochemistry). Both adrenals lie retroperitoneally and are incompletely divided ventrally into cranial and caudal parts by the cranial abdominal vein that lies in a deep transverse groove of the gland. The right adrenal is the more cranially situated and lies next to the caudal vena cava; the left adrenal abuts on the abdominal aorta.

Their **blood supply** is multiple and is from the suprarenal arteries and veins that originate from the aorta or the caudal vena cava, respectively. Branches may arise from the caudal phrenic artery and vein, from the cranial abdominal artery and vein, and from the renal artery and vein.

The adrenal capillaries arise from the suprarenal arteries that, one after the other, traverse the cortex and medulla. Suprarenal veins receive the blood from the central vein of the adrenal medulla.

The **lymph** flows to the lumbar aortic lymph nodes. **Autonomic innervation** is predominantly sympathetic by way of the suprarenal plexus, which communicates with the major splanchnic nerve and the celiacomesenteric plexus.

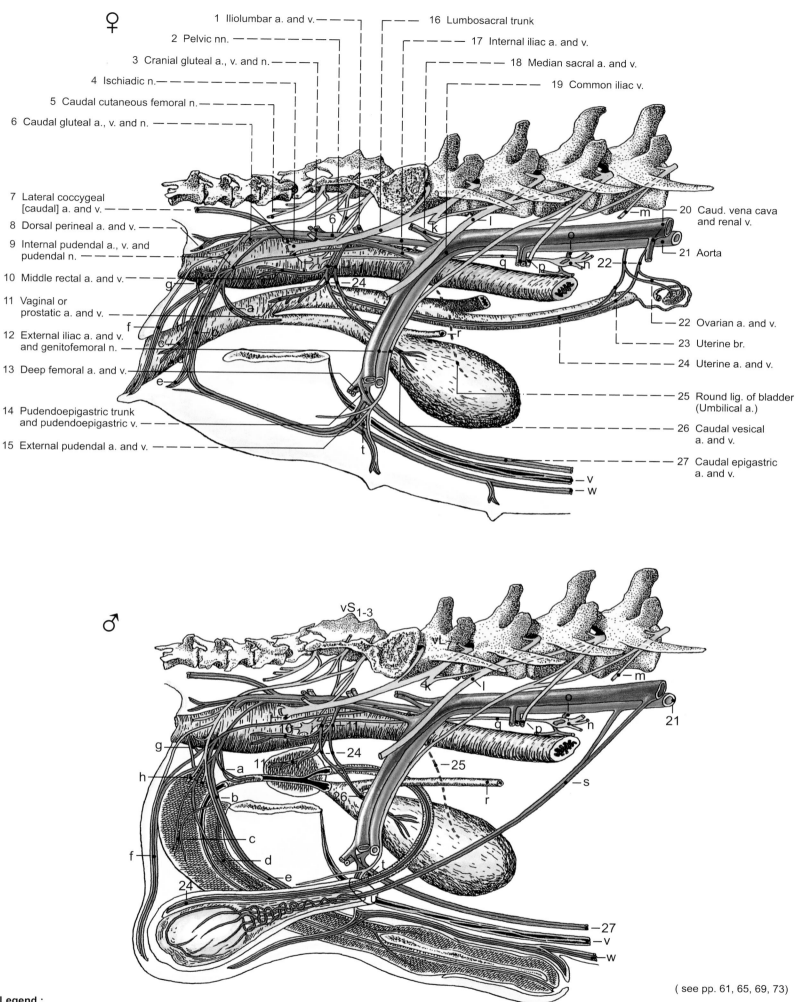

♀

1 Iliolumbar a. and v.
2 Pelvic nn.
3 Cranial gluteal a., v. and n.
4 Ischiadic n.
5 Caudal cutaneous femoral n.
6 Caudal gluteal a., v. and n.

7 Lateral coccygeal [caudal] a. and v.
8 Dorsal perineal a. and v.
9 Internal pudendal a., v. and pudendal n.
10 Middle rectal a. and v.
11 Vaginal or prostatic a. and v.
12 External iliac a. and v. and genitofemoral n.
13 Deep femoral a. and v.
14 Pudendoepigastric trunk and pudendoepigastric v.
15 External pudendal a. and v.

16 Lumbosacral trunk
17 Internal iliac a. and v.
18 Median sacral a. and v.
19 Common iliac v.

20 Caud. vena cava and renal v.
21 Aorta

22 Ovarian a. and v.
23 Uterine br.
24 Uterine a. and v.
25 Round lig. of bladder (Umbilical a.)
26 Caudal vesical a. and v.
27 Caudal epigastric a. and v.

♂

vS₁₋₃

vL

(see pp. 61, 65, 69, 73)

Legend :

a Urethral a. and v.
b A. and v. of clitoris or penis
c A. and v. of penile bulb
d Deep a., v. and n. of clitoris or penis
e Dorsal a., v. and n. of clitoris or penis

f Ventr. perineal a. and v. and supf. perineal n.
g Caud. rectal a., v. and n.
h Deep perineal nn.
i Pelvic ganglion
j Muscular brr. (rotator n.)
k Obturator n.

l Femoral n.
m Ilioinguinal n.
n Lumbar splanchnic nn.
o Caud. mesenteric a. and ggl.
p Deep circumflex iliac a. and v. and lat. cutaneous femoral n.

q Hypogastric n.
r Ureter
s Testicular a. and v.
t Supf. inguinal ln.
u Peritoneal vaginal process
v Rectus abdominis m.

w Caud. supf. epigastric a. and v.

71

6. PELVIC DIAPHRAGM, ISCHIORECTAL FOSSA; ASSOCIATED ARTERIES, VEINS AND NERVES

For the following dissection the skin is removed, making the incision around the anus and the vulvar lips (Labia pudendi s. Labia vulvae). After docking the tail, the remaining root of the tail is fixed dorsally. In this dissection, which is on the right side of the body, first the muscles, or stumps of the muscles as the case may be, are dissected, and this is followed by dissection of the arteries, veins and nerves. After this, also on the left side of the body, the arteries, veins and nerves are dissected and then the muscles.

The **pelvic outlet** in its middle region is closed off by the pelvic diaphragm which abuts the ischiorectal fossa on either side. The perineal region is superficial at the pelvic outlet and extends in the shape of a rhombus between the root of the tail, the ischiadic tubers of both sides and the caudal end of the pelvic symphysis. In the male dog, and in the bitch in which the vulva hangs considerably, the ventral border extends ventrally to the scrotum or to the ventral border of the vulva. In this expanded area of the perineal region, the body wall forms the perineum, so far as this is clinically useful and broadly defined. In the more narrow definition, the perineum is only the proper perineum between anus and vulva, which is formed superficially by the longitudinal perineal cutaneous muscle and, deeply, by a tendomuscular plate of insertion for neighboring muscles, the tendinous center of the perineum (perineal body).

a) The **PELVIC DIAPHRAGM** is the musculofascial closure of the pelvic outlet that is found internally and caudally at the pelvis. It is formed by the levator ani muscle of both sides with bilaterally adjacent coccygeus muscle and both lamellae of the diaphragmatic fasica of the pelvis. Looking into the pelvic cavity, a dorsoventrally arranged, longitudinal opening is recognizable in the slight depression between the bilateral levator ani muscles. This 'levator door' is closed dorsally in the anal part of the pelvic diaphragm by the anal canal with surrounding musculature and ventrally in the urogenital part of the pelvic diaphragm by the urogenital canal with surrounding musculature as well as in between by the proper perineum.

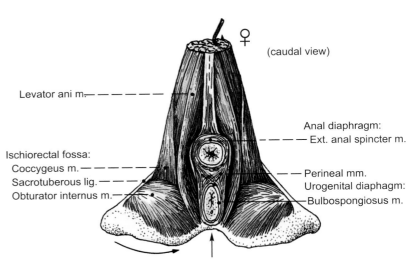

b) The **ISCHIORECTAL FOSSA** is the pyramidal pelvic outlet fossa with a cranial apex and a caudally situated, open, base. The lateral boundary is the ischiadic tuberosity and the sacrotuberous ligament that attaches there. The ventral boundary is the ischial arch including the internal obturator muscle, and the medial boundary, the pelvic diaphragm with the levator ani and coccygeus muscles. The ischiorectal fossa is filled by a pad of fat and arteries, veins, and nerves gathered in neurovascular bundles.

PELVIC DIAPHRAGM WITH COCCYGEUS AND LEVATOR ANI MUSCLES

Anal part of the pelvic diaphragm	Perineum proper	Urogenital part of the pelvic diaphragm
External anal sphincter muscle	Perineal muscles	Bulbospongiosus muscle
Internal anal sphincter muscle	Longitudinal cutaneous muscle of the perineum	Constrictor vestibuli muscle
Rectococcygeus muscle	Tendinous center of the perineum	Constrictor vulvae muscle
	(Perineal body)	Ischiocavernosus muscle
		Retractor penis or retractor clitoridis muscle

The **coccygeus muscle (13)** is situated medially beside the sacrotuberous ligament and courses between the ischiadic spine and the first four caudal vertebrae. The fibers of the **levator ani muscle (12,** —see also text-illustration) have a similar course; the muscle is located medial to the coccygeus. Its origin is linear and lies beside the pelvic symphysis at the ischiadic and pubic bones and ascends from here caudodorsally to the tail. Its tapering insertion is on the 4th to the 7th caudal vertebrae. Different from human beings, only a very few muscle fibers contact the sphincter ani externus muscle, so that in the dog, the function-related name of the muscle is a bit misleading. In bilateral contraction the tail is drawn ventrally, clamped down.

The **external anal sphincter muscle (14)**, together with the internal anal sphincter muscle, surrounds the anal canal. The sphincter ani internus muscle is the caudal continuation of the circular layer of smooth muscle of the rectum. The anal sac (paranal sinus) lies between the striated and smooth sphincter muscle of the anus.

Rectococcygeus muscle (11) and **retractor penis (clitoridis) muscle (19)**; see p. 74.

The **perineal muscles (15)** consist of longitudinally running bundles of muscle that extend between the external anal sphincter and the bulbospongiosus muscles or, resp., the constrictor vestibuli muscle.

The **bulbospongiosus muscle (20)** runs transversely across the bulb of the penis of the male dog. In the bitch, the muscle consists of the **constrictor vestibuli muscle (77)** with a roughly circular course of its fibers and the caudally following **constrictor vulvae muscle (18)** with a nearly longitudinal course of its fibers. The **ischiocavernosus muscle (16)** originates at the ischiadic arch and covers the crus of the clitoris or the crus penis.

The **innervation** of the coccygeus and levator ani muscles is by muscular branches of nSv 3. The other muscles are supplied by branches of the pudendal nerve; that is, the muscles of the anal part by the caudal rectal nerve, and the muscle of the urogenital part and those of the perineum by the deep perineal nerves.

c) NEUROVASCULAR BUNDLES traverse the pudendal canal to reach the fundus of the ischiorectal fossa.

The **pudendal nerve (2)** runs between the internal obturator muscle and the coccygeus muscle caudoventrally and medially into the ischiorectal fossa. It gives off the **caudal rectal nerve (3)** for the anal part of the pelvic diaphragm,

the long **superficial perineal nerve (7)** with originating dorsal labial or dorsal scrotal nerves for the skin and the short **deep perineal nerves (6)** for the muscle of the urogenital part of the pelvic diaphragm. The pudendal nerve ends on the dorsum of the clitoris (which, owing to the caudoventral course of the clitoris, is actually the ventral surface of the clitoris) as the **dorsal clitoridal nerve (5)** or, respectively, as the **dorsal nerve of the penis (10)** on the dorsum penis.

The **internal pudendal artery (2)** accompanies the pudendal nerve and gives off the urethral artery for the pelvic part of the urethra. It then gives off the **ventral perineal artery (8)** that, in turn, near its origin, gives off the caudodorsally directed **caudal rectal artery (3)**, and distally the caudoventrally directed dorsal labial or, respectively, dorsal scrotal branch. The internal pudendal is continued as the **artery of the clitoris (4)** or, respectively, **artery of the penis (9)**. The artery of the clitoris (4) gives off the large artery of the vestibular bulb and ends by dividing into the very small dorsal artery of the clitoris and the deep artery of the clitoris. The artery of the penis gives off the large artery of the bulb of the penis, the smaller deep artery of the penis, which enters the crus of the penis, and continues as the dorsal artery of the penis, which is usually of moderate size. The **dorsal perineal artery (1)** arises from the caudal gluteal artery.

The **internal pudendal vein** (see p. 71) accompanies only the caudal part of the same-named artery. It has a course similar to the artery but the sequence of its branches is different.

ARTERIES AND NERVES OF THE ISCHIORECTAL FOSSA

Internal pudendal artery	Pudendal nerve
Urethral artery	Caudal rectal nerve
Ventral perineal artery	Superficial perineal nerve
Caudal rectal artery	Dorsal labial nerves or
Dorsal labial branch or	Dorsal scrotal nerves
Dorsal scrotal branch	Deep perineal nerves
Artery of the clitoris or	Dorsal nerve of the clitoris or
Artery of the penis	Dorsal nerve of the penis
Artery of the vestibular bulb or	**Caudal cutaneous femoral nerve**
Artery of the bulb of the penis	
Deep artery of the clitoris or	
Deep artery of the penis	
Dorsal artery of the clitoris or	
Dorsal artery of the penis	

Ischiorectal fossa

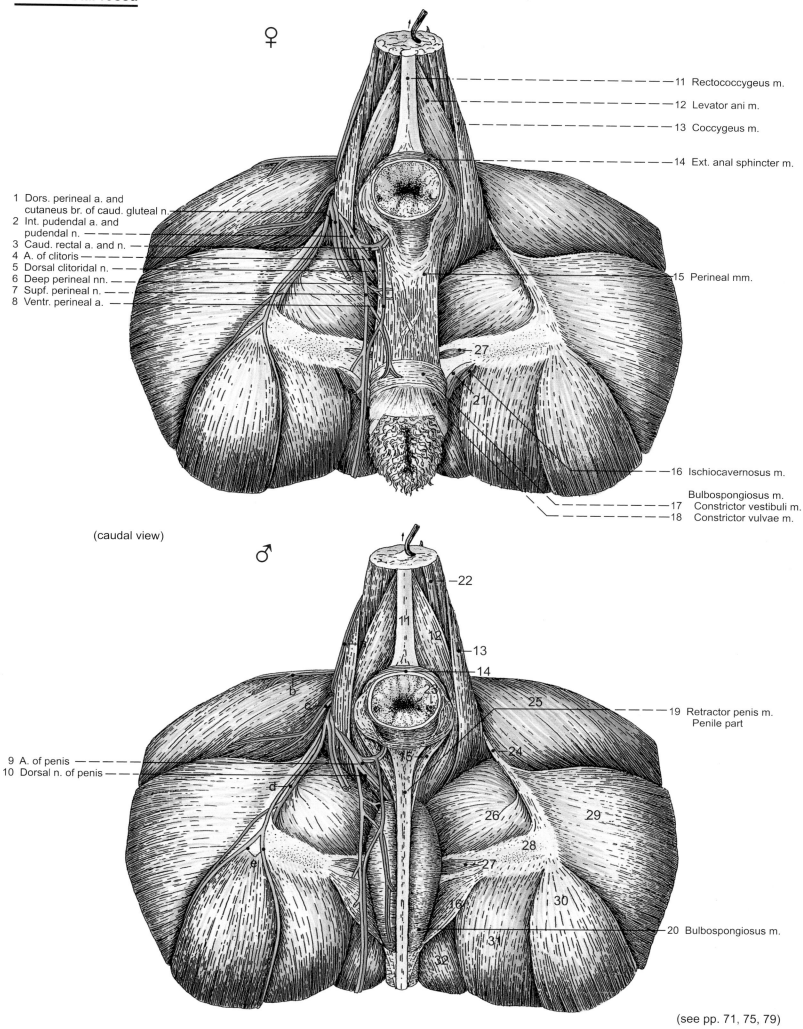

♀

(caudal view)

♂

1 Dors. perineal a. and
  cutaneus br. of caud. gluteal n.
2 Int. pudendal a. and
  pudendal n.
3 Caud. rectal a. and n.
4 A. of clitoris
5 Dorsal clitoridal n.
6 Deep perineal nn.
7 Supf. perineal n.
8 Ventr. perineal a.

9 A. of penis
10 Dorsal n. of penis

11 Rectococcygeus m.
12 Levator ani m.
13 Coccygeus m.
14 Ext. anal sphincter m.

15 Perineal mm.

16 Ischiocavernosus m.

Bulbospongiosus m.
17 Constrictor vestibuli m.
18 Constrictor vulvae m.

19 Retractor penis m.
   Penile part

20 Bulbospongiosus m.

(see pp. 71, 75, 79)

Legend :

21 Crus of Clitoris
22 Sacrocaudalis [-coccygeus] ventr.
   lat. and med. mm.
23 Ostium of paranal sinus
24 Sacrotuberous lig.

25 Supf. gluteal m.
26 Obturator int. m.
27 Ischiourethralis m.
28 Ischiatic tuberosity
29 Biceps femoris m.

30 Semitendinosus m.
31 Semimembranosus m.
32 Gracilis m.

a Lat. caudal [coccygeal] a.
b Cran. gluteal a. and
  middle clunial nn.
c Caud. gluteal a. (cutaneous brr.)
  and caud. (dors.) clunial nn.

d Caud. gluteal a. and
  caud. cutaneous femoral n.
e Caud. (lat. and med.)
  clunial nn.

73

7. SMOOTH MUSCLE OF THE PELVIC DIAPHRAGM AND THE BONY PELVIC GIRDLE

After cranial reflection of the free caudal border of the levator ani muscle and after caudal reflection of the anus with surrounding sphincter muscles, the smooth musculature can be seen in overall view.

a) The **SMOOTH MUSCLES OF THE PELVIC DIAPHRAGM** pass between the viscera and the skeletal system.

I. The unpaired **rectococcygeus muscle (A)** is a reinforcement of the longitudinal smooth muscle of the rectum, running ventromedian at the caudal vertebral column to the third caudal vertebra.

II. The paired **retractor clitoridis muscle** or **retractor penis muscle** begins under the levator ani muscle at the first caudal vertebra and divides caudolaterally on the rectum into three parts that lie next to each other in the following dorsoventral sequence: The strong **anal part (B)** inserts dorsolateral at the anus between the anal muscles. The moderately strong **penile part (C)** meets with the corresponding muscle of the opposite side caudomedian at the perineum and runs ventromedian on the penis cranially. The **clitoridal part (C)** of the bitch is weak and does not reach the clitoris. The **rectal part (D)** is weak or absent. If well developed, it loops around the rectum ventrally, which in the horse is very distinctly expressed and led to the naming of it as 'rectal loop.'

b) The **BONY PELVIC GIRDLE** (Cingulum membri pelvini, —see also text-illustration) consists of both hip bones (Ossa coxarum), the three individual bones of which are completely fused in the adult. The hip bones of both sides jointly form the ventromedian located **pelvic symphysis (1)** and are separated dorsally by the sacrum. Together with the sacrum and the first two caudal vertebrae, they form the bony pelvis. Of the three fused individual bones of the hip bone, the pubic bone and the ischiadic bone bound the **obturator foramen (2)** and both bones fuse with the third, the iliac bone, at the **acetabulum (3)**. In the depth of the acetabulum (**acetabular fossa, —4**) of fetuses and puppies a tiny fourth bone is found (acetabular bone) that fuses at an early age with the other components of the hip bone. The strong ligament of the femoral head courses between the acetabular fossa and the head of the femoral bone. The **acetabular notch (5)**, which is bridged over by the transverse acetabular ligament, is a ventromedial interruption of the **lunate surface (5)**. On the acetabular border the acetabular lip (Labrum acetabulare) is found. It is made up of fibrocartilage and deepens the acetabular fossa. Dorsal to the acetabulum in the dog the blunt-bordered **ischiadic spine (7)** is located. It is formed in the border area between the iliac and ischiadic bones, where they fuse. Cranially, the iliac bone borders the pubic bone at the **iliopubic eminence (34)**. The pubic bones of right and left sides unite to form the cranial part of the pelvic symphysis and the ischiadic bones of either side join to form the caudal part of the pelvic symphysis.

which, in the dog, is identical to the cranial ventral iliac spine. The **sacral tuber (14,** —lies opposite at the dorsocaudal border of the wing of the ilium and extends from the **cranial dorsal iliac spine (15)** to the **caudal dorsal iliac spine (16)**. The **gluteal surface (17)** is the surface of origin of the gluteal muscles laterally on the wing of the ilium, where at the level of the alar spine the indistinct **ventral gluteal line (17')** and at the level of the caudal ventral iliac spine the **caudal gluteal line (17")** begin. The medial surface of the wing of the ilium is the **sacropelvic surface (18)**, which is subdivided into the tuberculate, ear-shaped **auricular surface (Facies auricularis, —19)**, for the articulation with the sacrum, and into the dorsally continuing smooth-surfaced **iliac surface (20)** for the insertion of the longissimus dorsi and iliocostalis muscles. Cranioventrally at the ilium the **arcuate line (21)**, together with the dorsally located promontory of the sacrum and the ventrally located **pecten ossis pubis (33)**, participates in the formation of the terminal line. At midlevel, the arcuate line exhibits the very indistinct **psoas minor tubercle (22)**. Opposite to that, on the caudodorsal border of the iliac wing, is the **greater ischiadic notch (23)**. It extends from the caudal dorsal iliac spine of the sacral tuber to the ischiadic spine and furnishes the passage for the ischiadic nerve.

II. The **ischiadic bone** or **ischium** with its **body (24,** —Corpus ossis ischii) forms part of the acetabulum and passes over caudally into the horizontal **ischiadic table (25)**. The **symphysial branch of the ischium (26)**, which follows medially, participates with that of the opposite side in the formation of the caudal part of the pelvic symphysis. Laterodorsally opposite is the **lesser ischiadic notch (27)** that caudolaterally at the **ischiadic tuber (28,** —Tuber ischiadicum) passes over into the concave **ischiadic arch (29)**. Ischiadic arch and ischiadic tuber, jointly with the sacrotuberous ligament and the third caudal vertebra, border the pelvic outlet.

III. The **pubic bone** or **pubis** with its **body (30,** —Corpus ossis pubis) contributes to the formation of the acetabulum. From the body, as the **cranial ramus (32)**, it extends caudomedially in the direction of the pelvic symphysis and, at the symphysis, caudally as the **caudal ramus (symphysial ramus, —31)**. At the pelvic inlet the cranial ramus bears the **pecten ossis pubis (33)**, which extends from the laterally located **iliopubic eminence (34)** to the median situated **ventral pubic tubercle (35)**. On the internal surface of the pubic bone the direction of the course of the obturator nerve can be seen as the obturator sulcus.

c) The **PELVIC DIAMETERS** (see also text-illustration) are of importance in obstetrics in the evaluation of the natural birth passage. The **vertical diameter** is the vertical line from the cranial end of the pelvic symphysis to the vertebral column. The **conjugate diameter** extends from the cranial end of the pelvic symphysis to the promontory of the sacrum. Transverse diameters are present as a **dorsal transverse diameter** between the two ends of the sacral wings, as a **middle transverse diameter** between the right and left psoas minor tubercles, and as the **ventral transverse diameter** between the two iliopubic eminences.

Os coxae

(medial view)

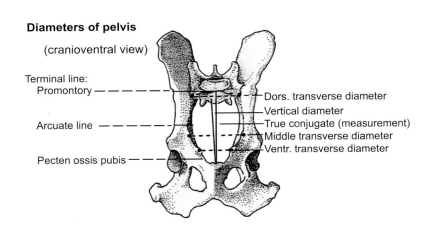

Diameters of pelvis

(cranioventral view)

Terminal line:
Promontory

Arcuate line

Pecten ossis pubis

Dors. transverse diameter
Vertical diameter
True conjugate (measurement)
Middle transverse diameter
Ventr. transverse diameter

I. The **body (8)** of the **iliac bone** or **ilium** takes part in the formation of the acetabulum (which is also true for the body of the pubic and ischiadic bones). The **caudal ventral iliac spine (9,** —area of origin of the rectus femoris muscle) is craniodorsal to the acetabulum; it is at the transition to the **wing of the ilium (10)**. The **alar spine (11,** —area of insertion of the caudal tendon of the quadratus lumborum muscle) is located at the cranioventral border of the wing of the ilium; that is, a thumbbreadth ventral to its transition into the dorsally situated, cartilage-covered **iliac crest (12)**. Here, at the transition, the **tuber coxae (13)** is found at the lateral angle of the ilium,

d) The **TERMINAL LINE** is the boundary between the abdominal and pelvic cavities. In human beings and domestic mammals the terminal line is formed by the promontory of the sacrum, the arcuate line of the ilium, and by the pecten ossis pubis.

e) Different from the situation in the erect human being, the **PELVIC FLOOR** is formed by the pubis and ischium with the obturator foramen that they contain.

Anal and urogenital muscles

(caudolateral view)

♀

Legend :

A Rectococcygeus m.
   Retractor clitoridis or penis m.
B   Anal part
C   Clitoridal or penile part
D   Rectal part
E   Sphincter ani ext. m.
F   Vertebral part
G   Paranal sinus
H   Longitudinal perineal
    cutaneous m.
I   Ischiourethralis m.
J   Ischiocavernosus m.
K   Bulbospongiosus m.
L   Constrictor vestibuli m.
M   Constrictor vulvae m.
N   Sacrocaudalis [-coccygeus]
    dors. lat. m.
O   Dorsal caud.
    intertransverse m.
P   Levator ani m.
Q   Coccygeus m.
R   Supf. gluteal m.
S   Middle gluteal m.
T   Sacrotuberous lig.
U   Obturator int. m.
V   Semimembranosus m.
W   Semitendinosus m.
X   Biceps femoris m.

(see pp. 73, 79)

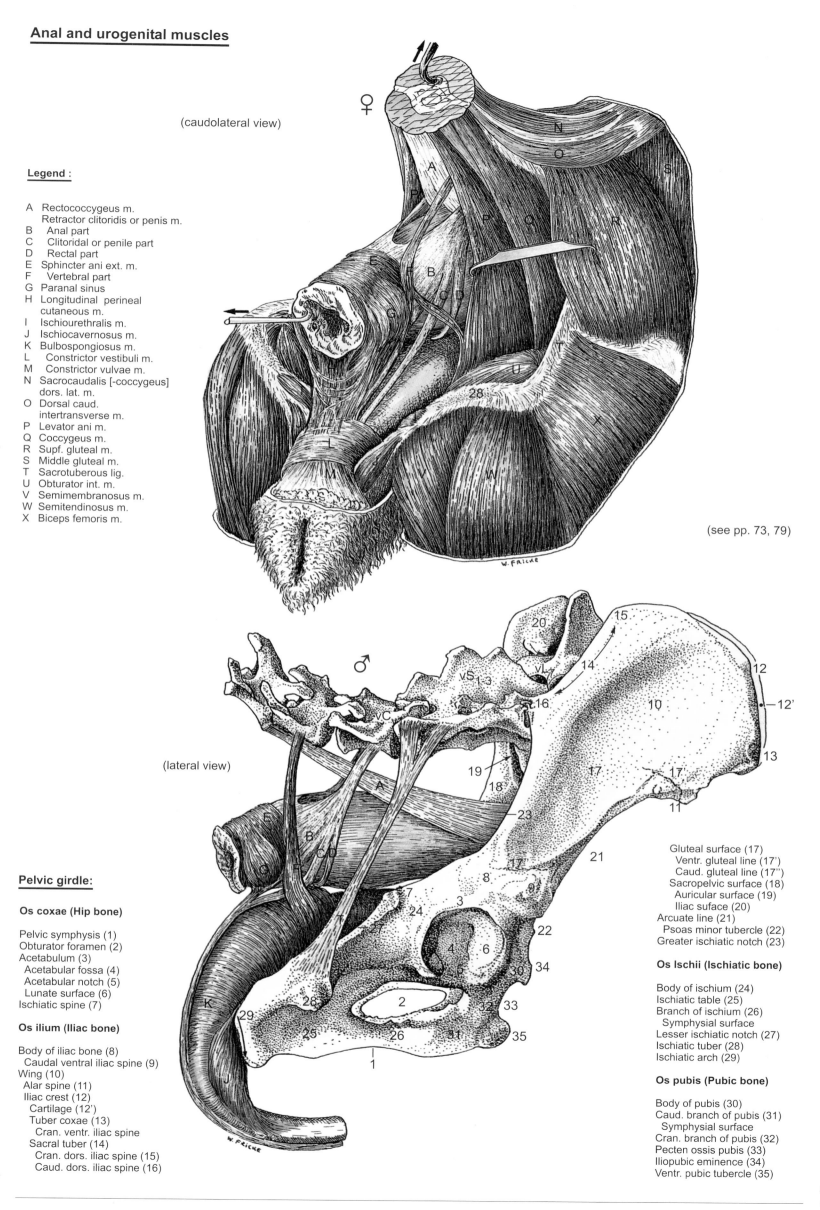

(lateral view)

♂

Pelvic girdle:

Os coxae (Hip bone)

Pelvic symphysis (1)
Obturator foramen (2)
Acetabulum (3)
  Acetabular fossa (4)
  Acetabular notch (5)
  Lunate surface (6)
Ischiatic spine (7)

Os ilium (Iliac bone)

Body of iliac bone (8)
Caudal ventral iliac spine (9)
Wing (10)
 Alar spine (11)
 Iliac crest (12)
   Cartilage (12')
  Tuber coxae (13)
   Cran. ventr. iliac spine
  Sacral tuber (14)
   Cran. dors. iliac spine (15)
   Caud. dors. iliac spine (16)

Gluteal surface (17)
  Ventr. gluteal line (17')
  Caud. gluteal line (17'')
Sacropelvic surface (18)
  Auricular surface (19)
  Iliac suface (20)
Arcuate line (21)
Psoas minor tubercle (22)
Greater ischiatic notch (23)

Os Ischii (Ischiatic bone)

Body of ischium (24)
Ischiatic table (25)
Branch of ischium (26)
  Symphysial surface
Lesser ischiatic notch (27)
Ischiatic tuber (28)
Ischiatic arch (29)

Os pubis (Pubic bone)

Body of pubis (30)
Caud. branch of pubis (31)
  Symphysial surface
Cran. branch of pubis (32)
Pecten ossis pubis (33)
Iliopubic eminence (34)
Ventr. pubic tubercle (35)

CHAPTER 8: PELVIC LIMB

1. THE SKELETON OF THE PELVIC LIMB

The **PELVIC LIMB** also includes the pelvic girdle. For the study of common characteristics in the structural plan of thoracic and pelvic limbs, the description of the thoracic limb should also be considered here.

a) The **FEMORAL BONE** (Os femoris, the bone of the thigh, commonly designated simply 'femur') consists proximally of a head, a thin neck, prominent muscular processes (trochanters) and a body or shaft that is continuous distally with the femoral trochlea and condyles. The **head of the femur (1)** bears an articular surface covered with cartilage except for a small, nearly central area, the **fovea capitis (2)**, which is the site of attachment of the ligament of the head of the femur. The ligament is attached to the acetabulum at the acetabular fossa. The **neck of the femur (3)** is a distinct narrowing of the bone between the head and the muscular processes. The lateral process, the **greater trochanter (4)**, is largest and is the site of attachment of the middle and deep gluteal muscles. Caudomedial to the base of the greater trochanter is the **trochanteric fossa (5)**, a deep depression that serves for the insertion of deep muscles of the coxal joint. Medial to the trochanteric fossa is the **lesser (or 'minor') trochanter (6)**, which is the insertion of the iliopsoas muscle. The **gluteal tuberosity** (not illustrated) is in the dog a small elevation of bone distal to the greater trochanter; it is the attachment of the superficial gluteal muscle. The **body (shaft) of the femur (8)** is long and exhibits caudally the **facies aspera (9)**, which is a rough area for insertion of the adductor magnus and adductor brevis muscles. The facies is bounded by a **lateral lip (labium, −10)** and a **medial lip (11)**. The **popliteal surface (12)** that follows the facies aspera distally is bordered laterally by the **lateral supracondylar tuberosity (13)**, a roughness for the origin of the lateral head of the gastrocnemius and the superficial digital flexor muscles. A **medial supracondylar tuberosity** is the origin of the medial head of the gastrocnemius. The **medial femoral condyle (14)** bears caudally a smooth **articular surface for the medial sesamoid bone (15)** for articulation with the **sesamoid bone of the gastrocnemius (64)** and a prominent **medial epicondyle (16)** for the attachment of the medial collateral ligament of the femorotibial joint. The **lateral femoral condyle (17)** with its **articular surface for the lateral sesamoid bone (18)** and **lateral epicondyle (19)** has a corresponding configuration. The **intercondylar fossa (20)** cranially abuts on the **femoral trochlea (21)**, which acts as a gliding surface for the **patella (69)** between the two ridges of the trochlea.

b) The tibia and fibula are the **BONES OF THE CRUS (LEG)** and articulate proximally and distally with each other. At the tarsus, the distal ends of the tibia and fibula project abaxially beyond the articular surface as the medial or, respectively, lateral malleolus.

I. The menisci of the femorotibial joint are attached by ligaments to the **proximal articular surface of the tibia (22)**. The **medial tibial condyle (23)** is set off from the **lateral condyle (26)** by the **intercondylar eminence (24)**, a proximomedian projection. The lateral condyle bears the **fibular articular surface (26)** for the joint with the head of the fibula. Cranial to this joint is the **extensor groove (27)** for the tendon of the long digital extensor muscle, which takes origin at the extensor fossa, a small depression that is lateral at the margin of junction of the trochlea and lateral condyle. The **body of the tibia (28)** continues distally from the condyles. Proximally, on its cranial aspect, it bears the **tibial tuberosity (29)**, which is the site of termination of the patellar ligament (tendon of the quadriceps). The **cranial margin of the tibia (29')** is distal to the tuberosity. At the distal end of the tibia the **tibial cochlea (30)** is surmounted by the **medial malleolus (31)**.

II. On the fibula, the **head (32)** with its **articular surface (33)** is continued by the long **body (34)**, which is again followed distally by the **lateral malleolus (35)**. The two crural bones enclose the **crural interosseous space (36)** between them.

c) The **TARSAL BONES** are arranged in three rows. Of the two bones of the proximal row, the medial one, the **talus (37)**, has proximally a **body (38)** and a **trochlea (39)**, a **neck (40)** following, and distally a **head (41)**. The laterally located **calcaneus (42)** projects far proximally with its **tuber calcanei (43)**, which facilitates its function as a lever for the tarsal extensors. The tendon of the lateral digital flexor muscle runs over the **sustentaculum tali (44)** before it unites distally with the tendon of the medial digital flexor muscle to form the deep digital flexor tendon. The **central tarsal bone (45)** is the one bone of the middle row, into which the especially large fourth tarsal bone projects. The **tarsal bones I – IV (46)** form the distal row of the tarsal bones.

d) The **METATARSAL BONES I – V** consist of a proximal **base (47)**, a middle **body (48)** and a distal **head (49)**. The short first metatarsal bone can be absent. Occasionally, it is divided into two bones, in which case the proximal part can fuse with the first tarsal bone.

e) For the most part, the description of the digital bones of the thoracic limb (see thoracic limb) holds for the **DIGITAL BONES** of the pelvic limb.

The **proximal phalanx (50)** and **middle phalanx (51)** have a **base (52)** proximally (with an indistinct flexor tuberosity of the middle phalanx), a middle **body (54)** and a distal **head (55)**. The indistinct **flexor tuberosity (53)** is located proximoplantarly on the base of the middle phalanx; it is the area of insertion of the superficial digital flexor tendon. The **distal phalanx or unguicular bone (56)** has its **articular surface (57)** proximally and proximodorsally an indistinct **extensor process (58)** on which the digital extensor inserts. The **flexor tubercle (59)**, on which the deep digital flexor tendon inserts, is proximoplantar. The sharp **unguicular crest (60)** surmounts the **unguicular sulcus (61)**. The distal part of the unguicular bone is the **unguicular process (62)**, which is surrounded by the horn of the claw.

When, on the first digit only, the claw is retained and the central bony supporting skeleton is lacking, the term 'wolf's claw' (Paraunguicula, −60) is sometimes used.

f) Of the **SESAMOID BONES**, the sesamoid bones of the gastrocnemius muscle (64) were discussed in the context of the femoral condyles. The sesamoid bone of the popliteus muscle (65) is caudolateral at the stifle joint, at the transition of the tendon of origin of the muscle into its belly. The **proximal sesamoid bones (66)** are plantar at the metatarsophalangeal joint. The **distal sesamoids (67)**, which are plantar at the distal interphalangeal joints, and the **dorsal sesamoids at the proximal interphalangeal joints** are cartilaginous. The **dorsal sesamoids at the metatarsophalangeal joints (68)** are usually osseous. The **patella (69)** is the largest sesamoid bone of the body and lies in the tendon of insertion of the quadriceps femoris muscle. It bears a cartilage-covered articular surface for articulation with the trochlea of the femur.

Pelvic limb

(Artesien-Normand Basset)

(medial view)

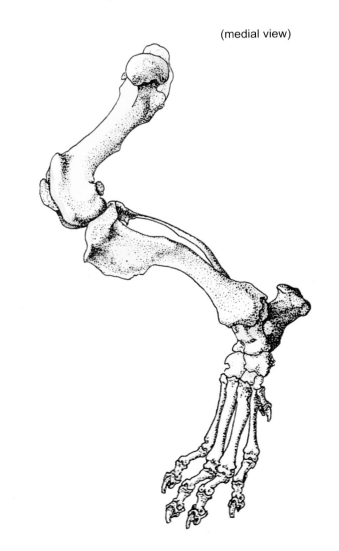

Bones of pelvic limb

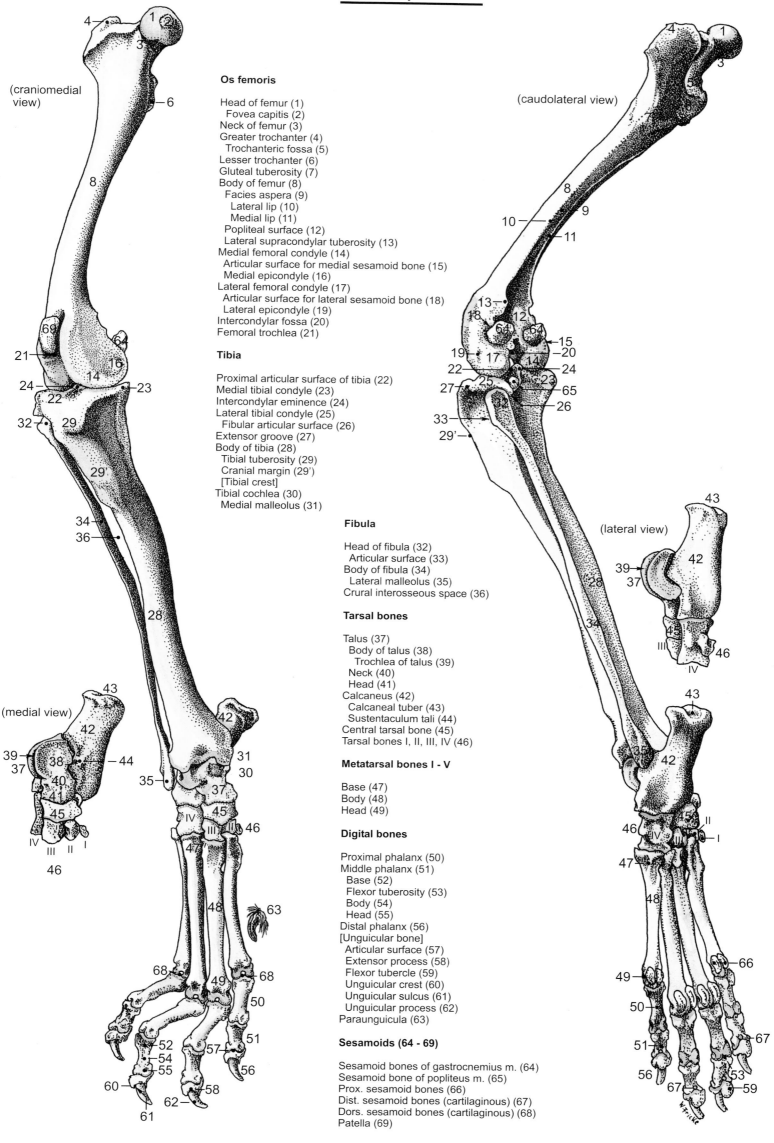

(craniomedial view)

(caudolateral view)

(medial view)

(lateral view)

Os femoris

Head of femur (1)
Fovea capitis (2)
Neck of femur (3)
Greater trochanter (4)
Trochanteric fossa (5)
Lesser trochanter (6)
Gluteal tuberosity (7)
Body of femur (8)
Facies aspera (9)
Lateral lip (10)
Medial lip (11)
Popliteal surface (12)
Lateral supracondylar tuberosity (13)
Medial femoral condyle (14)
Articular surface for medial sesamoid bone (15)
Medial epicondyle (16)
Lateral femoral condyle (17)
Articular surface for lateral sesamoid bone (18)
Lateral epicondyle (19)
Intercondylar fossa (20)
Femoral trochlea (21)

Tibia

Proximal articular surface of tibia (22)
Medial tibial condyle (23)
Intercondylar eminence (24)
Lateral tibial condyle (25)
Fibular articular surface (26)
Extensor groove (27)
Body of tibia (28)
Tibial tuberosity (29)
Cranial margin (29')
[Tibial crest]
Tibial cochlea (30)
Medial malleolus (31)

Fibula

Head of fibula (32)
Articular surface (33)
Body of fibula (34)
Lateral malleolus (35)
Crural interosseous space (36)

Tarsal bones

Talus (37)
Body of talus (38)
Trochlea of talus (39)
Neck (40)
Head (41)
Calcaneus (42)
Calcaneal tuber (43)
Sustentaculum tali (44)
Central tarsal bone (45)
Tarsal bones I, II, III, IV (46)

Metatarsal bones I - V

Base (47)
Body (48)
Head (49)

Digital bones

Proximal phalanx (50)
Middle phalanx (51)
Base (52)
Flexor tuberosity (53)
Body (54)
Head (55)
Distal phalanx (56)
[Unguicular bone]
Articular surface (57)
Extensor process (58)
Flexor tubercle (59)
Unguicular crest (60)
Unguicular sulcus (61)
Unguicular process (62)
Paraunguicula (63)

Sesamoids (64 - 69)

Sesamoid bones of gastrocnemius m. (64)
Sesamoid bone of popliteus m. (65)
Prox. sesamoid bones (66)
Dist. sesamoid bones (cartilaginous) (67)
Dors. sesamoid bones (cartilaginous) (68)
Patella (69)

2. THE MUSCLES OF THE HIP JOINT AND THEIR NERVE SUPPLY

Reflect the skin of the limb distally to the level of the tarsal joint, preserving the large subcutaneous veins (see pp. 81 and 83). Following their dissection and examination, the superficial gluteal, middle gluteal and biceps femoris muscles should be transected at the junction of their middle and distal thirds. Different from the usual procedure, the nerve supply can be studied only after sectioning the muscles. For this reason, the nerve supply of a muscle will be described after the description of its muscle group. The tensor fasciae latae muscle and the three muscle groups, croup muscles, hamstring muscles, and deep muscles of the coxal joint comprise the muscles of the hip joint.

a) The **SUPERFICIAL FASCIA** of the gluteal region is the **gluteal fascia (14)**. It passes from the thoracolumbar fascia and, in the direction of the femur, is continued as the multilaminated fascia lata, which is tensed by the tensor fasciae latae muscle.

The **tensor fasciae latae muscle (3)** originates at the tuber coxae and neighboring part of the ilium and radiates with its cranial main portion into the superficial lamina of the fascia lata, which fuses distally with the patellar ligament (quadriceps tendon). Its caudal, fan-shaped, part passes over into the deep portion of the fascia lata, that ends on the lateral lip of the rough area of the femur (*Facies aspera ossis femoris*). **Function**: Tensor of the fascia lata and flexor of the hip joint. **Nerve supply**: cranial gluteal nerve.

b) The **CROUP MUSCLES** arise from the gluteal surface of the ilium (middle and deep gluteal muscles) or from the sacrum and sacrotuberous ligament (piriformis and superficial gluteal muscle). All croup muscles end on the greater trochanter of the femur. **Function**: Extension of the hip joint and abduction of the limb. The deep gluteal turns the cranial face of the thigh (and limb) medially.

The **superficial gluteal muscle (2)** lies most caudally and terminates most distally at the base of the greater trochanter on the gluteal tuberosity. The latter attachment is clearly seen after section and reflection of the muscle stumps.

The **middle gluteal muscle (1)** originates dorsally at the gluteal surface between the ventral gluteal line and the iliac crest.

The **piriformis muscle (6)** (Henning 1965) lies deep to the middle gluteal muscle and ends jointly with it on the caudal part of the greater trochanter of the femur.

The **deep gluteal muscle (7)** has an extended area of origin between the ventral and caudal gluteal lines. Its fibers converge to insert on the cranial part of the greater trochanter.

Innervation of the croup muscles is by the cranial and caudal gluteal nerves, both of which emerge at the major ischiadic notch. The **caudal gluteal nerve (17)** enters the medial aspect of the superficial gluteal muscle and in exceptional cases also the piriformis muscle. The **cranial gluteal nerve (5)** passes between the middle and deep gluteal muscles. It supplies these muscles and, usually, the piriformis muscle, and a branch passes through the lateral part of the deep gluteal to end in the tensor fasciae latae muscle.

c) The **HAMSTRING MUSCLES** (long ischiatic muscles) are the biceps femoris, semitendinosus, and semimembranosus. They arise from the ischiadic tuber and additionally (biceps femoris) from the neighboring part of the sacrotuberous ligament. The caudal crural abductor, which may be described with this group, has its origin only from the sacrotuberous ligament. **Function**: Extension of the hip joint, flexion of the stifle joint, and also extension of the hock joint insofar as they end in a calcanean tract (biceps femoris and semitendinosus muscles).

The **biceps femoris muscle (4)** terminates with a broad aponeurosis on the patellar ligament (quadriceps tendon) and on the crural fascia. Moreover, it terminates on the calcanean tuber by the lateral calcanean tract, which at the distal third of the crus fuses with the medial calcanean tract from the semitendinosus and gracilis muscles. After section of the biceps femoris muscle, it becomes clear that the lateral calcanean tract gets a fascial reinforcement from the lateral lip of the facies aspera of the femur (and it is for this reason that the term 'tract' is used instead of 'tendon').

The straplike **caudal crural abductor muscle (20)** originates from the distal part of the sacrotuberous ligament, deep to the biceps femoris muscle, and its insertion radiates into the crural fascia with the caudal border of the biceps.

The caudolaterally located **semitendinosus muscle (16)** ends proximomedially on the tibia and, together with the tendon of the gracilis muscle, is continued by the medial calcanean tract.

The caudomedially placed **semimembranosus muscle (15)** has two strong muscle bellies. The cranial one terminates on the medial condyle of the femur, and the caudal one distal to the femorotibial joint space on the medial condyle of the tibia.

The **innervation** of the hamstring muscles is by muscular branches that proceed from the proximal part of the **ischiatic nerve (18)**, which ends at midthigh by dividing into the **tibial nerve (13)** and the **common peroneal (fibular) nerve (11)**. The cranial part of the biceps femoris muscle originates from the sacrotuberous ligament and receives additionally a branch of the caudal gluteal nerve (thus the term *gluteobiceps* may properly be used to designate the biceps femoris). The caudal crural abductor muscle is innerva-

ted by a **musculocutaneous branch (12)** of the common peroneal (fibular) nerve. After the muscular branch is given off, this small nerve ends as a cutaneous branch.

Proximal to its branching, the **ischiadic nerve (18)** crosses the greater ischiadic notch, and then passes over the neck of the femur where the neck is covered by the deep muscles of the hip joint. It innervates the hip joint and divides between the biceps femoris and adductor magnus muscles into the strong tibial nerve (13) and the smaller common peroneal (fibular) nerve (11). The division of the ischiadic nerve into tibial and common peroneal nerves becomes distinct only in the distal half of the thigh; because, in the proximal thigh, the two nerves are held together in a common connective tissue envelope.

d) The **DEEP HIP JOINT MUSCLES** (see text-illustration) are supinators of the limb. They turn the cranial face of the thigh (and limb) laterally.

The **origin** of the deep muscles of the hip joint is from the hip bone in the vicinity of the obturator foramen. Their **insertion** is in the trochanteric fossa of the femur and (quadratus femoris only) just distal to the fossa on the caudal surface of the femur. In craniocaudal sequence, the four muscles are:

The **gemelli muscles (8)** originate in the region of the lesser ischiadic notch and bound on the caudal border of the deep gluteal muscle.

The **internal obturator muscle (19)** has its origin internally on the medial border of the obturator foramen and passes with a strong tendon dorsal to the fanlike gemelli muscles, which form a central sulcus where the tendon passes over them.

The **external obturator muscle (9)** has a similar area of origin on the medial border of the obturator foramen, but it lies externally on the bony pelvis (see also text-illustration p. 80). From this muscle, only a more deeply located strong terminal tendon is visible at the caudal border of the gemelli muscles. **Innervation**: obturator nerve.

The **quadratus femoris muscle (10)** begins ventromedially at the ischiadic tuber and ends at the distal border of the trochanteric fossa.

Innervation is by the muscular branches of the ischiadic nerve (rotator nerve), which originates at the caudal border of the deep gluteal muscle from the ischiadic nerve. An exception is the external obturator muscle, which is supplied only by the obturator nerve.

Deep muscles of hip joint

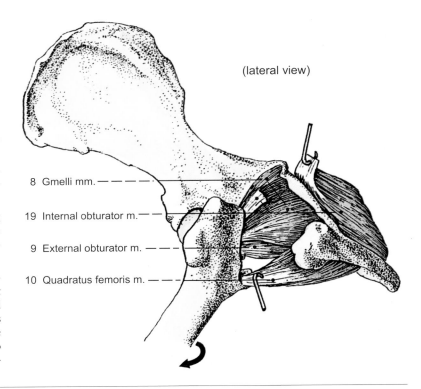

(lateral view)

8 Gemelli mm.

19 Internal obturator m.

9 External obturator m.

10 Quadratus femoris m.

Muscles of the hip joint

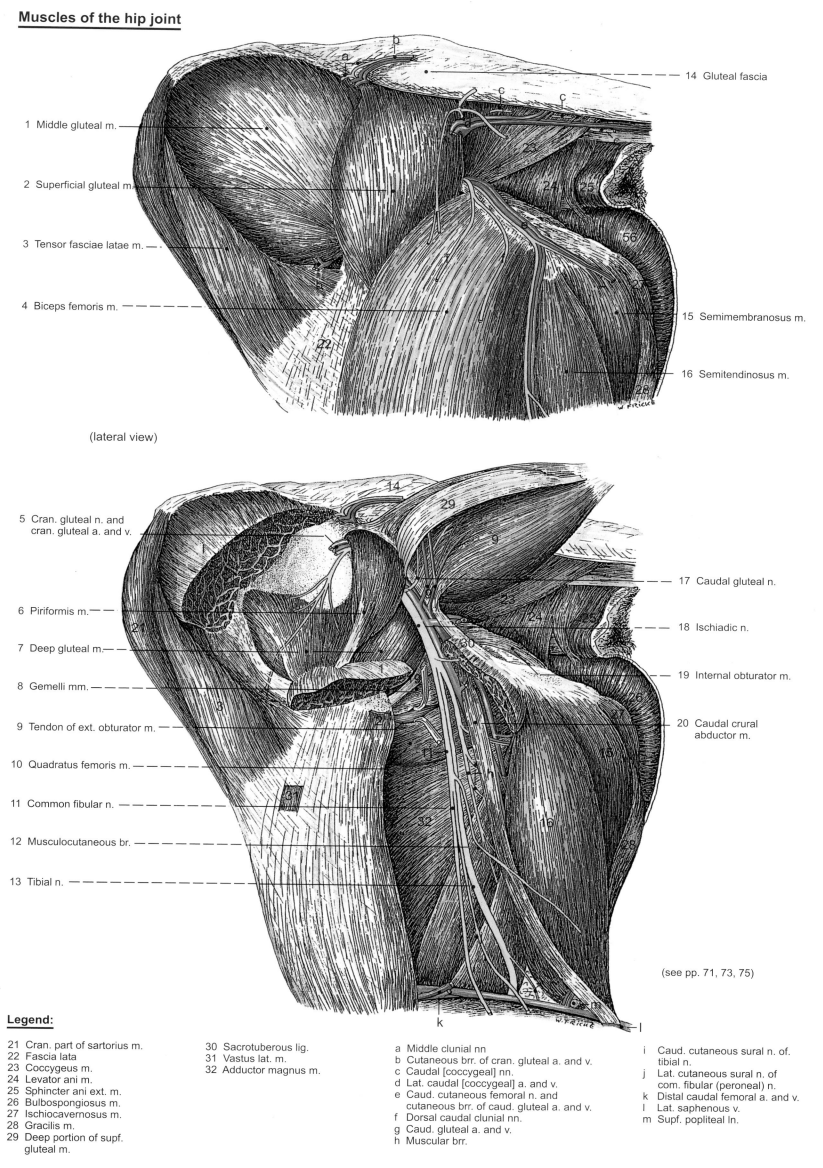

1 Middle gluteal m.

2 Superficial gluteal m.

3 Tensor fasciae latae m.

4 Biceps femoris m.

14 Gluteal fascia

15 Semimembranosus m.

16 Semitendinosus m.

(lateral view)

5 Cran. gluteal n. and cran. gluteal a. and v.

6 Piriformis m.

7 Deep gluteal m.

8 Gemelli mm.

9 Tendon of ext. obturator m.

10 Quadratus femoris m.

11 Common fibular n.

12 Musculocutaneous br.

13 Tibial n.

17 Caudal gluteal n.

18 Ischiadic n.

19 Internal obturator m.

20 Caudal crural abductor m.

(see pp. 71, 73, 75)

Legend:

21 Cran. part of sartorius m.
22 Fascia lata
23 Coccygeus m.
24 Levator ani m.
25 Sphincter ani ext. m.
26 Bulbospongiosus m.
27 Ischiocavernosus m.
28 Gracilis m.
29 Deep portion of supf. gluteal m.

30 Sacrotuberous lig.
31 Vastus lat. m.
32 Adductor magnus m.

a Middle clunial nn
b Cutaneous brr. of cran. gluteal a. and v.
c Caudal [coccygeal] nn.
d Lat. caudal [coccygeal] a. and v.
e Caud. cutaneous femoral n. and cutaneous brr. of caud. gluteal a. and v.
f Dorsal caudal clunial nn.
g Caud. gluteal a. and v.
h Muscular brr.

i Caud. cutaneous sural n. of tibial n.
j Lat. cutaneous sural n. of com. fibular (peroneal) n.
k Distal caudal femoral a. and v.
l Lat. saphenous v.
m Supf. popliteal ln.

79

3. THE MEDIAL SAPHENOUS VEIN, OBTURATOR NERVE, FEMORAL NERVE, MEDIAL MUSCLES OF THE THIGH AND THE FEMORAL SPACE (FEMORAL CANAL)

> After exposing the quadriceps femoris and identifying its four heads, sever the rectus femoris head a fingerbreadth distal to its origin from the ilium. Reflect the distal stump to obtain an overview of the four heads. To do this, the caudal part of the sartorius must be displaced caudally or cut.

a) The **MEDIAL SAPHENOUS VEIN (6)** originates from the femoral vein at the tip of the femoral triangle. With the **saphenous artery (6)** and the **saphenous nerve (12)**, it runs distally to the crus, crossing the stifle joint medially. In the proximal third of the crus, it divides into a **cranial branch (8)** and a **caudal branch (7)**.

b) The **OBTURATOR NERVE (1)** courses on the internal surface of the pelvis, through a gap of the levator ani muscle and, following in the obturator sulcus of the pubic bone, continues to the obturator foramen. It passes through the obturator foramen, supplies the **external obturator muscle (G)** and gives off muscular branches for the adductor muscles of the thigh (adductor magnus, adductor brevis, pectineus muscles). Emerging medially between the pectineus adductor muscles, it enters the deep surface of the gracilis muscle, which also acts as an adductor. The obturator nerve ends medially at the stifle joint with a very weak sensory branch.

1 The **gracilis muscle (5)** has its ultimate origin from the pelvic symphysis. The aponeuroses of origin of the ipsi- and contralateral muscles arise from a median tendinous double-plate, the **symphysial tendon (2)**, which lies between right and left adductor muscles, and to which it gives origin. The symphysial tendon can be observed after the removal of the fleshy fibers of origin of the adductor magnus muscle. At the level of the stifle joint, the gracilis muscle is continued by the crural fascia and joins the formation of the medial calcanean tract.

The **adductor magnus muscle (4)** originates in an extended area from the lateral surface of the symphysial tendon and from the pubic and ischiadic bones along the pelvic symphysis. It has a broad-surfaced 'fleshy' insertion at the facies aspera of the femur.

The **adductor brevis muscle (3)** arises from the ventral pubic tubercle and ends, together with the adductor magnus, proximally on the facies aspera. It can be identified on the basis of a typical nerve branch that crosses over the adductor brevis before it enters the adductor magnus.

2 The **pectineus (13, F) muscle** must be considered as a double muscle according to its phylogenetic development, because it is fused with the adductor longus muscle. In the dog, the m. pectineus incorporates the m. adductor longus. In addition to its supply by the obturator nerve it often has an additional innervation by the saphenous nerve or the femoral branch of the genitofemoral nerve. The muscle originates at the iliopubic eminence and at the caudal angle of the superficial inguinal ring and ends at the medial lip of the facies aspera.

c) The **FEMORAL NERVE (9)** in the abdominal region is embedded in the iliopsoas muscle and courses together with it through the neuromuscular lacuna. It then emerges from the ventral surface of the iliopsoas muscle. Here it gives off the **saphenous nerve (12)**, which supplies the stifle joint and runs as a sensory nerve on the medial surface of the limb distally to the first and second digits. After release of the saphenous nerve, the femoral nerve supplies the sartorius muscle and the four heads of the quadriceps femoris muscle. The branch to the sartorius may arise from the saphenous nerve.

The **sartorius muscle (10)** is split into a cranial and a caudal part, which originate at the iliac crest and, respectively at the cranial margin of the wing of the ilium, and radiate into the medial femoral and crural fasciae. Function: Adductor of the limb and extensor of the stifle joint.

The **quadriceps femoris muscle** (see text-illustration) consists of the **vastus lateralis (A)**, **vastus intermedius (B)** and **vastus medialis (11, C)** muscles, which originate proximally from the femur, and of the **rectus femoris muscle (D)**, which originates craniodorsal to the acetabulum at the caudal ventral iliac spine. Owing to its origin from the bony pelvis, the rectus femoris muscle can act as an extensor of the stifle joint and at the same time as a flexor of the hip joint. After reflection of the cut rectus femoris muscle all four heads of the muscle become visible. The strong tendon of insertion of the quadriceps femoris muscle invests the patella and terminates with the **patellar ligament (E**; this ligament is better named the quadriceps tendon, *Tendo m. quadricipitis*) on the tibial tuberosity where the insertion tendon is underlain by the distal infrapatellar (subtendinous) bursa (see p. 87).

d) The **FEMORAL SPACE** or **FEMORAL CANAL*** lies in the *femoral triangle*, which is bounded basally by the inguinal ligament, cranially by the caudal sartorius muscle and caudally by the pectineus muscle. Deeply, the groove-like femoral space is bounded by the iliopsoas muscle and superficially it is covered by the medial femoral fascia. The space contains the femoral artery and vein and the saphenous nerve. Its access from the abdominal cavity is the femoral ring, which is closed only by peritoneum and the transversalis fascia. At the distal tip of the femoral triangle the femoral vessels pass deeply onto the caudal surface of the femur and reach the popliteal region. They pass from the femoral space caudodistally between the adductor magnus and semimembranosus muscles or by a cleft in the adductor magnus that sometimes occurs.

3

Muscles of hip and knee joints

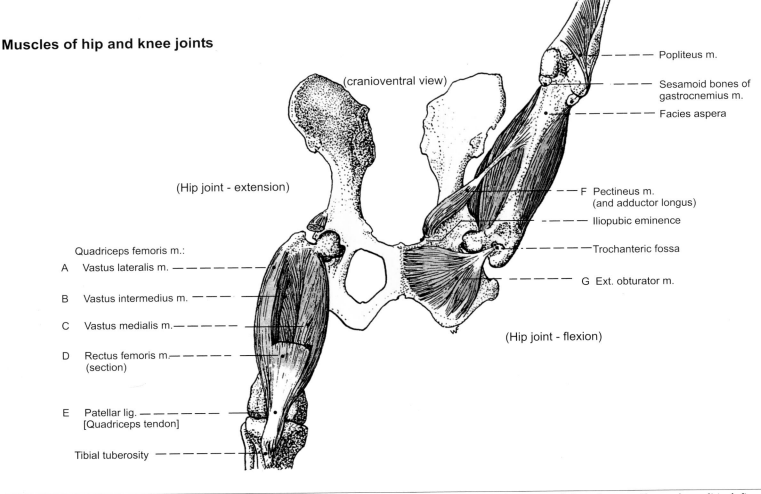

(cranioventral view)

Popliteus m.

Sesamoid bones of gastrocnemius m.

Facies aspera

(Hip joint - extension)

F Pectineus m. (and adductor longus)

Iliopubic eminence

Trochanteric fossa

G Ext. obturator m.

(Hip joint - flexion)

Quadriceps femoris m.:
A Vastus lateralis m.
B Vastus intermedius m.
C Vastus medialis m.
D Rectus femoris m. (section)
E Patellar lig. [Quadriceps tendon]
Tibial tuberosity

*) Femoral space and femoral canal are understood as synonyms by many veterinary anatomists. In human medicine, the term 'femoral canal' is defined quite differently as the 'hernial canal', the site of femoral hernia.

Pelvic limb

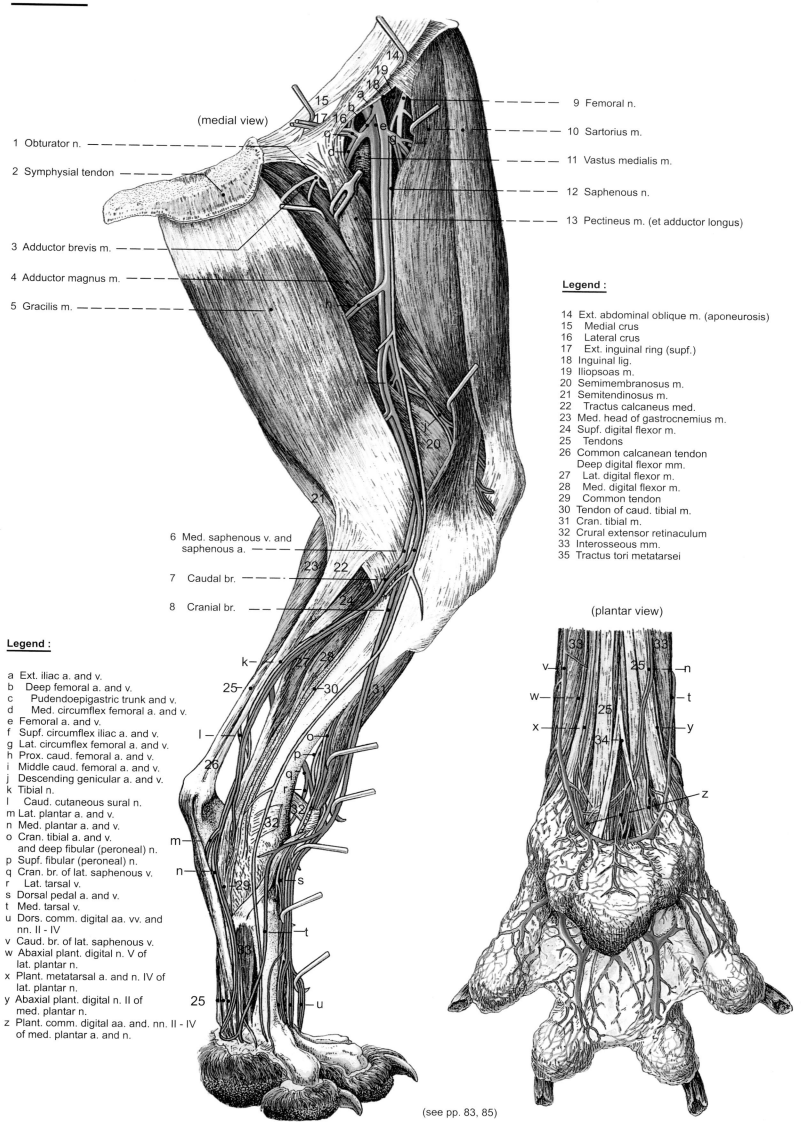

(medial view)

1 Obturator n.

2 Symphysial tendon

3 Adductor brevis m.

4 Adductor magnus m.

5 Gracilis m.

6 Med. saphenous v. and saphenous a.

7 Caudal br.

8 Cranial br.

9 Femoral n.

10 Sartorius m.

11 Vastus medialis m.

12 Saphenous n.

13 Pectineus m. (et adductor longus)

(plantar view)

(see pp. 83, 85)

4. THE LATERAL SAPHENOUS VEIN, COMMON PERONEAL NERVE AND TIBIAL NERVE, CRURAL (LEG) MUSCLES AND POPLITEUS MUSCLE

> The skin of the limb is reflected to the distal end of the metatarsus and the second digit. To dissect the origins of the muscles of the leg, the semitendinosus and gracilis muscles are cut at the transition to their insertion tendons. To demonstrate the common peroneal nerve and the origins of the digital extensors and the tarsal flexors the broad tendon of insertion of the biceps femoris muscle has to be fenestrated as shown in the accompanying illustration, so that only two terminal tendinous strips remain preserved, each about a fingerbreadth in width: (1) the proximal tendon ending on the patellar ligament; and (2) the distal tendon ending in the crural facia. The lateral calcanean tract should be preserved.

1 a) The **LATERAL SAPHENOUS VEIN (25)** originates in the popliteal region from the distal caudal femoral vein. It divides in the distal third of the crus into a **cranial branch (26)** and a **caudal branch (27)**. The cranial branches of the lateral and medial saphenous veins anastomose on the dorsum pedis (see p. 85), on the flexor aspect of the tarsus. From their union the large common trunk of dorsal common digital veins II – IV is formed. The caudal branches of the lateral and medial saphenous veins also anastomose proximal to the plantar tarsus. Each vein continues distally. The caudal branch of the lateral saphenous vein is large. It runs distally on the lateral plantar aspect of the hock and, at the level of the proximal border of the metatarsal pad, forms the superficial plantar venous arch. It is this arch that receives plantar common digital veins II – IV.

2 b) The **COMMON PERONEAL (FIBULAR) NERVE (21)*** originates as the lateral division of the ischiadic nerve. Before crossing the lateral head of the gastrocnemius muscle it gives off the **lateral cutaneous sural nerve (22)**, which at popliteal level penetrates between the main and accessory portions of the biceps femoris muscle and reaches the skin. After this, the common peroneal nerve enters the crural musculature laterally and divides here into the **superficial peroneal (fibular) nerve (8)** and **deep peroneal (fibular) nerve (9)**. It is these nerves that provide the distal muscular branches for the tarsal flexors and digital extensors. Both nerves pass distally onto the flexor aspect of the tarsus. The superficial peroneal nerve is craniolateral and the deep peroneal nerve runs craniomedially through the ringlike opening of the crural extensor retinaculum. After this, the superficial peroneal nerve dispatches the dorsal common digital nerves II – IV (the first and second digits are supplied dorsally by the saphenous nerve). The deep peroneal nerve gives off a muscular branch for the **extensor digitalis brevis muscle (15)** and ends by dividing into the dorsal metatarsal nerves II – IV (see p. 85).

3 c) The **CRANIOLATERAL CRURAL (LEG) MUSCLES** are flexors of the tarsus and extensors of the digits. In craniocaudal sequence these muscles are the following:

I. The **cranial tibial muscle (4)** originates laterally on the cranial border of the tibia. It extends together with the long digital extensor and digiti I muscle, and with the deep peroneal nerve, through the crural extensor retinaculum and ends proximally on the first and second metatarsal bones.

4 **II.** The **long digital extensor muscle (7)** originates at the extensor fossa of the femur (for this reason long[!] digital extensor muscle) and, after the division of its tendon of insertion, ends on the distal phalanx of all digits. With the tibialis cranialis and the extensor of digit I, it passes deep to the crural extensor retinaculum and, after this, as the only muscle, passes within the ringlike opening of the tarsal extensor retinaculum.

III. The **extensor muscle of digit I** lies as an inconspicuous muscle at the distal two thirds of the tibia deep to the long digital extensor muscle. It originates proximally from the fibula and ends on the first and second digits.

IV. The **peroneus (fibularis) longus muscle (3)*** takes origin from the head of the fibula and the proximal tibia. It crosses the tendons of the peroneus brevis and lateral digital extensor muscles. It attaches plantarly with a transversely running tendon on the proximal ends of the metatarsal bones and ends medially on the first tarsal bone.

V. The **lateral digital extensor muscle (10)** originates at the proximal third of the fibula and joins the long digital extensor on the proximal phalanx of the fifth digit.

VI. The **peroneus (fibularis) brevis muscle (11)*** originates at the distal two thirds of the fibula and ends proximally on the fifth metatarsal bone.

d) Before the **TIBIAL NERVE (23)** passes deeply between the two heads of the gastrocnemius muscle, it releases the distal muscular branches for the tarsal extensors and the digital flexors and gives off the **caudal cutaneous sural nerve (24)**. This cutaneous nerve crosses the lateral head of the gastrocnemius muscle and crosses or penetrates the lateral calcanean tract. It innervates the caudal cutaneous area of the leg (crus) and, a fingerbreadth proximal to the calcanean tuber, joins again with the tibial nerve. After this, the tibial nerve crosses the sustentaculum tali deep to the flexor retinaculum and upon the plantar aspect of the lateral digital flexor tendon (see below). It divides here into the medial and lateral plantar nerves. The **medial plantar nerve (19)** gives off the plantar common digital nerves II – IV, and the **lateral plantar nerve (18)** gives off the plantar metatarsal nerves II – IV.

3 e) The **CAUDAL CRURAL (LEG) MUSCLES** are extensors of the hock joint and/or flexors of the digit.

I. The **gastrocnemius muscle** is the extensor muscle of the hock joint. In the tendon of origin of its **lateral head (1)** and of its **medial head (2)** are the sesamoid bones of the gastrocnemius muscle that articulate with the underly-

ing lateral or, respectively, medial condyle of the femur. The insertion of the gastrocnemius is by tendon, also called the calcanean or Achilles tendon, on the calcanean tuber.

II. The **superficial digital flexor muscle (6)** originates from the lateral supracondylar tuberosity of the femur and is proximally surrounded by the gastrocnemius muscle. After section of the medial head of the gastrocnemius muscle, the superficial digital flexor muscle can be taken out of its muscular investment. Its continuation as the superficial digital flexor tendon is called *tendo plantaris* up to the calcanean tuber and, together with the calcanean tract and the gastrocnemius (calcanean) tendon, forms the **common calcanean tendon (12)**. From a position that is initially cranial to the gastrocnemius tendon, the **superficial digital flexor tendon (17)** crosses the medial side of the gastrocnemius tendon and arrives caudal to the gastrocnemius tendon at the hock. It broadens at the calcanean tuber to form an expanded **calcanean 'cap' (Galea calcanea, —16)**. The tendon branches on the plantar metatarsus and each of its branches, after forming the tunnel-like manica flexoria (see p. 23) at metatarsophalangeal joint level, runs plantarly to insert on the middle phalanx of the digit. The calcanean cap is fixed to the calcanean tuber laterally and medially by retinacula. Upon the calcanean cap lies the inconstant (acquired) subcutaneous calcanean bursa and, deep to the calcanean cap, the **subtendinous calcanean bursa (13)** that is opened after severing the lateral part of the **flexor retinaculum (14)** and reflecting the calcanean cap to the medial side.

III. The **deep digital flexor muscle** (see also text-illustration) is composed of the large **lateral digital flexor muscle (5)** and the smaller **medial digital flexor muscle (C)****. The very slight **caudal tibial muscle (B)** originates from the head of the fibula and, in the dog, terminates with a very long and thin tendon on the central tarsal bone. In the domestic ungulates, the muscle is larger and its tendon contributes to the deep flexor tendon. The two muscles that together make up the deep digital flexor originate proximocaudally from the tibia and fibula. Their tendons pass separately upon the flexor aspect of the tarsal joint and join in the proximal plantar metatarsus to form the **deep digital flexor tendon (20)**. The branches of the deep digital flexor tendon course through the tunnel-like manica flexoria of the superficial digital flexor tendon-branches and extend to the unguicular bones.

f) The **SPECIAL FLEXOR MUSCLE OF THE STIFLE JOINT** (see text-illustration) is the **popliteus muscle (A)**. This muscle also acts to rotate the tibia on the femur, turning the cranial face of the crus (leg) medially, an action analogous to pronation of the thoracic limb. The innervation of the popliteus is by the tibial nerve. The muscle originates by tendon at the *popliteal fossa* of the lateral condyle of the femur. Its belly lies in the popliteal region deep to the gastrocnemius muscle and is attached to the proximomedial part of the caudal surface of the tibia. The sesamoid bone of the popliteus muscle (see also p. 87) is within the tendon of origin at its transition to the belly of the muscle.

Deep digital flexor muscles and popliteus muscle

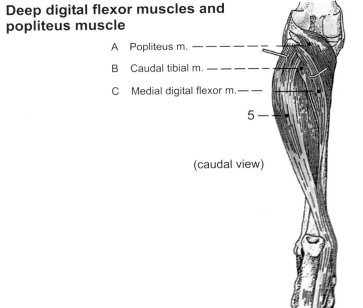

A Popliteus m. ― ― ― ―
B Caudal tibial m. ― ― ― ―
C Medial digital flexor m. ― ―

5 ―

(caudal view)

20 ―

*) In the NAV (1994) the terms *peronaeus* and *peroneus* are given as synonyms for fibularis.
**) The medial digital flexor muscle is also designated *long digital flexor muscle* and the lateral digital flexor muscle is also designated the *long digital flexor* of digit I.

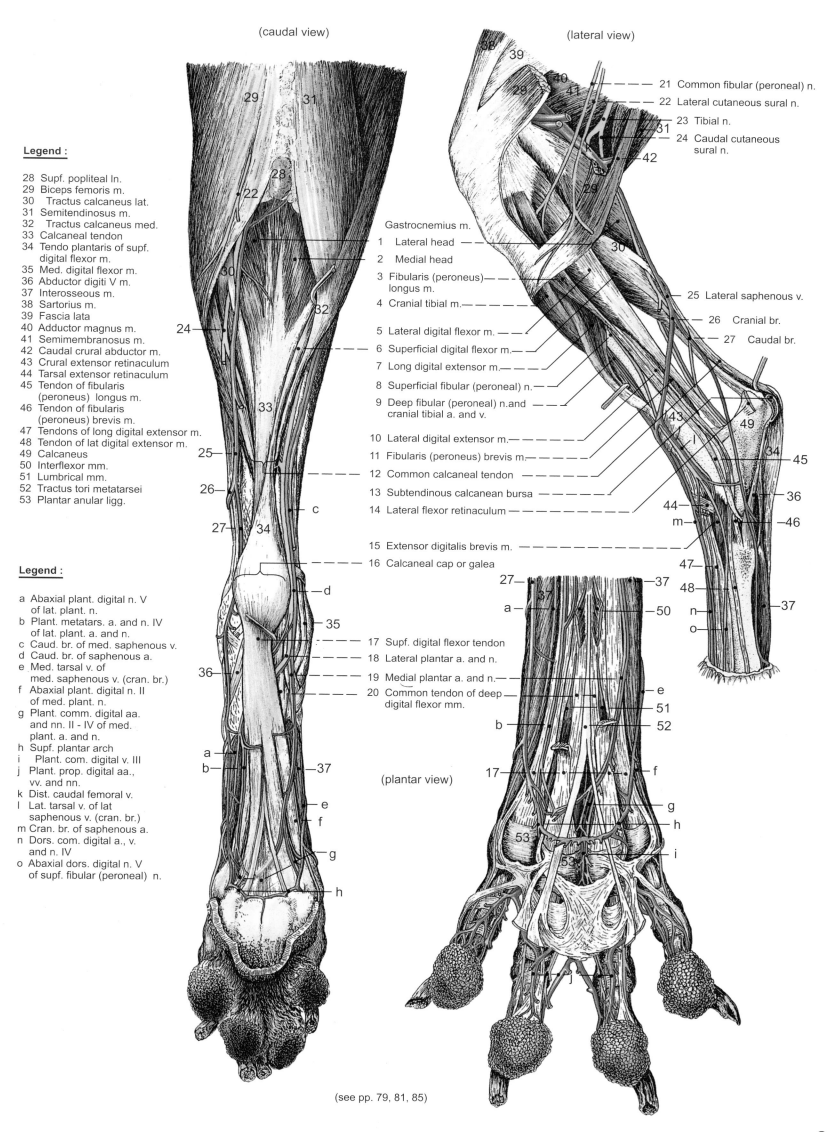

(caudal view)

(lateral view)

Legend :

28 Supf. popliteal ln.
29 Biceps femoris m.
30 Tractus calcaneus lat.
31 Semitendinosus m.
32 Tractus calcaneus med.
33 Calcaneal tendon
34 Tendo plantaris of supf. digital flexor m.
35 Med. digital flexor m.
36 Abductor digiti V m.
37 Interosseous m.
38 Sartorius m.
39 Fascia lata
40 Adductor magnus m.
41 Semimembranosus m.
42 Caudal crural abductor m.
43 Crural extensor retinaculum
44 Tarsal extensor retinaculum
45 Tendon of fibularis (peroneus) longus m.
46 Tendon of fibularis (peroneus) brevis m.
47 Tendons of long digital extensor m.
48 Tendon of lat digital extensor m.
49 Calcaneus
50 Interflexor mm.
51 Lumbrical mm.
52 Tractus tori metatarsei
53 Plantar anular ligg.

Legend :

a Abaxial plant. digital n. V of lat. plant. n.
b Plant. metatars. a. and n. IV of lat. plant. a. and n.
c Caud. br. of med. saphenous v.
d Caud. br. of saphenous a.
e Med. tarsal v. of med. saphenous v. (cran. br.)
f Abaxial plant. digital n. II of med. plant. n.
g Plant. comm. digital aa. and nn. II - IV of med. plant. a. and n.
h Supf. plantar arch
i Plant. com. digital v. III
j Plant. prop. digital aa., vv. and nn.
k Dist. caudal femoral v.
l Lat. tarsal v. of lat saphenous v. (cran. br.)
m Cran. br. of saphenous a.
n Dors. com. digital a., v. and n. IV
o Abaxial dors. digital n. V of supf. fibular (peroneal) n.

21 Common fibular (peroneal) n.
22 Lateral cutaneous sural n.
23 Tibial n.
24 Caudal cutaneous sural n.

Gastrocnemius m.
1 Lateral head
2 Medial head
3 Fibularis (peroneus) longus m.
4 Cranial tibial m.
5 Lateral digital flexor m.
6 Superficial digital flexor m.
7 Long digital extensor m.
8 Superficial fibular (peroneal) n.
9 Deep fibular (peroneal) n.and cranial tibial a. and v.
10 Lateral digital extensor m.
11 Fibularis (peroneus) brevis m.
12 Common calcaneal tendon
13 Subtendinous calcanean bursa
14 Lateral flexor retinaculum
15 Extensor digitalis brevis m.
16 Calcaneal cap or galea

17 Supf. digital flexor tendon
18 Lateral plantar a. and n.
19 Medial plantar a. and n.
20 Common tendon of deep digital flexor mm.

25 Lateral saphenous v.
26 Cranial br.
27 Caudal br.

(plantar view)

(see pp. 79, 81, 85)

5. ARTERIES AND ACCOMPANYING VESSELS AND NERVES OF THE PELVIC LIMB

> With the dissection of the arteries, the satellite, same-named, veins are considered and the accompanying nerves are recapitulated. In this dissection, the popliteus muscle is severed at its insertion at the medial margin of the tibia to permit examination of the popliteal vessels.

a) The **REGION OF THE CROUP AND LATERAL THIGH** is supplied by parietal branches of the internal iliac artery (see p. 79). The **cranial gluteal artery (2)** with its cutaneous branches and in the company of the middle clunial nerves appears superficially at the proximal cranial border of the superficial gluteal muscle. Its deeper branches accompany branches of the **cranial gluteal nerve (1)** between the middle and deep gluteal muscles, which are supplied with arteries or, respectively, nerves. With its lateral (caudal) coccygeal artery (see p. 79) and the accompanying caudal clunial nerves the large **caudal gluteal artery (3)** passes proximally under the skin at the caudal border of the superficial gluteal muscle. With deeply lying branches the caudal gluteal artery accompanies the ischiadic nerve caudally and supplies the superficial gluteal muscle as well as the heads of origin of the hamstring muscles.

b) **THIGH AND CRUS** are supplied by the distal continuations of the external iliac artery.

Just proximal to the vascular lacuna, the **external iliac artery (8)** ends by dividing into the **femoral artery (10)** and the **deep femoral artery (9)**. The deep femoral artery gives off the pudendoepigastric trunk, a short common trunk of the caudal epigastric and external pudendal arteries, or the caudal epigastric and external pudendal arteries arise separately from the deep femoral with no trunk being formed. After dispatching the pudendoepigastric trunk or the separate vessels, the deep femoral continues as the medial circumflex artery, which passes caudally deep to the pectineus muscle. It passes upon the cranial surface of the adductor magnus, which it supplies. A branch runs caudally between the adductor magnus and the obturator externus muscles and anastomoses here with the lateral circumflex femoral artery. The **lateral circumflex femoral artery (12)** and the **superficial circumflex iliac artery (11)** originate a fingerbreadth distal to the lacuna vasorum by a common stem or individually from the cranial wall of the femoral artery. The superficial circumflex iliac artery runs between the sartorius and tensor faciae latae muscles to reach the rectus femoris muscle. The **proximal caudal femoral artery (4)** originates at the half-length of the femoral triangle from the caudal wall of the femoral artery and goes deep (lateral) to the gracilis muscle into the the musculature of the medial thigh. At the distal tip of the femoral triangle, the femoral artery gives off craniodistally the **descending genual artery (13)** to the vastus medialis and the stifle joint, and caudodistally the deeply lying **middle caudal femoral artery (5)** to the cranial part of the semimembranosus muscle. Proximal to the descending genual artery, the femoral gives off the saphenous artery, which is superficially located and accompanies the medial saphenous vein. With its satellite vein, the **saphenous artery (16)** divides at the proximal third of the crus into cranial and caudal branches. Its **cranial branch (17)** courses distally on the cranial tibial muscle and, on the dorsum of the pes, releases dorsal common digital arteries I – IV. The caudal branch of the saphenous artery passes distally upon the medial head of the gastrocnemius muscle and divides on the medial plantar aspect of the hock joint into a **medial plantar artery (19)** and a **lateral plantar artery (18)**. The medial plantar artery gives off the plantar common digital arteries II – IV, and the lateral plantar artery joins with the perforating metatarsal artery and a deep branch of the medial plantar to form the deep plantar arch, which lies deep to the flexor tendons in relation to the proximal parts of the plantar muscles of the paw. Plantar metatarsal arteries II – IV take origin from the deep plantar arch. The **distal caudal femoral artery (6)** and the **popliteal artery (14)** are the end branches of the femoral artery. In the popliteal region, the distal caudal femoral artery supplies the hamstring muscles and the gastrocnemius. (The accompanying distal caudal femoral vein is continuous here with the lateral saphenous vein that, unaccompanied by a corresponding artery, runs distally on the lateral head of the gastrocnemius muscle. The lateral saphenous divides at the distal third of the crus into a cranial branch and a caudal branch.)

The **popliteal artery (14)** is the continuation of the femoral artery and lies deep to the popliteal muscle. It gives off several branches for the stifle joint and divides deep to the popliteus muscle into the shorter and somewhat smaller caudal tibial artery and the longer and larger cranial tibial artery. The **cranial tibial artery (15)** passes craniolaterally through the crural interosseous space and, with the same-named vein and joined by the deep peroneal nerve, passes distally on the cranial surface of the tibia. On the distal crus, it passes beneath the crural extensor retinaculum, lying next to the tibia and deep to the cranial tibial and long digital extensor muscles. On the dorsum of the pes, the cranial tibial is continued as the **dorsal pedal artery (7)** that, on the distal tarsus, ends as the arcuate artery with the dorsal metatarsal arteries II – IV that arise from the latter.

c) The **VESSEL AND NERVE SUPPLY OF THE FOOT** is predominantly by the superficially running dorsal common digital arteries, veins and nerves and the respective plantar common digital arteries, veins and nerves as well as by the deeply situated dorsal metatarsal and plantar metatarsal arteries, veins, and nerves.

I. On the **dorsum of the pes**, the dorsal common digital arteries I – IV pass from the cranial branch of the saphenous artery. The dorsal common digital veins II – IV arise from the large common trunk that is formed by the union of the cranial branches of the medial and lateral saphenous veins. The dorsal common digital nerves are branches of the superficial peroneal nerve. Dorsal metatarsal veins II – IV arise from the deep dorsal venous arch that is satellite to the arcuate artery and is continued proximally by the dorsal pedal vein. Dorsal metatarsal nerves II – IV are branches of the deep peroneal nerve.

II. On the **plantar surface of the foot (Planta)**, plantar common digital arteries II – IV pass from the medial plantar artery. Plantar metatarsal arteries II –IV arise from the deep plantar arch, which is supplied by the lateral plantar artery, a deep branch of the medial plantar artery, and a perforating branch ('perforating metatarsal artery') from dorsal metatarsal artery II. The plantar common digital veins II – IV pass to the superficial plantar venous arch, which is formed by the caudal branch of the lateral saphenous vein and a medial tributary of the dorsal pedal vein and dorsal common digital venous trunk. Plantar metatarsal veins II – IV pass to the deep plantar venous arch, which is satellite to the deep plantar arch formed by the arteries. At its lateral end, the deep plantar venous arch runs to the caudal branch of the lateral saphenous vein. Plantar common digital nerves II – IV are branches of the medial plantar nerve. Plantar metatarsal nerves II – IV are branches of the lateral plantar nerve. Medial and lateral plantar nerves are terminal branches of the tibial nerve.

d) The **LYMPH VESSELS** begin distally in the region of the digits and the digital and metatarsal pads with a well developed net of lymphatic capillaries, which are suitable for direct lymphography. (The applied radiopaque contrast media reach the lymph vessels indirectly from the connective tissue.) From the distal region of the pelvic limb the superficial lymph vessels go to the **superficial popliteal lymph node** (see p. 83) that lies in the popliteal region between the biceps femoris and semitendinosus muscles. After that, the superficial lymph vessels run predominantly to the superficial inguinal lymph nodes and from there through the inguinal canal to the medial iliac lymph nodes. The deep lymph vessels also reach the popliteal lymph node and from there in a variable manner to the medial iliac lymph nodes. On the one hand they course in company with the tibial and ischiadic nerves to the sacral lymph nodes and from there to the medial iliac lymph nodes. Otherwise they pass with the femoral artery and vein and by way of the femoral space and ring the inconstant iliofemoral lymph node and finally the medial iliac lymph nodes. From the medial iliac lymph nodes the lymph flows to the cisterna chyli and may pass by way of the aortic lumbar lymph nodes. The cranial continuation of the cisterna chyli is the thoracic duct, which transports the lymph to the venous angle between the external and internal jugular veins.

Legend (see opposite page)

20 Lumbosacral trunk
21 Caudal gluteal n.
22 Ischiadic n.
23 Rotator n.
24 Tibial n.
25   Muscular branch (of ischiadic n.)
26   Caudal cutaneous sural n. (of tibial n.)
27 Common peroneal (fibular) n.
28   Musculocutaneous branch
29   Lateral cutaneous sural n.
30   Deep peroneal (fibular) n.

31   Superficial peroneal (fibular) n.
32 Lateral saphenous v.
33   Caudal branch
34   Anatomosis with caudal branch of medial saphenous v.
35   Cranial branch
36   Anastomosis with cranial branch of medial saphenous v.
37 Medial saphenous v. and saphenous a., caudal branch
38 Pudendoepigastric trunk

39 Femoral n.
40   Saphenous n.
41 Cranial tibial a., superficial branch
42 Medial tarsal v.
43 Dorsal abaxial a., v., and n. of digit V
44 Arcuate a.
45 Deep dorsal (plantar) arch
46 Superficial dorsal (plantar) arch
47 Dorsal (plantar) metatarsal aa., vv., nn.
48 Dorsal (plantar) common digital aa., vv., nn.
49   Dorsal (plantar) proper digital aa., vv., nn.
50 Plantar abaxial n. of digit V
51 Plantar abaxial n. of digit II

Arteries, veins and nerves of pelvic limb

(Atresien - Normand Basset)

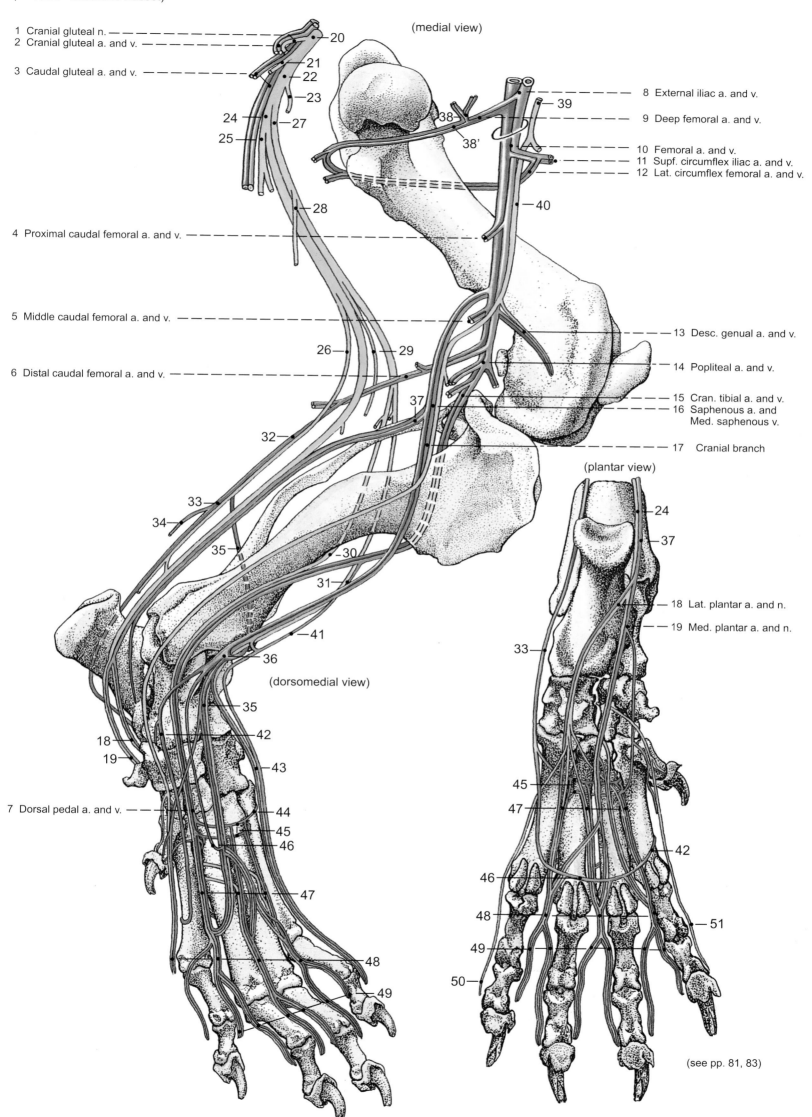

1 Cranial gluteal n.
2 Cranial gluteal a. and v.
3 Caudal gluteal a. and v.

20
21
22
23
24
25
27
28

(medial view)

8 External iliac a. and v.
9 Deep femoral a. and v.
10 Femoral a. and v.
11 Supf. circumflex iliac a. and v.
12 Lat. circumflex femoral a. and v.

39
38
38'
40

4 Proximal caudal femoral a. and v.

5 Middle caudal femoral a. and v.

6 Distal caudal femoral a. and v.

26
29

13 Desc. genual a. and v.
14 Popliteal a. and v.
15 Cran. tibial a. and v.
16 Saphenous a. and Med. saphenous v.
17 Cranial branch

37
32

(plantar view)

24
37

33
34

35
30
31

41
36

(dorsomedial view)

35
42

18
19

43

18 Lat. plantar a. and n.
19 Med. plantar a. and n.

33

45
47

42

7 Dorsal pedal a. and v.

44
45
46

46
48
49

51

47

50

48

49

(see pp. 81, 83)

85

6. SYNOVIAL STRUCTURES OF THE PELVIC LIMB

a) JOINTS OF THE PELVIC LIMB

NAME	Participating BONES	FORM/COMPOSITION	FUNCTION	REMARKS
I. Sacroiliac joint	Auricular surfaces of the sacrum and ilium	Plane joint, Simple joint	Amphiarthrosis	This tight joint is the connection of the pelvic limb to the trunk
II. Hip joint	Acetabulum formed by ilium, ischium, pubis and acetabular bone/ Head of the femur	Spheroid joint, Compound joint	Free joint (all movements possible)	The ligament of the head of the femur anchors the head of the femur to the acetabulum and, at least in young dogs, conducts blood vessels (A. epiphysialis) to the femoral head.
III. Stifle joint (genual joint, knee joint) Femorotibial joint	Lateral and medial condyles of the femur and tibia Sesamoid bones of the gastrocnemius and popliteal muscles	Spiral joint, Compound joint	Ginglymus with braking action, chiefly uniaxial with slight abduction and adduction as well as rotation of the tibia on its long axis	Two fibrocartilaginous menisci compensate for the incongruent surfaces of femur and tibia and act also to absorb shock. The menisci are attached by meniscal ligaments to each other and to the tibia. The meniscofemoral ligament produces a connection of the lateral meniscus to the femur. The form of the menisci is altered with the movements of the joint.
Femoropatellar joint	Trochlea of the femur/ Patellar articular surface	Sliding joint, Simple joint	Gliding movement	The patella is a sesamoid bone that is embedded in the end-tendon of the quadriceps femoris muscle and by way of its insertion (patellar ligament) is attached to the tibial tuberosity.
IV. Proximal tibiofibular joint	Tibia/Head of the fibula	Plane joint, Simple joint	Tight joint without movement	Communicates with the stifle joint.
V. Distal tibiofibular joint	Distal ends of tibia and fibula	Plane joint, Simple joint	Tight joint without movement	Communicates with the tarsocrural joint.
VI. Tarsal joint (hock joint)		Compound joint		For a) and b) there is a large common joint cavity. Within b), between the trochlea of the talus and the sustentaculum tali, there is a small, separate joint cavity that does not communicate with the common joint cavity. c) and d) possess their own joint cavities.
a) Tarsocrural joint	Cochlea of the tibia/ Trochlea of the talus/ Articular surface of the lateral malleolus	Cochlear joint, Compound joint	Ginglymus, slight rotation mainly in a), less in b)	The ligaments of the hock joint consist of long ligaments, which bridge over several joints, and short ligaments that bridge over single joints. The long lateral collateral tarsal ligament extends from the lateral malleolus to the proximal end of metatarsal bone V. It is superficial to the short ligaments. The long medial collateral tarsal ligament extends from the tibia to metatarsal bones I and II. The long plantar ligament extends from the calcaneus to metatarsal bone IV. Other ligaments can be studied in the accompanying illustrations (below).
b) Proximal intertarsal joint*	Between talus, calcaneus, and the central tarsal bone and tarsal bone IV	Plane joint, Compound joint		
c) Distal intertarsal joint*	Between the central tarsal bone and tarsal bones I – III	Plane joint, Compound joint	In c) – e) little mobility	
d) Tarsometatarsal joint	Between tarsal bones I – IV and metatarsal bones II – V	Plane joint, Compound joint		

e) Intertarsal (perpendicular) joints: tight perpendicular joints between the tarsal bones.

VI. The **JOINTS OF THE DIGITS** are similar to those of the manus.

The tight joint capsule and the ligaments (sacrotuberous, dorsal and ventral sacroiliac ligaments) of the **sacroiliac joint** are loosened at the end of pregnancy and permit some dilatation of the birth canal.

At the **hip joint** the transverse acetabular ligament bridges over the acetabular notch, and the labrum of the acetabulum, which is fibrocartilage, deepens the joint cavity without projecting beyond the 'equator' of the femoral head. For this reason, in the dog, the hip joint is a spheroid joint and not an enarthrosis.

The **stifle (knee) joint** is composed of the femorotibial and the femoropatellar joints. The first has two joint sacs that communicate openly and that again communicate with the femoropatellar and the proximal tibiofibular joints as well as the articulations of the sesamoid bones of the gastrocnemius muscle with the femoral condyles. The capsule of the stifle joint also invests the tendons of origin of the popliteal and long digital extensor muscles as a capsular tendinous sheath by which these tendons are integrated into the joint. The joint capsule attaches to the convexity of the menisci (cruciate ligaments; see clinical-functional anatomy 86.2)

b) SYNOVIAL BURSAE

The **ischiadic bursa of the internal obturator muscle** lies between the muscle and the lesser ischiadic notch.

The **trochanteric bursa of the superficial gluteal muscle** is present in about one-third of specimens. It is between the insertion tendon of the muscle and the greater trochanter.

The **trochanteric bursa of the biceps femoris muscle** is found between the muscle and the tendon of insertion of the superficial gluteal.

The **distal infrapatellar bursa** is located deep to the patellar ligament upon the tibial tuberosity.

The **subtendinous calcanean bursa of the superficial digital flexor muscle** lies deep to the calcanean cap of that muscle, upon the calcanean tuber.

c) SYNOVIAL SHEATHS

In crossing the hock joint the tendons are protected by synovial sheaths. An exception is the superficial digital flexor tendon in which its subtendinous bursa serves a similar function. The tendinous sheaths of the digital articulations are similar to those of the thoracic limb.

*) In the nomenclature instead of proximal intertarsal joint, the terms talocalcaneocentral joint and calcaneoquartal joint are used; and, instead of distal intertarsal joint, the term centrodistal joint is employed.

Joints, synovial bursae and sheaths

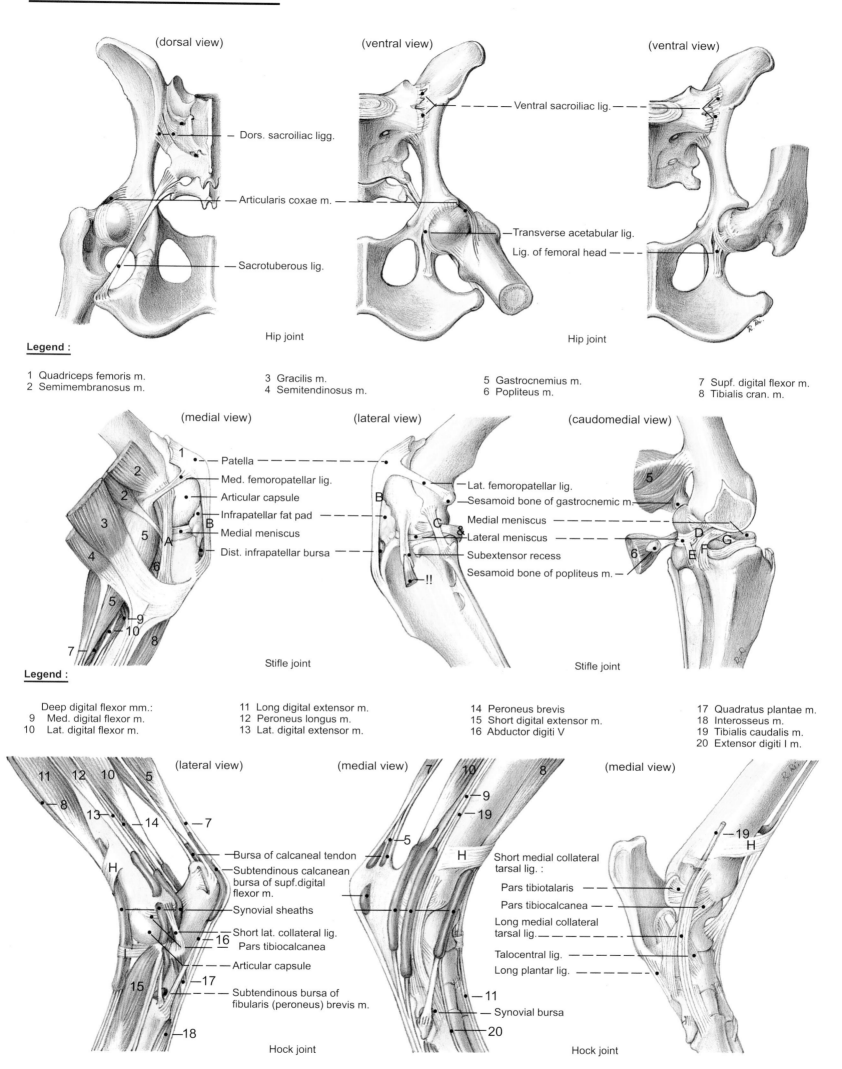

(dorsal view)

Dors. sacroiliac ligg.

Articularis coxae m.

Sacrotuberous lig.

Hip joint

(ventral view)

Ventral sacroiliac lig.

Transverse acetabular lig.

Lig. of femoral head

Hip joint

(ventral view)

Ventral sacroiliac lig.

Legend :

1 Quadriceps femoris m.
2 Semimembranosus m.

3 Gracilis m.
4 Semitendinosus m.

5 Gastrocnemius m.
6 Popliteus m.

7 Supf. digital flexor m.
8 Tibialis cran. m.

(medial view)

1 Patella
Med. femoropatellar lig.
2 Articular capsule
Infrapatellar fat pad
3 Medial meniscus
4 Dist. infrapatellar bursa
5 B
A
6

5
9
10
8
7

Stifle joint

(lateral view)

B
C
&

!!

Lat. femoropatellar lig.
Sesamoid bone of gastrocnemic m.
Medial meniscus
Lateral meniscus
Subextensor recess
Sesamoid bone of popliteus m.

(caudomedial view)

5

D
G
F
6
E

Stifle joint

Legend :

Deep digital flexor mm.:
9 Med. digital flexor m.
10 Lat. digital flexor m.

11 Long digital extensor m.
12 Peroneus longus m.
13 Lat. digital extensor m.

14 Peroneus brevis
15 Short digital extensor m.
16 Abductor digiti V

17 Quadratus plantae m.
18 Interosseus m.
19 Tibialis caudalis m.
20 Extensor digiti I m.

(lateral view)

11 12 10 5
8
13 14 7
H

Bursa of calcaneal tendon
Subtendinous calcanean bursa of supf.digital flexor m.
Synovial sheaths
Short lat. collateral lig.
16 Pars tibiocalcanea
Articular capsule
17 Subtendinous bursa of fibularis (peroneus) brevis m.
15
18

Hock joint

(medial view)

7 10 8
9
19
5
H

11
Synovial bursa
20

Short medial collateral tarsal lig. :
Pars tibiotalaris
Pars tibiocalcanea
Long medial collateral tarsal lig.
Talocentral lig.
Long plantar lig.

Hock joint

(medial view)

19
H

(see pp. 81,83,143)

Legend :

A Med. collateral lig.
B Patellar lig.

C Lat. collateral lig.
D Meniscofemoral lig.

E Caudal tibial lig. of lat. meniscus
F Caudal cruciate lig.

G Cranial cruciate lig.
H Crural extensor retinaculum
I Tarsal extensor retinaculum

Chapter 9: HEAD

1. SKULL, INCLUDING THE HYOID APPARATUS

1 The **skull** is the skeleton of the head, organized into a **cranial part (cranium)** and a **facial part**. Of the seven bones of the (neuro)cranium, those numbered I to III and IVc are membranous bones forming the roof of the skull or calvaria. Individual bones numbered **IVa and b, V to VII** are replacement or primordial bones which replace the cartilaginous primordial skeleton at the base of the skull.

2 a) With regard to the **CRANIUM** the calvaria has a **temporal fossa (j)** which one can regard as the site of origin of the m. temporalis and which is bounded by the **external frontal crest (k)**, the **external sagittal crest (l)**, the **nuchal crest (m)** and the **temporal crest (m')**. The carotid canal housing the internal carotid a. begins at the **caudal carotid foramen (n)** deep to the jugular foramen at the base of the skull. It terminates at the **internal carotid foramen (o)** within the cranial cavity rostrally, and at the **external carotid foramen (p)** on the base of the skull. The **jugular foramen (q)** gives passage to cranial nerves IX, X and XI. The parts of the **cranial cavity** are described on p 90.

I. Caudodorsal to the orbit, the **frontal bone** possesses the **zygomatic process (1)** from which the orbital ligament runs to the frontal process of the **zygomatic bone (56)**. The external ethmoid a. and v. and the ethmoid n. passs through the **ethmoidal foramina (2)**. The **frontal sinuses** are described on p. 90.

II. The **parietal bone** and

III. the **interparietal bone** project into the cranial cavity by means of their tentorial processes (4 and 5 on p. 91).

IV. The **temporal bone** consists of petrosal, tympanic and squamous parts.

a. Of the **petrosal part (6)** only the following features are visible externally: the **mastoid process (7)** for the attachment of tendons of the sternocleidomastoideus, the **stylomastoid foramen (10)** for the exit of the facial n., the external opening of the **canaliculus of the chorda tympani (11)**, and the **petrotympanic fissure (12)**. (Nos. 8, 9, 13, and 14 are described on p. 90.)

b. The **tympanic part (15)** lies caudal to the temporomandibular articulation on the base of the skull. The external acoustic meatus, commencing at the **external acoustic pore (16)**, is separated from the **bulla tympanica (17)** medially by the tympanic membrane. The bulla contains the tympanic cavity of the middle ear into which opens the tympanic ostium of the auditory tube. The other end of the auditory tube, the pharyngeal ostium, opens into the pharynx.

c. The **squamous part (18)** belongs to the roof of the skull, its **zygomatic process (19)** participating in the formation of the zygomatic arch. Caudoventrally, at the base of the arch, are located the **mandibular fossa (20)** and its **articular surface (21)**, and the well-defined **retroarticular process (22)** caudal to these.

Temporal bone

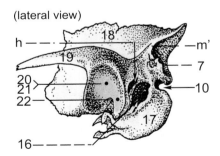

(lateral view)

V. The **ethmoid bone** and its parts (23 to 29) are discussed with the paranasal sinuses and nasal cavity (see p. 90).

VI. The **occipital bone** of the fetus has recognizable sutures between its squamous, lateral and basilar parts.

The **squamous part (30)** has a conspicuous **external occipital protuberance (31)** situated mid-dorsally, which is continuous on either side with the nuchal crest.

The **lateral part (32)** bears an **occipital condyle (33)** on each side of the foramen magnum for participation in the atlanto-occipital articulation. Within the foramen magnum and occipital condyle is the **condylar canal (34)** for the passage of emissary vv. from the skull. Rostroventral to this lies the opening at the commencement of the **hypoglossal canal (35)**. The external opening of the canal is caudal to the jugular foramen between the occipital condyle and the **jugular process (36)**. The **basilar part (37)** borders the **foramen magnum (38)** ventrally. Midventrally between the jugular foramina it possesses an indistinct unpaired **pharyngeal tubercle (39)** for the origin of pharyngeal muscles. Adjacent and medial to the tympanic bulla of either side, the basilar part has a **muscular tubercle (40)** for the insertion of the longus capitis muscle.

Occipital bone

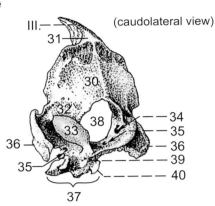

(caudolateral view)

VII. The **sphenoid bone** consists of two bones, the basisphenoid and the presphenoid. Each of these has a (horizontal) body situated medially, and a (vertical) wing laterally.

The **basisphenoid bone** bears the **sella turcica (42)** on the inner surface of the **body (41)**. Internally, the **wing (43)** bears the **foramen rotundum (44)** for the entrance of the maxillary n. (V2), while externally the **foramen ovale (45)** for the passage of the mandibular n. is seen medial and adjacent to the mandibular fossa. The **pterygoid crest (46)**, the osseous ridge of origin of the extrinsic muscles of the ocular bulb, commences ventrally at the **alar canal (47)**. The maxillary a. and n. leave the alar canal at the **rostral alar foramen (48)**, having entered it at the **caudal alar foramen (49)** and the foramen rotundum, respectively.

The **body (95)** of the **presphenoid bone**, which is median in position, merges with the **wing (51)** laterally. The **optic canal (52)**, the passage of the **optic n.**, is situated cranially on the wing at the base of the orbit. Caudally, the **orbital fissure (53)** affords passage to cranial nerves III, IV, V1, and VI.

b) Rostroventral to the orbit, the **FACE** houses the **pterygopalatine fossa (A)**. The greater palatine canal, containing the greater palatine n., begins in the fossa at the **caudal palatine foramen (B)** and ends at the **greater palatine foramen (C)** on the hard palate. Lesser palatine canals, containing lesser palatine nn., branch from within the greater palatine canal and terminate likewise at **lesser palatine foramina (D)**. The **sphenopalatine foramen (E)**, lying dorsal to the caudal palatine foramen, contains the caudal nasal n. (from V2) going to the nasal cavity. At the **choanae (F)** the nasopharyngeal canal is continuous with the nasopharynx. The **orbit (G)** is closed caudally by the orbital ligament. The paired **palatine fissures (H)**, housing the incisive ducts, are located in the hard palate caudal to the upper incisor teeth. Pit-like excavations, the **dental alveoli (J)**, accommodate the roots of the teeth and are responsible for the external prominences of the **alveolar juga (K)**. Alveolar canals (L) begin in the depth of the alveoli and conduct arteries, veins and nerves to the teeth. **Interalveolar septa (M)** are osseous ridges between the alveoli; whereas, a **diastema (N)** or gap between the teeth is rostral and caudal to the canine tooth.

VIII. to XVII. are described on p. 90.

3 XVIII. The **hyoid bone**, also designated **hyoid apparatus**, has cartilaginous precursors in the branchial arches and is therefore classified as a bone of the skull. The unpaired **basihyoid (90)** element lies transversely at the base of the tongue, and is flanked on both sides by the paired **ceratohyoid (91)** elements. From the basihyoid, the two **thyrohyoid (92)** elements are directed caudodorsally to articulate with the thyroid cartilage of the larynx. The **epihyoid (93)** elements extend caudodorsally from the ceratohyoids and these are followed by **stylohyoid (94)** elements directed towards the base of the skull. A cartilaginous **tympanohyoid (95)** connects each stylohyoid to the mastoid process of the temporal bone of the same side.

Cranium

External lamina (a)
Diploë (b)
Internal lamina (c)
Osseous tentorium cerebelli (d)
Temporal meatus (e)
Transverse sinus canal (f)
Sulcus of transverse sinus (g)
Retroarticular foramen (h)●
Temporal fossa (j)●
  External frontal crest (k)★
  External sagittal crest (l)★●
  Nuchal crest (m)★●
  Temporal crest (m')★●
Carotid canal
  Caudal carotid foramen (n)●
  Internal carotid foramen (o)●
  External carotid foramen (p)●
Jugular foramen (q)●

Ossa neurocranii
I. Os frontale ★ ●
Zygomatic process (1)★●
Ethmoidal foramina (2)★●
Rostral frontal sinus (3a)
Lateral frontal sinus (3b)
Medial frontal sinus (3c)
II. Os parietale ★ ●
Tentorial process (4)
III. Os interparietale ★ ●
Tentorial process (5)
IV. Os temporale ★ ●
a. Petrous part (6)★●
Mastoid process (7)★●
Internal acoustic meatus
  Internal acoustic pore (8)
Facial canal (9)
  Stylomastoid foramen (10)●
  Canaliculus of chorda tympani (11)●
  Petrotympanic fissure (12)●
Cerebellar (floccular) fossa (13)
Canal of trigeminal nerve (14)

b. Tympanic part (15)●
External acoustic meatus
  External acoustic pore (16)★
Bulla tympanica (17)●
Ostium tympanicum tubae auditivae (17')●

c. Squamous part (18)★●
Zygomatic process (19)★●
Mandibular fossa (20)●
Articular surface (21)●
Retroarticular process (22)★●

VI. Os occipitale ●
Squama occipitalis (30)●
External occipital protuberance (31)●
  Tentorial process (31')●
Lateral part (32)●
  Occipital condyle (33)★●
  Condylar canal (34)●
  Hypoglossal canal (35)●
  Jugular (paracondylar) process (36)★●
Basilar part (37)●
  Foramen magnum (38)●
  Pharyngeal tubercle (39)●
  Muscular tubercle (40)●

VII. Os sphenoidale ●
Os basisphenoidale
Body (41)●
  Sella turcica (42)
Wing (43)★●
  Foramen rotundum (44)
  Foramen ovale (45)●
  Pterygoid crest (46)★●
Alar canal (47)●
  Rostral alar foramen (48)★●
  Caudal alar foramen (49)●

Os presphenoidale
Body (50)●
Wing (51)★●
  Optic canal (52)★●
  Orbital fissure (53)★●

Face

Pterygopalatine fossa (A)●
Greater palatine canal
  Caudal palatine foramen (B)★●
  Greater palatine foramen (C)●
Lesser palatine canals
  Caudal palatine foramen (B)★●
  Lesser palatine foramina (D)●
Sphenopalatine foramen (E)★●
Choanae (F)●
Orbit (G)★●
Palatine fissures (H)★●
Dental alveoli (J)●
  Alveolar juga (K)★●
Alveolar canals (L)●
Interalveolar septa (M)●
Diastema (N)★

Bones of face
VIII. Lacrimal bone ★ ●
Fossa of lacrimal sac (54)★●
IX. Zygomatic bone ●
Temporal process (55)●
Frontal process (56)●

X. Nasal bone ★
XI. Maxilla ★
Body of maxilla (57)★
  Infraorbital canal
    Maxillary foramen (58)★●
    Infraorbital foramen (59)★
  Lacrimal canal (60)
  Lacrimal groove (61)
Frontal process (62)★
Zygomatic process (63)★●
Palatine process (64)●
Alveolar process (65)●
Maxillary recess (65')

XII. Incisive bone ★ ●
Body of incisive bone (66)
Alveolar process (67)●
Palatine process (68)●
Nasal process (69)★

XIII. Palatine bone ●
Perpendicular lamina (70)●
Horizontal lamina (71)●

XIV. Pterygoid bone ★●
Pterygoid hamulus (72)★●

XV. Vomer ●
Septal groove (73)

XVII. Hyoid bone ★
Basihyoid (90)★
Ceratohyoid (91)★
Thyrohyoid (92)★
Epihyoid (93)★
Stylohyoid (94)★
Tympanohyoid (95)★

Thyroid cartilage

$I_1 - I_3$ Incisor teeth
C   Canine tooth
$L(P_1)$ Wolf tooth
$P_2 - P_4$ Premolar teeth
$M_1 - M_2$ Molar teeth

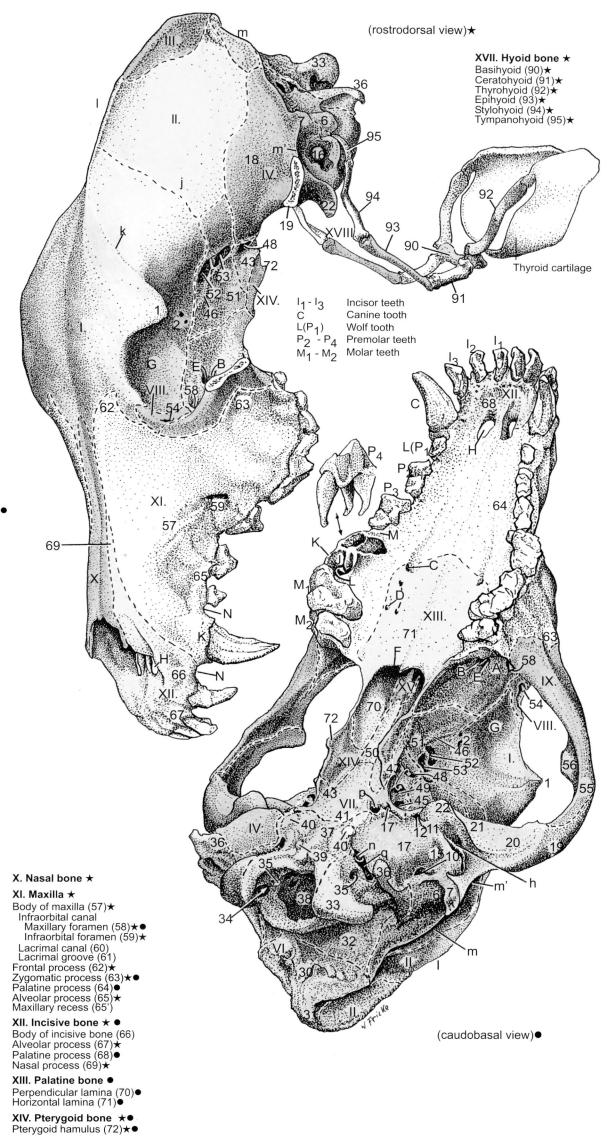

(caudobasal view)●

89

2. SKULL, PARANASAL SINUSES

1 a) The **WALL OF THE SKULL** consists of an **outer cortical layer of bone, the external lamina (a)**, a middle, reduced layer of **spongiosa, the diploë (b)**, and an **inner cortical layer of bone, the lamina interna (c)**. Dorsally, the spongy substance of the frontal bone is lost and the two cortical layers of bone diverge from one another, forming the frontal sinuses. The paired fron-

2 tal sinuses are paranasal sinuses and are in open communication with the nasal cavity. The **rostral frontal sinus (3a)** lies between the median osseous septum of the frontal sinus and the orbit. The **lateral frontal sinus (3b)** is the largest of the frontal sinuses and extends into the zygomatic process of the frontal bone. The **medial frontal sinus (3c)** is very small and lies between the other two. Occasionally it is absent. In some cases a sphenoidal paranasal sinus is developed.

The **osseous tentorium cerebelli (d)** is formed from the fused **tentorial processes (4, 5, and 31')** of the parietal, interparietal and occipital bones. It is the bony basis of the membranous tentorium cerebelli that separates the cerebrum from the cerebellum within the cranial cavity.

The exit passages for the dorsal system of sinuses of the dura mater lies in part internal to the skull wall. It begins in a dorsal median position at the base of the osseous tentorium cerebelli as the **canal of the transverse sinus (f)** which is continued laterally at the petrous temporal bone into the **sulcus of the transverse sinus (g)** and, following that, into the **temporal meatus (e)**. The temporal meatus ends externally at the **retroarticular foramen (h)**.

3 b) The **CRANIAL CAVITY** is bounded by the internal surfaces of the cranial bones. Rostral, middle and caudal fossae of the cranium are present at the base of the cranial cavity. The **rostral fossa (r)** begins with the paired **ethmoidal fossae (s)** and ends at the **chiasmatic sulcus (t)** at which the two optic nerves cross caudal to the entrance into the **optic canal (52)**. On the midline, the **middle cranial fossa (u)** houses the **sella turcica (42)** formed by the basisphenoid. Cranial to the dorsum sellae, a median **hypophyseal fossa (v)** is present to seat the hypophysis. Laterally, the paired **piriform fossae (w)** accommodate the pear-shaped olfactory lobes. The **caudal fossa of the cranium (x)** has a shallow **pontine impression (y)** on the midline rostrally for the pons of the metencephalon and, caudally, the **medullary impression (z)** for the medulla oblongata. In the dog the **petro-occipital fissure (z')** is a very narrow space between the petrous part of the temporal bone and the basioccipital bone. It is occasionally lacking.

IV. a. The **petrous part of the temporal bone (6)** has only the **mastoid process (7)** on the external surface of the skull while the petrous pyramid limits the cranial cavity basolaterally. In the middle of the medial surface of the petrous pyramid, the **internal acoustic pore (8)** marks the beginning of the internal acoustic meatus into which cranial nerves VII and VIII enter. The **facial canal (9)**, housing the facial nerve, proceeds deeply rostrodorsally from the internal acoustic meatus and ends externally at the **stylomastoid foramen (10)**. Centrally, within the petrous temporal bone, the **canaliculus of the chorda tympani (11)** arises from the facial canal and terminates externally at the **minute petrotympanic fissure (12)**. The **cerebellar fossa (13)**, situated dorsocaudally on the petrosal pyramid, receives a small appendage, the ventral paraflocculus of the cerebellum. Rostroventrally, the pyramid is pierced by the **canal of the trigeminal nerve (14)**.

Temporal bone

(medial view)

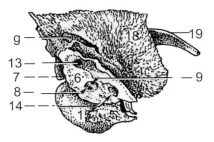

V. The **lamina cribrosa (23)** and the **median crista galli (24)** of the **ethmoid bone** lie at the boundary with the nasal cavity. The **ethmoidal labyrinth (25)** and its ethmoturbinates project into the nasal cavity. The smaller ethmoturbinates situated externally are called **ectoturbinates (26)**. The larger, internal **endoturbinates (27)**, situated near the nasal septum, are numbered I to IV in series dorsoventrally. Endoturbinate I forms the osseous base for the **dorsal nasal concha (28)** while endoturbinate II is similarly associated with the **middle nasal concha (29)**. The **ventral nasal conchal bone (XVI)** is the osseous basis of the ventral nasal concha and belongs properly to the facial bones, not to the ethmoid bone.

Ethmoidal bone

(rostral view)

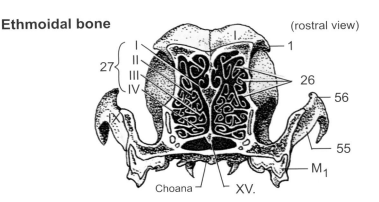

c) The **FACIAL PART OF THE SKULL** is formed by the **facial bones (VIII to XVII)**. It takes part in the external form of the nose or, respectively, of the nasopharyngeal inlet and of the nasal pharynx.

VIII. The small **lacrimal bone** bears in its center the **fossa of the lacrimal sac (54)**, which receives the lacrimal sac.

IX. With its **temporal process (55)**, the zygomatic bone participates in forming the zygomatic arch. Its **frontal process (56)** is the site of attachment of the orbital ligament.

X. The **nasal bone** lies dorsal on the nose.

4 **XI.** The **maxilla** has an infraorbital canal situated centrally in its **body (57)**. The canal is the passage for the infraorbital a. and n. Coming from the pterygopalatine fossa caudally, these structures enter the canal through the **maxillary foramen (58)** and leave it by the **infraorbital foramen (59)** rostrolaterally. The lacrimal sac passes over into the nasolacrimal duct which passes through the **lacrimal canal (60)** and, rostrally, the **lacrimal groove (61)**. The **frontal (62)**, **zygomatic (63)** and **palatine (64)** processes respectively, border the bones of like name. The **alveolar process (65)** bears dental alveoli. In contrast to the other domestic mammals, the canine maxilla has no paranasal sinus, but rather a laterally directed outpouching, the **maxillary recess (65')**.

XII. The **incisive bone** consists of a **body (66)**, an **alveolar process (67)**, a **palatine process (68)**, and a **nasal process (69)**.

XIII. The **palatine bone**, by means of the medial surface of its **perpendicular lamina (70)**, participates in the formation of the nasopharyngeal meatus. Its lateral surface enters into the formation of the orbit. In common with the palatine process of the maxilla, the **horizontal lamina (71)** forms the osseous base of the hard palate.

XIV. The pterygoid bone bounds the nasopharynx laterally and features a **hamulus (72)** caudoventrally.

XV. The vomer has a dorsomedian **septal groove (73)** for the reception of the nasal septum.

XVI. The ventral nasal conchal bone was mentioned previously as the osseous base of the ventral concha. It is joined by suture to the medial surface of the maxilla.

5 **XVII.** The mandible consists of a vertical ramus and a horizontal body. The long mandibular canal (for the inferior alveolar a., v. and n.) begins caudally on the ramus at the **mandibular foramen (74)** and terminates rostrally on the body with several **mental foramina (75)**. The **body of the mandible (76)** has a **ventral margin (77)**, an **alveolar margin (78)**, and medially a very faint **mylohyoid line (79)** for the origin of the m. mylohyoideus. Caudoventrally, the **ramus of the mandible (80)** exhibits an **angle of the mandible (81)** with an **angular process (82)**. The **masseteric fossa (83)** is a triangular fossa on the lateral surface of the mandible for the attachment of the m. masseter; whereas, an indistinct **pterygoid fossa (84)** is present medially, providing insertion to the m. pterygoideus. The **condylar process (85)** participates with its **head of the mandible (86)** in the formation of the temporomandibular articulation and, with the **neck of the mandible (87)** passes over into the concave **mandibular notch (88)** situated caudal to the **coronoid process (89)**. The temporalis muscle inserts on the coronoid process.

Cranium

External lamina (a) ▶
Diploë (b) ▶
Internal lamina (c) ▶
Osseous tentorium cerebelli (d) ▶
Temporal meatus (e) ▶
Transverse sinus canal (f) ▼
Sulcus of transverse sinus (g) ▶
Retroarticular foramen (h) ▶
Temporal fossa (j)
  External frontal crest (k)
  External sagittal crest (l)
  Nuchal crest (m)
  Temporal crest (m')
Carotid canal
  Caudal carotid foramen (n) ▶
  Internal carotid foramen (o) ▶
  External carotid foramen (p) ▶
Jugular foramen (q) ▶
Cranial cavity
Rostral fossa of cranium (r) ▶
  Ethmoidal fossae (s) ▶
  Sulcus chiasmatis (t) ▶
Middle fossa of cranium (u) ▶
  Hypophyseal fossa (v) ▶
  Piriform fossa (w) ▶
Caudal fossa of cranium (x) ▶
  Pontine impression (y) ▶
  Medullary impression (z) ▶
Petrooccipital fissure (z') ▶

Ossa neurocranii

I. Os frontale ▶
Zygomatic process (1)
Ethmoidal foramina (2)
Rostral frontal sinus (3a)
Lateral frontal sinus (3b)
Medial frontal sinus (3c)

II. Os parietale
Tentorial process (4)

III. Os interparietale
Tentorial process (5)

IV. Os temporale
a. Petrous part (6)
Mastoid process (7)
Internal acoustic meatus
  Internal acoustic pore (8) ▶
Facial canal (9) ▶
  Stylomastoid foramen (10)
Canaliculus of chorda tympani (11)
  Petrotympanic fissure (12)
Cerebellar (floccular) fossa (13) ▶
Canal of trigeminal nerve (14) ▶

b. Tympanic part (15)
External acoustic meatus
  External acoustic pore (16)
Bulla tympanica (17)
Ostium tympanicum tubae auditivae (17')

c. Squamous part (18)
Zygomatic process (19) ▼
Mandibular fossa (20)
  Articular surface (21)
Retroarticular process (22)

V. Ethmoidal bone ▶
Lamina cribrosa (23) ▶
Crista galli (24) ▶
Ethmoidal labyrinth (25) ▶
Ethmoturbinates
  Ectoturbinates (26) ▶
  Endoturbinates (27) ▶
    Dorsal nasal concha (28) ▶
    Middle nasal concha (29) ▶

VI. Os occipitale ▶
Squama occipitalis (30) ▶
  External occipital protuberance (31) ▶
  Tentorial process (31') ▶
Lateral part (32) ▶
  Occipital condyle (33) ▶
  Condylar canal (34) ▶
  Hypoglossal canal (35) ▶
  Jugular (paracondylar) process (36) ▶
Basilar part (37) ▶
  Foramen magnum (38) ▶
  Pharyngeal tubercle (39) ▶
  Muscular tubercle (40) ▶

VII. Os sphenoidale ▶
Os basisphenoidale
Body (41) ▶
  Sella turcica (42) ▶
Wing (43) ▶
  Foramen rotundum (44) ▶
  Foramen ovale (45) ▶
  Pterygoid crest (46) ▶
Alar canal (47) ▶
  Rostral alar foramen (48) ▶
  Caudal alar foramen (49)

Os presphenoidale
Body (50) ▶
Wing (51) ▶
  Optic canal (52) ▶
  Orbital fissure (53) ▶

Face

Bones of face ▶

VIII. Lacrimal bone ▶
Fossa of lacrimal bone (54) ▶

IX. Zygomatic bone ▶
Temporal process (55) ▶
Frontal process (56) ▶

X. Nasal bone ▶

XI. Maxilla ☆
Body of maxilla (57) ☆
  Infraorbital canal
    Maxillary foramen (58) ☆
    Infraorbital foramen (69) ☆
  Lacrimal canal (60) ☆
  Lacrimal groove (61) ☆
  Frontal process (62) ☆
  Zygomatic process (63) ☆
  Palatine process (64) ☆
  Alveolar process (65) ☆
  Maxillary recess (65')

XII. Incisive bone ▶
Body of incisive bone (66) ▶
Alveolar process (67) ▶
Palatine process (68) ▶
Nasal process (69) ▶

XIII. Palatine bone ▶
Perpendicular lamina (70) ▶
Horizontal lamina (71) ▶

XIV. Pterygoid bone ▶
Pterygoid hamulus (72) ▶

XV. Vomer ▶
Septal groove (73) ▶

XVI. Bone of ventral nasal concha ▶ ☆

XVII. Mandible ☐
Mandibular canal
  Mandibular foramen (74) ☐
  Mental foramina (75) ☐
Body of mandible (76) ☐
  Ventral border (77) ☐
  Alveolar border (78) ☐
  Mylohyoid line (79) ☐
Ramus of mandible (80) ☐
  Angle of mandible (81) ☐
    Angular process (82) ☐
  Masseteric fossa (83) ☐
  Pterygoid fossa (84) ☐
  Condylar [articular] process (85) ☐
    Head of mandible (86) ☐
    Neck of mandible (87) ☐
  Mandibular notch (88) ☐
  Coronoid [muscular] process (89) ☐

(paramedian section) ▶

XI. Maxilla ☆

XVII. Mandible ☐

3. LYMPHATIC SYSTEM, SUPERFICIAL VEINS OF THE HEAD, FACIAL NERVE (VII)

The skin is removed from the left side of the head taking care to preserve superficial arteries, veins and nerves, and cutaneous muscles. The external ear is severed at its base and removed. Following this, the m. cutaneus faciei, a part of the platysma, is exposed, detached from underlying structures and reflected rostrally, keeping intact the mm. malaris, zygomaticus and parotidoauricularis. To display arteries, veins and nerves, each of the facial muscles is either retracted or its coarse muscle bundles are pushed aside serially along the course of the veins and nerves. After its exposure the m. levator nasolabialis is transected and both parts reflected. The maxillary v. and facial n. are displayed by removing all of the parotid gland except for a small remnant at the beginning of the parotid duct.

a) The **LYMPHATIC SYSTEM** of the head (see also text-illustration) includes the palpable parotid and mandibular lymph nodes, which are situated superficially, and the deeper medial retropharyngeal and inconstant lateral retropharyngeal lymph nodes.

The **parotid lymph node (24)** lies at the level of the temporomandibular joint deep to the rostral border of the parotid gland. Afferent lymphatic vessels come from the superficial head regions dorsal to a line joining the eye and the base of the ear. Efferent vessels go to the medial retropharyngeal lymph node.

The **mandibular lymph nodes (29)** lie rostroventral to the mandibular gland. Afferent lymphatic vessels come from the deeper regions of the head and from superficial regions of the head ventral to the line joining the eye and the base of the ear. Efferent vessels also pass to the medial retropharyngeal lymph node.

The **medial retropharyngeal lymph node (30)** lies deep to and caudal to the mandibular gland, dorsolaterally and caudal to the pharynx. Lymph is derived from the deeper regions of the head, and from the mandibular and parotid lymph nodes. Its efferent vessels unite to form the jugular trunk (tracheal lymphatic trunk). An inconstant lateral retropharyngeal lymph node may be intercalated in the path of lymph vessels passing to the medial retropharyngeal node. The lateral node then also receives a part of the lymph from the parotid node. When present, the lateral retropharyngeal node lies at the caudal border of the parotid gland, on a level with the wing of the atlas. Its efferent vessels run to the medial retropharyngeal node.

Lymph nodes of head

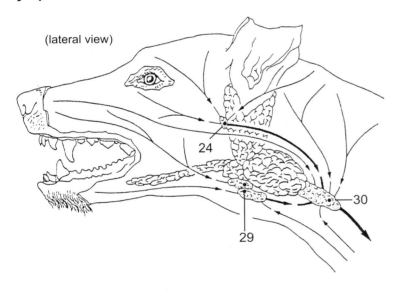

(lateral view)

b) The **SUPERFICIAL VEINS** arise from the **external jugular v. (18)** that, caudal to the mandibular gland, bifurcates into a maxillary v. dorsally and a linguofacial v. ventrally. (The superficial arteries of the external ear and face stem from the external carotid and the facial a. respectively, and will be considered with the veins.)

The **maxillary v. (8)** collects blood from the external ear and in particular from the deeper head regions such as palate, cranial cavity, eye and mandible. Within the parotid gland, it gives off the **caudal auricular v. (7)** to the caudal contour of the ear, and a thumbs breadth rostral to that the **superficial temporal v. (6)**, which arches across the temporal region. At the base of the ear, the large **rostral auricular v. (5)** branches from the latter to reach the cranial border of the external ear. The maxillary v. continues deeply medial to the temporomandibular joint. After forming the pterygoid, palatine and ophthalmic plexuses, the maxillary v. anastomoses at the medial angle of the eye with a terminal branch of the facial v. and deep facial v. (see below).

The **linguofacial v. (17)** provides for the venous drainage of the tongue and face. Ventral to the mandibular gland it bifurcates into the lingual v. directed ventrorostrally and the facial v., which extends dorsorostrally. Shortly after

its origin, the **lingual v. (15)** dispatches the hyoid venous arch that passes transversely to anastomose with the lingual v. of the opposite side. After that, the lingual v. crosses the caudal border of the m. mylohyoideus dorsally, and just before entering the tongue gives off the **sublingual v. (11)**. The latter vein is seen by displacing the caudal border of the m. stylohyoideus rostrally.

Initially, the **facial v. (14)** runs ventrolaterally along the mandible where it gives off the **submental v. (10)**. This vein is directed ventrally across the insertion of the m. digastricus and continues ventromedial to the body of the mandible as far as the chin (mental region). The facial vein, after providing the **inferior labial v. (9)** to the lower lip, and then the **angular v. of the mouth (12)** to the oral commissure, continues obliquely, curving over the face to the medial angle of the eye. On the caudal aspect of the facial v. at the level of the angle of the mouth, the **deep facial v. (13)** runs deeply under the zygomatic arch to the pterygopalatine fossa and orbit. From the rostral aspect of the facial v. the **superior labial v. (1)** branches to the upper lip and the small **lateral nasal v. (2)** is directed rostrally on the lateral aspect of the nose. The facial v. also anastomoses with the infraorbital v. This vein takes origin from the termination of the deep facial v. at the pterygopalatine fossa and runs rostrally through the infraorbital canal. (The **facial a. (14)** ends here by anastomosing with the infraorbital a.) Finally, reaching the *dorsum nasi*, the facial v. divides in the form of a 'T.' The **dorsal nasal v. (3)** runs rostrally toward the tip of the nose, while the **angular v. of the eye (4)** runs in the opposite direction to the medial angle of the eye where it anastomoses with branches of the deep facial and maxillary vv.

c) The **FACIAL NERVE (VII, INTERMEDIOFACIAL NERVE, —26)** consists of two parts, the facial n. and the intermediate n. The still undivided facial n. enters the facial canal at the internal acoustic pore of the petrous part of the temporal bone. At the sensory geniculate ganglion, it discharges the intermediate n. from which the chorda tympani runs through the petrotympanic fissure to join the lingual n. (from V3). The greater petrosal nerve, a parasympathetic nerve, also arises from the facial nerve. After uniting with the deep petrosal nerve, a sympathetic nerve, the greater petrosal n. continues as the n. of the pterygoid canal to the pterygopalatine ganglion (see p. 137). Still within the facial canal the facial n. proper gives off the n. stapedius to the m. stapedius. With the exception of its predominantly sensory internal auricular branches, the facial n. proper conveys exclusively motor fibers. The sensory fibers of its internal auricular branches are conveyed to the facial n. by the auricular branch of the vagus n. (X). After the facial n. emerges from the stylomastoid foramen, the internal auricular branches leave the facial n. and subsequently pierce the auricular cartilage to supply the external acoustic meatus, reaching nearly to the tympanic membrane. The facial n. continues by running around the osseous external acoustic meatus in a ventrally convex arch, deep to the parotid gland. From the convexity of the facial n. terminal branches arise in a caudorostral sequence and are described below. These are combined with sensory portions of the fifth cranial nerve and second cervical n. and innervate deep and superficial facial muscles, including the platysma and the caudal belly of the m. digastricus.

The **caudal auricular n. (23)** innervates the caudal auricular muscles and provides the **r. platysmatis (21)** for the cervical platysma. Consecutive digastric and stylohyoid branches supply the respective muscles. From the convexity of the facial n., the common trunk of the ramus colli and ventral buccal branch (labeled *R. buccolabialis ventr.* in the figure) passes ventrally. The **ramus colli (27)** is directed caudally. It innervates the m. parotidoauricularis and provides motor fibers to the transverse cervical n. of the second cervical n. The **ventral buccal branch (28, —labeled *R. buccolabialis ventr.* in the figure)**, accompanies the facial v. rostrally. At the level of the eye, it communicates with the dorsal buccal branch (labeled *R. buccolabialis dors.* in the figure) and the two nerves innervate the muscles of the cheek, lips and nose. The **dorsal buccal branch (25, —labeled *R. buccolabialis dors.* in the figure)** continues the rostral course of the facial nerve, passing upon the masseter about 2 cm. dorsal and parallel to the parotid duct. Its origin from the facial n. is deep to the parotid gland, and it emerges at the rostral border of the gland a little ventral to the parotid lymph node. With the dorsal buccal branch, the **auriculopalpebral n. (22)** is a terminal branch of the facial n. Its **rostral auricular branches (19)** supply the rostral and dorsal auricular muscles and its **palpebral branch (20)** forms a broadly ramifying plexus in the temporal region caudal to its entry into the muscles of the eyelids and nose.

Lymph nodes, arteries and veins of head and facialis n. (VII)

(lateral view)

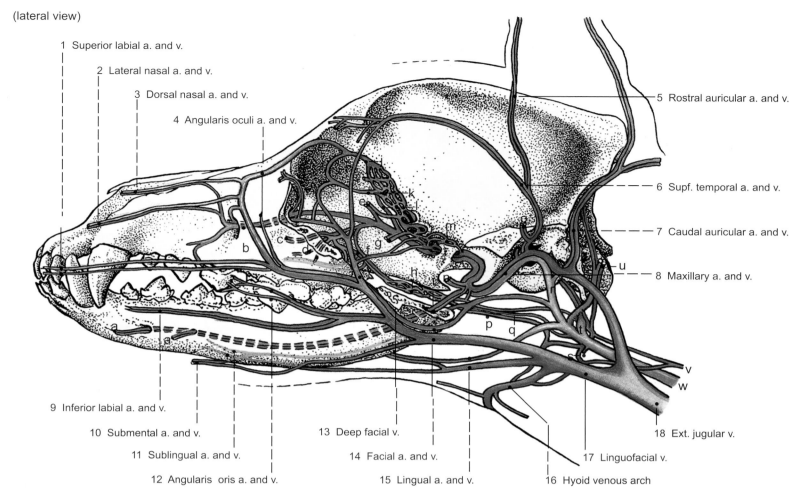

1 Superior labial a. and v.
2 Lateral nasal a. and v.
3 Dorsal nasal a. and v.
4 Angularis oculi a. and v.
5 Rostral auricular a. and v.
6 Supf. temporal a. and v.
7 Caudal auricular a. and v.
8 Maxillary a. and v.
9 Inferior labial a. and v.
10 Submental a. and v.
11 Sublingual a. and v.
12 Angularis oris a. and v.
13 Deep facial v.
14 Facial a. and v.
15 Lingual a. and v.
16 Hyoid venous arch
17 Linguofacial v.
18 Ext. jugular v.

Legend :

a Mental br.
b Infraorbital a. and v.
c Sphenopalatine a. and v.
d Greater palatine a. and v.
e Rostr. deep temporal a. and v.
f Lesser palatine a. and v.
g Buccal a. and v.
h Palatine plexus
i Inferior alveolar a. and v.
j Dors. ext. ophthalmic v.
k Ventr. ext. ophthalmic v.
l Ophthalmic plexus and ext. ophthalmic a.
m Pterygoid plexus
n Deep temporal a. and v.
o Transverse facial a. and v.
p Ascending pharyngeal a. and v.
q Pharyngeal v.
r Ext. carotid a.
s Cran. thyroid a. and v.
t Int. carotid a. and carotid sinus
u Occipital a. and v.
v Int. jugular v.
w Com. carotid a.

19 Rostr. auricular brr.
20 Palpebral br.
21 Platysmal br.
22 Auriculopalpebral n.
23 Caud. auricular n.
24 Parotid ln
25 Dors. buccolabial br.
26 Intermediofacial n.
27 Ramus colli
28 Ventr. buccolabial br.
29 Mandubular lnn.
30 Med. retropharyngeal ln.

(see pp. 95, 103)

Legend :

31 Levator nasolabialis m.
32 Levator labii superioris m.
33 Caninus m.
34 Mentalis m.
35 Orbicularis oris m.
36 Levator anguli oculi med. m.
37 Orbicularis oculi m.
38 Retractor anguli oculi lat. m.
39 Malaris m.
40 Zygomaticus m.
41 Frontoscutularis m.
42 Interscutularis m.
43 Scutuloauricularis supf. m.
44 Occipitalis m.
45 Cervicoscutularis m.
46 Cervicoauricularis medius m.
47 Cervicoauricularis supf. m.
48 Cervicoauricularis prof. m.
49 Parotidoauricularis m.
50 Mylohyoideus m.
51 Cleidocervicalis m.
52 Sternocleidomastoideus m.
53 Sternohyoideus m.
a Infraorbital n. (V2)
b Transverse facial br. (V3)
c Parotid duct
d Int. auricular br. (VII)
e Great auricular n.
f Transverse cervical n.

4. FACIAL MUSCLES AND MANDIBULAR MUSCLES

The superficial facial muscles in the masseteric and temporal regions will be dissected on the left half of the head and the mandibular muscles will be demonstrated on the right half of the head, where the skin is removed. The innervation by the mandibular nerve (V3) will be identified later after the removal of the mandible (see page 97).

The FACIAL MUSCLES and MANDIBULAR MUSCLES are two of six muscle groups on the head. The division into muscle groups is according to the genesis of the muscles and therefore according to their innervation. The facial muscles are supplied by the facial nerve (VII) and the masticatory muscles and mylohyoideus by the mandibular division (V3) of the trigeminal nerve (V). The muscles that manipulate the eyeball are innervated by cranial nerves III, IV and VI. The pharyngeal muscles belong to the area of innervation of the IX and X cranial nerves and the laryngeal muscles to the area of innervation of cranial nerve X. The hypoglossal nerve innervates the muscles of the tongue.

a) Corresponding to their innervation by the facial nerve, the MUSCLES OF FACIAL EXPRESSION are also called FACIAL MUSCLES and subdivided into superficial and deep muscles. The deep facial muscles (the mm. stapedius, occipitohyoideus and stylohyoideus) are either not demonstrated or are discussed with the muscles of the mandibular space (m. digastricus). In the main, the superficial facial muscles have the characteristics of cutaneous muscles. Arising chiefly on smooth bony areas or from fascia, they either radiate in the skin or are arranged in a sphincter-like manner around facial openings by a looping course of their fibers. Facial muscles are not antagonistic to one another but determine facial expression by their disposition and are therefore also called mimic muscles. In lower animals the facial muscles are stratified into three more or less uniform layers, one upon the other, from which, in phylogenetically advanced development, the individual facial muscles have derived.

The transverse muscle fibers of the very weak **m. sphincter colli superficialis** (24) lie in the ventral neck region and are most distinct in the laryngeal region. No facial muscles are derived from this muscle.

The caudal auricular muscles have split off from the longitudinal muscle fibers of the platysma. By means of its **m. cutaneus faciei** (23), the platysma radiates into the lips.

In the phylogenetic sense, the m. sphincter colli profundus consisted originally of a transverse cutaneous muscle layer which, even yet, is evident in the direction of the muscle fibers of the mm. malaris, zygomaticus and parotidoauricularis. In the course of phylogenesis, the original uniform muscle layer, seen for example in the mole, has split up into the individual ear muscles, the muscles of the eyelid and nose as well as the muscles of the lips and cheeks.

Of the **auricular muscles** with caudal, dorsal, rostral and ventral groups, two each of the most superficial muscles are represented. **Functionally** the auricular muscles are classified into tensors of the scutiform cartilage, muscles that turn the funnel-shaped opening of the external ear laterally, muscles that elevate the ear, muscles that depress the external ear, and muscles that turn the opening of the external ear medially. Each muscle derives its name from its origin and insertion. Innervation: Facial nerve with its auricular and cervical branches. The **scutiform cartilage** (11) lies rostrodorsal to the external ear between individual ear muscles, and is a moveable site of attachment for several muscles.

Of the **caudal auricular muscles**, the **m. cervicoauricularis superficialis** (9) and the muscle with which it is continuous rostrally, the **m. cervicoscutularis** (12), are fused at their origin at the nuchal midline, separating only at their insertions on the auricular and scutiform cartilages, respectively. (The underlying mm. cervicoauricularis medius and cervicoauricularis profundus turn the auricular opening laterally; see page 93.)

Of the **dorsal auricular muscles**, the weak **m. occipitalis** (13) runs rostrally in an arch from the external sagittal crest of the parietal bone, contacting the lateral side of the scutiform cartilage on its lateral side. The **m. interscutularis** (14) is in association with the occipitalis rostrally. Its transverse fibers extend between right and left scutiform cartilages.

Of the **rostral auricular muscles**, the **m. frontoscutularis** (4) which is continuous with the interscutularis, runs in a rostrally convex arch across the midline, connecting the scutiform cartilages of both sides. Rostrally, muscle bundles separate from the m. frontoscutularis and, without reaching the midline, radiate into the upper eyelid. The **m. scutuloauricularis superficialis** (10) runs from the scutiform cartilage to the rostral border of the auricular cartilage.

Of the **ventral auricular muscles**, the **m. parotidoauricularis** (8) extends from the region of the larynx across the lateral surface of the parotid gland to the base of the ear. The m. mandibuloauricularis (26) runs deeply between the mandible and the base of the ear. It can vary considerably in size or even be lacking.

II. Muscles of the eyelids and of the nose are supplied by the auriculopalpebral n., a branch of the facial nerve.

The **m. orbicularis oculi** (2) is the anular muscle that closes the palpebral fissure.

The **m. retractor anguli oculi lateralis** (3) radiates into the lateral angle of the eye.

The **m. levator anguli oculi medialis** (15) extends into the upper eyelid near the medial angle of the eye.

The **m. levator nasolabialis** (1) begins at the medial angle of the eye and is expanded before it radiates into the upper lip.

The **m. malaris** (6) is interwoven with muscle fibers of the platysma and, with very delicate bundles of muscle fibers, extends from the cheek into the lower eyelid.

III. The muscles of the lips and cheek are innervated by dorsal and ventral buccal branches of the facial nerve.

The **m. orbicularis oris** (5) surrounds the opening of the mouth in a circular manner with a median interruption in both the upper and lower lip.

Rostrally the **m. buccinator** (17) is situated deep to the m. orbicularis oris and is interwoven with it. From the upper lip it crosses over the cheek to the alveolar border of the mandible, and from the lower lip to the alveolar border of the maxilla. The intercrossing of muscle fibers on the cheek gives rise to a longitudinal muscle raphe.

The **m. zygomaticus** (7) courses between the angle of the mouth and the scutiform cartilage. From its caudal border transverse muscle bundles pass toward the mandibular space.

The **m. caninus** (see p. 93) arises ventral to the infraorbital foramen and radiates into the upper lip at the level of the canine tooth.

The **m. levator labii superioris** (see p. 93) arises rostral to the infraorbital foramen and enters the upper lip dorsoparallel to the m. caninus.

b) From a functional-topographical point of view, and corresponding to their position on the mandible, the **MANDIBULAR MUSCLES** are subdivided into superficial muscles of the throat and external and internal muscles of mastication. Each group consists of two muscles. As muscles that act to close the mouth, the muscles of mastication, particularly in carnivores, are very strong with tendinous tissue permeating through them. Their place of origin or insertion is marked on the bones of the skull by more or less distinct fossae: Temporal fossa, masseteric fossa, pterygoid fossa and fovea for the correspondingly named muscles. Of the muscles of the mandibular space (the space between right and left halves of the mandible), only the digastricus in contracting acts to open the mouth, and the m. mylohyoideus as a levator of the tongue advances the ingesta to a position between the cheek teeth and in that way supports the masticatory process.

I. Of the **superficial muscles of the mandibular space**, the **m. digastricus** (20) runs from the jugular process to the ventral border of the body of the mandible. A slight, indistinct, intermediate tendon separates its two muscle bellies. Only the rostral belly is innervated by the mandibular nerve, the caudal belly being supplied by the facial nerve. The **m. mylohyoideus** (18) has a linear origin from the very weak mylohyoid line on the medial side of each half of the body of the mandible, and its transverse muscle fibers run to a median muscle raphe. Its caudal fibers attach to the basihyoid bone. The hammock-like muscle elevates and supports the tongue as well as the floor of the mouth.

II. Of the **external muscles of mastication**, the **m. temporalis** (16) arises from the circumference and the base of the temporal fossa to the coronoid process of the mandible. An accessory portion with a completely divergent muscle fiber direction commences at the caudal end of the zygomatic arch and courses dorsoparallel to the latter as far as the rostral border of the coronoid process. The varying fiber direction can be seen after removal of the temporal fascia. The **m. masseter** (19) consists of a superficial and a deep part, which arise laterally or, respectively, medially from the zygomatic arch and insert at the masseteric fossa or, respectively, at its circumference.

Muscles of head

Regions of face

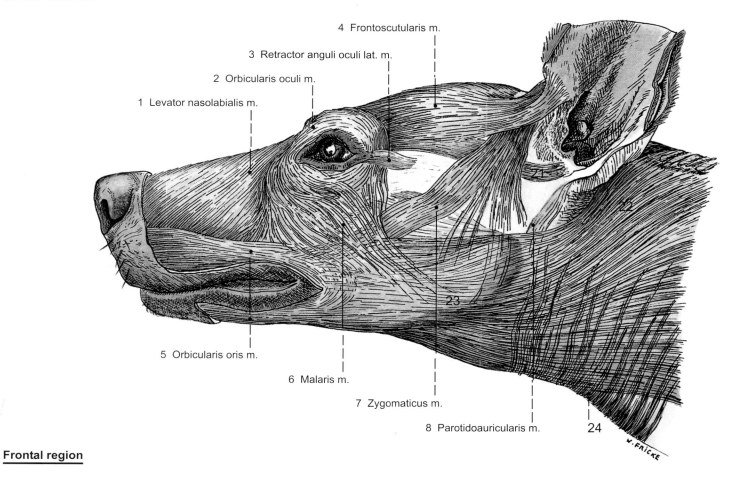

4 Frontoscutularis m.

3 Retractor anguli oculi lat. m.

2 Orbicularis oculi m.

1 Levator nasolabialis m.

5 Orbicularis oris m.

6 Malaris m.

7 Zygomaticus m.

8 Parotidoauricularis m.

23

24

W. FRICKE

Frontal region

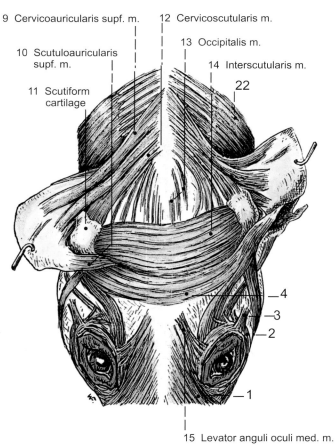

9 Cervicoauricularis supf. m.

10 Scutuloauricularis supf. m.

11 Scutiform cartilage

12 Cervicoscutularis m.

13 Occipitalis m.

14 Interscutularis m.

22

— 4

— 3

— 2

— 1

15 Levator anguli oculi med. m.

Masseteric and temporal regions

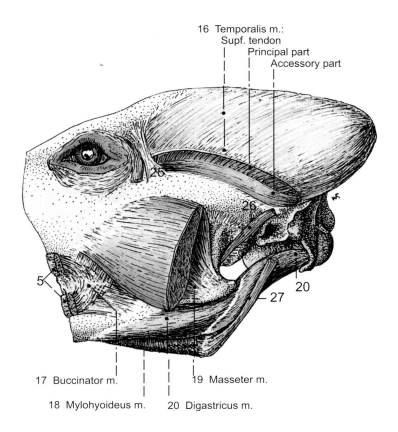

16 Temporalis m.:
Supf. tendon
Principal part
Accessory part

26

26

20

5

27

17 Buccinator m.

18 Mylohyoideus m.

19 Masseter m.

20 Digastricus m.

Legend :

21 Zygomaticoauricularis m.
   Platysma:
22   Cutaneus colli m.
23   Cutaneus faciei m.

24 Sphincter colli supf. m.
25 Orbital lig.
26 Mandibuloauricularis m.
27 Stylohyoideus m.

(see pp. 93, 97)

5. INTERNAL (DEEP) MUSCLES OF MASTICATION, TRIGEMINAL NERVE (V), MAXILLARY NERVE (V2) AND MANDIBULAR NERVE (V3)

The head is bisected midsagittally. The right half is used for the present dissection and involves the disarticulation of the right side of the mandible and subsequent demonstration of internal muscles of mastication, and the mandibular and maxillary nn. The masseter muscle is removed in layers so that one is able to observe the different fiber directions of the superficial and deep parts of the muscle and its strong central tendons. Two centimeters rostral to the temporomandibular articulation, the terminal branches of the masseteric n. (3) are then demonstrated on the cut surface of the muscle after the nerve courses laterally over the mandibular notch. The zygomatic arch is sawn through at the temporomandibular articulation and rostral to the attachment of the orbital ligament. The isolated piece of arch is then removed. The m. digastricus is detached at its insertion onto the ventral border of the body of the mandible, taking care to preserve the branch of the mylohyoid n. innervating it. Subsequently the m. mylohyoideus is incised at its origin along the mylo-hyoid line in common with the oral mucous membrane lying deeper. With a strong sideways movement of the mandible it is possible to transect: a) the insertion of the m. temporalis onto the medial and lateral surfaces of the coronoid process of the mandible; and b) the mm. pterygoideus medialis and latera-lis at the pterygoid fossa. Following this, the inferior alveolar a., v., and n. are cut through at the mandibular foramen, the entrance to the mandibular canal. The preparation is completed by disarticulating the mandible after transecting associated ligaments. The articular cavity is subdivided into two 'storeys' by the articular disc. To widen the field of dissection, the m. temporalis is removed in part as far as the dorsal contour of the periorbita. The **deep temporal nn.** (2) within the m. temporalis are preserved and followed retrogressively to their ramification from the masticatorius n. in common with the masseteric n. To demonstrate the branches of the maxillary n., the zygomatic gland is retracted from the pterygopalatine fossa.

a) The **INTERNAL MUSCLES OF MASTICATION** include the strong m. pterygoideus medialis and the weak m. pterygoideus lateralis. They extend from the pterygoid and adjacent bones to the indistinct pterygoid fossa on the medial surface of the ramus of the mandible. The mm. pterygoideus medialis and pterygoideus lateralis are innervated by the deeply situated nerves of like name. They leave the mandibular n. (V 3) immediately after its emergence from the foramen ovale.

The origin of the **m. pterygoideus medialis (8)** exhibits a conspicuous, glistening tendon on its external surface and is crossed superficially by the mandibular n.

The **m. pterygoideus lateralis (18)** is significantly smaller. It lies dorsal to the caudal border of the medial muscle, in the bifurcation between the buccal n. and the parent mandibular n.

b) The **TRIGEMINAL N.** (V; see also text-illustration) has a large sensory root and a smaller motor root. After leaving the brain but before passing through the skull, the sensory fibers of the large root are associated with the trigeminal ganglion (see p. 137). At the ganglion, the peripheral processes of the nerve cells form the three branches of the trigeminal n. The first branch, the sensory ophthalmic n. (V1), passes through the orbital fissure. The second branch, the sensory maxillary n. (V2), passes from the alar canal to ramify in the pterygopalatine fossa. The third branch, the mandibular n. (V3), joins the motor root before passing through the foramen ovale.

1 I. The **mandibular n. (V3, −5)** passes from the foramen ovale medial to the temporomandibular articulation and gives off the following nerve branches:

The **n. masticatorius (4)** supplies purely motor branches, the *deep temporal nn.* and the *masseteric n.* (see p. 95), to the like-named muscles of mastication.

With the n. masticatorius, the **buccal n. (1)** passes rostrodorsolaterally over the m. pterygoideus lateralis. Its sensory fibers supply the oral mucous membrane, and its autonomic fibers pass to the zygomatic and buccal glands.

The **lingual n. (10)** is the direct continuation of the mandibular n. The chorda tympani of the facial nerve passes rostroventrally from the tympanic fissure, crosses the external carotid artery medially and joins the commencement of the lingual n. at an acute angle. The special sensory fibers of the chorda tympani supply the taste buds of the rostral two-thirds of the tongue. Its autonomic fibers reach the mandibular gland and, rostrally, the sublingual gland. Sensory fibers of the lingual n. supply the rostral two-thirds of the tongue. A branch, the **sublingual n. (11)**, supplies the mucosa of the floor of the mouth.

The **auriculotemporal n. (7)** branches near the emergence of the mandibular n. from the foramen ovale and runs caudally around the temporomandibular articulation in a ventrally convex arch. Its autonomic fibers supply the parotid gland, and a sensory branch, the n. of the external acoustic meatus, supplies the meatus as far as the tympanic membrane. Its sensory rostral auricular branches pass on the rostral border of the external ear, and its sensory transverse facial branch supplies the face.

The **mylohyoid n. (9)** supplies motor innervation to the mylohyoideus muscle and the rostral belly of the m. digastricus; whereas, its sensory submental branches ramify in the chin region.

The **inferior alveolar n. (6)** enters the mandibular canal at the mandibular foramen (where it was previously transected). Here, it provides sensory fibers to the teeth of the lower jaw, and the skin of the chin by way of the mental branches that emerge through mental foramina.

2

II. The **maxillary n. (V2, −16)** passes through the foramen rotundum (round foramen) into the alar canal. This purely sensory nerve ramifies with three main nerve branches:

The **zygomatic n. (14)** proceeds to the ocular bulb and bifurcates within the periorbita into a ventral **zygomaticofacial ramus (13)** and a dorsal **zygomaticotemporal ramus (12)**. The latter receives autonomic fibers from the pterygopalatine ganglion and conveys these to the lacrimal gland. After leaving the orbit both rami supply the skin of the face dorsolateral to the eye.

The **infraorbital n. (15)**, a sensory nerve, continues the rostral course of the maxillary n. and, in the pterygopalatine fossa, enters into the infraorbital canal through the maxillary foramen. Within the pterygopalatine fossa it gives off alveolar branches that enter alveolar foramina of the maxilla to reach the caudal cheek teeth, and within the infraorbital canal it supplies branches to the remaining teeth of the upper jaw. After leaving the infraorbital foramen, the infraorbital nerve furnishes sensory branches to the external nose and the upper lip.

3

The **pterygopalatine n. (17)** leaves the maxillary n. rostroventrally. On its dorsal border, medial to the infraorbital n., the pterygopalatine n. exhibits the brownish pterygopalatine ganglion (m). This ganglion receives its parasympathetic and sympathetic fibers from the slender nerve of the pterygoid canal from VII and the sympathetic trunk respectively. The parasympathetic fibers synapse here with second neurons of the ganglion, and from the ganglion both sympathetic (without synapse) and parasympathetic fibers then pass to the end-branches of the pterygopalatine nerve. The following three end-branches, in dorsoventral sequence, supply sensory fibers to the mucous membrane and autonomic fibers to the glands of their area of supply, the palatine and nasal glands:

The **caudal nasal n. (21)** passes through the sphenopalatine foramen to the lateral nasal gland and the nasal conchae.

The **greater palatine n. (20)** reaches the hard palate through the greater palatine canal.

The **lesser palatine n. (19)** extends rostroventrally and medially around the rostral border of the medial pterygoid muscle to reach the soft palate.

Trigeminal n. (V)

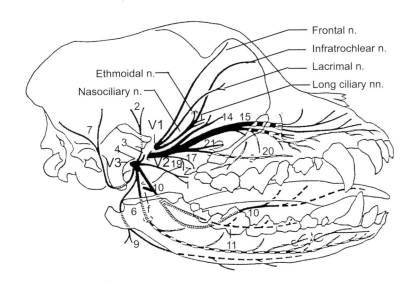

Frontal n.
Infratrochlear n.
Lacrimal n.
Long ciliary nn.
Ethmoidal n.
Nasociliary n.

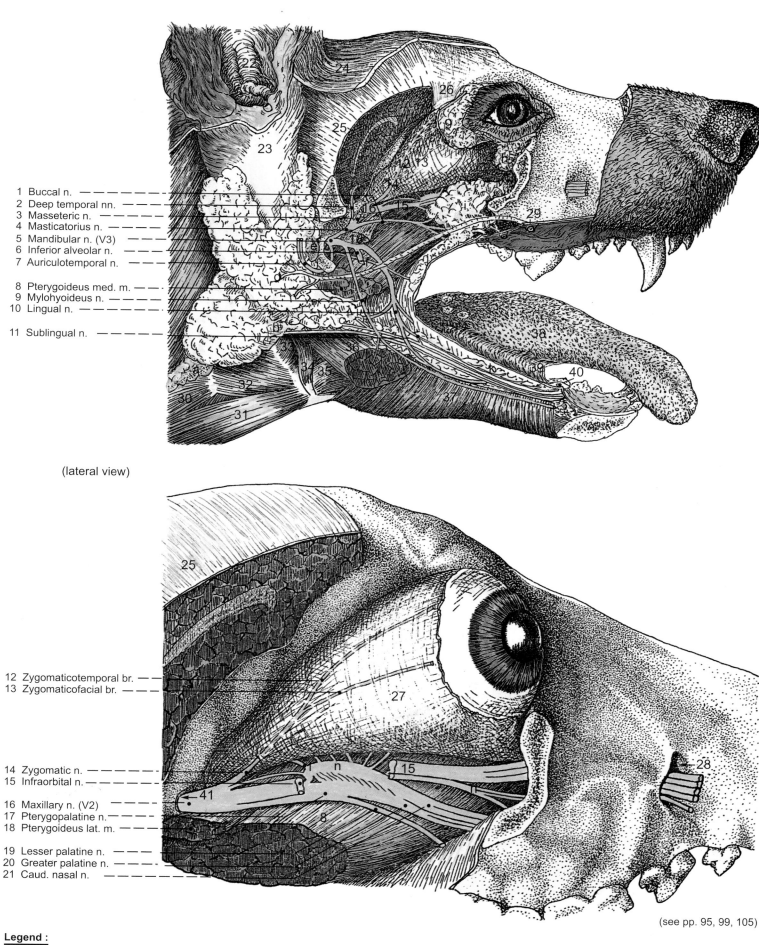

1 Buccal n.
2 Deep temporal nn.
3 Masseteric n.
4 Masticatorius n.
5 Mandibular n. (V3)
6 Inferior alveolar n.
7 Auriculotemporal n.

8 Pterygoideus med. m.
9 Mylohyoideus n.
10 Lingual n.

11 Sublingual n.

(lateral view)

12 Zygomaticotemporal br.
13 Zygomaticofacial br.

14 Zygomatic n.
15 Infraorbital n.

16 Maxillary n. (V2)
17 Pterygopalatine n.
18 Pterygoideus lat. m.

19 Lesser palatine n.
20 Greater palatine n.
21 Caud. nasal n.

(see pp. 95, 99, 105)

Legend :

22 Auricle (Scapha)	30 Sternothyreoideus m.	38 Tongue	a Med. retropharyngeal ln.	h Supf. gl. of third eyelid
23 Auricular cartilage	31 Sternohyoideus m.	39 Frenulum	b Mandibular gl. and duct	i Zygomatic gl. and duct
24 Frontascutularis m.	32 Thyreohyoideus m.	40 Sublingual caruncle	c Monostomatic sublingual	j Buccal gll.
25 Temporalis m.	33 Hyopharyngeus m.	41 Rostral alar foramen	gl. and duct	k Polystomatic sublingual gl.
26 Orbital lig.	34 Stylohyoideus m.		d Parotid gland and duct	l N. of pterygoid canal
27 Periorbita	35 Hyoglossus m.		e Parotid ln.	m Pterygopalatine ggl. and
28 Infraorbital for.	36 Digastricus m.		f Chorda tympani	orbital branches
29 Parotid papilla	37 Mylohyoideus m.		g Lacrimal gl.	n Superior alveolar branches

6. LACRIMAL APPARATUS, OPTIC NERVE (II), OPHTHALMIC NERVE (V1), NERVES AND MUSCLES OF THE EYE, AND EXTERNAL NOSE

With the separation of upper and lower eyelids, parts of the lacrimal apparatus are exposed as a result. Following this, the apex of the triangular cartilage supporting the third eyelid is freed from its site of attachment in the orbital cavity. On the lateral surface of the cartilage, the cutaneous covering is removed to expose the accessory lacrimal glands, namely the superficial gland of the third eyelid, while numerous lymph nodules are observed on the medial surface of the third eyelid. To expose and dissect the ocular bulb, more of the m. temporalis is ablated, the remaining periorbita removed, and the cone of eye muscles retracted ventrolaterally away from the osseous part of the orbital cavity. At this stage, one can see the **trochlea (21)** dorsomedial to the ocular bulb and should detach it from its site of attachment to the orbit. The optic n. lies centrally in the cone of extrinsic eye muscles and is surveyed by retracting them.

a) The **LACRIMAL APPARATUS** (see also text-illustration) includes the lacrimal glands and their system of excretory ducts. The **lacrimal gland (16)**, which lies medial to the orbital ligament and the **superficial gland of the third eyelid (20)** secrete the lacrimal fluid. This flows from the glands through narrow ductules into the **superior conjunctival fornix (A)** of the conjunctival sac. With movement of the eyelids, the cornea is moistened by a film of lacrimal fluid. This collects within the depth of the medial angle of the eye at the **lacrimal lake (B)** in the middle of which is the **lacrimal caruncle (C)** appearing above the surrounding fluid. A few millimeters away from the medial angle of the eye, the **lacrimal puncta (17)** lie near a margin of pigmented epithelium on the bulbar surface of the upper and lower eyelids. Lacrimal fluid flows through these small openings to superior and inferior **lacrimal canaliculi (18)**, which, in turn, unite at the **lacrimal sac (19)**. The nasolacrimal duct, which begins here, lies at first in the osseous lacrimal canal and then more rostrally in the lacrimal groove of the maxilla. The duct conveys the lacrimal fluid to the **nasolacrimal ostium**, a millimeter-sized opening in the nasal vestibule about one centimeter caudal to the ventral angle of the naris. The opening is found one centimeter caudal to the ventral angle of the naris at the beginning of the ventral nasal meatus where a distinct pigmented border is visible.

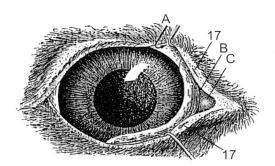

b) The **OPTIC N. (II, —13)** consists of a large bundle of nerve fibers that begins at the retina and the fibers of which, proceeding from the eyeball, receive medullary sheaths. The nerve passes to the optic chiasm, where the optic tract, the continuation to the diencephalon, begins. Developmentally, the optic nerve is to be regarded as a part of the brain. It is surrounded by a continuation of the three meninges, and the myelin sheaths of its fibers are formed by glial cells (oligodendroglia) of the central nervous system.

c) The **OPHTHALMIC N. (V1,** see text-illustration p.96) is the first branch of the trigeminal n. (V). Its branches are the lacrimal, frontal and nasociliary nerves.

The **lacrimal n. (5)** is slender; it accompanies the artery of like name and the previously discussed ramus zygomaticotemporalis (V2). Its autonomic fibers, which pass from the pterygopalatine ganglion, supply the lacrimal gland; and its sensory fibers, the upper eyelid.

The **frontal n. (4)** leaves the orbit lateral to the trochlea. It supplies sensory innervation to the skin of the frontal region.

The **nasociliary n. (10)** branches into the infratrochlear, ethmoidal and long ciliary nerves. The **infratrochlear n. (22)** leaves the orbit ventromedial to the trochlea and supplies the skin at the medial angle of the eye. The **ethmoidal n. (8)** contains sensory and autonomic fibers. It passes through the ethmoidal foramen (and is most easily identified here in the dissection) and then through the lamina cribrosa to the fundus of the nasal cavity. It can be followed between the m. rectus medialis and the m. obliquus dorsalis to its origin from the nasociliary n. Likewise, the **long ciliary nn. (9)** branch here from the nasociliary n. and accompany the optic n. laterally. Their sympathetic fibers innervate the m. dilatator pupillae and their sensory fibers supply the cornea.

d) The **NERVES and MUSCLES OF THE EYE** are discussed together. In the ongoing dissection, the nerves to the extrinsic eye muscles (III, IV and VI) are used to identify the muscles themselves and the nerves are also followed in

retrograde fashion to their origins. The muscles of the ocular bulb (eyeball) include the mm. rectus dorsalis, —medialis, —ventralis, and –lateralis, the mm. obliquus dorsalis and –ventralis, the m. levator palpebrae superioris; and the m. retractor bulbi, which surrounds the optic n. like a cloak. In the main, the rectus muscles move the eyeball medially toward the nose or laterally toward the temporal region, as well as dorsally and ventrally. The mm. obliquus dorsalis and ventralis produce inward and outward rotation of the bulb respectively.

I. The **oculomotor n. (III)** innervates all extrinsic muscles of the eye except the mm. obliquus dorsalis and rectus lateralis. (Some authors exclude the retractor bulbi muscle.)

II. The **trochlear n. (IV)** supplies only the m. obliquus dorsalis.

III. The **abducent n. (VI)** innervates the m. rectus lateralis and the lateral portion of the m. retractor bulbi. (Some authors include the entire retractor bulbi muscle.)

The **oculomotor n.** terminates with its **ventral ramus (12)** passing distally into the **m. obliquus ventralis (23)**. The ramus can be followed in retrograde fashion between the mm. rectus lateralis and ventralis and finally through the m. retractor bulbi to the lateral aspect of the optic n. The **ciliary ganglion (15)** can be seen there as a brownish body the size of a millet seed. Fine short ciliary nn. from the ganglion accompany the optic n. and penetrate the sclera. They supply parasympathetic fibers to the mm. ciliaris and sphincter pupillae and sympathetic fibers to the m. dilatator pupillae. The **dorsal ramus (11)** of the oculomotor n. innervates the **m. rectus dorsalis (3)** and the more superficial **m. levator palpebrae superioris (2)**, both of which are crossed over in succession by the frontal n. (from V1). The **trochlear n. (6)** enters the **m. obliquus dorsalis (1)** at the junction of its caudal and middle thirds. The tendon of insertion of the latter muscle passes over the trochlear cartilage, turning here from a longitudinal to a transverse direction and ending on the eyeball ventral to the insertion of the m. rectus dorsalis. The **m. rectus medialis (14)**, which lies ventromedial to the dorsal rectus, is supplied by the oculomotor n. The **m. rectus lateralis (24)**, an abductor of the eyeball (turns the anterior pole of the eyeball laterally), is entered on its dorsal border by the **abducens n. (7)**.

e) The **EXTERNAL NOSE** (see text-illustration) extends from the **root of the nose (D)** over the **dorsum nasi (E)** up to the **apex of the nose (G)**. At the apex, each of the nares is bounded laterally by the **wing of the nostril (H, —ala nasi)** and medially by the **planum nasale (F)**. These rostral features are supported by the cartilages of nose and septum. The planum nasale is formed by hairless, modified skin in the region of the nares and exhibits a median **philtrum (I)**. The nasal septum is membranous in the region of the nares and cartilaginous in its rostral two-thirds and supported by bone in its caudal third.

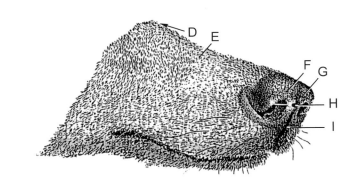

Lacrimal apparatus, accessory organs of eye and cranial nn. II, III, IV, V1, V2 and VI

(lateral view)

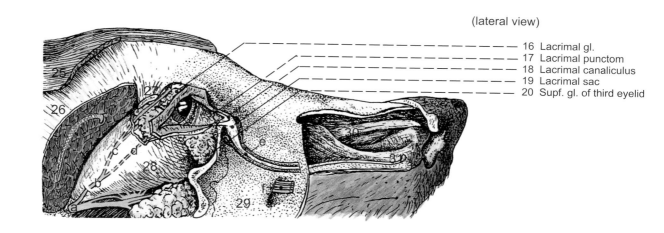

(dorsolateral view)

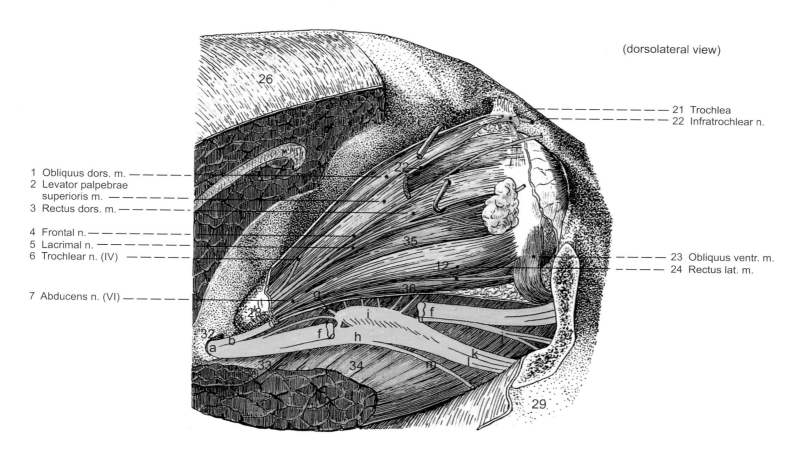

(dorsolateral view)

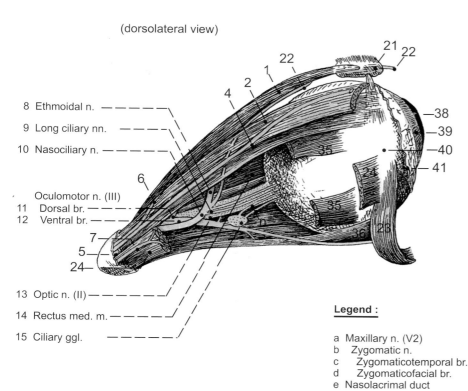

(rostral view)

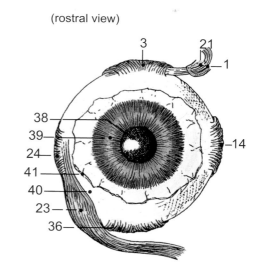

(see pp. 97, 103, 105)

7. NOSE, LARYNX, ORAL CAVITY AND PHARYNX

a) NOSE:

1 I. The **nasal cavity** begins at the naris with the **nasal vestibule (1)**, which is covered by a pigmented cutaneous mucous membrane. The vestibule houses the **straight fold (4)** dorsally, a mucosal fold extending rostrally from the dorsal nasal concha; the **alar fold (3)** a cartilage-supported mucosal fold extending rostrally from the ventral nasal concha; and an indistinct **basal fold (2)** ventral to the alar fold. The nasal cavity proper is covered with respiratory mucous membrane and contains the dorsal and ventral nasal conchae (see p. 90). The middle nasal concha coming from the caudal part of the nasal cavity inserts between them. The lateral nasal gland lies in the maxillary recess of the maxilla and, like the nasolacrimal duct, opens into the nasal vestibule. Both the secretion from the gland and the lacrimal fluid moisten the planum nasale. The **fundus nasi (9)** houses the ethmoidal labyrinth which is in part clothed with olfactory mucous membrane.

II. Four **nasal meatuses** extend through the nasal cavity. The **dorsal nasal meatus (8)** is between the dorsal nasal concha and the nasal bone and leads to the olfactory organ (therefore, the *olfactory meatus*). The **middle nasal meatus (6)** first lies between the dorsal and ventral nasal conchae and then, at the middle nasal concha, splits into a dorsal passage and a ventral passage that lead to paranasal sinuses. Hence it is also called the *sinus meatus*. The **ventral**
2 **nasal meatus (5)** is also called the *respiratory meatus*. It lies between the ventral nasal concha and the palate and reaches to the fundus nasi where it is continued by the nasopharyngeal meatus to the choanae. Olfactory, sinus and respiratory meatuses merge medially into the **common nasal meatus (7)**, which is the narrow passage alongside the nasal septum the entire dorsoventral extent of the nasal cavity.

III. The **olfactory organ** lies in the fundus nasi, its olfactory mucous membrane clothing here part of the ethmoidal labyrinth.

IV. The **vomeronasal organ** (see p. 123) is also lined with olfactory mucous membrane. It is on the floor of the nasal vestibule at the transition to the nasal cavity proper and lies directly on the cartilaginous nasal septum. It communicates with the roof of the oral cavity through the incisive (or nasopalatine) duct. Functionally it serves as an oral olfactory- or scent-organ for the reception of odors, especially pheromones.

V. The **olfactory nn. (I)** are composed of the processes of olfactory cells running chiefly from the olfactory organ in the fundus nasi and also from the vomeronasal organ in the nasal vestibule (vomeronasal n.). The nerves pass through the cribriform plate of the ethmoid bone into the olfactory bulb of the telencephalon (see p. 137).

b) The **LARYNX** is palpable ventral at the boundary of head and neck, forming part of the respiratory pathway and serving in phonation. Its entrance can be sealed off from the pharynx and from the path of food as occurs in swallowing. From within outwards the wall of the larynx consists of mucous membrane, cartilage and laryngeal muscles.

3 I. The **laryngeal mucosa** lines the lumen of the larynx. At the entrance of the larynx, on the vocal folds, and in the laryngeal ventricles it is a cutaneous mucosa with a stratified squamous epithelium; whereas in the remaining areas a ciliated respiratory mucosa is present.

II. The **cavity of the larynx** includes the vestibule of the larynx, the *rima glottis* with its vocal apparatus *(glottis)*, and the infraglottic cavity.

The **vestibule of the larynx (E)** extends from the free margin of the epiglottis to the **vestibular folds (F'')**. The **vocal apparatus (glottis, —F)** is formed by
4 both **vocal folds (F)** whose free borders bound the intermembranous part of the rima glottidis. The intercartilaginous part of the rima glottidis is formed by the arytenoid cartilages and their lining of mucous membrane. The muco-
5 sa of the vocal folds is underlain by the vocal ligament and is supported laterally by the vocalis muscle. Between the vestibular fold and the vocal fold is
6 the entrance to the **laryngeal ventricle (F')**. The infraglottic cavity extends from the vocal folds to the first tracheal ring.

7 III. Of the four **laryngeal cartilages**, portions of the arytenoid cartilages and the **epiglottic cartilage (21)** are elastic cartilage. The remaining laryngeal cartilages are hyaline. With its laminae, which are open dorsally, the **thyroid cartilage (20)** extensively encloses and protects the remaining parts of the larynx. The rostral cornu of the thyroid lamina is attached to the thyrohyoid element of the hyoid apparatus, the caudal cornu to the cricoid cartilage. The **arytenoid cartilage (19)** is paired. It has a muscular process caudally, a vocal process ventrally for attachment of the vocal ligament and vocalis muscle, a

wedge-shaped cuneiform process rostrodorsally, and a corniculate process caudodorsally. The unpaired **cricoid cartilage (22)** supports the laryngeal lumen dorsally between the laminae of the thyroid cartilage.

8 IV. Of the **laryngeal muscles** the m. cricoarytenoideus dorsalis is the only one that functions to widen the rima glottidis and is important clinically. It extends from the cricoid cartilage to the muscular process of the arytenoid cartilage and by lever action tenses the vocal ligament, which is attached to the vocal process. (For muscles that narrow the rima glottidis, see Table of Muscles.)

The **innervation** of the laryngeal muscles and mucous membrane is by the vagus n. Its caudal laryngeal n. innervates all laryngeal muscles except the m. cricothyroideus, which is the most caudal and external of them. The cricothyroideus m. is supplied by the cranial laryngeal n., which is also a branch of the vagus (see p. 103). Cranial to the rima glottidis sensory innervation is provided by the internal ramus of the cranial laryngeal n. and caudal to it by the caudal laryngeal n.

c) The **ORAL CAVITY** comprises the **vestibule (11)**, which is the space between cheeks and lips and the dental arcades, and the **oral cavity proper (10)**, **9** which is the space internal to the dental arcades. Caudal to the last cheek teeth, the oral cavity passes over into the oral pharynx. The roof of the oral cavity is formed by the hard palate whose transverse **palatine rugae (13)** are **10** bisected by a median **palatine raphe** (not illustrated). Caudal to the upper central incisor teeth, is the median **incisive papilla (12)**, on either side of which is the opening of an incisive (nasopalatine) duct. Each duct passes through the palatine fissure of its side and before opening into the nasal cavity is connected to the ipsilateral vomeronasal organ. The floor of the oral cavity proper contains the tongue and its frenulum.

d) The **PHARYNX** surrounds the pharyngeal cavity. Within it, an intrapharyngeal ostium is the opening between the nasal pharynx and the laryngeal part of the pharynx **(Pars laryngea pharyngis)**.

I. Oral and laryngeal parts of the pharynx form a part of the digestive pathway, **pars digestoria (B – D)**. The **oropharynx** (oral pharynx) is also called the *isthmus faucium*. The oral pharynx (Pars oralis, —B) extends from the last cheek teeth to the base of the epiglottis. The floor of the oral pharynx is formed by the base of the tongue, its lateral walls by the palatoglossal arches, which house the palatine tonsil within the tonsillar sinus, and the roof by the soft palate. The **laryngopharynx (Pars laryngea pharyngis, —C)** commences at the intrapharyngeal ostium into which the rostral part of the larynx projects. The caudal part of the laryngopharynx is the esophageal vestibule. This passes over into the esophagus at a distinct prominence of the mucosa, the **limen pharyngoesophageum (18)**.

II. The **nasopharynx (Pars nasalis pharyngis, —A)** extends from the choanae to the intrapharyngeal ostium. The intrapharyngeal ostium is bounded by the caudal free border of the soft palate, **arcus veli palatini (16)**, and the **palatopharyngeal arch (17)**. The paired **pharyngeal ostia of the auditory tubes (14)** **11** open into the nasopharynx about halfway along its length. Each auditory tube opens into the middle ear.

The **tonsils** surround ring-like the oro- and nasopharynx. In the tonsils there are tonsillar lymphatic nodules and diffusely distributed lymphatic tissue in close relationship to the overlying epithelium of the oral mucous membrane. Lymphocytes and also granulocytes migrate from the underlying lymphoreticular tissue into the epithelium, in which they widen the intercellular spaces and give it a reticular appearance. Deeply, the tonsils are separated from neighboring tissues by a fibrous capsule. The tonsils are richly vascularized and have only efferent vessels. No afferent vessels pass to the tonsils.

The lymphatic 'pharyngeal ring' is formed by the pharyngeal tonsil on the roof of the nasopharynx, by the **palatine tonsil (15)** on the sides of the oro- **12** pharynx, and by the lingual tonsil on its floor.

Pharyngeal cavity { Nasopharynx / Oropharynx | — Intrapharyngeal ostium / — Laryngopharynx / Esophageal vestibule } Pars digestoria

Median section of head

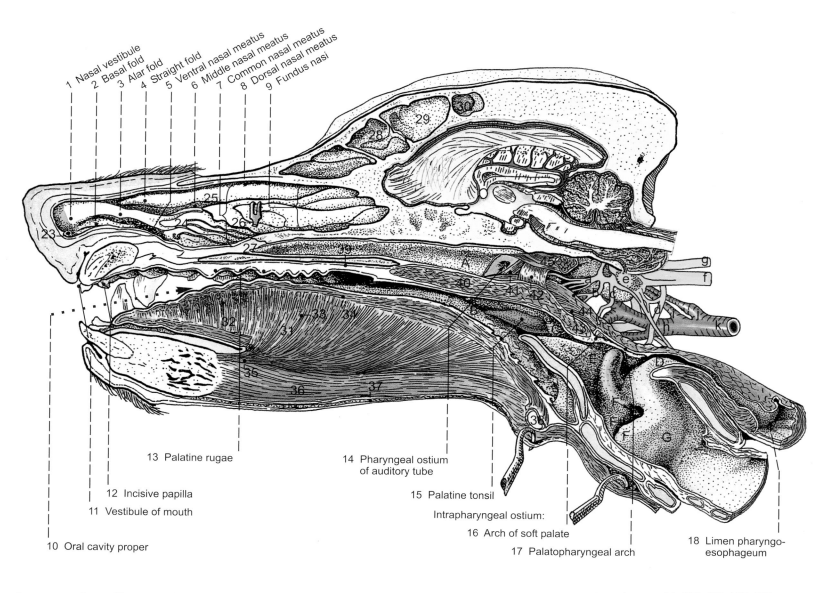

1 Nasal vestibule
2 Basal fold
3 Alar fold
4 Straight fold
5 Ventral nasal meatus
6 Middle nasal meatus
7 Common nasal meatus
8 Dorsal nasal meatus
9 Fundus nasi

13 Palatine rugae

12 Incisive papilla

11 Vestibule of mouth

10 Oral cavity proper

14 Pharyngeal ostium of auditory tube

15 Palatine tonsil

Intrapharyngeal ostium:

16 Arch of soft palate

17 Palatopharyngeal arch

18 Limen pharyngo-esophageum

Laryngeal cartilages

(craniolateral view)

19 Arytenoid cartilage
20 Thyroid cartilage
21 Epiglottic cartilage
22 Cricoid cartilage

(see pp. 91, 103, 106, 107, 111)

Cavity of pharynx

A   Pars nasalis
B - D Pars digestoria
B   Pars oralis
C   Pars laryngea
D   Vestibule of esophagus

Cavity of larynx

E   Vestibule of larynx
F   Glottis (vocal fold)
F'   Laryngeal ventricle
F'' Vestibular fold
G   Infraglottic cavity

Legend :

23 Nasolacrimal ostium
   Nasal cavity proper:
24   Ventr. nasal concha
25   Dors. nasal concha
26   Middle nasal concha
27 Nasal septum (section)
28 Rostr. frontal sinus
29 Med. frontal sinus
30 Lat. frontal sinus
31 Lingualis proprius m.:
32   Transverse fibers
33   Perpendicular fibers
34   Longitudinal fibers

35 Genioglossus m.
36 Geniohyoideus m.
37 Mylohyoideus m.
38 Basihyoid
39 Hard palate
40 Soft palate
   (Velum palatinum)
41 Tensor veli palatini m.
42 Levator veli palatini m.
43 Palatopharyngeus m.
44 Pterygopharyngeus m.
45 Longus capitis m. (section)

46 Cuneiform process
47 Corniculate process
48 Muscular process
49 Vocal process
50 Rostral cornu
51 Caudal cornu
52 Arch of cricoid cartilage
53 Lamina of cricoid cartilage
54 Thyrohyoid articulation
55 Cricothyroid articulatin
56 Trachea

Glossopharyngeal n. (IX):
a   Lingual br.
b   Pharyngeal br.
c Pharyngeal br. of n. vagus (X)
d Cran. laryngeal n.
e Cran. cervical ggl.
f Vagosympathetic trunk
g Accessory n. (XI)
h External carotid a.
i Occipital a.
j Internal carotid a.
k Com. carotid a.

101

8. PHARYNGEAL MUSCLES, CRANIAL NERVES OF THE VAGUS GROUP (IX, X, XI), AUTONOMIC NERVOUS SYSTEM OF THE HEAD, ARTERIES OF HEAD, EXTERNAL ACOUSTIC MEATUS

The dissection is performed simultaneously on medial and lateral sides of the specimen. The respiratory mucosa of the nasopharynx, from the pharyngeal ostium of the auditory tube as far as the intrapharyngeal ostium, is dissected away from underlying tissue in order to display muscles of the soft palate, the rostral constrictor muscles of the pharynx and cranial nerves IX − XI. The m. longus capitis is also detached from its insertion on the muscular tubercle of the occipital bone (see p. 101). To demonstrate the external acoustic meatus a wedge-shaped piece of tissue is excised from the auricular cartilage and removed, beginning cranial and caudal to the quadrangular tragus (J). This is similar to the technique used in the surgical treatment of otitis externa. For this purpose one begins the rostral incision at the pretragic incisure and the caudal incision at the intertragic incisure. Both incisions converge to the osseous external acoustic meatus.

1 a) The **PHARYNGEAL MUSCLES** include dilator of the pharynx (I), muscles of the soft palate (II), and rostral, middle and caudal constrictors of the pharynx (III-V).

I. The **m. stylopharyngeus caudalis (14)** is the only **dilator of the pharynx**. It extends from the caudal aspect of the stylohyoid element to the dorsolateral wall of the pharynx. II. Both muscles of the soft palate arise rostral to the tympanic bulla at the base of the skull. The **m. tensor veli palatini (2)** proceeds rostroventrally around the hamulus of the pterygoid bone to the soft palate. The **m. levator veli palatini (7)** extends perpendicularly into the soft palate. III. Of the two **rostral constrictors of the pharynx**, the **m. pterygopharyngeus (5)** arises on the hamulus of the pterygoid bone and crosses lateral to the m. levator veli palatini before attaching to the wall of the pharynx. The **m. palatopharyngeus (6)** runs between the aponeurosis of the soft palate and the wall of the pharynx. IV. The **middle constrictor of the pharynx**, the **m. hyopharyngeus (18)**, extends from the basihyoid and thyrohyoid elements dorsally to the rostral part of the pharyngeal raphe. V. Of the two **caudal constrictors of the pharynx**, the **m. thyropharyngeus (19)** arises from the thyroid cartilage and the **m. cricopharyngeus (17)**, which is not clearly set off from the thyropharyngeus, from the cricoid cartilage. Both insert into the dorsal wall of the pharynx at the pharyngeal raphe, caudal to the hyopharyngeus.

The **innervation** of most of the pharyngeal muscles is by the pharyngeal branches of the glossopharyngeal and vagus nerves, which form the pharyngeal plexus on the dorsolateral wall of the pharynx. The m. tensor veli palatini, supplied by the mandibular n. (V3), is an exception, as is the m. stylopharyngeus caudalis, which is innervated only by the glossopharyngeal n.

b) The **CRANIAL NERVES OF THE VAGUS GROUP** all pass through the jugular foramen and, except for the accessory n. (XI), are crossed laterally by the hypoglossal n. (XII).

2 The **glossopharyngeal n. (IX, −9)**, shortly after its emergence from the jugular foramen, gives off the parasympathetic tympanic n. which is continued as the minor petrosal n. and extends across the otic ganglion to reach the mandibular n. (V3; see p. 137). After that, the glossopharyngeal n. innervates the m. stylopharyngeus caudalis and, medial to the tympanic bulla, divides into lingual and pharyngeal branches. The **lingual branch (13)** crosses the stylohyoid element, and the m. styloglossus arising from it, medially. It supplies general sensory innervation to the base of the tongue and special sensory innervation to the taste buds of the vallate and foliate papillae. With the pharyngeal branch of the vagus n., and sympathetic fibers from the cranial cervical ganglion, the **pharyngeal branch (10)** forms the pharyngeal plexus on the dorsolateral pharynx. The plexus furnishes the motor and sensory supply to the pharynx.

2 The **vagus n. (X, −8)**, after passing through the jugular foramen, gives off a sensory part to the facial n., which as the internal auricular ramus, supplies the external acoustic meatus (see p. 93). Its **pharyngeal branch (10)** communicates with the same-named branch of the glossopharyngeal n., forming the pharyngeal plexus. The vagus n. bends around caudally, exhibiting here the distinct distal (nodose) ganglion, where the **cranial laryngeal n. (15)** begins. With its external branch, the cranial laryngeal nerve supplies the m. cricothyroideus and with its sensory internal branch passes through the thyroid notch to supply the laryngeal mucosa cranial to the rima glottidis. The vagus n. runs in the vagosympathetic trunk dorsoparallel to the common carotid a. and, within the thoracic cavity (see p. 49), gives off the recurrent laryngeal n. The recurrent laryngeal n. ascends the neck applied to the lateral surface of the trachea. After supplying tracheal and esophageal rami, it continues as the **caudal laryngeal n. (20)**, proceeding to the larynx deep to the m. cricopharyngeus. With the exception of the cricothyroideus m., the caudal laryngeal n. innervates all intrinsic laryngeal muscles and the laryngeal mucosa caudal to the rima glottidis.

The **accessory n. (XI, −11)** runs dorsolateral to the distal ganglion (X) to innervate the mm. trapezius and sternocleidomastoideus.

c) The **AUTONOMIC NERVOUS SYSTEM OF THE HEAD** (see p. 137) includes: the parasympathetic division, whose nerve cells of origin lie in the mesencephalon and rhombencephalon; and the sympathetic division, which has origin from the thoracic spinal cord.

3 I. The **sympathetic trunk** (see p. 49), containing preganglionic nerve fibers, passes to the junction of head and neck in the vagosympathetic trunk (18). There the vagosympathetic trunk bifurcates, the vagus n. lying dorsally, the sympathetic trunk and its cranial cervical ganglion ventrally. After synapsing in the **cranial cervical ganglion (12)** unmyelinated postganglionic sympathetic fibers pass as perivascular plexuses in the adventitia of the larger vessels of the head (e.g., Plexus caroticus internus, Plexus caroticus externus) to their areas of supply (e.g., glands, mucosae and internal muscles of the eye).

4 II. Emerging from the brain with their parent cranial nerve, preganglionic **parasympathetic fibers** continue with those cranial nerves (III, VII, IX and X) for the first part of their course. They soon however branch to their respective parasympathetic ganglia where synapse occurs and the excitatory state is then carried by postganglionic fibers. These reach their areas of innervation in common with branches of other cranial nerves. Only the vagus, cranial nerve X, conducts itself differently in that it extends with its parasympathetic fibers into the large body cavities. It gives off no parasympathetic fibers to other cranial nerves.

d) The **ARTERIES OF THE HEAD** arise from the **common carotid a. (33)** which dispatches the cranial thyroid artery (34) to the thyroid gland and at the junction of head and neck bifurcates (the carotid bifurcation) into the small internal carotid a., which extends rostrodorsally, and a large external carotid a. that continues the rostral direction of the common carotid. At its origin, the **internal carotid a. (27)** exhibits a localized swelling, the **carotid sinus (27)**, which contains pressor receptors. The glomus caroticum, which contains chemoreceptors, lies in the carotid bifurcation. The internal carotid a. passes through the carotid canal in a typical loop-formation, and gives off several cerebral arteries within the cranial cavity. The **external carotid a. (29)** reaches the temporomandibular joint where it passes over into to the maxillary a. At its origin, still at the carotid bifurcation, the external carotid gives off the **occipital a. (28)**, which initially runs parallel to the internal carotid a. and then continues dorsally to the occipital region. At about the same level, the **cranial laryngeal a. (30)** leaves the ventral aspect of the external carotid a. to enter the thyroid notch along with the same-named nerve. The lingual a. and the facial a. also proceed from the ventral aspect of the external carotid artery about a fingerbreadth rostral to the cranial thyroid artery. The **lingual a. (32)** passes between the mm. ceratohyoideus and hyoglossus to reach the tongue and tonsils. At first, the **facial a. (31)** extends medial to and alongside the mandible and gives off here the **sublingual a. (41)** (the accompanying sublingual v. arises from the lingual v.). The facial a. then runs between the insertion of the m. digastricus and the ventral border of the mandible, and arches dorsally onto the lateral surface of the mandible. Its further course on the face is described on p. 93. The **caudal auricular a. (23)** and the **superficial temporal a. (22)**, with its branch, the **rostral auricular a. (21)**, proceed from the dorsal convexity of the terminal curve of the external carotid a. They supply the external ear and the temporal region. As the rostral continuation of the external carotid a., the **maxillary a. (24)** passes medially, ventral to the temporomandibular joint, giving off here the **inferior alveolar a. (26)** into the mandibular canal and the **caudal deep temporal a. (25)** to the m. temporalis. After its passage through the alar canal, the maxillary a. gives off the **external ophthalmic a. (35)** to the ocular bulb and the **rostral deep temporal a. (36)** to the m. temporalis. The terminal branches of the maxillary a. (infraorbital a., −37, greater palatine a., −39, lesser palatine a., −40, and sphenopalatine a., −38) run, with the exception noted below, with like-named nerves through appropriately denoted osseous canals or foramina to the areas that they supply. (The sphenopalatine a. traverses the sphenopalatine foramen with the caudal nasal n.)

e) The **EXTERNAL ACOUSTIC MEATUS (3)** is supported proximally by the scrolled **auricular cartilage (1)** followed by the anular cartilage and finally by the osseous external acoustic meatus. The external acoustic meatus is subdivided into a long auricular (perpendicular) part and a short tympanic (horizontal) part, which can be observed after it is opened. Between the two parts is an approximate right-angled bend (about 100 degrees in breeds with erect ears and more than 110 degrees in breeds with pendant ears). As extensions of the auricular cartilage in the formation of the tympanic (horizontal) part, the ringlike **anular cartilage (4)** and the osseous external acoustic meatus (which extends only a few millimeters up to the tympanic membrane that closes off the canal) take part.

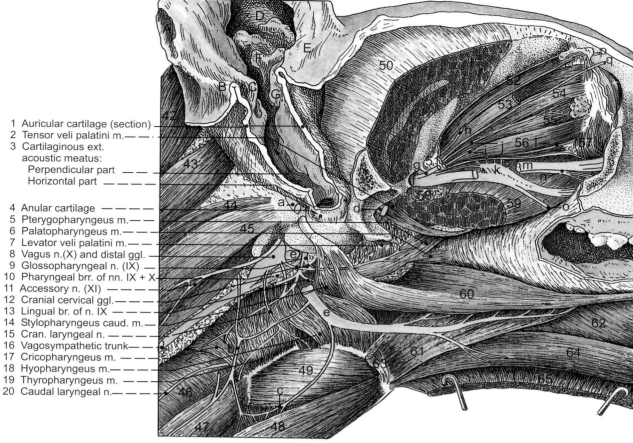

1 Auricular cartilage (section)
2 Tensor veli palatini m.
3 Cartilaginous ext. acoustic meatus:
   Perpendicular part
   Horizontal part
4 Anular cartilage
5 Pterygopharyngeus m.
6 Palatopharyngeus m.
7 Levator veli palatini m.
8 Vagus n.(X) and distal ggl.
9 Glossopharyngeal n. (IX)
10 Pharyngeal brr. of nn. IX + X
11 Accessory n. (XI)
12 Cranial cervical ggl.
13 Lingual br. of n. IX
14 Stylopharyngeus caud. m.
15 Cran. laryngeal n.
16 Vagosympathetic trunk
17 Cricopharyngeus m.
18 Hyopharyngeus m.
19 Thyropharyngeus m.
20 Caudal laryngeal n.

Legend :

42 Cleidocervical m.
   Sternocleidomastoid m.:
43   Sternooccipital m.
44   Sternomastoid m.
45   Cleidomastoid m.
46 Esophagus
47 Sternothyroideus m.
48 Sternohyoideus m.
49 Thyrohyoideus m.
50 Temporal m.
51 Periorbita
52 Dors. oblique m.
53 Levator palpebrae
   superioris m.
54 Dorsal rectus m.
55 Retractor bulbi m.
56 Lat. rectus m.
57 Ventral oblique m.
58 Lat. pterygoideus m.
59 Med. pterygoideus m.
60 Styloglossus m.
61 Hyoglossus m.
62 Genioglossus m.
63 Stylohyoideus m.
64 Geniohyoideus m.
65 Mylohyoideus m.
66 Digastricus m.

(lateral view)

Legend :

A Cutaneous marginal sac
B Lat. process of antitragus
C Med process of antitragus
D Scapha

E Helix
F Med. crus of helix
G Lat. crus of helix
H Antitragus

I Incisura intertragica
J Tragus
K Pretragic incisure

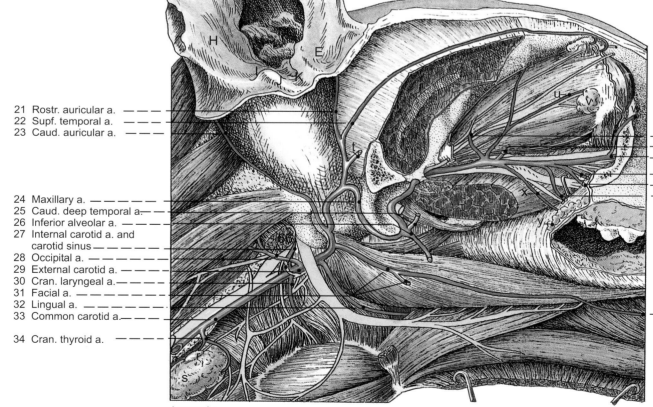

21 Rostr. auricular a.
22 Supf. temporal a.
23 Caud. auricular a.

24 Maxillary a.
25 Caud. deep temporal a.
26 Inferior alveolar a.
27 Internal carotid a. and
   carotid sinus
28 Occipital a.
29 External carotid a.
30 Cran. laryngeal a.
31 Facial a.
32 Lingual a.
33 Common carotid a.

34 Cran. thyroid a.

35 Ext. ophthalmic a.
36 Rostr. deep temporal a.
37 Infraorbital a.
38 Sphenopalatine a.
39 Greater palatine a.
40 Lesser palatine a.

41 Sublingual a.

(see pp. 93, 95, 99)

Legend :

a Facial n. (VII)
b Cervical n. (C1)
c Ansa cervicalis
d Mandibular n. (V3)
e Hypoglossal n. (XII)
f Maxillary n. (V2)
g Zygomatic n.
h Trochlear n. (IV)
i Abducens n. (VI)

j Lacrimal n.
k Pterygopalatine n. and
   pterygopalatine ggl.
l Ventr. br. of oculomotor n. (III)
m Infraorbital n.
n Superior alveolar n.
o Lesser palatine n.
p Infratrochlear n.
q Frontal n.

r Parathyroid gl.
s Thyroid gl.
t Transverse facial a.
u Lacrimal a.
v Lacrimal gl.
w Malar a.
x Buccal a.
y Buccal gll.

103

a) The **TONGUE** with its **frenulum (17)** occupies the floor of the mouth and contains in its **root (Radix linguae)** the basihyoid element and is flanked on either side by the ceratohyoid elements; whereas, the **body** and **apex** of the tongue project rostrally into the oral cavity. The mucous membrane of the **dorsum of the tongue (Dorsum linguae)** bears **mechanical papillae**, that is to say, the entire dorsum being covered by fine, thread-like, **filiform papillae (13)** and on the root of the tongue the strikingly larger and more plump special forms as **conical papillae (10)**. The **gustatory papillae** bear taste buds and are innervated by special sensory fibers. These include vallate, foliate, and some of the fungiform papillae. The four to six **vallate papillae (11)** lie at the root of the tongue. Each is surrounded by a wall and by a groove. At the same level, a less distinct leaf-shaped **foliate papillae (12)** is present on either side of the tongue. The mushroom-shaped **fungiform papillae (14)** are present over the entire dorsum of the tongue. **Marginal papillae** are present only in the newborn pup. For general sensation (pain, touch, and temperature) the mucous membrane of the tongue is supplied by the lingual nerve (from V3) and the lingual branch of the glossopharyngeal n. The chorda tympani (from VII) supplies the fungiform papillae in the rostral two-thirds of the tongue, while the glossopharyngeal nerve (IX) innervates the vallate and foliate papillae in the caudal third of the tongue with special sensory fibers. The parasympathetic part of the chorda tympani innervates the lingual glands, to which the irrigating glands of the vallate papillae belong (these glands secrete into the groove surrounding the papilla). The **lyssa** is a rod-shaped formation with a maximum length of 4 cm. It is a morphological characteristic of carnivores and is ventromedian at the apex of the tongue. The lyssa consists of an envelope of connective tissue containing striated muscle cells, fat and cartilaginous tissue.

b) The **TONGUE MUSCLES** include the proper or intrinsic muscle of the tongue, the extrinsic tongue muscles, which come from outside the organ and radiate within it, and the hyoid muscles that insert into the basihyoid element.

I. The **m. lingualis proprius**, the proper muscle of the tongue, contains longitudinal, transverse and perpendicular fibers (see page 101).

II. The extrinsic tongue muscles radiate into the tongue from the stylohyoid element of the hyoid apparatus (**m. styloglossus, 9**), from the basihyoid element (**m. hyoglossus, 8**) and from the body of the mandible lateral to the intermandibular joint (**m. genioglossus, 16**).

III. Of the **hyoid muscles**, the **m. geniohyoideus (18)** runs from the body of the mandible near the intermandibular joint to the basihyoid element and the **m. thyrohyoideus (7**, as the cranial continuation of the m. sternothyroideus) from the thyroid cartilage to the basihyoid element. (Long hyoid muscles: mm. sternohyoideus and sternothyroideus, see p. 14). The mm. stylohyoideus, occipitohyoideus and ceratohyoideus are not given attention in the dissection.

The **innervation** of the muscles of the tongue is by the **hypoglossal n. (XII)**; except for the hyoid muscles, which are supplied predominantly by way of the ansa cervicalis that joins the hypoglossal n. and first cervical nerve. After its emerging from the hypoglossal canal, the **hypoglossal nerve (XII, −6)** crosses the sympathetic trunk and glossopharyngeal nerve laterally and communicates with the first cervical nerve by the ansa cervicalis before it reaches the lingual muscles. Although the vagus nerve participates in the innervation of the canine tongue, its role is not absolutely clear. As a branchial arch nerve, it takes part in the genesis of the tongue. In human beings, its innervation of the root of the tongue near the base of the epiglottis is proven.

c) The SALIVARY GLANDS of the oral cavity are divided into those lying in the surrounding wall, which have many short ducts, and accessory glands more or less far removed from the oral cavity and connected to it by a relatively long excretory duct. The accessory glands that open into the oral vestibule are the parotid and zygomatic glands. Those that open into the oral cavity proper are the mandibular and monostomatic sublingual glands. The **parotid gland (3)** is triangular. It lies laterally at the base of the ear and ends with its **parotid duct (3)** on the **parotid papilla (2)** dorsal to the sectorial tooth (P 4) of the upper jaw. The **zygomatic gland (1)** lies ventrolaterally in the orbit under the rostral end of the zygomatic arch. It opens with one large and several small excretory ducts caudal to the upper sectorial tooth (p. 4).

The **mandibular gland (5)** and the **monostomatic sublingual gland (4)** that is applied to it rostrodorsally discharge with parallel coursing excretory ducts rostrally on the **caruncula sublingualis (19)**. The caruncle lies on the floor of the oral cavity rostral to the lingual frenulum. At the level of the lingual frenulum, the **polystomatic sublingual gland (15)** opens into the oral cavity with many short excretory ducts and is thus a gland of the oral wall. This is true also for the buccal and palatine glands.

The **parasympathetic nerve supply** of the palatine glands (see p. 137) is by the nerve of the pterygoid canal, whose neurons synapse in the pterygopalatine ganglion. The zygomatic, buccal and parotid glands are innervated by way of the minor petrosal nerve of the glossopharyngeal nerve (IX) and the otic ganglion. The mandibular and sublingual glands are innervated by the chorda tympani from (VII).

d) With respect to the **DENTITION** of the upper and lower jaws, the individual teeth of the upper and lower dental arcades can be identified on the basis of a dental formula. In mammals this is derived from a full dentition numbering forty-four teeth, which among the domestic mammals is complete only in the pig.

Temporary dentition (deciduous teeth)
$$\frac{\text{iii c oppp oo0}}{\text{iii c oppp ooo}} = (7+7) \times 2 = 28 \text{ deciduous teeth}$$

Permanent dentition (permanent teeth)
$$\frac{\text{III C LPPPMM0}}{\text{III C LPPPMMM}} = (10+11) \times 2 = 42 \text{ permanent teeth}$$

To interpret the dental formula, the numerator represents the teeth of the upper arcade; the denominator, the teeth of the lower arcade. Symbols in lower case represent deciduous teeth; symbols in capitals, permanent teeth. Small zeros (o) symbolize that in this place a tooth will be present in the permanent dentition. A large zero (0) symbolizes a total absence of a tooth in the canine dentition. The permanent teeth either replace the deciduous teeth or develop without having temporary precursors; e.g., the first premolar (P1 = L) and all molars (M). The **incisor teeth (I)** of the upper jaw are larger than those of the lower. In the upper jaw, a distinct **diastema (20)** or interdental space is present between the third incisor and the **canine tooth (C)**; whereas in the lower arcade the diastema is between the canine and the first premolar. The first **premolar tooth (P1)** of each arcade is sometimes referred to as a **wolf tooth (Dens lupinus, L)**. Like the incisor and canine teeth, it has only one root. The remaining three **premolar teeth (P2 – P4)** of each arcade are cutting teeth, each having two roots. An exception to this is P4 of the upper arcade, which has three roots. It is the strongest tooth of the upper jaw and is also called a **sectorial tooth**. The sectorial tooth of the lower jaw is the first molar (M1). The **molar teeth (M)** have surfaces used for crushing. They have three roots in the upper jaw, two roots in the lower jaw.

In animals, the **eruption** and wear of the teeth permit an approximate estimation of age of the animal. Both criteria however are related to breed and the maintenance of the animal. Regarding the eruption of the teeth, the following approximations are worth noting:

> Up to the third week of age: edentulous;
> From the sixth week: complete deciduous dentition;
> From the third month: commencement of growth of permanent incisors;
> From the sixth month: complete permanent dentition.

Three hard substances, enamel, cementum, and dentin, participate in **tooth structure**. Enamel (22) covers the free part of the tooth, the crown. It is a very hard, conspicuously white, layer approximately one millimeter thick. Cementum (27) consists of interwoven osseous tissue, approximately one millimeter thick, surrounding the whole **root of the tooth (28)** and extending to the **neck (24)** to the beginning of the enamel layer and the crown. **Dentin (21)** is a tissue free of cells and resembling bone. It consists of a calcified ground substance and collagenous fiber bundles. Internal to the covering layers of enamel and cementum, it forms the bulk of the tooth and surrounds the **pulp cavity (29)**. The pulp cavity contains the dental pulp, nerves, blood and lymph vessels. These enter the cavity through the **apical foramen (31)** and the **root canal (30)**. On the **crown of the tooth (23)**, five contact surfaces are distinguished; namely, the occlusal surface or masticatory surface, the vestibular surface, the lingual surface, the contact surface with mesial (rostral) and distal (caudal) surfaces. From the anatomical point of view, the neck of the tooth is regarded as the site of contact between enamel and cementum; whereas, clinically, the term encompasses the region between the alveolus and the **gingiva (25)**. In that view, the crown projects beyond the gingiva and the clinical root is that portion of the tooth fixed in the alveolus and covered by gingiva.

Teeth are 'wedged' into the osseous alveoli by means of the **parodontium (26)**, which produces a resilient, springy, fibrous union (gomphosis). The term *parodontium* embraces the alveolus, the *periodontium* and the cementum. Collagen fibers of the periodontium run in varying directions between the cementum and the alveolus.

Tongue, lingual mm., hypoglossal n. (XII) and salivary glands

(lateral view)

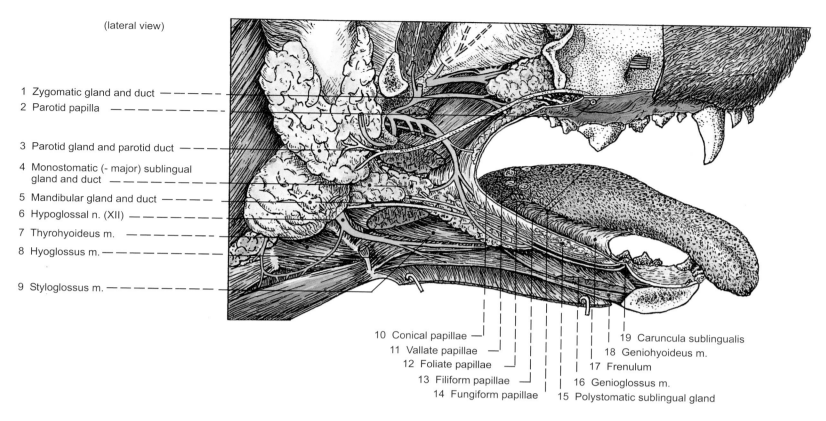

1 Zygomatic gland and duct
2 Parotid papilla
3 Parotid gland and parotid duct
4 Monostomatic (- major) sublingual gland and duct
5 Mandibular gland and duct
6 Hypoglossal n. (XII)
7 Thyrohyoideus m.
8 Hyoglossus m.
9 Styloglossus m.

10 Conical papillae
11 Vallate papillae
12 Foliate papillae
13 Filiform papillae
14 Fungiform papillae
15 Polystomatic sublingual gland
16 Genioglossus m.
17 Frenulum
18 Geniohyoideus m.
19 Caruncula sublingualis

Maxillary dental arch

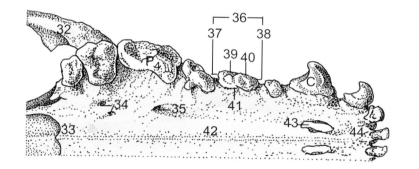

Legend :

32 Zygomatic arch
33 Horizontal lamina of palatine bone
34 Lesser palatine forr.
35 Greater palatine forr.
36 Contact surface:
37   Distal surface
38   Mesial surface
39 Vestibuar surface
40 Occlusal surface
41 Lingual surface
42 Palatine process of maxilla
43 Palatine fissure
44 Palatine process of incisive bone
45 Cuticle
46 Anatomical root of tooth
47 Alveolar canal

Permanent teeth

(lateral view)

Canine tooth

(median section)

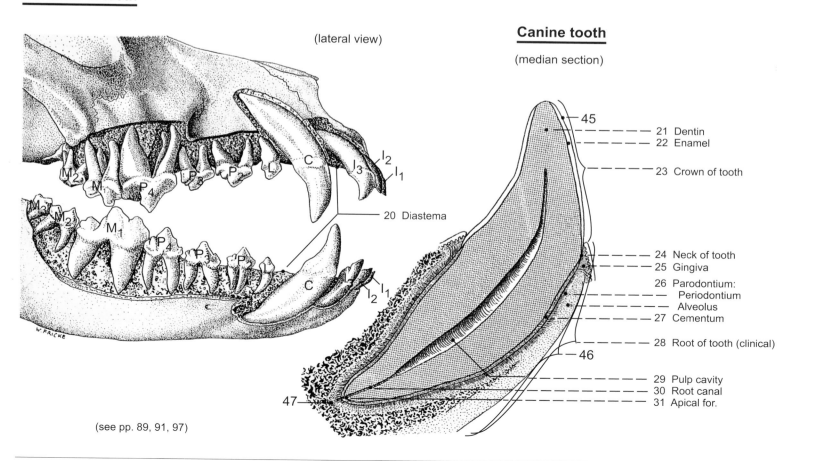

20 Diastema

21 Dentin
22 Enamel
23 Crown of tooth
24 Neck of tooth
25 Gingiva
26 Parodontium:
  Periodontium
  Alveolus
27 Cementum
28 Root of tooth (clinical)
29 Pulp cavity
30 Root canal
31 Apical for.

(see pp. 89, 91, 97)

10. JOINTS OF THE HEAD

NAME	BONES forming the joint	TYPE/COMPO-SITION	FUNCTION	COMMENT
1 **I. Temporomandibular joint:**	Condylar process of the mandible and the mandibular fossa of the temporal bone;	Condylar joint/ simple joint;	Hinge joint;	A fibrocartilaginous articular disc subdivides the joint cavity into dorsal and ventral cavities.

2   **II. Intermandibular symphysis (articulation):** This joint connects right and left halves of the mandible.

III. Hyoid bone (hyoid apparatus): The hyoid bone is connected with the temporal bone by the tympanohyoid (consists of connective tissue), and its thyrohyoid element forms a synovial joint with the rostral cornu of the thyroid cartilage. Except for the union of the tympanohyoid with the stylohyoid, the individual elements of the hyoid apparatus are joined by synovial joints.

The **temporomandibular joint** is an incongruent condylar joint which is subdivided by a fibrocartilaginous articular disc into two compartments, lying one above the other. The dorsal compartment is the larger. The transversely located condylar process of the mandible is smaller than the articular depression that is formed by the mandibular fossa of the temporal bone at the temporal base of the zygomatic arch. Caudally the fossa is supported by the retroarticular process, which limits caudal displacement of the mandible. The joint capsule attaches to the margins of the articular surfaces of the temporal bone and mandible and at the circumference of the cartilaginous articular disc. The capsule is reinforced laterally by dense connective tissue, the **lateral ligament.** The locomotor activity, which takes place synchronously on right and left sides, is restricted in the dog chiefly to the hinge-like opening and closing of the mouth. Some side-to-side movement is possible when the mouth is not fully opened. Canine breeds with a relatively large coronoid process, as, for example, the Basset, tend to 'lock' the jaw in the case of extreme opening of the mouth. The joint is fixed and there is an inability to close the mouth.

The **intermandibular symphysis** (in the most recent nomenclature it is designated an *intermandibular articulation*) joins right and left halves of the mandible. The joint consists of a cartilaginous part **(intermandibular synchondrosis)** and a larger fibrous connective tissue portion **(intermandibular suture)**. The tight connection permits only a little movement that allows alignment of the upper and lower dental arcades. A traumatic separation of the intermandibular symphysis is possible. Ossification of the joint may occur in old age.

The **sutures of the upper jaw** (this term includes the cranial and facial bones excepting the hyoid bone, mandible, and ear ossicles) are located between the individual bones of the neuro- and viscerocranium, which are partially interdigitated in a zigzag line. In the area of the cranial vault, the connective tissue portions of the cranial sutures are the remnant potential of the membranous ossification which after the final breed-specific development of the skull is finished by the formation of a bony growth zone. Broad connective tissue parts are present perinatally as fontanelles.

The **temporohyoid articulation** fixes the tympanohyoid to the mastoid process of the petrosal part. Between individual elements of the hyoid bone (tympano-, stylo-, epi-, cerato-, basi-, and thyrohyoid) are also articulations (see III. above).

At the thyrohyoid articulation the thyrohyoid is connected with the rostral horn of the thyroid cartilage by a synovial joint.

Articulations and Ligaments of the Larynx

Articulations, ligaments and muscles connect all laryngeal cartilages with each other and enable intralaryngeal movements.

The **cricothyroid joint** is located between a small articular surface of the cricoid cartilage at the dorsal part of the arch and an articular surface on the medial aspect of the caudal cornu of the thyroid cartilage. It permits a hinge-like rocking movement between cricoid and thyroid cartilages.

The **cricoarytenoid joint** lies between the base of each arytenoid cartilage and the rostral margin of the lamina of the cricoid cartilage. The chief movement is one in which the muscular process of the arytenoid cartilage is drawn caudomedially as its vocal process is moved craniolaterally. The reverse movement also takes place. Some axial rotation (the axis passes through the arytenoid caudal to rostral) of the arytenoid at its joint with the cricoid is also possible. A cricoarytenoid ligament reinforces the joint capsule.

The **ligaments of the larynx** (see text-illustration) become visible after removal of the mucous membrane of the larynx. Broad-surfaced ligamentous connections are called membranes.

The **vocal ligament** contains predominantly elastic fibers and is drawn between the internal surface of the thyroid cartilage and the vocal process of the arytenoid.

The **vestibular ligament** is the connective tissue basis of the vestibular fold and courses between the ventral extremity of the cuneiform process of the arytenoid cartilage and the internal surface of the thyroid cartilage.

The **thyrohyoid membrane** stretches between the rostral border of the thyroid cartilage and the basihyoid.

The **hyoepiglottic ligament** connects the basihyoid with the epiglottic cartilage.

The **cricothyroid ligament** joins the ventral part of the rostral border of the cricoid cartilage to the caudal margin of the thyroid cartilage.

The **laryngeal fibroelastic membrane** is the broad-surfaced lateral continuation of the cricothyroid ligament.

The **thyroepiglottic ligament** connects the epiglottic cartilage with the rostral border of the thyroid cartilage.

The **cricotracheal ligament** is the fibrous connection between the cricoid cartilage and the first tracheal cartilage.

The **transverse arytenoid ligament** extends between the apposed medial borders of the two arytenoid cartilages and fixes here the roughly millet-sized interarytenoid cartilage and the sesamoid cartilage (not depicted), which is about the same size.

Larynx
(median section)

(medial view)

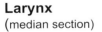

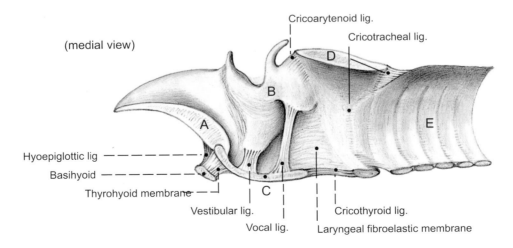

Cricoarytenoid lig.

Cricotracheal lig.

Hyoepiglottic lig

Basihyoid

Thyrohyoid membrane

Vestibular lig.

Vocal lig.

Cricothyroid lig.

Laryngeal fibroelastic membrane

Legend :

A Epiglottic cartilage
B Arytenoid cartilage
C Thyroid cartilage
D Cricoid cartilage
E Trachea

(lateral view)

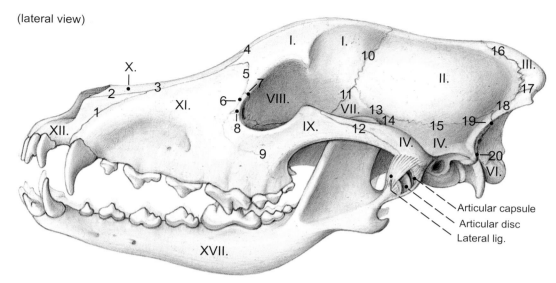

Articular capsule
Articular disc
Lateral lig.

Temporomandibular joint and sutures of skull

(medial view)

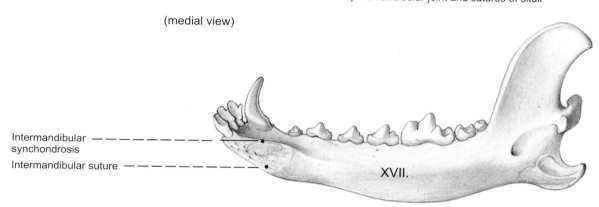

Intermandibular synchondrosis

Intermandibular suture

Intermandibular symphysis (articulation)

(see pp. 89, 91, 101, 105)

Legend:

I.	Frontal bone
II.	Parietal bone
III.	Interparietal bone
IV.	Temporal bone
V.	Ethmoidal bone (see p. 91)
VI.	Occipital bone
VII.	Sphenoid bone
VIII.	Lacrimal bone
IX.	Zygomatic bone
X.	Nasal bone
XI.	Maxilla
XVII.	Mandible

Joints of head and sutures of skull

(lateral view)

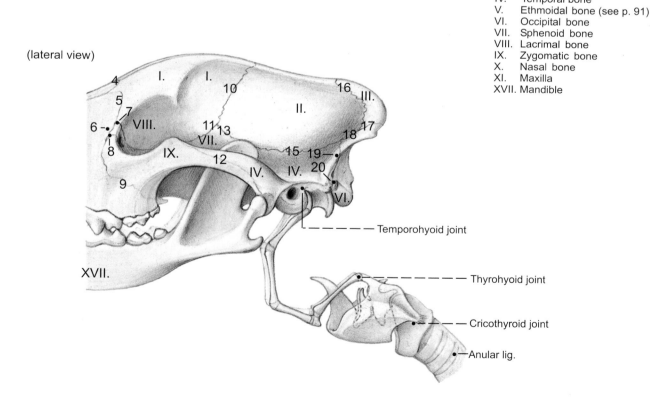

Temporohyoid joint

Thyrohyoid joint

Cricothyroid joint

Anular lig.

Legend:

1 Maxilloincisive suture	6 Lacrimomaxillary suture	11 Sphenofrontal suture	16 Parietointerparietal suture
2 Nasoincisive suture	7 Frontolacrimal suture	12 Temporozygomatic suture	17 Occipitointerparietal suture
3 Nasomaxillary suture	8 Lacrimozygomatic suture	13 Sphenoparietal suture	18 Lambdoid suture
4 Frontonasal suture	9 Zygomaticomaxillary suture	14 Sphenopetrosal synchondrosis	19 Occipitosquamous suture
5 Frontomaxillary suture	10 Coronal suture	15 Squamous suture	20 Occipitomastoid suture

CHAPTER 10: CENTRAL NERVOUS SYSTEM

1. SPINAL CORD AND MENINGES

a) At the foramen magnum, the **THREE SPINAL MENINGES** are continuous with the three cerebral meninges. The external *ectomeninx* invests the arachnoidea, and the soft pia mater, which is closely applied to the spinal cord. The arachnoidea and pia mater are also designated *endomeninx* or *leptomeninx* (see corresponding relations of the cerebral meninges, p. 110).

The *ectomeninx* consists of two layers. The external layer is identical in structure and function to the periosteal lining of the vertebral canal (**periosteum, –1**). The tough internal layer is the **dura mater (3)**. It envelops the spinal cord and the roots of the spinal nerves up to the spinal ganglion and is continuous with the external covering of the first part of the spinal nerve, the epineurium. Cranial to the fourth cervical vertebra the dorsal and ventral roots of the spinal nerve have a common dural sheath; whereas, caudal to it, each root has its own dural sheath (middle figure, opposite page).

The **epidural space (2)** is between the two layers of the ectomeninx; it contains adipose tissue, lymph vessels and large calibered venous plexuses. The fat tissue cushions the spinal cord which is passively deformed by the curvatures of the vertebral column.

The endo- or leptomeninx is internal to the dura mater and also consists of two layers. The **arachnoidea (31)** is outermost of the two layers. It consists superficially of a layer of epithelioid cells that is continued as the neurothelial inner lining of the *perineurium internum* upon the peripheral nerves (not illustrated). The deeper layer of the arachnoidea is a connective tissue layer that is relatively avascular. From it there radiates a loosely arranged trabecular network of connective tissue that contains within its meshes the **subarachnoid space (32)**. The subarachnoid space is filled with cererospinal fluid (see corresponding relations of the brain, p. 111). The subarachnoid space extends to the spinal ganglion and is remarkably enlarged between the cerebellum and the beginning of the spinal cord as the **cerebellomedullary cistern** (see p. 111). It is also relatively wide around the *conus medullaris* and the *filum terminale* (see below) and at these sites is suitable for puncture to obtain cerebrospinal fluid. The **pia mater (33)** is a vascular membrane and is closely attached to the surface of the spinal cord. Externally the pia mater forms the **denticulate ligaments (22)** that are fixed with a broadened base between the roots of the spinal nerves. The ligaments penetrate the arachnoidea and taper here, attaching with their apical part to the internal surface of the dura mater. They attach the spinal cord to its surrounding tunics.

The arterial supply of the spinal cord is chiefly by the **ventral spinal artery (6)** that runs along the ventral **median fissure** the entire length of the spinal cord.

The venous **ventral internal vertebral plexus (29)** is on the floor of the vertebral canal embedded in epidural fat tissue. (The **ventral external vertebral plexus (30)** runs externally, ventrally along the vertebral column.)

b) The **SPINAL CORD** (see also text-illustration) proceeds from the myelencephalon at the level of the first cervical vertebra. At the junction of neck and thorax, it exhibits the **cervical enlargement (4)**, the origin of the nerves of the brachial plexus, and, in the lumbar part of the spinal cord, the **lumbar enlargement (14)**, the origin of the nerves of the lumbosacral plexus. Caudal to the lumbar enlargement, at the level of the fifth lumbar vertebra, it narrows like a cone (**Conus medullaris, –15**) and is continued by the **filum terminale (16)** at the level of the seventh lumbar vertebra. The filum terminale and the accompanying roots of the caudal lumbar, sacral, and caudal (coccygeal) spinal nerves altogether form within the vertebral canal the **cauda equina (17)**. The roots of the spinal nerves in the cervical and thoracic region run approximately transversely and, after a brief course, exit the vertebral canal at an **intervertebral foramen (5)**. In the lumbar region, and even more distinctly in the sacral region, the roots of the spinal nerves leave the vertebral canal only after a long course and one increasingly parallel to the spinal cord. In the embryo, in all regions of the spinal cord, the origins of the spinal nerves and the passage of the nerves through the intervertebral foramina are approximately at the same level. With increasing age, the reduced growth of the spinal cord relative to the vertebral canal results in a difference in the level of the spinal cord segment from which the roots of the spinal nerve take origin, and the level at which the nerve exits the vertebral canal. This result is the *ascensus medullae* ('ascent of the spinal cord'). In the cervical spinal cord, the **spinal roots of the accessory nerve (23)** arise. They lie along the lateral surface of the cord, dorsal to the denticulate ligaments, and run cranially between the dorsal and ventral roots of the cervical spinal nerves. After passing through the foramen magnum, they join the medullary roots of the nerve. The accessory nerve is formed by the union of its spinal and medullary roots and leaves the cranial cavity at the jugular foramen. On the surface of the spinal cord, and in cross-section, the dorsal **median sulcus (25)** can be seen on the dorsal midline and a **dorsal lateral sulcus (24)** can be seen at the origin of the dorsal roots of the spinal nerves. These sulci form the medial and lateral boundaries, respectively, of white substance (white matter), the longitudinally coursing **dorsal funiculus (19)**. In the cervical spinal cord a **dorsal intermediate sulcus (18)** can be observed between the dorsal median and dorsal lateral sulci. The **fasciculus gracilis (20)** lies medial to the dorsal intermediate sulcus and the **fasciculus cuneatus (21)** is lateral to it. The **lateral funiculus** (see text-illustration) is the white substance between the dorsal lateral sulcus

dorsally and the less distinct **ventral lateral sulcus ventrally**. The ventral lateral sulcus, is indistinct or lacking and is demarcated by the origin of the ventral roots of the spinal nerves. Ventromedial to the ventral root filaments is the white matter designated the **ventral funiculus**; it is bounded medially by the ventral median fissure. The ventral funiculus consists of several fiber-tracts, not named here, that connect different parts of the spinal cord and the brain and that cannot be precisely distinguished gross anatomically.

c) On **CROSS-SECTION OF THE SPINAL CORD** (see text-illustration), internal to the **white substance** with its myelinated nerve tracts, the **gray substance** can be located as a 'butterfly figure.' It exhibits a **dorsal horn** and **ventral horn** and, in the thoracic and lumbar regions of the spinal cord, there is in addition, a **lateral horn**. The gray substance is present the length of the spinal cord and, considered in three dimensions, the horns are more correctly designated columns. Between the dorsal and ventral horns there are scattered groups of cells and white substance that are part of the **reticular formation**, which is continuous up to the brain. In the central area of the gray substance, the **central canal** pierces the spinal cord.

d) The **ROOTS OF THE SPINAL NERVES** are dorsal and ventral. Axons of the **motor (efferent) neurons (37)** are situated in the **ventral root (28)**, and have their origin in the large cells of the ventral horn of the gray substance.

C3   T3

Legend :

a White substance
  Gray substance
b Dorsal horn
c Lateral horn
d Ventral horn
e Substantia gelatinosa
f Reticular formation
g Dorsal median septum
h Central canal
i Median fissure [ventr.]
j Dorsal funiculus
k Lateral funiculus
l Ventral funiculus
m Dorsolateral sulcus
n Ventrolateral sulcus

Axons of **sympathetic neurons (38)** arise from nerve cells in the lateral horn of the thoracic and lumbar part of the spinal cord and also pass in the ventral root. (Parasympathetic neurons have their cell bodies in the intermediocentral cellular column of the gray substance of the sacral part of the spinal cord, which is also called lateral horn (column) by some authors; their axons pass in the ventral root of sacral spinal nerves.) The **dorsal root (26)** of the spinal nerve contains the axons (central processes) of **afferent (sensory) neurons (36)** whose peripheral processes, dendrites, (some authors refer to these peripheral processes also as axons or axis cylinders) proceed from receptors in the skin, muscle, fascia, etc. of the particular body segment. The perikarya of these sensory neurons are located in the **spinal ganglion (27)**.

e) From their perikarya of origin in the lateral horn, the axons of **SYMPATHETIC NEURONS** (see also p. 149) leave the thoracic and lumbar spinal cord in the ventral root. At the origin of the spinal nerve from the union of its dorsal and ventral roots, these axons leave the spinal nerve in myelinated **white communicating rami (7)** and reach the **sympathetic trunk (35)**. Within the trunk, the axons pass especially to the **sympathetic trunk ganglia (34)**, where most synapse on a second neuron. From some of the perikarya of the trunk ganglia (second neurons), axons return in the non-myelinated **gray communicating rami (8)** to the segmental (somatic) spinal nerve. Those myelinated sympathetic fibers that pass within the sympathetic trunk without synapsing in the trunk ganglia leave the trunk and extend to the more distal paravertebral ganglia; e.g., the **celiac ganglion (10)**. They reach the paravertebral ganglia in the **major splanchnic nerve** (see p. 49) and **minor splanchnic nerve (9)** and in the lumbar splanchnic nerves and synapse on perikarya within the paravertebral ganglia. The unmyelinated axons of the second neurons of the paravertebral ganglia pass to the viscera in the adventitia of the visceral arteries. They form a periarterial plexus extending to the stomach, duodenum, jejunum, etc. Within the viscera, they pass to intramural plexuses, which are designated, according to their position as **subserosal (11)**, **myenteric (12)** and **submucosal plexuses (13)**. (The ganglion cells in the intramural plexuses belong predominantly to the parasympathetic nervous system.) Nerve fibers of **parasympathetic neurons (39)** within the **dorsal vagal trunk (40)** and **ventral vagal trunk** (see p. 49) are axons of first neurons. They reach the different abdominal viscera by way of the celiacomesenteric (solar) plexus and the perivascular plexuses surrounding the branches of the celiac and mesenteric arteries to reach the different parts of the gut.

Spinal cord

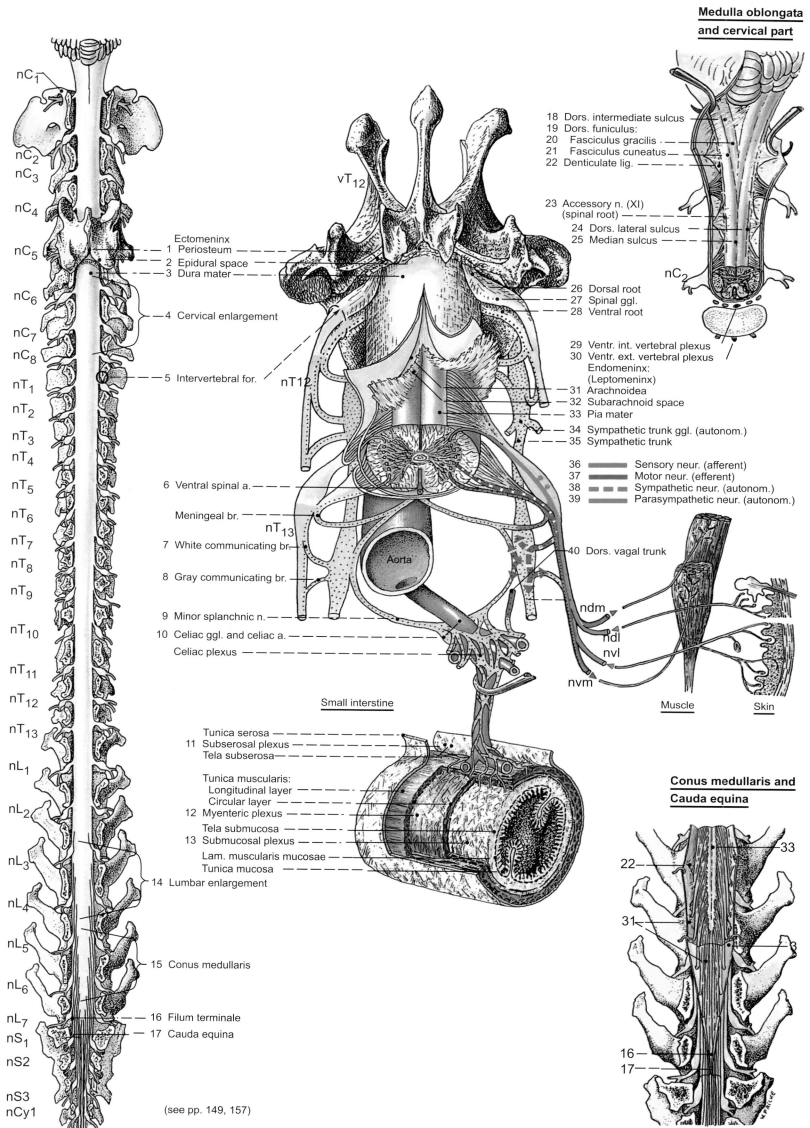

nC₁
nC₂
nC₃
nC₄
nC₅
nC₆
nC₇
nC₈
nT₁
nT₂
nT₃
nT₄
nT₅
nT₆
nT₇
nT₈
nT₉
nT₁₀
nT₁₁
nT₁₂
nT₁₃
nL₁
nL₂
nL₃
nL₄
nL₅
nL₆
nL₇
nS₁
nS2
nS3
nCy1

Ectomeninx
1 Periosteum
2 Epidural space
3 Dura mater
4 Cervical enlargement
5 Intervertebral for.
6 Ventral spinal a.
Meningeal br.
7 White communicating br.
8 Gray communicating br.
9 Minor splanchnic n.
10 Celiac ggl. and celiac a.
Celiac plexus

Tunica serosa
11 Subserosal plexus
Tela subserosa
Tunica muscularis:
Longitudinal layer
Circular layer
12 Myenteric plexus
Tela submucosa
13 Submucosal plexus
Lam. muscularis mucosae
Tunica mucosa
14 Lumbar enlargement
15 Conus medullaris
16 Filum terminale
17 Cauda equina

(see pp. 149, 157)

vT₁₂
nT12
nT₁₃
Aorta

Small interstine

Medulla oblongata and cervical part

18 Dors. intermediate sulcus
19 Dors. funiculus:
20 Fasciculus gracilis
21 Fasciculus cuneatus
22 Denticulate lig.
23 Accessory n. (XI) (spinal root)
24 Dors. lateral sulcus
25 Median sulcus
26 Dorsal root
27 Spinal ggl.
28 Ventral root
29 Ventr. int. vertebral plexus
30 Ventr. ext. vertebral plexus
Endomeninx: (Leptomeninx)
31 Arachnoidea
32 Subarachnoid space
33 Pia mater
34 Sympathetic trunk ggl. (autonom.)
35 Sympathetic trunk
36 Sensory neur. (afferent)
37 Motor neur. (efferent)
38 Sympathetic neur. (autonom.)
39 Parasympathetic neur. (autonom.)
40 Dors. vagal trunk

nC₂

ndm
ndl
nvl
nvm

Muscle   Skin

Conus medullaris and Cauda equina

33
22
31
3
16
17

2. BRAIN (ENCEPHALON) AND ITS MENINGEAL COVERINGS

1 a) The **CEREBRAL MENINGES** are continuous with the spinal meninges.

I. The **external meninges (Ectomeninx)** consist of the periosteal lining of the endocranium (periosteum, −24) and the dura mater (pachymeninx). Both layers are separated in the vertebral canal by the epidural space; but in the cranial cavity they fuse to form the united ectomeninx. The layers are separated in two places: (1) in the formation of the **diaphragma sellae (33)** of the hypophysis; and (2) where the **sinuses of the dura mater (26)** are present. At the hypophysis the periosteal layer lines the *sella turcica* and surrounds the hypophysis, which projects into the 'saddle-space' here. The dura mater itself separates from the margins of the sella turcica and covers the hypophysis dorsally as the diaphragm of the sella turcica. Within the diaphragm is a central opening for the stalk of the hypophysis, which connects the hypophysis with the hypothalamus of the brain. In the removal of the brain from the cranial cavity, this stalk is usually ruptured at the diaphragm. The ectomeninx covers the entire internal surface of the cranial cavity with the two fused layers. The **dura mater (25)** separates from the periosteum on the dorsal midline between right and left cerebral hemispheres and, transversely, at the border between the cerebral hemispheres and the cerebellum. On the dorsal midline, it extends as a dorsal median fold, the **falx cerebri (27)** and, between the cerebrum and cerebellum as a dorsal membranous transverse fold, the **tentorium cerebelli membranaceum**. The falx cerebri extends from the ethmoid bone rostrally to the occipital bone caudally. The membranous tentorium cerebelli is supported dorsally by a thin transverse plate of bone, the **tentorium cerebelli osseum (28)**. The osseous part of the tentorium projects rostroventrally from the interparietal and occipital bones; it lies within the base of the membranous tentorium, which projects over the cerebellum like a tent and thus separates the cerebellum from the cerebrum.

II. The **internal, soft meninges (Endomeninx, Leptomeninx)** consist of the arachnoidea and the pia mater. With its neurothelium, the **arachnoidea (21)** is applied to the internal surface of the dura mater and is separated from the pia mater by the **subarachnoid space (22)**. A network of connective tissue trabeculae pass from the deep surface of the arachnoidea, cross the subarachnoid space and join the pia mater. Within the meshes of the arachnoid trabeculae, the subarachnoid space is an expansive chamber that contains the cerebrospinal fluid. The space with its cerebrospinal fluid invests the brain, which in a certain manner floats in a fluid environment. The subarachnoid space is variably wide in relation to the different parts of the brain. On the superficial convexities of the cerebral gyri it is very narrow and here the dura and pia mater are closely attached. On the other hand, the subarachnoid space is very wide at the cerebral sulci where the pia mater passes deeply. The dura mater passes over the sulcus at a considerable distance and the meshes of the arachnoidea fill the wide space between them. The wide passages of the subarachnoid space are designated cisterns. The **cerebellomedullary cistern (31)** is 2 dorsolateral between the cerebellum and the spinal cord. The **intercrural cistern (34)** is ventromedian between the two cerebral peduncles. The arachnoidea with its **arachnoid granulations (20)** projects into the sinuses of the dura mater and at other sites into openings into the internal surface of the cranial bones. The arachnoid granulations were thought to be sites of resorption of cerebrospinal fluid. That is placed in doubt on the basis of more recent investigations (see p. 116). The **pia mater (23)** is tightly attached to the surface of the brain and follows into the depth of the cerebral sulci.

3 b) The **STRUCTURE OF THE INDIVIDUAL PORTIONS OF THE BRAIN** is considered in rostral-caudal sequence on median section of the brain. The parts of the brain develop embryologically from the neural tube and the three cerebral vesicles (according to another opinion, two cerebral vesicles), which differentiate into the five parts of the brain:

prosencephalon ⟨ telencephalon / diencephalon

mesencephalon ——— mesencephalon

rhombencephalon ⟨ metencephalon / myelencephalon

I. The **rhombencephalon (46)** is subdivided into the metencephalon and myelencephalon. It contains the **fourth ventricle (40)** and is distinctly similar in its basic plan to the spinal cord. This is also valid, with increasing limitation, for the mesencephalon and diencephalon. The nuclei and the place of departure of the hypoglossal nerve (XII) is ventromedial (see p. 115), which is comparable to the relations of the ventral motor column of the spinal cord. The exits of the sensory nerves (such as VIII) are dorsolateral, which is comparable to the relations of the dorsal sensory column of the spinal cord. Nuclei and the place of exit of nerves with predominant parasympathetic

portions (such as X) are located in between, which is comparable to the relations of the lateral horn of the spinal cord. Cranial nerves V – XII arise from the rhombencephalon. (XI has an additional root from the spinal cord, and V has additionally sensory nuclei in the mesencephalon and spinal cord.) In the rhombencephalon as well as the mesencephalon and spinal cord there is the **reticular formation (42)**. It consists of scattered concentrations of nerve cells 4 in the meshes of irregularly arranged nerve fibers and, as a superior center of nervous function, coordinates sensory, motor and autonomic functions (e.g, cardiovascular and respiratory centers). Moreover, it serves as a functional coordinator of the cranial nerves with each other and with adjacent parts of the central nervous system. Important nerve tracts traverse the ventral area of the rhombencephalon. One of these, the **pyramidal tract (43)**, exhibits the pyramidal decussation at the transition to the spinal cord.

The **metencephalon (44)** is the rostral part of the rhombencephalon. Its ventral part is the **pons (45)**; its dorsal part is the cerebellum. The ventral part of the pons consists predominantly of transverse fiber tracts that are continued dorsally into the cerebellum as the middle cerebellar peduncle (see p. 115). Longitudinal nerve tracts, the pyramidal and other tracts that connect the brain and spinal cord traverse the central area of the pons.

The **cerebellum** is the dorsal part of the metencephalon and is connected to 5 the other parts of the central nervous system by the cerebellar peduncles (see text-illustration, p. 112). The rostral cerebellar peduncle leads to the mesencephalon, the middle cerebellar peduncle to the pons of the metencephalon and the caudal cerebellar peduncle to the medulla oblongata. Rostrally the cerebellum is separated from the cerebral hemispheres by the tentorium cerebelli. The unpaired cerebellar vermis (see p. 113) is median and flanked by the paired cerebellar hemispheres or lateral lobes. This is seen most clearly on dorsal view of the brain. On median section can be seen the external gray substance of the **cerebellar cortex (29)** and the internal white substance of the **corpus medullare** (medullary body). The cerebellar cortex is much more finely divided and subdivided than the cerebral cortex and the white substance of the medullary body is so strongly branched that it appears as the **arbor vitae (30)** or 'tree of life.'

The **myelencephalon** (medulla oblongata, −41) extends from the pons to the roots of the first cervical nerves.

II. Three main parts of the **mesencephalon (16)** are described: The **tectum** 6 **(35)** with the **lamina tecti quadrigemina (Corpora quadrigemina −36)** forms the roof of the **mesencephalic aqueduct (39)**. The **rostral colliculus (37)** is associated with the visual pathway and the **caudal colliculus (38)** with the auditory pathway. The **tegmentum (17)** is ventral to the mesencephalic aqueduct. It contains the motor nuclei of the oculomotor (III) and trochlear (IV) nerves and a part of the reticular formation as well as the *nucleus ruber* (red nucleus) and the *substantia nigra*. The paired **cerebral peduncle (crus cerebri, −18)** lies ventrally separated by the median **intercrural fossa (19)**.

III. Of the **diencephalon (2)**, thalamus, epithalamus and hypothalamus are described here. The **thalamus (3)** bounds laterally the circular **third ventricle** 7 **(15)**. The paired parts contact each other on the midline at the **interthalamic adhesion (4)** and bear laterally the geniculate bodies. The **lateral geniculate body** (see p. 115) lies at the end of the optic tract and is connected with the rostral colliculus of the corpora quadrigemina. The **medial geniculate body** (see p. 115) is connected to the caudal colliculus of the corpora quadrigemina. Functionally the thalamus is the last site of synapse of all tracts ascending to the cerebral cortex with the exception of the olfactory tract. Thus the thalamus is the 'door to consciousness', the door to the cerebral cortex; for it is in the cerebral cortex that the phenomenon of consciousness, awareness of the stimulus, is chiefly realized. The epithalamus bears the **epiphysis (pineal** 8 **body, −1)**, which, as an appendage of the roof of the third ventricle, bounds the corpora quadrigemina rostrally. It is homologus to the parietal eye of lower vertebrates. The **hypothalamus (5)** is ventrolateral to the third ventricle and has predominant autonomic function. The **hypophysis (7)** is ven- 9 tral to the hypothalamus and connected to it by a narrow stalk. Its neural part, the **posterior lobe (9)**, develops as a ventral extension of the hypothalamus and its **anterior lobe (8)** has origin from the roof of the pharynx. Caudal 10 to the attachment of the stalk of the hypophysis to the hypothalamus is the **mammillary body (32, −** see also p. 115). It is partly divided and rounded and forms the floor of the third ventricle at the boundary of the diencephalon with the mesencephalon. Rostral to the attachment of the hypophyseal stalk, the **optic nerve (6)** arises from the diencephalon.

IV. The **telencephalon (10)** consists of the **cerebral hemispheres (11)** and their commissures. The **rhinencephalon (12)** is the olfactory part of the hemisphere. Right and left cerebral hemispheres are separated on the midline by the falx cerebri of the dura mater. The central commissures of the **corpus callosum (13)** and the **rostral commissure (14)** remain undivided.

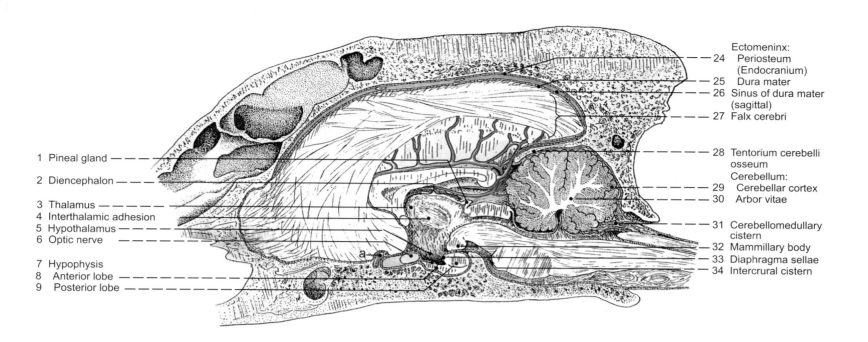

Ectomeninx:
24 Periosteum (Endocranium)
25 Dura mater
26 Sinus of dura mater (sagittal)
27 Falx cerebri

28 Tentorium cerebelli osseum

Cerebellum:
29 Cerebellar cortex
30 Arbor vitae

31 Cerebellomedullary cistern
32 Mammillary body
33 Diaphragma sellae
34 Intercrural cistern

1 Pineal gland
2 Diencephalon
3 Thalamus
4 Interthalamic adhesion
5 Hypothalamus
6 Optic nerve
7 Hypophysis
8   Anterior lobe
9   Posterior lobe

(Median section)

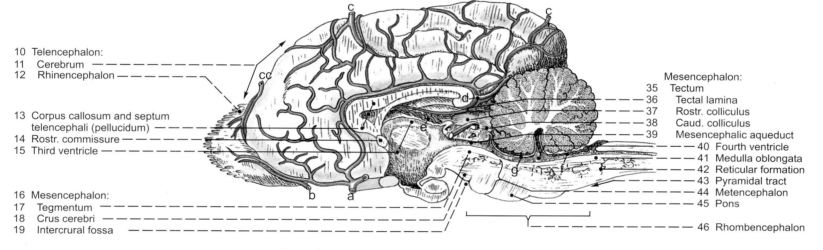

10 Telencephalon:
11   Cerebrum
12   Rhinencephalon

13 Corpus callosum and septum telencephali (pellucidum)
14 Rostr. commissure
15 Third ventricle

16 Mesencephalon:
17   Tegmentum
18   Crus cerebri
19   Intercrural fossa

Mesencephalon:
35 Tectum
36   Tectal lamina
37   Rostr. colliculus
38   Caud. colliculus
39   Mesencephalic aqueduct
40 Fourth ventricle
41 Medulla oblongata
42 Reticular formation
43 Pyramidal tract
44 Metencephalon
45 Pons

46 Rhombencephalon

Legend :

a Rostr. cerebral a.
b Ventr. cerebral v.
c Dors. cerebral vv.
d Great cerebral v.

e Choroid plexus of third ventricle
f Choroid plexus of fourth ventricle
g Rostr. medullary velum
h Parietal diploic v.

(see pp. 113, 115, 116, 117)

(Transverse section)

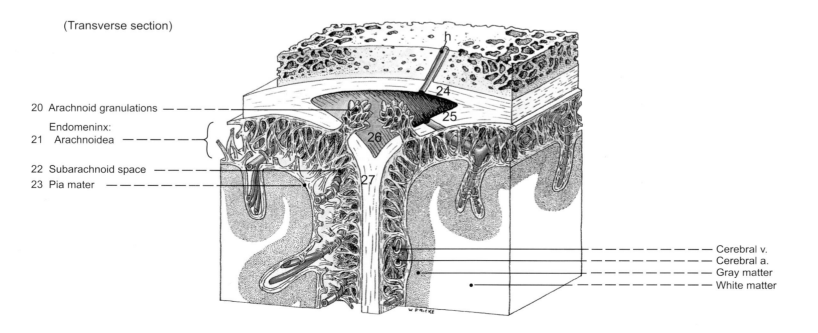

20 Arachnoid granulations

Endomeninx:
21   Arachnoidea

22 Subarachnoid space
23 Pia mater

Cerebral v.
Cerebral a.
Gray matter
White matter

111

3. CEREBRUM (TELENCEPHALON), BRAIN STEM AND LIMBIC SYSTEM

> Examination and study of the brain is done after removal of the brain from the cranial cavity. In doing this, the cranial nerves are cut at the base of the brain proximal to their perforating the meninges. Cross-sections of the brain at the level of the optic chiasm are drawn on for study.

The **telencephalon** is further classified according to phylogenetic criteria. In phylogenesis there are three phases of cerebral development. The phylogenetically oldest part of the cerebral cortex, the **paleopallium** and the part of the cortex whose development soon follows, the **archipallium**, form the rhinencephalon in the broader sense. In mammals, the archipallium has lost most of its olfactory function and the paleopallium has taken on additional functions. For this reason, some authors no longer use the term 'rhinencephalon.' However, by international agreement the term is employed further in the Nomina Anatomica Veterinaria. The phylogenetically youngest part of the cerebral cortex, the **neopallium**, in the dog develops as a gyrencephalic brain.

a) In the process of ontogenesis, the **CEREBRUM** (the term 'cerebrum' is used here to designate the cerebral hemispheres and their commissures), as the largest part of the brain, grows from rostral to dorsal to caudoventral, and covers over the rest of the brain excepting only the cerebellum, pons, and medulla oblongata. This process of development is called dorsal rotation in which parts of the hemispheres, including cerebral ventricles I and II, actually 'roll in.' This is seen distinctly in lateral view of the brain, and also in casts demonstrating the cerebral ventricles (see text-illustration, p. 116).

I. On account of the hemispherical form of the cerebrum, its two halves, the **cerebral hemispheres (1)**, are, *e.g.*, in brachycephalic breeds, not hemispheres but rather 'quarter-spheres' separated from each other on the midline by the falx cerebri. On section of the hemispheres, it is clear that there is, similar to the cerebellum, a segregation into a peripheral **cerebral cortex or gray substance (4)** and a more centrally located **medulla or white substance (5)**. In ontogenesis, the great majority of neuroblasts of the telencephalic vesicle emigrates to the periphery in a process in which the peripheral gray of the cortex or pallium develops with accumulations of perikarya and the central, white, medulla with myelinated fibers.

II. The **cerebral sulci (2)** and **cerebral gyri (3)** of the hemisphere are, in their degree of development, a reflection of the developmental level of the particular species. Primitive mammals and birds do not yet have gyri and sulci and for this reason are designated lissencephalic (smooth brain). Different from this, our domestic mammals are gyrencephalic (a brain with gyri and sulci). The regularly appearing gyri can be seen in the accompanying figures (top figure, opposite page) and in the lower figure, p. 117. In addition to the constant gyri there are also accessory ones that occur in a broad range of variation and can be observed as differences in the two hemispheres of an individual.

III. The **lobes of each hemisphere** are located in relation to bones of the same-name: **frontal lobe, occipital lobe, temporal lobe** and **parietal lobe**. Some authors differentiate additionally a rhinencephalic (olfactory) lobe (see illustration, p. 117).

IV. The **cerebral cortex** is of varying thickness. According to their specific cytoarchitecture, a number of **cortical areas** are distinguished (in human beings, areas 1 – 52), which are drawn on to designate certain details of the brain.

A **somatotopic division** into sensory and motor areas divides the cortex according to functional aspects. A certain sensation at a restricted area of the body or a certain movement of parts of the body can be assigned to a circumscribed sensory or motor projection-area of the cerebral cortex. Research into the somatotopic classification could be done because a peripheral loss of function could be assigned to a certain area of cerebral cortical damage, e.g., traumatic injuries. In addition, specific peripheral reactions could be elicited by electrical stimulation of a certain area of the cerebral cortex.

The sensory and motor regions of the cerebral cortex are connected with one another and with deep parts of the central nervous system by afferent and efferent fiber-tracts, groups of fibers of similar function, that compose the central white substance of the hemisphere.

V. The white substance of the hemisphere consists of three systems of fibers:

Association fibers are fibers that extend between different parts of the hemisphere of the same side.

Commissural fibers are transverse connections extending between the two hemispheres. They are represented by the **rostral commissure** (see p. 111), **corpus callosum (6)** and **commissural fibers of the fornix (7)**.

Projection fibers are connections of the cerebral cortex with other deep, more caudal parts of the central nervous system such as the brain stem and spinal cord. Projection fibers are arranged fan-like and converge to the dien-

cephalon. The fan-like part penetrates the area of the basal nuclei (basal ganglia), passing between the caudate nucleus and the lentiform nucleus, and is designated the **internal capsule (9)**. A thinner fiber-tract lateral to the lentiform nucleus is designated the **external capsule (13)**. From the diencephalon the projection fibers pass in the cerebral peduncle of the mesencephalon. In the area of the basal ganglia, at the site of penetration of the internal and external capsules, the alternating bands of gray and white substance give the cut surface of the brain a striate appearance and for this reason this area is named the **striate body** or **corpus striatum**.

b) The **BRAIN STEM** is defined differently by the individual textbook authors. Without doubt, the mesencephalon, pons and medulla oblongata belong to the brain stem. Beyond this, some authors include the diencephalon, and some include the basal nuclei (basal ganglia), which were named accordingly the 'stem ganglia.'

(dorsal view)

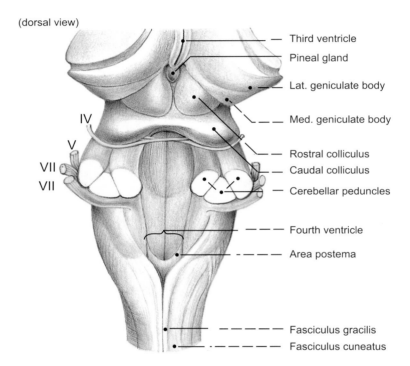

Third ventricle
Pineal gland
Lat. geniculate body
Med. geniculate body
Rostral colliculus
Caudal colliculus
Cerebellar peduncles
Fourth ventricle
Area postema
Fasciculus gracilis
Fasciculus cuneatus

I. The **basal nuclei** of the corpus striatum are gray substance, consisting of neurons that do not migrate to the peripheral cortex during ontogenesis. They remain in the area bordering the diencephalon. The basal nuclei are the **caudate nucleus (8)**, the **lentiform nucleus**, the **claustrum (14)** and the **amygdaloid body (12)**. The caudate nucleus projects into the lateral ventricle. The **lentiform nucleus** consists of the **putamen (10)**, which is lateral, and the **pallidum (Globus pallidus)**, which is medial. Many authors do not account the pallidum as part of the cerebral hemisphere but consider it a part of the diencephalon, and in this area the two parts of the brain cannot be sharply separated from one another. Topographically, the amygdaloid body belongs to the basal nuclei, but functionally to the rhinencephalon. The function of the basal nuclei has not been completely resolved. In human beings, they are involved in pathways that coordinate the pattern of movements, and they modify the output from motor areas of the cerebral cortex, especially the program of slow movements. Some of the basal nuclei take part in the functions of the limbic system.

c) The **LIMBIC SYSTEM** is the imprecisely defined border zone (limbus = border) between the diencephalon and telencephalon and, within the telencephalon, between the neopallium and the rhinencephalon. The limbic system consists of limbic cortical parts such as the **piriform lobe** and the **hippocampus** and more deeply placed parts of the hemisphere. Of the more deeply placed parts, the following are mentioned: septal nuclei of the **telencephalic septum** (previously designated the **Septum pellucidum**) and parts of the corpus striatum: **caudate nucleus, putamen** and the **amygdaloid body**. There is extensive communication (connection) between the parts of the limbic system and other regions of the brain. Many functions of the limbic system are unclear. The system is involved in the control of 'feelings', of moods, of 'drives' as well as other emotional behavior and, for this reason, this part of the nervous system is also called the 'visceral' or 'emotional' brain.

Brain (Neopallium)

(dorsal view)

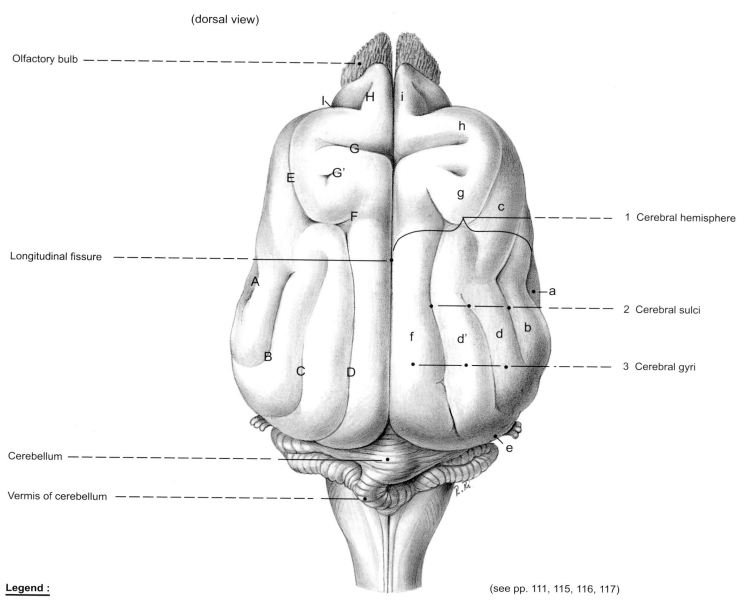

Olfactory bulb

Longitudinal fissure

Cerebellum

Vermis of cerebellum

1 Cerebral hemisphere

2 Cerebral sulci

3 Cerebral gyri

(see pp. 111, 115, 116, 117)

Legend :

A Caudal ectosylvian sulcus
B Suprasylvian sulcus
C Ectomarginal sulcus
D Marginal sulcus
E Coronal sulcus

F Ansate sulcus
G Cruciate sulcus
G' Postcruciate sulcus
H Prorean
I Presylvian sulcus

a Sylvian gyrus
b Caud. ectosylvian gyrus
c Rostr. ectomarginal gyrus
  Middle ectomarginal gyrus:
d Lateral part
d' Medial part

e Caud. ectomarginal gyrus
f Marginal gyrus
g Postcruciate gyrus
h Precruciate gyrus
i Prorean gyrus

Thalamus (section) and striate body

(transverse section)

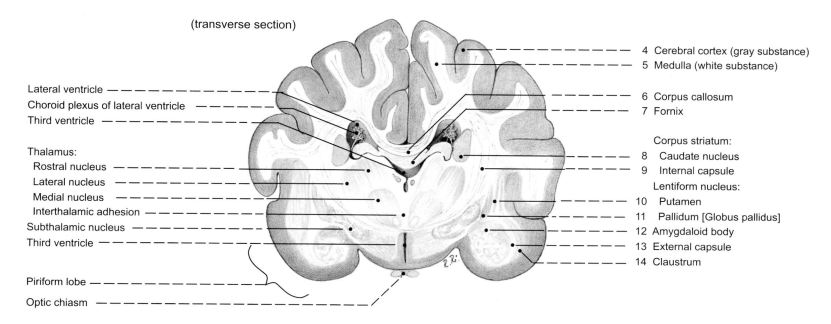

Lateral ventricle
Choroid plexus of lateral ventricle
Third ventricle

Thalamus:
Rostral nucleus
Lateral nucleus
Medial nucleus
Interthalamic adhesion
Subthalamic nucleus
Third ventricle

Piriform lobe

Optic chiasm

4 Cerebral cortex (gray substance)
5 Medulla (white substance)

6 Corpus callosum
7 Fornix

Corpus striatum:
8 Caudate nucleus
9 Internal capsule
  Lentiform nucleus:
10 Putamen
11 Pallidum [Globus pallidus]
12 Amygdaloid body
13 External capsule
14 Claustrum

113

4. RHINENCEPHALON, SITES OF EGRESSION OF THE CRANIAL NERVES, ARTERIAL SUPPLY OF THE BRAIN

> With the assistance of the instructors, the dorsal part of the cerebral hemispheres and all of the cerebellum are removed by horizontal section of the brain across the corpus callosum, opening the lateral ventricles of the brain. To demonstrate the area of the geniculate bodies and the optic tract, the hippocampus is lifted off to give the view shown by the lower figure on the opposite page.

a) The **RHINENCEPHALON**, a part of the telencephalon, begins with its **basal part (2)** rostrally at the **olfactory bulb (3)**. Here the fibers of the olfactory nerve (**Fila olfactoria**, —1) end. The perikarya and dendrites of these olfactory neurons are in the olfactory mucous membrane of the nasal fundus and of the vomeronasal organ. The second neurons of the olfactory pathway begin in the olfactory bulb. They course at first in the short **olfactory peduncle (4)** and, after its division, in the **lateral (5)**, **intermediate**, and **medial (6) olfactory tracts**. In the lateral olfactory tract, after synapse on another neuron, this olfactory pathway reaches the primary olfactory cortex of the **piriform lobe (9)** and, beyond the piriform lobe, the limbic system, in particular, the amygdaloid body. Following synapse of some fibers in the **septal part of the rhinencephalon**, neurons of the medial olfactory tract run chiefly to the septal nuclei of the telencephalic septum (*Septum pellucidum*). The olfactory trigone is the triangular area bounded by the medial and lateral olfactory tracts. Many of the fibers of the intermediate olfactory tract end in the **olfactory trigone**.

b) The **HIPPOCAMPUS (28)** is a nuclear area of the limbic system and, in human beings, takes part in memory function. It lies caudally on the floor of the **lateral ventricle (25)**. Its common name, 'Ammon's horn', is derived from its smooth surface and its form, which is curved like a ram's horn. A transverse section through the hemisphere at the level of the **epiphysis (27,** —see also pp. 111 and 117) reveals the coiled course of the hippocampus. The hippocampus covers the lateral and medial geniculate bodies like a shell and, with its dorsomedial *fimbria hippocampi*, lies beneath the **choroid plexus (26)** of the lateral ventricle.

c) Of the **CONDUCTION PATHWAYS (FIBER-TRACTS)** leading to and from the brain, only two descending (motor) tracts and two ascending (sensory) tracts are considered here.

I. The pyramidal and extrapyramidal systems are **motor pathways**.

The **pyramidal system** is responsible for fine coordinated movements and in human beings is of more importance than in the domestic mammals. It begins with projection fibers in the motor cortex of the neopallium and continues in the internal capsule to the cerebral peduncle. After traversing the peduncle, its fibers follow different paths. One bundle of fibers crosses to the motor nuclei of the contralateral cranial nerves. Another bundle (collateral branches) courses to the pons and, further, by way of the middle cerebellar peduncle, to the cerebellum. The largest group of fibers continues ventromedially on the medulla oblongata as the **pyramid (17)** where caudally most of the fibers cross the median plane in the **pyramidal decussation (22)**. These fibers reach motor nuclei of the spinal cord directly or by multisynaptic pathways.

The **extrapyramidal system** is responsible for coarser movements and dominates as the motor system in our domestic mammals. It begins in the cerebral cortex. Synapses onto lower neurons take place in the **caudate nucleus (24)**, in the **tegmentum of the mesencephalon** (see p. 111), especially in the substantia nigra and the nucleus ruber, and in the **olive (21)** of the medulla oblongata. Fibers from these nuclei pass in the lateral funiculus of the spinal cord to motor neurons of the ventral horn. The extrapyramidal system has numerous feed-back mechanisms that pass to the cerebellum in the **caudal cerebellar peduncle (33)** and, by way of the cerebellar circuitry, bring about excitatory and inhibitory impulses. The **rostral and middle cerebellar peduncles (33)** furnish the connection between the cerebellum and the midbrain or the pons of the metencephalon.

II. Sensory pathways run in the fasciculus gracilis and fasciculus cuneatus.

The **fasciculus gracilis (34)** ascends dorsomedially in the dorsal funiculus of the spinal cord. Its fibers conduct sensory proprioceptive (muscle and joint sense) impulses from receptors in the pelvic limb and caudal trunk regions to the dorsocaudal area of the medulla oblongata. Here, synapses take place in the nucleus gracilis (at the tubercle of the nucleus gracilis) with further conduction to the cerebral cortex.

The **fasciculus cuneatus (35)** runs dorsolaterally in the dorsal funiculus of the spinal cord. It is composed of sensory proprioceptive fibers from the thoracic limb and cranial thoracic region to the nucleus cuneatus at the tubercle of the nucleus cuneatus. The cuneate tubercle is dorsocaudal in the medulla oblongata, cranial and lateral to the tubercle of the nucleus gracilis. Synapses take place in the cuneate nucleus from which the pathway is continued to the cerebral cortex.

d) **EMERGENCE OF THE CRANIAL NERVES FROM THE BRAIN** (see pp. 136/137)

The **olfactory nerves (I)** pass through the foramina of the cribriform plate of the ethmoid bone to reach the olfactory bulb of the rhinencephalon.

The **optic nerve (II)** extends from the ganglion cell layer of the retina to the **optic chiasm (7)** by way of the optic canal (see p. 91). At the chiasm, about 75% of the fibers cross the midline. They are predominantly those from the nasal half of the retina; whereas, 25% of the fibers, especially those from the temporal half of the retina, continue on the same side. Beyond the optic chiasm, optic nerve fibers from the same and contralateral side continue as the **optic tract (8)** and end with synapse in the **lateral geniculate body (29)**. From the lateral geniculate body, the optic pathway passes by way of the internal capsule to the visual cortex in the occipital lobe of the hemisphere, where conscious visual perception takes place. Collateral branches from fibers of the optic tract and from the lateral geniculate body reach the mesencephalon and the **rostral colliculus (31)**, the oculomotor nucleus and the parasympathetic nucleus of the oculomotor nerve. These connections regulate the movements of the ocular and some other muscles and, by way of the parasympathetic nucleus, the diameter of the pupil.

The **oculomotor nerve (III)** emerges from the mesencephalon caudolateral to the **mamillary body (11)**.

The **trochlear nerve (IV)** originates from the dorsal mesencephalon at the caudal border of the caudal colliculus. Right and left nerves cross the midline and then curve laterally and rostroventrally between the hemisphere and the cerebellum to the base of the brain, then to the orbital fissure (see pp. 89 and 91) to reach the apex of the periorbita and the dorsal oblique muscle of the eye.

The **trigeminal nerve (V)** emerges from the brain with its large sensory root and its small motor root laterally between the **pons (14)** and the **trapezoid body (15)** of the rhombencephalon. The perikarya of the sensory, afferent, neurons lie in the strikingly large trigeminal ganglion, which is subdural between the rostal end of the petrous temporal bone and the foramina by which its three branches leave the cranial cavity.

The **abducens nerve (VI)** passes from the rhombencephalon caudal to the pons, in the angle between the **pyramid (17)** and the **trapezoid body (15)**.

The **facial nerve (VII)** emerges from the rhombencephalon, laterally from the trapezoid body at its junction with the medulla oblongata. It enters the *porus acusticus internus* from which it then passes in the osseous facial canal to the stylomastoid foramen.

The **vestibulocochlear nerve (VIII)** emerges from the brain at the trapezoid body, dorsal to the facial nerve, and, like that nerve, also enters the porus acusticus internus. The **auditory pathway** is multisynaptic, beginning in the internal ear and ending in the cerebral cortex. Peripheral processes of nerve cells of the spiral ganglion lead from the cochlear duct of the internal ear. Central processes (axons) of the ganglion cells pass in the vestibulocochlear nerve to the cochlear nuclei. From the cochlear nuclei, fibers pass both ipsilaterally and contralaterally in the trapezoid body to nuclei of the trapezoid body, to the nuclei of the **caudal colliculus (32)** and to the **medial geniculate body (30)**. From the medial geniculate body, fibers pass in the internal capsule to the auditory cortex of the temporal lobe of the hemisphere. The vestibular pathway leads from the vestibular ganglia of the internal ear to vestibular nuclei of the floor of the fourth ventricle and, from there by diverse pathways to the cerebellum, the spinal cord, and the cerebral cortex.

The **glossopharyngeal nerve (IX)** leaves the medulla oblongata from the lateral aspect of the medulla oblongata and runs to the jugular foramen (see pp. 89 and 91).

The roots of the **vagus nerve (X)** arise from the lateral aspect of the medulla oblongata caudal to the roots of the glossopharyngeal nerve. With the glossopharyngeal and accessory nerves, it passes from the cranial cavity through the jugular foramen.

The **accessory nerve (XI, —18)** has a thick part that arises from the spinal cord and a thin part that arises from the medulla oblongata of the brain. The **spinal roots (20)** arise from the cervical spinal cord. They pass cranially on the lateral contour of the cord between the dorsal and ventral roots of the cervical nerves, entering the cranial cavity at the foramen magnum. The **medullary roots (19)** arise from the medulla oblongata caudal to the vagus nerve. Both parts pass together through the jugular foramen. The medullary part joins the vagus as the *internal ramus*. The spinal part, as the *external ramus*, innervates the trapezius, sternocleidomastoid and cleidocervical muscles.

The **hypoglossal nerve (XII)** passes from the brain ventrally at the caudal end of the medulla oblongata, its numerous nerve fibers emerging near the lateral border of the **olive (21)**. Its fibers unite to a single bundle that leaves the skull through the hypoglossal canal and peripherally extends to the muscles of the tongue.

e) The **ARTERIAL SUPPLY OF THE BRAIN** proceeds from the **cerebral arterial circle (12)**, which is fed laterally by the **internal carotid artery (10)** and caudally by the unpaired **basilar artery (13)**. The basilar artery originates at the level of origin of the first cervical nerves from the confluence of right and left **vertebral arteries (23)**.

Brain and cranial nerves

Base of brain (ventral view)

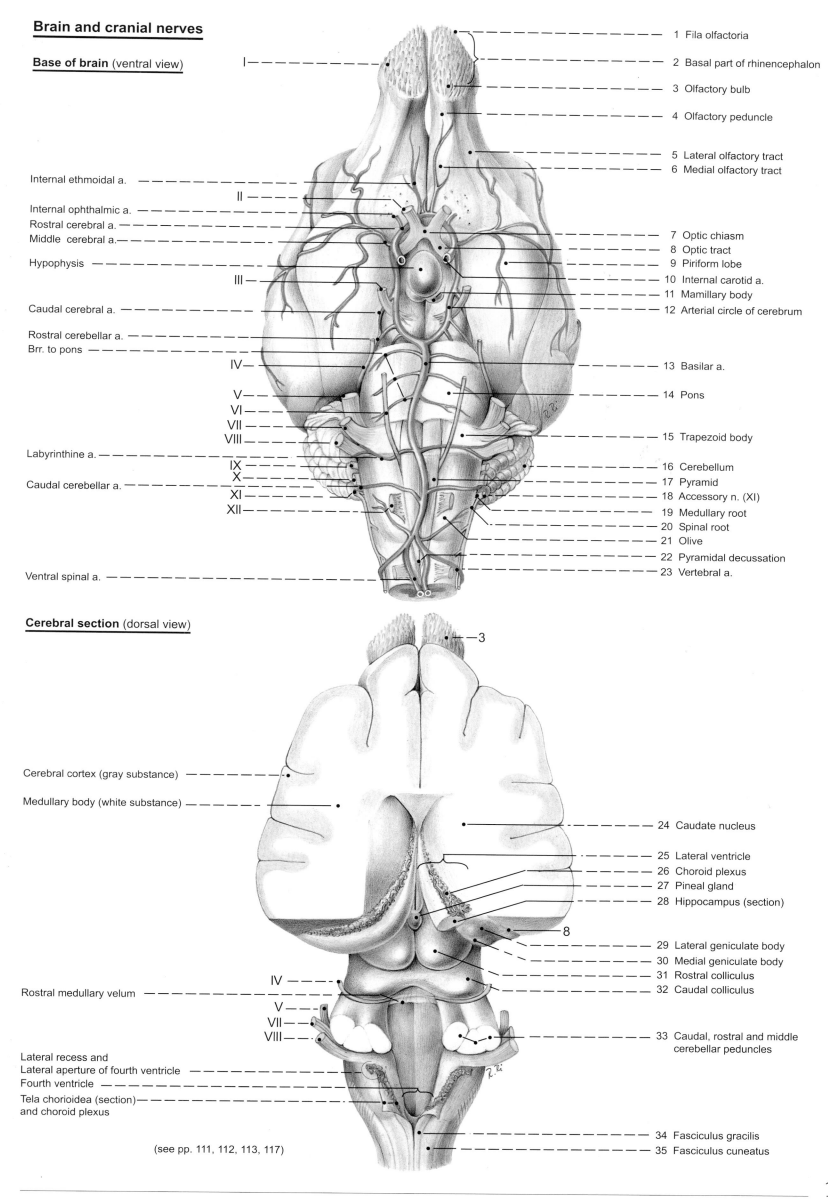

1 Fila olfactoria
2 Basal part of rhinencephalon
3 Olfactory bulb
4 Olfactory peduncle
5 Lateral olfactory tract
6 Medial olfactory tract

Internal ethmoidal a.
Internal ophthalmic a.
Rostral cerebral a.
Middle cerebral a.
Hypophysis

7 Optic chiasm
8 Optic tract
9 Piriform lobe
10 Internal carotid a.
11 Mamillary body
12 Arterial circle of cerebrum

Caudal cerebral a.

Rostral cerebellar a.
Brr. to pons

13 Basilar a.

14 Pons

15 Trapezoid body

Labyrinthine a.

16 Cerebellum
17 Pyramid
18 Accessory n. (XI)
19 Medullary root
20 Spinal root
21 Olive
22 Pyramidal decussation
23 Vertebral a.

Caudal cerebellar a.

Ventral spinal a.

Cerebral section (dorsal view)

3

Cerebral cortex (gray substance)

Medullary body (white substance)

24 Caudate nucleus

25 Lateral ventricle
26 Choroid plexus
27 Pineal gland
28 Hippocampus (section)

8

29 Lateral geniculate body
30 Medial geniculate body
31 Rostral colliculus
32 Caudal colliculus

Rostral medullary velum

33 Caudal, rostral and middle cerebellar peduncles

Lateral recess and
Lateral aperture of fourth ventricle
Fourth ventricle
Tela chorioidea (section)
and choroid plexus

34 Fasciculus gracilis
35 Fasciculus cuneatus

(see pp. 111, 112, 113, 117)

5. CEREBRAL VEINS, SINUSES OF THE DURA MATER, CEREBRAL VENTRICLES AND CHOROID PLEXUSES

a) The **CEREBRAL VEINS**, unaccompanied by arteries, discharge into the sinuses of the dura mater. Like the sinuses they have no valves and are without smooth muscle in their walls. Superficial and deep cerebral veins are distinguished.

Of the superficial veins of the brain, two to four **dorsal cerebral veins (1)** open into the dorsal sagittal sinus. The ventral cerebral veins (lower illustration on opposite page, A and B) are superficial at the base of the brain and laterally on the temporal lobe; they open at different places into the ventral sinus system of the dura mater.

The deep cerebral veins come chiefly from the corpus callosum, the area of the basal nuclei and the choroid plexuses of the lateral ventricles (see below) and unite to form the **great cerebral vein (6)**. As the straight sinus, the latter continues caudodorsally between the hemispheres and the cerebellum within the membranous tentorium cerebelli.

b) The **SINUSES OF THE DURA MATER** are modified venous channels within the ectomeninx (see p. 111) that run predominantly between its periosteal and dura mater layers. Owing to their position in the ectomeninx or in osseous canals of the cranial bones, the width of their lumens is kept constant even in the absence of a muscular coat. The absence of venous valves facilitates a blood flow in different directions. The dural sinuses take up mainly the above- mentioned cerebral veins and the **veins of the wall of the cranium (diploic veins, —2)**. By way of emissary veins, they drain the blood to the veins of the head and to the **internal jugular vein (15)**. Corresponding to their position with respect to the brain, dorsal and ventral systems of dural venous sinuses are distinguished.

I. The **ventral system of dural venous sinuses** begins with right and left **cavernous sinuses (8)**, both of which are connected rostrally with the **ophthalmic plexus (17)** of the orbit. Rostral to the hypophysis, the cavernous sinuses are connected by a variably present intercavernous sinus and, caudal to the hypophysis, by a constant **intercavernous sinus (14)**. Caudally, each cavernous sinus is continued in the petro-occipital canal by the **ventral petrosal sinus (12)**. The latter is connected to the internal jugular vein by the emissary vein of the jugular foramen. Caudal to the emissary vein, the ventral petrosal sinus anastomoses with the **sigmoid sinus (11)** before joining the **basilar sinus (10)**. After passing through the condylar canal and the foramen magnum, the basilar sinus joins the **ventral internal vertebral plexus (9)**. The dorsal petrosal sinus (7) passes in the membranous tentorium cerebelli to the transverse sinus.

II. The **dorsal system of dural venous sinuses** begins rostrally with the **dorsal sagittal sinus (3)**, which takes up venous branches from the nasal cavity. Caudally, after having taken up the **straight sinus (4, —the continuation of the great cerebral vein)**, it bifurcates dorsal to the osseous tentorium cerebelli into the paired **transverse sinuses (5)**. The transverse sinus runs laterally in the osseous canal and sulcus of the transverse sinus. Here it gives off the sigmoid sinus, an anastomosis to the ventral system of dural venous sinuses, and, in the temporal meatus passes over into the **temporal sinus (13)**. The temporal sinus is continued by the emissary vein of the retroarticular foramen, which opens into the **maxillary vein (16)**.

c) The **VENTRICLES OF THE BRAIN** (see text-illustration) develop during ontogenesis from the lumen of the neural tube. The right and left **lateral ventricles (S)** lie within the corresponding cerebral hemisphere (see also p. 113).

The **interventricular foramen (W)** connects the lateral ventricles with the unpaired **third ventricle (Y)** that centrally surrounds ring-like the interthalamic adhesion of the diencephalon. The third ventricle outpouches ventrally in the direction of the optic chiasm and the neurohypophysis, forming a **recess (Z, Z')** at each. The narrow **mesencephalic aqueduct (X)** proceeds from the third ventricle at the transition to the mesencephalon and joins the spacious **fourth ventricle (V)** at the transition to the rhombencephalon. The fourth ventricle is continuous caudally with the narrow **central canal (U)** of the spinal cord. The floor of the fourth ventricle (see p. 115) appears rhomboid in dorsal view, which is responsible for the naming of this part of the surrounding brain. The roof of the fourth ventricle is formed rostrally in the metencephalon by the very thin rostral medullary velum and, in the myelencephalon, by the caudal medullary velum and the tela choroidea. (With fixation, the rostral medullary velum tends to collapse and adhere to the floor of the fourth ventricle, which blocks the connection to the mesencephalic aqueduct.) The very thin caudal medullary velum is closely attached to the cerebellum and to the cerebellar peduncles. It bears the tela choroidea (see p. 115) with the choroid plexus. In the **lateral recess (T)** on each side of the fourth ventricle is a lateral aperture by which the fourth ventricle communicates with the subarachnoid space.

d) The **CHOROID PLEXUSES** (see pp. 111 and 115) that lie in all four cerebral ventricles, but not in the mesencephalic aqueduct, produce cerebrospinal fluid. In addition to the choroid plexuses, cerebrospinal fluid is formed by the blood vessels of the pia mater. To form the choroid plexuses, the pia mater with its contained blood vessels projects garland-like into the lumen of the ventricle and is covered here by a modified cuboidal ependyma, the internal lining of the ventricle.

The **cerebrospinal fluid** originates from the blood and passes into the ventricle through the pores of the capillary endothelium, the basal membrane and the modified ependymal cells, while at the same time retaining the blood cells and plasma proteins. The fluid fills the ventricles, including the mesencephalic aqueduct and the central canal of the spinal cord. These internal chambers are connected to the subarachnoid space (see p. 111) which is external to the brain and spinal cord. The connection is by the lateral aperture at the lateral end of each lateral recess of the fourth ventricle (see p. 115). Cerebrospinal fluid is formed in considerable amounts, in the dog about 350 ml per day. However, the total amount of fluid within the ventricles, aqueduct, central canal and subarachnoid space remains constant, and there is a balance between fluid formation and fluid resorption (lower illustration, p. 111). Sites of resorption are the arachnoid granulations and the extensions of the subarachnoid space upon the first part of the spinal nerves, and upon the afferent and efferent blood vessels of the brain. Also the meningeal coats of the olfactory (I) and optic (II) nerves are sites of absorption of cerebrospinal fluid. By means of the meningeal coats of the olfactory nerves, cerebrospinal fluid reaches from the brain to the olfactory mucous membrane of the nasal fundus by way of the lamina cribrosa of the ethmoid bone. The fluid is taken up and removed by nasal lymph vessels. In a similar manner, the cerebrospinal fluid reaches the tissues surrounding the optic nerve, passing from the subarachnoid space by pores and microcanals into the retrobulbar loose connective tissue of the eye from which it is drained by lymph and blood vessels. In the case of an imbalance between formation and absorption, an internal hydrocephalus may develop after excessive formation or reduced or blocked drainage. In such a case, depending on the site of blockage, the cerebral ventricles are enlarged and the surrounding brain tissue compressed and thin. The head is disproportionately large and the cranial bones are abnormally thin. Pathological increases in volume, especially in the narrow passages of the internal spaces, are regarded as the cause.

In healthy animals the cerebrospinal fluid has in addition to nutritive functions also thermoregulatory functions, but its function is chiefly mechanical in providing a protective fluid covering. In the case of trauma to the head, the movement of the brain is retarded by the cerebrospinal fluid. At the site of the trauma, lesions develop and after a certain time also on the opposite side. With violent rotation of the head, there arise shearing forces at the passage of vessels and nerves upon the skull, which can lead to hemorrhage at the openings of the cerebral veins into the venous sinuses.

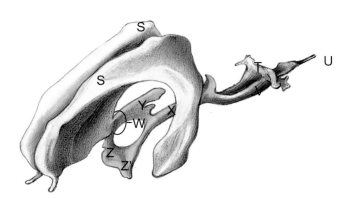

Legend:

S Lateral ventricle	**V** Fourth ventricle
T Lateral recess of the fourth ventricle	**W** Interventricular foramen
	X Mesencephalic aqueduct
U Central canal of the spinal cord	**Y** Third Ventricle
	Z Optic recess
	Z' Neurohypophyseal recess

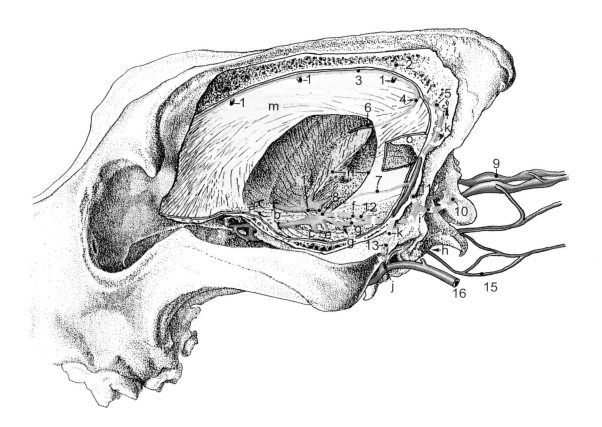

Sinuses of dura mater

1 Dors. cerebral vv.
2 Diploic v.
3 Dors. sagittal sinus
4 Straight sinus
5 Transverse sinus
6 Great cerebral v.
7 Dors. petrosal sinus
8 Cavernous sinus
9 Ventr. int. vertebral plexus
10 Basilar sinus
11 Sigmoid sinus
12 Ventr. petrosal sinus
13 Temporal sinus
14 Intercavernous sinus
15 Internal jugular v.
16 Maxillary v.
17 Ophthalmic plexus

Cranial cavity and
sinuses of dura mater

a Optic canal
b Orbital fissure
c Foramen rotundum
d Alar canal
e Foramen ovale
f Petrooccipital canal
g Carotid canal
g' Ext. carotid for.
h Jugular foramen
i Condylar canal
j Retroarticular foramen
k Canal of temporal sinus
l Temporal meatus
m Falx cerebri
n Membranous tentorium cerebelli
o Tentorial process

Brain (lateral view)

A Ventr. cerebral vv. (rostr.)
B Ventr. cerebral vv. (caud.)
C Dors. cerebellar vv.
D Int. carotid a.
E Rostr. cerebellar a.
F Labyrinthine a.
G Caud. cerebellar a.
H Presylvian sulcus
J Lat. rhinal sulcus
K Cruciate sulcus
L Marginal sulcus
L' Marginal gyrus
M Suprasylvian sulcus
M' Middle ectosylvian gyrus
N Caud. ectosylvian sulcus
N' Caudal ectosylvian gyrus
O Rostr. ectosylvian sulcus
P Pseudosylvian fissure
Q Rostr. sylvian gyrus
R Caud. sylvian gyrus

(see pp. 111, 113, 115)

CHAPTER 11: SENSE ORGANS

1. THE EYE

The **sense organs** receive adequate sensory stimuli of physical or chemical nature by way of their receptor cells that, with supporting cells and one or more afferent neurons, form the receptor organ. Sensory cells are classified into primary and secondary according to morphological criteria. Primary sensory cells are modified nerve cells with a short dendritic receptor and a long axon that leads to the central nervous system. Secondary sensory cells are non-neural receptor cells of certain sense organs that by way of synapses with investing nerve fibers conduct stimuli to the central nervous system.

The **ORGAN OF VISION** consists of the **eye (eyeball, bulb or globe of the eye)**, including the optic nerve with its coverings (**external sheath of the optic nerve, −25**), the central **visual pathways** and the **visual centers** of the brain.

The **globe of the eye (*Bulbus oculi*)** is nearly spherical and for that reason directional terms such as **equatorial** or **meridional** can be used without misunderstanding. With accessory structures such as the external ocular muscles and including the periorbita, orbital structures have a pyramidal form that extends from the base at the orbital margin to the apex at the openings of the optic canal and orbital fissure. Directional terms with respect to the eye correspond to terms used in human anatomy and, if logically used, misunderstandings can be avoided. The terms **anterior** and **posterior**, which are not used in other regions of the animal body, refer to the rostral aspect of the globe of the eye or, respectively, to the ocular fundus. Also, the terms **superior** and **inferior** can be applied to the eye if they relate, for example, to the upper or, respectively, lower eyelid. The bulb of the eye is an outpouching of the brain and the meninges. The external, fibrous, coat of the eyeball can be understood as the continuation of the dura mater and the middle, vascular, coat as a continuation of the leptomeninx. The internal coat of the eyeball is a continuation of the nerve cell-rich cerebral surface.

Functionally, the eyeball can be compared to the five main constituents of a photo camera.

1   The **eyelids** or **palpebrae (superior palpebra, −1, and inferior palpebra, −9)** are auxiliary, protective organs that bring about the closure of the palpebral fissure, the space between the eyelids, and correspond to the shutter of the
2   camera (1). The **third eyelid (8)** lies in the medial angle of the eye.

I. The external coat of the eyeball is the **fibrous tunic.** It consists posteriorly of the **sclera** that, at the **limbus of the cornea (15)**, is continuous with the **cornea**, which is anterior. The fibrous tunic gives form to the eyeball and corresponds to the box of the camera with the cornea as the lens (2).

3   The transparent **cornea (2)** maintains its transparency with a certain normal degree of moisture, which is provided anteriorly by the lacrimal fluid and posteriorly by the aqueous humor (see below). Light rays are refracted at the external surface of the cornea, but refraction is negligible at its internal surface. The corneal epithelium, which forms the superficial layer of the cornea, is not cornified.

4   In the **sclera (22)** the direction of the tensile fibers corresponds to mechanical stresses; that is, to the considerable internal ocular pressure and to the traction of the external ocular muscles. At the site of the optic disc, the sclera is modified to a cribrosal area for the passage of the optic nerve axons. Scleral pigment cells are predominantly at the boundary with the middle coat of the eyeball and serve to darken the internal chamber of the eye (comparable to the box of the camera).

5   **II.** The middle coat is the **vascular tunic** of the eyeball. The part designated the **choroid (23)** is approximately coextensive with the sclera of the fibrous tunic. It is rich in melanin pigment and has a limiting internal membrane, the basal lamina of the choroid (BRUCH'S membrane) that forms the surface next to the internal coat of the eyeball, the nervous tunic. A well-developed network of coarse vessels permeates the pigmented choroid and a finer capillary network is between this coarse vessel layer and the internal limiting membrane. The **tapetum lucidum (21)** is a circumscribed layer of cells within the choroid that reflects the incident light, increasing the stimulation of the photoreceptors of the internal tunic. Carnivores have a **tapetum cellulosum**, its cells containing a latticework of microscopic rodlets that reflect and scatter the light. (Other domestic mammals with a tapetum lucidum have at this site a *tapetum fibrosum* that contains special fibers.) Owing to its reflection by the tapetum, the incident light acts twice on the photoreceptors. Its reflected colors, which vary with species, are produced by interference phenomena, much like the colors produced by a thin film of oil on water. In the area of the tapetum, the choroid has little or no pigment. Depending on breed and the size of the dog, the tapetum occupies a roughly triangular area dorsal to the 'blind spot' of the retina, the optic disc.

6   The **iris (3)** corresponds to the diaphragm (3) of a photo camera. It belongs to the vascular tunic and is anterior to the lens, located between the anterior and posterior chambers of the eye. Its central opening is the **pupil (4)**. It regulates the passage of light by means of two smooth muscles that have their ori-

gin in the neuroectoderm. The circular **m. sphincter pupillae (11)** surrounds the pupil with a circular fiber course; whereas, the **m. dilatator pupillae (12)** with radial fibers lies in the posterior part of the iris. The posterior surface of the iris is covered by a heavily pigmented epithelium that is the cecal part of the retina (see below). Also the stroma of the iris contains pigments that are responsible for its genetically determined color.

The **ciliary body** is also a constituent of the vascular tunic and forms a circular thickening around the lens. In accomodation, it functions by contraction of its **ciliary smooth muscle (17)** with mediation by the **zonular fibers (14)** that extend from the ciliary body to the elastic lens capsule. Varying the tension on the lens capsule alters the form of the ocular lens. In this regard, the lens and ciliary body with the zonular fibers can be compared to a variable objective lens (4) of a photo camera, which permits the focusing of light on the retina (film). At its base, the surface of the ciliary body forms the **orbiculus ciliaris (7)** and is enlarged in the area of the **corona ciliaris (6)** by about 80 **ciliary processes (6)**. The ciliary processes, with the zonular fibers that pass from them, produce the connection to the ocular lens. With contraction of the meridional fibers of the ciliary muscle, the ciliary processes are brought nearer to the lens, relaxing the tension on the zonular fibers. In so doing, the lens capsule, which is elastic and surrounds the lens, acts to 'round off' (increase the curvature of) the lens. The greater curvature increases the refractive power of the lens, making the final correction to bring near objects into focus on the retina. Accomodation is achieved most easily in younger animals in which the lens is more pliable and its form more easily altered by varying the tension on the elastic lens capsule. With far vision, the ciliary muscle is relaxed and the ciliary processes farther from the lens capsule with increased tension of the zonular fibers. The lens is 'flatter' with its curvature reduced and its focal length increased.

7   **III.** The internal coat is the nervous tunic of the globe of the eye, the **retina**. It is composed of 10 layers (see histology) and, in the 9th layer − the layers are numbered from internal to external − contains the photoreceptors, the cone cells and rod cells. The retina is for this reason comparable to the film (image-carrier, −5) of a photo camera. The light sensitive **optic part of the retina (19)** extends from the ocular fundus to the base of the ciliary body where, at the **ora serrata (20)**, it is continued by the part of the retina that is free of photoreceptors and heavily pigmented. This is the **blind part of the retina or pars ceca (18)** of the retina, which covers the internal aspect of the ciliary body and the posterior surface of the iris. The photoreceptors consist of about 95% rods and only 5% cones. The sensitivity to light, which in the photo camera is determined by different light-sensitive films (= DIN number), in the retina is regulated by the pigment epithelium. With light stimulation, the processes of the pigment epithelium project into the area of the photoreceptors and actually 'embrace' them. In darkness, the pigment epithelium retracts from the area of the rods and cones.

In the **blind spot (optic disc, −27)** there are no photoreceptors. It is the site of penetration of the sclera by the **optic nerve (26)** and the **retinal blood vessels (24)**, which can be seen in the examination of the fundus of the eye. A few millimeters dorsolateral to the disc, is the macula, the place of most acute vision. Compared to primates, the macula is underdeveloped in the dog and scarcely visible. The concentration of cones is only slightly increased here. The corresponding area in human beings is especially rich in cones for which, because of its color, it is designated the 'yellow spot' *(Macula lutea)*.

8   **IV.** The **lens (5)** does not originate from the brain but from the cutaneous ectoderm. It lies posterior to the pupil and iris. The lens is contained within the elastic lens capsule, a product of the lens epithelium that is the attachment of the zonular fibers. In ontogenesis, the anterior surface of the lens is monolayered (lens epithelium); whereas, the cells of the posterior lens epithelium, with loss of their nuclei, elongate and form lens fibers. They have a length up to 1 cm and fill the hollow space of the original lens vesicle. The lens fibers have a course that is roughly hemispherical, their ends meeting at the anterior and posterior surfaces of the lens in two 'lens stars' that have an upright or, respectively, upside-down 'Y' form.

9   **V.** In the **interior of the eye** there is an **anterior chamber of the eye (10)** that is anterior to the iris and a **posterior chamber (13)** that is posterior to the iris and anterior to the lens. Behind the lens there is a **vitreous chamber of the eye (28)** occupied by the **vitreous body**. The anterior and posterior chambers contain a clear fluid, the aqueous humor, which is secreted by the 'pars ceca cells of the retina that cover the anterior surface of the ciliary body, the surface that faces the posterior chamber. Absorption of the aqueous humor is by way of the sponge-like trabecular system of spaces formed by the pectinate ligament at the **iridocorneal angle (16)**. In the depth of these spaces, the aqueous humor is absorbed into the scleral venous plexuses, which are equivalent to SCHLEMM'S canal (scleral venous sinus) of the human being. The plexuses are drained by ciliary veins. In case of a blockage of the drainage system, the interior pressure of the eye increases and, depending on its extent, results in the condition of glaucoma.

Organn of vision

Right eye

(nasal view)

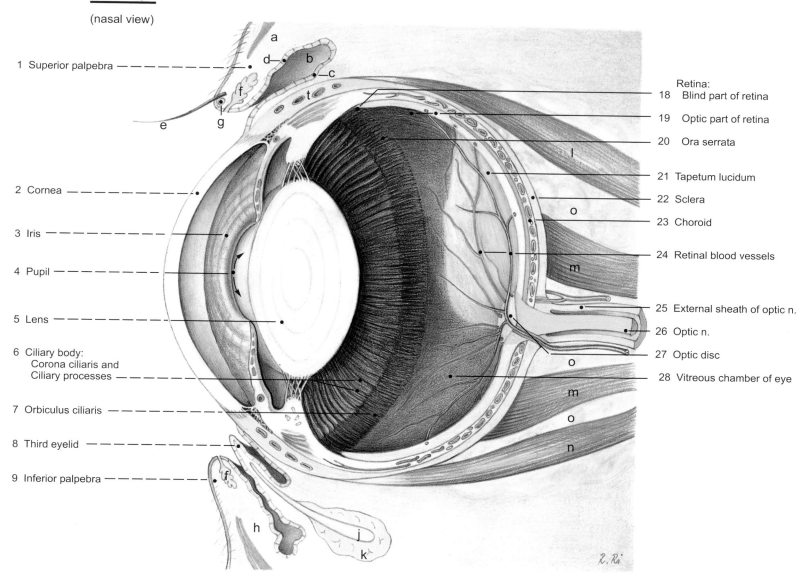

1 Superior palpebra
2 Cornea
3 Iris
4 Pupil
5 Lens
6 Ciliary body:
   Corona ciliaris and
   Ciliary processes
7 Orbiculus ciliaris
8 Third eyelid
9 Inferior palpebra

Retina:
18 Blind part of retina
19 Optic part of retina
20 Ora serrata
21 Tapetum lucidum
22 Sclera
23 Choroid
24 Retinal blood vessels
25 External sheath of optic n.
26 Optic n.
27 Optic disc
28 Vitreous chamber of eye

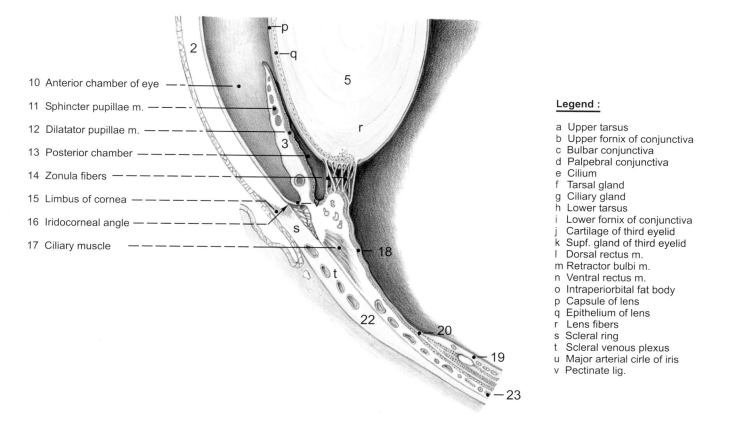

10 Anterior chamber of eye
11 Sphincter pupillae m.
12 Dilatator pupillae m.
13 Posterior chamber
14 Zonula fibers
15 Limbus of cornea
16 Iridocorneal angle
17 Ciliary muscle

Legend :

a Upper tarsus
b Upper fornix of conjunctiva
c Bulbar conjunctiva
d Palpebral conjunctiva
e Cilium
f Tarsal gland
g Ciliary gland
h Lower tarsus
i Lower fornix of conjunctiva
j Cartilage of third eyelid
k Supf. gland of third eyelid
l Dorsal rectus m.
m Retractor bulbi m.
n Ventral rectus m.
o Intraperiorbital fat body
p Capsule of lens
q Epithelium of lens
r Lens fibers
s Scleral ring
t Scleral venous plexus
u Major arterial cirle of iris
v Pectinate lig.

2. THE EAR

The **ear** (Auris) is a double sense-organ, serving as an auditory organ for the perception of sound and as an organ of equilibration for the perception of the position of the body in its environment; that is, the relation of the body to the force of gravity. The ear consists of the external, middle and the internal ear. Whereas the structures serving the function of hearing are found in all parts of the ear, the vestibulocochlear organ is found only in the internal ear.

a) The **EXTERNAL EAR** (see also pp. 102 and 103) serves to receive and conduct sound waves to the tympanic membrane (eardrum). It is composed of the **auricle (1)** and the **external acoustic meatus**. The basis of the auricle is formed by an **elastic auricular cartilage (3)** covered by a thin cutis. Externally, the ear is covered by dense hairs, internally by relatively sparse hairs, and at the beginning of the external acoustic meatus there are coarser, protective hairs. In some breeds in which the ear hangs down (*e.g.*, Basset), the hairs may reach a considerable length. At the caudal border of the auricle, the skin is folded to form a marginal **cutaneous pouch (2)**. The auricular cartilage is curved to form the horn-like concha auriculae, which at its base is continued by the **external acoustic meatus**. The meatus begins as the **cartilaginous external acoustic meatus (4)**, which at first descends and runs perpendicularly (perpendicular part), then turns medially and horizontally (horizontal part, –see p. 103). At the level of the turn, the auricular cartilage is continued by the semi-ringlike **cartilage of the acoustic meatus (5)**, which is followed by the **anular cartilage (6)**. The latter covers the short tubular **osseous external acoustic meatus (7)** of the tympanic part of the temporal bone. The osseous external acoustic meatus ends at the tympanic anulus, which attaches the tympanic anulus.

Auricular muscles (see pp. 93 – 95).

b) The **TYMPANIC MEMBRANE (8)** lies at the boundary between the external acoustic meatus and the middle ear. Its cutaneous external surface is free of hair and glands, and is without pigment; its internal surface is the aglandular mucous membrane of the tympanic cavity. Centrally, between the two layers, is a vascular connective tissue, which is attached by a **ring of fibrocartilage** to the **tympanic anulus**. The tympanic membrane bulges into the tympanic cavity with its *pars tensa* (tense part). A dorsal, flaccid part (*Pars flaccida*) closes the gap in the bracelet-like tympanic anulus.

c) The **MIDDLE EAR** consists of the tympanic cavity, the auditory ossicles which are within the cavity, and the auditory tube. The walls of the tympanic cavity and the surface of the auditory ossicles are covered by a mucous membrane with a monolayered squamous epithelium and, in part, by a ciliated epithelium.

I. Laterally, the tympanic membrane projects into the **tympanic cavity (9)** and, medially, the promontory of the petrous temporal bone. The dorsal part of the cavity with the auditory ossicles and chorda tympani is called the **epitympanicum**; the middle part, the **mesotympanicum**; and the ventral part or floor, which corresponds to the **tympanic bulla (9)**, the **hypotympanicum**. There are two openings in the medial wall. The more dorsal opening is oval and is designated the **vestibular window (13)**; it is closed off from the vestibule of the internal ear by the foot-plate of the stapes, which is attached by ligament to the margin of the window. The more ventral opening is the round **cochlear window (14)**, which is closed off by membrane.

II. The **auditory ossicles** (malleus, incus, and stapes) form a chain reaching from the tympanic membrane laterally to the vestibular window medially. The tympanic membrane and auditory ossicles together represent the sound conducting apparatus.

The **malleus** (hammer, –10) lies farthest laterally and is anchored to the fibrous layer of the tympanic membrane by its handle, the **manubrium (A)**. The **neck of the malleus (B)** is followed by the **head of the malleus (C)**, which articulates by a synovial joint with the **body (D)** of the **incus (11)**. The incus has a **long (E)** and a **short (F)** crus. A small **lenticular bone (E')** fits on the long crus at a right angle and articulates with the **head (G)** of the **stapes (12)**. The **rostral crus (H)** and **caudal crus (I)** of the stapes rest upon the oval **foot-plate (Basis stapedis, –J)** of the stapes, which closes the vestibular window. The auditory ossicles are held in place by ligaments. The intensity of the sound is regulated by two antagonistic muscles that act reflexly. Their function is still not definitively established. In contracting, the **tensor tympani muscle** draws the malleus toward the tympanic cavity, thus tensing the tympanic membrane. It is innervated by the tensor tympani nerve, a branch of the mandibular nerve (V3). The **stapedius muscle** alters the position of the base of the stapes in the vestibular window; it is supplied by the stapedial nerve, a branch of the facial nerve (VII).

III. The **auditory tube (15)** connects the middle ear with the nasal pharynx. It serves to equalize the pressure in the tympanic cavity with the pressure external to the tympanic membrane. It also provides drainage for the secretion of glands that are in the region of the pharyngeal ostium of the tube. The auditory tube consists of an **osseous part** and a **cartilaginous part**. It is trough-like, open ventrally and lined by a tubular mucous membrane bearing a ciliated epithelium. It is compressed from side to side and ends in the nasal pharynx at the pharyngeal ostium of the auditory tube.

d) The **INTERNAL EAR** consists of a closed system of thin-walled membranous vesicles and channels, the **membranous labyrinth**. It is surrounded by a bony capsule, the **osseous labyrinth**, the spaces of which correspond to the different parts of the membranous labyrinth that each contains. The cross-section of the entire internal ear measures about 12 mm in the dog. The bony labyrinth contains a clear fluid **perilymph** (cerebrospinal fluid) that surrounds the membranous labyrinth as a water-cushion. The **perilymphatic spaces (20)** are connected to the subarachnoid space of the cranial cavity by the perilymphatic duct (23). A viscous **endolymph** is within the membranous labyrinth. The **endolymphatic duct (27)** lies within the vestibular aqueduct, a narrow passage that leads from the vestibule of the osseous labyrinth to the interior of the cranial cavity. The endolymphatic duct ends blindly in the endolymphatic sac, which lies between the two layers of the ectomeninx.

The bony labyrinth consists of the vestibule, the osseous semicircular canals and the cochlea.

I. The undivided **vestibule (16)** occupies the center of the osseous labyrinth and contains two membranous sacs, the dorsal **utriculus (25)** and the ventral **sacculus (24)**.

Caudodorsally, the osseous semicircular canals lead from the vestibule; rostroventrally, the bony cochlea. The membranous **semicircular ducts (26)** originate from the utriculus, the membranous **cochlear duct (28)** from the sacculus by way of the ductus reuniens.

II. The **osseous semicircular canals (17)** and the membranous **semicircular ducts (26)** that they contain are oriented to one another roughly at right angles. The anterior canal and duct lie transversely, the posterior ones sagittally, and the lateral ones horizontally. At one end of the attachment of the semicircular duct to the utriculus and the associated communication of the semicircular canal with the vestibule, there is formed an enlargement, the membranous ampulla, and, in the canal, the osseous ampulla. The anterior and posterior osseous semicircular canals unite posteriorly to form a short common canal, and there is a corresponding union of the associated semicircular ducts.

Sacculus, utriculus and the semicircular ducts contain the **vestibular apparatus**, which functions in equilibration (orientation of the head with respect to the force of gravity, linear and angular acceleration of the body). The sensory cells are found on circumscribed areas that, according to their position and shape are called **macula sacculi, macula utriculi** and **ampullary crests**. Afferent sensory nerve fibers lead from synapse with the hair cells to the superior and inferior **vestibular ganglia (d)**, then to the brain by the **vestibular nerve (6)**. The vestibular nerve joins the cochlear nerve (see below) to form the **vestibulocochlear nerve (VIII, –a)**.

III. The **cochlea (18)** winds rostro-ventrolaterally around the **modiolus** and, in the dog, has three coils. From the modiolus, the **osseous spiral lamina** projects into the cochlea and with the cochlear duct divides the cochlear space into an upper spiral chamber, the **scala vestibuli (21)** and a lower spiral chamber, the **scala tympani (22)**. The scala vestibuli begins in the vestibule, and the scala tympani ends at the cochlear window. The scalae communicate at the **helicotrema** of the cochlear cupula. In a cross-section of the cochlea, the scalae are separated centrally by the osseous spiral lamina, peripherally by the triangular **cochlear duct (28)**. The dorsal separation of the cochlear duct from the scala vestibuli is formed by REISSNER'S membrane (**vestibular membrane, –K**); its ventral separation from the scala tympani is formed by the **spiral membrane (L)**. The peripheral wall of the cochlear duct is formed by the vascular, thickened **spiral ligament of the cochlea (M)**, which is fused with the periosteum lining the cochlear wall. The spiral organ (**ORGAN OF CORTI, –N**) lies within the cochlear duct; it consists of sensory hair cells that rest on the basilar (spiral) membrane. Afferent sensory nerve fibers synapse with the hair cells and pass centrally to the **spiral ganglion (O)** at the base of the osseous spiral lamina. Their peripheral axons unite within the central axis of the modiolus to form the **cochlear nerve (c)**. Efferent nerve fibers also pass in the vestibulocochlear nerve and synapse on the sensory hair cells.

Vestibulocochlearorgan [ear]

(Petrosal part of the petrous
temporal bone, rostral view)

External ear

1 Auricle
2 Cutaneous pouch
3 Auricular cartilage and concha
4 Cartilaginous external acoustic meatus
5 Auricular cartilage
6 Anular cartilage
7 Osseous external acoustic meatus

(see p. 103)

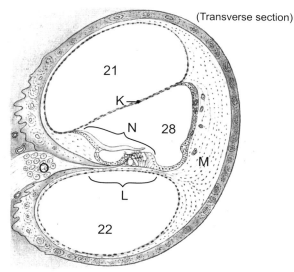

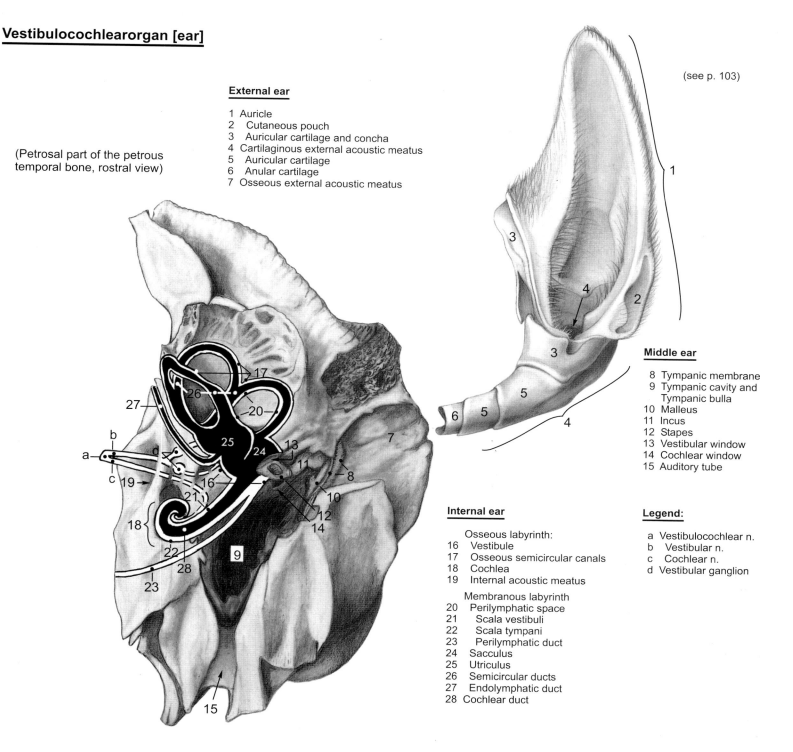

Middle ear

8 Tympanic membrane
9 Tympanic cavity and
   Tympanic bulla
10 Malleus
11 Incus
12 Stapes
13 Vestibular window
14 Cochlear window
15 Auditory tube

Internal ear

Osseous labyrinth:
16 Vestibule
17 Osseous semicircular canals
18 Cochlea
19 Internal acoustic meatus

Membranous labyrinth
20 Perilymphatic space
21 Scala vestibuli
22 Scala tympani
23 Perilymphatic duct
24 Sacculus
25 Utriculus
26 Semicircular ducts
27 Endolymphatic duct
28 Cochlear duct

Legend:

a Vestibulocochlear n.
b Vestibular n.
c Cochlear n.
d Vestibular ganglion

Tympanic membrane and auditory ossicles

(medial view)

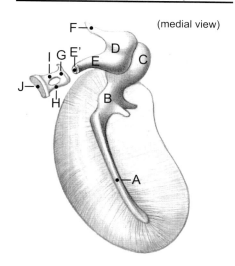

Canalis spiralis cochleae

(Transverse section)

Legend:

Malleus:
A Manubrium
B Neck
C Head

Incus:
D Body
E Long crus
E' Lenticular bone
F Short crus

Stapes:
G Head
H Rostral crus
I Caudal crus
J Basis

K Vestibular membrane
L Spiral membrane
M Spiral ligament of cochlea
N Organ of corti
O Spiral ganglion of cochlea

3. OLFACTORY AND GUSTATORY (CHEMICAL) SENSES; SUPERFICIAL, DEEP, AND VISCERAL SENSIBILITY

a) The **OLFACTORY ORGAN** is especially well developed in the dog and, with the olfactory sense (sense of smell), serves for orientation in the environment.

The nasal fundus is clothed with an **olfactory mucous membrane** and is designated the **olfactory region or olfactory area**. It is lined by an **olfactory epithelium** in which the **olfactory neurosensory epitheliocytes (b)** are flanked by **supporting cells (a)** and **basal cells (c)**. With the olfactory glands, they give the entire olfactory region a yellow-brown tint. The difference in color with respect to the adjacent respiratory mucous membrane does not permit a precise identification of the olfactory area with the naked eye. The olfactory cells live only a short time (about 30 – 60 days in human beings) and are regularly replaced. This is remarkable in that the olfactory cells are nerve cells and their replacement in the adult is a special case. The dog as a macrosmatic animal has an olfactory region of considerable size, fifteen times larger in a medium-sized dog than in human beings. The dog is able to perceive olfactory stimuli in very low concentrations, far beyond the capability of a human being.

b) The **VOMERONASAL ORGAN** is also called JACOBSON'S organ according to its discoverer. The organ lies directly on the cartilaginous nasal septum and extends from the **incisive papilla (1)** to the level of the second premolar tooth. It communicates with the roof of the oral cavity by a **vomeronasal duct (2)** and an **incisive duct (3)**. In the case of the vomeronasal organ, we are dealing with a tube, the vomeronasal duct, a few millimeters thick, that on its inner surface is lined with a modified olfactory epithelium and externally is supported by cartilage (**vomeronasal cartilage, –4**). The **function** of the organ is still not entirely clear. But it is certain that it functions as an accessory olfactory organ. It perceives olfactory stimuli from the food, and pheromones by which an impact on reproduction is recognized. The vomeronasal organ is a receptor for non-volatile substances that do not reach the olfactory region of the nasal fundus. Sensory innervation of the organ is by the **vomeronasal nerve (5)**, which is accounted as one of the *fila olfactoria*. In human beings and many mammals, the organ undergoes involution early in ontogenesis.

c) The **GUSTATORY ORGAN** serves with the **sense of taste (gustatory sense)** for perception of gustatory substances by means of special **gustatory cells (e)**. With **supporting, sustentacular, cells (f)** and **basal cells (g)** the gustatory cells are integrated in a barrel-like **gustatory bud (taste-bud)** that reaches the surface at a **gustatory pore (d)**. The taste-buds are in the surface epithelium of the tongue in association with certain lingual papillae designated **gustatory papillae**. The gustatory papillae are the **foliate (6)**, **vallate (7)** and **fungiform papillae (8, –** see also p. 105). The **gustatory cells** are **secondary sensory cells** from which the stimulus is conducted to the brain by synaptic contact of the receptor cell with a sensory nerve fiber.

d) **SUPERFICIAL, DEEP AND VISCERAL SENSIBILITY** is not bound to specific sense organs as is the case with the visual, vestibulocochlear, gustatory and olfactory sense organs in which there is a great concentration of the receptor cells. The density of receptors and their associated afferent nerves can be relatively high or low; or receptors may be entirely absent. From the peripheral receptors, long dendrites (in some textbooks, these long dendrites may be denominated 'axons') extend centrally to their perikarya, which are located near the central nervous system in the spinal and cranial ganglia. From the perikarya, an axon enters the brain or spinal cord.

I. **Superficial (surface) sensibility** is provided by touch, pressure, pain and temperature receptors in the skin. The receptors are either **free nerve endings** of afferent neurons, which function as pain receptors and, with loss of their myelin sheaths, penetrate the deeper layers of the epidermis, or they are receptor-corpuscles. The latter are club-shaped, lamellar or disc-like and are found predominantly in the dermis or subcutis. **Club-shaped corpuscles** are

probably temperature receptors. **Lamellar corpuscles** attain a remarkable size, up to 3 mm, and consist of flattened cells that form cone-shaped lamellae wrapped around a central afferent nerve-ending. They are sensitive to pressure stimuli. **Disc-shaped nerve-endings (tactile menisci)** act presumably as touch (tactile) receptors (see also p. 5).

Sinus hairs with their associated nerve endings are very sensitive to tactile stimuli (see also p. 5).

II. **Deep sensibility** is mediated by proprioceptors that are sensitive to stretch. They are found in skeletal muscle, tendons, joint capsules and joint ligaments. The term 'proprioceptor' is based on the fact that the exciting stimulus does not have its origin from outside the body but instead from the animal's own 'proper' body. **Joint receptors** are sensitive to the **angulation of the joint** and the **rapidity of movement**. Deep receptors are **neuromuscular spindles**, neurotendinous spindles, and according to many authors lamellar corpuscles. The neuromuscular spindle is a receptor in skeletal muscle. The receptors are located near the transition of the muscle to its tendon. They are up to 3 mm long and up to 0.5 mm thick. Wrapped in a connective tissue capsule, they are composed of modified, especially thin, skeletal muscle fibers, the cell nuclei of which are arranged chain-like one-after-the-other (chain fiber) or in which the cell nuclei are in a central cluster within the muscle fiber (cluster fiber or nuclear bag fiber).

Afferent and efferent nerve fibers pass onto the neuromuscular spindle in different formations. Efferent (gamma) motor neurons end with motor end-plates at both ends of the muscle spindle and regulate the resting tone of these modified spindle fibers. Afferent nerve endings proceed from the central region of the muscle spindle and are stimulated by distension of the modified muscle fibers. The stimulus is conducted to the spinal cord and here there is a direct synapse with the normal (alpha) motor neurons, effecting a monosynaptic reflex. The alpha motor neurons pass peripherally to the hilus of the muscle, ending with motor end-plates on normal skeletal muscle fibers and thus giving rise to contraction of the muscle. In addition to carrying out a monosynaptic reflex, the afferent neuron ascends the spinal cord with synapse on multisynaptic pathways. In examining reflexes, *e.g.*, the patellar reflex, the function of other conducting tracts of certain segments of the spinal cord is also evaluated.

The **neurotendinous spindle** is structured similar to the neuromuscular spindle. But the spindles are thinner and shorter. They are within the tendon where it passes over into the muscle belly. They should be considered as tension-receptors and cooperate in their function with the neuromuscular spindles. In addition, they are present in low numbers in the joint ligaments, *e.g.*, in the cruciate ligaments of the stifle joint. Functionally they regulate the coordination of movements.

Information passes by the afferent limb of a reflex arc to the central nervous system and, from here, following synapse(s), the efferent limb of the arc activates the pertinent muscle groups. When the muscles (or the nervous system) tire, the activity is slowed and may result in instability of movement (*e.g.*, stumbling). Running parallel to the afferent neurons of the deep receptors are pain-conducting nerve fibers that pass to the spinal ganglion and finally to the central nervous system.

III. **Visceral sensibility** having its origin in stimuli resulting from distension of the internal organs gives rise to a deep, dull and imprecisely localized pain. The intramural receptors of the viscera are sensitive to stretch, and to strong contractions and spasms, *e.g.*, in the case of colics. The smooth muscle of the viscera and the striated musculature of the body wall react with a reduced respiratory movements and reflex contraction of the striated muscle of the body wall (the tension of the abdominal muscles is significant for diagnosis). Visceral pain is projected by spinal cord mechanisms onto cutaneous regions (referred pain).

Olfactory and gustatory organs

Vomeronasal organ

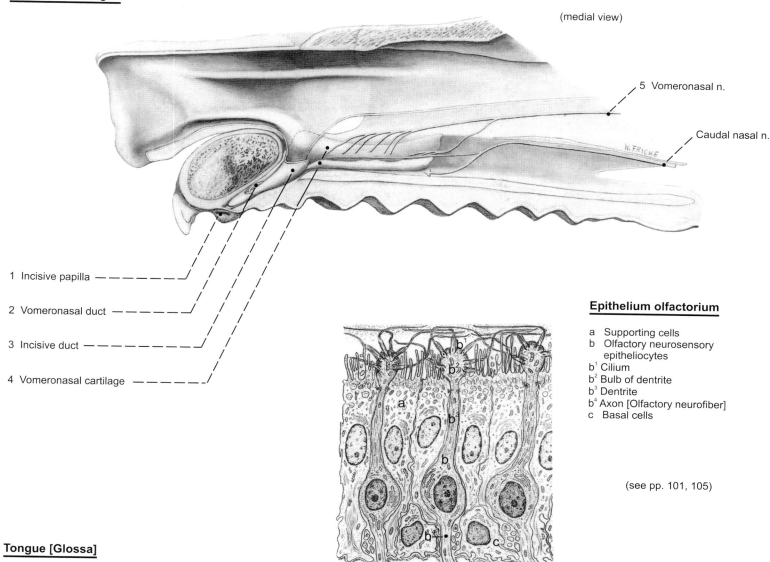

(medial view)

5 Vomeronasal n.

Caudal nasal n.

N. FRICKE

1 Incisive papilla

2 Vomeronasal duct

3 Incisive duct

4 Vomeronasal cartilage

Epithelium olfactorium

a   Supporting cells
b   Olfactory neurosensory
    epitheliocytes
b¹ Cilium
b² Bulb of dentrite
b³ Dentrite
b⁴ Axon [Olfactory neurofiber]
c   Basal cells

(see pp. 101, 105)

Tongue [Glossa]

(dorsal view)

6 Foliate papillae

Conical papillae

7 Vallate papillae

Filiform papillae

8 Fungiform papillae

Caliculus gustatorius [Gemma gustatoria]

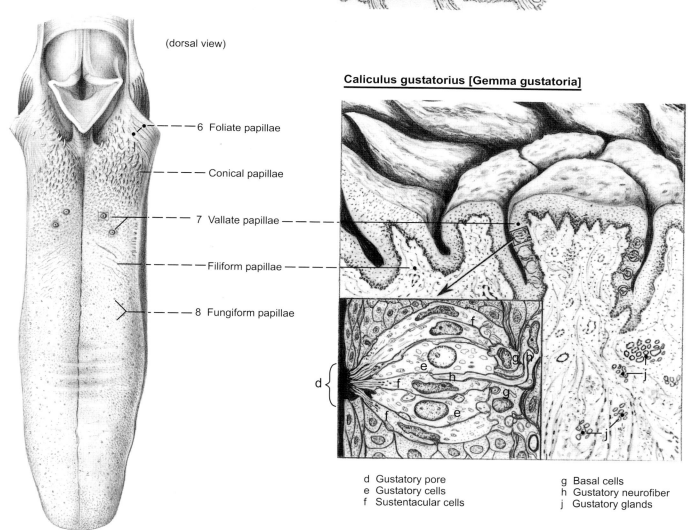

d Gustatory pore
e Gustatory cells
f Sustentacular cells

g Basal cells
h Gustatory neurofiber
j Gustatory glands

123

TABLES

1. MYOLOGY

MUSCLE	ORIGIN	INSERTION	INNERVATION	FUNCTION	COMMENTS
DORSAL MUSCLES CONNECTING THE TRUNK AND THORACIC LIMB – SUSPENSION OF THE TRUNK (turn to p. 12)					
M. trapezius	Dorsal median raphe of the neck from the 3rd cervical vertebra to the spinous processes of thoracic vertebrae 1 – 9	**Cervical part:** Dorsal two-thirds of the scapular spine **Thoracic part:** Dorsal third of the scapular spine	Dorsal branch of accessory n. (XI)	Acting together, draw the scapula dorsally. Cervical part: draws the scapula craniodorsally. Thoracic part: draws the scapula caudodorsally	Together, muscles of right and left sides form a trapezium.
M. cleidocervicalis	Dorsal median raphe of the neck cranial to trapezius	Clavicular intersection	Dorsal branch of accessory n. (XI)	Draws the thoracic limb forward	Homologous to clavicular trapezius of human beings.
M. omotrans-versarius	Acromion of scapula	Wing of atlas	Ventral branch of fourth cervical n.	Draws thoracic limb forward, bends neck to one side	Covers superficial cervical lymph nodes.
M. rhomboideus, —capitis, —cervicis, —thoracis	Nuchal crest (capital part), dorsal median raphe of the neck from second cervical to first thoracic vertebra (cervical part), cranial thoracic spines (thoracic part)	Medial surface of scapular cartilage	Ventral branches of cervical nerves	Fixation of thoracic limb, elevates scapula and draws it forward	Muscles of right and left sides are rhomboid in form in human beings; covered by m. trapezius.
M. latissimus dorsi	Thoracolumbar fascia	Teres major tuberosity with the m. teres major tendon	Thoracodorsal n.	Draws the thoracic limb caudally; flexor of shoulder joint; with limb fixed, draws the trunk forward	
VENTRAL MUSCLES CONNECTING THE TRUNK AND THORACIC LIMB – SUSPENSION OF TRUNK (turn to p. 14)					
Mm. pectorales superficiales: M. pectoralis descendens, M. pectoralis transversus	Manubrium and cranial part of body of the sternum	Crest of the greater tubercle	Cranial pectoral nn.	Trunk-limb attachment; adductor, protractor and retractor of thoracic limb	Forms the lateral pectoral groove with the clavicular part of m. deltoideus (m. cleidobrachialis).
M. pectoralis profundus	Body of the sternum	Greater and lesser tubercles of humerus; brachial fascia	Caudal pectoral nn.	Supports trunk; retractor of thoracic limb; fixes shoulder joint	Divided into a principal and an accessory part.
M. serratus ventralis, —cervicis, —thoracis	Transverse processes of cervical vertebrae 2 – 7 (cervical part), ribs 1 – 7 (10)	Facies serrata of scapula	Ventral branches of cervical nn. (cervical part), long thoracic n. (thoracic part)	Most important muscle supporting trunk; raises neck; when thoracic limb is fixed, an auxiliary inspiratory muscle	A serrated muscle; the dorsal scapular a. courses on the deep face of the muscle, between its two parts.
M. sternocleidomastoideus: M. cleidomastoideus, M. sternomastoideus, M. sterno-occipitalis	Clavicular intersection (m. cleidomastoideus), manubrium of sternum (m. sternomastoideus and m. sterno-occipitalis)	Mastoid process of temporal bone (m. cleidomastoideus, m. sternomastoideus), nuchal crest (m. sterno-occipitalis)	Accessory n. (XI)	Protractor of thoracic limb; draws the head ventrally and to the side of the muscle acting; turns the head and neck to the side of the muscle acting	The external jugular v. crosses the lateral side of the muscle.
M. brachiocephalicus (M. cleidobrachialis, M. cleidocervicalis, and M. cleidomastoideus, —see p. 14)					
M. deltoideus	(see *Lateral Shoulder and Arm Muscles*)				
LONG HYOID MUSCLES (turn to p. 14)					
M. sternohyoideus	Manubrium of sternum and first costal cartilage	Basihyoideum	Ventral branch of first cervical n.	Draws the hyoid apparatus and tongue caudally	Right and left muscles are joined at their medial borders.
M. sternothyroideus	Manubrium of sternum and first costal cartilage	Thyroid cartilage of larynx	Ventral branch of first cervical n.	Synergist of m. sternohyoideus, draws the larynx caudally	At its origin, connected to m. sternohyoideus.

MUSCLE	ORIGIN	INSERTION	INNERVATION	FUNCTION	COMMENTS
MEDIAL SHOULDER AND ARM MUSCLES (turn to p. 18)					
M. teres major	Caudal margin of the scapula	Teres major tuberosity	Axillary n.	Flexor of shoulder joint	
M. subscapularis	Subscapular fossa	Lesser tubercle of the humerus	Subscapular (main part) and axillary nn. (caudal part)	Adductor of the shoulder joint	Serves as a contractile medial collateral 'ligament' of the shoulder joint.
M. coracobrachialis	Coracoid process of the scapula	Caudomedial area of proximal humerus	Musculocutaneous n.	Extensor and adductor of shoulder joint; rotates humerus and distal limb, turning the cranial face of the limb laterally	Its tendon of origin is enveloped by a synovial sheath.
M. biceps brachii	Supraglenoid tubercle of the scapula	Radial tuberosity and proximomedial ulna	Musculocutaneous n.	Flexor of the elbow joint	In human beings, this muscle has two heads of origin.
M. tensor fasciae antebrachii	Caudal margin of the scapula and m. latissimus dorsi	Olecranon and antebrachial fascia	Radial n.	Extension of elbow joint, tensor of forearm fascia	
LATERAL SHOULDER AND ARM MUSCLES (turn to pp. 14 and 20)					
M. deltoideus: P. scapularis, P. acromialis, P. clavicularis (M. cleidobrachialis)	Clavicular intersection (clavicular part), spine of the scapula by aponeurosis (scapular part), acromion (acromial part)	Humeral crest (clavicular part), deltoid tuberosity (scapular and acromial parts)	Axillary n. (scapular and acromial parts), accessory axillary n.* (clavicular part), *This nerve may also be called the n. brachiocephalicus.	Scapular and acromial parts, flexors of the shoulder joint; clavicular part, as part of the brachiocephalicus m., draws the limb forward	A surgical approach to the humeral head is between the acromial part and the supraspinatus m.
M. teres minor	Infraglenoid tubercle and distal infraspinous fossa	Teres minor tuberosity	Axillary n.	Flexor of the shoulder joint	Lies deep to the scapular part of the deltoideus m.
M. supraspinatus	Supraspinous fossa and spine of the scapula	Greater tubercle of the humerus	Suprascapular n.	Extends and 'fixes' the shoulder joint	
M. infraspinatus	Infraspinous fossa and spine of the scapula	Infraspinatus m. surface of the humerus	Suprascapular n.	Flexor and abductor of the shoulder joint	Strong muscle lying deep to the scapular part of the deltoid m.; a bursa underlies its tendon of insertion.
M. triceps brachii: Caput longum, —laterale, —mediale, —accessorium	Caudal margin of the scapula (long head), proximal lateral humerus, (lateral head), medial humerus (medial head), caudal neck of the humerus (accessory head)	Olecranon	Radial n.	Extensor of the elbow joint; the long head also flexes the shoulder joint	Fills the triangle between scapula, humerus and olecranon. Its caudal contour forms the tricipital margin (Margo tricipitalis) from the withers descending to the olecranon; a bursa underlies the common tendon of insertion.
M. anconeus	Margin of the olecranon fossa	Fleshy; laterally with the triceps tendon on the olecranon.	Radial n.	Extensor of the elbow joint	Can be regarded as a fifth head of the triceps brachii m.
CAUDOMEDIAL MUSCLES OF THE FOREARM (most are flexors arising on the medial epicondyle of the humerus; turn to p. 22):					
M. flexor digitalis superficialis	Medial epicondyle of the humerus	Flexor tuberosity of the middle phalanx of digits II – V	Median n.	Flexor of the digital and carpal joints	The superficial flexor tendon is formed in the distal forearm. The manica flexoria of each tendon-branch envelops the corresponding deep flexor tendon.
M. flexor digitalis profundus: Caput humerale, —radiale, —ulnare	Medial epicondyle of the humerus, radius, ulna	Flexor tuberosity of the distal phalanx of digits I – V	Ulnar and median nn. (humeral head), median n. (radial head), ulnar n. (ulnar head)	Flexor of the digital and carpal joints	Tendons of its 3 heads unite in the distal forearm to form the deep flexor tendon, which passes through the manica flexoria of the superficial flexor tendon.
M. flexor carpi ulnaris	Medial epicondyle of the humerus (humeral head), olecranon (ulnar head)	Accessory carpal bone	Ulnar n.	Flexor of the carpal joints	The two heads of the muscle are separated throughout.
M. flexor carpi radialis	Medial epicondyle of the humerus	Mc II and III	Median n.	Flexor of the carpal joints	Its tendon of insertion is divided.
M. pronator teres	Medial epicondyle of the humerus	Proximal craniomedial radius	Median n.	Pronator of the antebrachium and manus (turns the cranial face of the forearm and distal limb medially)	Lies medial at the elbow joint.
M. pronator quadratus	Bridges over the interosseous space between radius and ulna		Median n.	Pronator of the antebrachium and manus (turns the cranial face of the forearm and distal limb medially)	Constant only in the carnivores.

MUSCLE	ORIGIN	INSERTION	INNERVATION	FUNCTION	COMMENTS
CRANIOLATERAL MUSCLES OF THE FOREARM (most are extensors arising on the lateral epicondyle of the humerus; turn to p. 22):					
M. extensor digitalis communis	Lateral epicondyle of the humerus	Distal phalanx of digits II – V	Radial n.	Extensor of the digital and carpal joints	
M. extensor digitalis lateralis	Lateral epicondyle of the humerus	Distal phalanx of digits III – V	Radial n.	Extensor of the digits III – V	
M. abductor pollicis longus	Craniolateral surface of radius and ulna	Proximal extremity of Mc I, superficial part of flexor retinaculum	Radial n.	Extensor and abductor of digit I, extensor of carpus	A sesamoid bone in the tendon as it crosses over the caudomedial aspect of the radial carpal bone.
M. extensor digiti I et II	Middle third of cranial surface of ulna	Distal end of Mc I, joins common digital extensor tendon to digit II	Radial n.	Extensor of digits I and II	Constant only in carnivores.
M. extensor carpi ulnaris (M. ulnaris lateralis)	Lateral epicondyle of humerus	Mc V and accessory carpal bone	Radial n.	Extensor of carpal joints	Due to its attachment to the accessory carpal bone, the muscle can function as a flexor and abductor of the carpal joints.
M. supinator	Lateral collateral ligament of elbow joint	Proximal craniolateral surface of radius	Radial n.	Supinator of antebrachium and manus (turns the cranial face of the forearm and distal limb laterally)	Lies deep to mm. ext. carpi radialis and ext. dig. com.
M. brachioradialis	Lateral supracondylar crest	Distomedial radius	Radial n.	Flexor of the elbow joint and supinator of the antebrachium and manus	Absent in about 50 per cent of cases.

MUSCLES OF THE VERTEBRAL COLUMN
A. DORSAL VERTEBRAL MUSCLES (turn to p. 28)

MUSCLE	ORIGIN	INSERTION	INNERVATION	FUNCTION	COMMENTS
M. splenius	Spinous processes of vT1 – vT3	Nuchal crest	Dorsal branches of cervical and thoracic nn.	Extension and lateral flexion of head and neck	The form of this muscle resembles a spleen or strap.
M. iliocostalis, —lumborum, —thoracis	Ilium (lumbar part); several adjacent ribs beginning several segments caudal to rib of insertion, and transverse process of vC7(6) (thoracic part)	Transverse processes of lumbar vertebrae and caudal ribs (lumbar part); caudal margin of rib several segments cranial to ribs of origin, and transverse process of vC7(6) (thoracic part)		Fixation of lumbar vertebrae and ribs, erection and lateral flexion of vertebral column (lumbar part); draws ribs caudally in expiration, attachments to transverse processes of vC7(6) draw corresponding ribs cranially in inspiration (thoracic part)	M. iliocostalis thoracis and m. iliocostalis lumborum form a continuous muscle.
M. longissimus, —lumborum, —thoracis, —cervicis, —capitis	Spinous processes of sacral, lumbar and thoracic vertebrae; wing of ilium (lumbar and thoracic parts); transverse processes of thoracic vertebrae, articular processes of cervical vertebrae (cervical and capital parts)	Transverse and accessory processes of lumbar and thoracic vertebrae, ribs at the angle (lumbar and thoracic parts); transverse processes of the cervical vertebrae (cervical part), mastoid process of temporal bone (capital part)	Dorsal branches of lumbar, thoracic, and cervical spinal nerves	Fixation and extension of the vertebral column; erection of the upper body; elevation of head and neck; lateral flexion of trunk and neck when only one side is acting	Deep to the thoracolumbar fascia, medial to the adjacent m. iliocostalis; the longest muscle of the vertebral column.
M. spinalis et semispinalis thoracis et cervicis	Lumbar spinous and mamillary processes (thoracic spinalis et semispinalis), cranial thoracic spinous processes (cervical spinalis)	Spinous processes of cranial thoracic vertebrae (thoracic spinalis et semispinalis), spinous processes of cervical vertebrae up to the axis (cervical spinalis)	Dorsal branches of lumbar, thoracic, and cervical spinal nn.	Fixation of dorsum and neck, bends the trunk and neck to the side of the muscle acting	
M. semispinalis capitis, M. biventer cervicis, M. complexus	Transverse processes of cranial thoracic vertebrae, articular processes of cervical vertebrae 3 – 7	Nuchal surface of squamous occipital bone ventral to nuchal crest	Dorsal branches of cranial thoracic and cervical spinal nerves	Elevation and lateral flexion of head and neck	M. biventer is dorsal and has transverse tendinous intersections; m. complexus is ventral.
Mm. multifidi, —multifid. cervicis, —multifid. thoracis, —multifid. lumb.	Mamillary (lumbar and thoracic multifidi) and articular (cervical multifidi) processes from sacrum to the axis	Spinous process of vertebra three segments cranial to vertebra of origin (lumbar and thoracic multifidi); spine of axis (cervical multifidi)	Dorsal branches of segmental spinal nerves	Fixation and rotation of the vertebral column	A series of individual muscles extending from the axis to the sacrum. The lumbar series is particularly strong and lies next to the vertebral spines medial to the m. longissimus and m. sacrocaudalis dorsalis lateralis.
Mm. intertransversarii	Bundles passing between transverse, mamillary, articular and accessory processes of adjacent vertebrae		Dorsal branches of segmental spinal nerves	Fixation of vertebrae, lateral flexion of the vertebral column with unilateral action	In the neck and tail, the muscles are in dorsal and ventral series.
Mm. interspinales	Bundles passing between adjacent spinous processes of lumbar, thoracic and cervical vertebrae		Dorsal branches of segmental spinal nerves	Fixation, dorsal and lateral flexion of vertebral column	
M. sacrocaudalis (-coccygeus) dorsalis medialis	Mamilloarticular processes of more caudally situated vertebrae and, caudally, their small vestigial eminences	Spinous processes of sacral and caudal vertebrae	Dorsal branches of segmental spinal nerves	Elevation and lateral flexion of tail	Caudal continuation of the mm. multifidi.
M. sacrocaudalis (-coccygeus) dorsalis lateralis	Mamillary processes of lumbar, sacral, and the more cranial of the caudal (tail) vertebrae	Mamillary processes of the more caudal of the caudal (tail) vertebrae	Dorsal branches of the segmental spinal nerves	Elevation and lateral flexion of the tail	Caudomedial continuation of the m. longissimus.

MUSCLE	ORIGIN	INSERTION	INNERVATION	FUNCTION	COMMENTS
MUSCLES OF THE VERTEBRAL COLUMN **B. VENTRAL VERTEBRAL MUSCLES** (turn to p. 28)					
Mm. scaleni: M. scalenus dorsalis, —ventralis, —medius,	Transverse processes of the last four cervical vertebrae	Ribs 3 – 9 (scalenus dorsalis), the middle of the cranial margin of rib 1 (scalenus ventralis), the dorsal part of rib 1 (scalenus medius)	Ventral branches of cervical spinal nn.	Draw the ribs cranially in inspiration, ventral flexion of the neck	
M. longus capitis	Transverse processes of cervical vertebrae 2 – 6; the separate bundle arising from the ventral tubercle of the atlas is designated *rectus capitis ventralis*.	Muscular tubercle at the base of the skull	Ventral branches of cervical spinal nn.	Ventral flexion of the head and neck, lateral flexion if only the muscles of one side are acting	
M. longus colli	Transverse processes of cervical vertebrae 2 – 6	Caudal prominence of the ventral median crest of the vertebrae two segments cranially, the most cranial insertion is on the ventral tubercle of the atlas.	Ventral branches of cervical spinal nn.	Ventral flexion of the neck	The muscle is in serial segments in a 'herringbone' pattern on the ventral surface of the neck. Surgical access to the cervical intervertebral disk is between right and left muscle bundles.
MUSCLES OF THE VERTEBRAL COLUMN **C. DORSAL MUSCLES OF THE ATLANTO-OCCIPITAL AND ATLANTO-AXIAL JOINTS** (turn to p. 28)					
M. rectus capitis dorsalis major	Dorsal margin of the spine of the axis	Ventral to the nuchal crest	Dorsal branch of the first cervical n.	Dorsal flexor of the atlanto-occipital joint	A deep part of this muscle can be separated off as a *m. rectus capitis dorsalis intermedius*.
M. rectus capitis dorsalis minor	Dorsal tubercle of the atlas	Nuchal surface of the skull (occipital bone)	Dorsal branch of the first cervical n.	Dorsal flexor of the atlanto-occipital joint	Lies deep to the m. rectus capitis dorsalis major (pars intermedia).
M. obliquus capitis caudalis	Lateral surface of the spine of the axis	Dorsal surface of the wing of the atlas	Dorsal branch of the second cervical n.	Rotates the atlas (and head) around the dens of the axis	
M. obliquus capitis cranialis	Lateral margin of the wing of the atlas	Nuchal surface of the skull (occipital bone)	Dorsal branch of the first cervical n.	Acting together with its fellow, dorsal flexion of the atlanto-occipital joint; acting separately, a lateral flexor of the atlanto-occipital joint	Occupies much of the atlanto-occipital space.
RESPIRATORY MUSCLES (EXPIRATORY MUSCLES) (All of the muscles listed below are expiratory, drawing the ribs caudally and inward, reducing the transverse diameter of the thorax; turn to p. 30.)					
M. serratus dorsalis caudalis	Thoracolumbar fascia	Caudal margin of the last 3 ribs	Intercostal nn.	Expiratory	The costal attachment passes deep to the mm. intercostales externi.
Mm. intercostales interni	Caudal margin of the more cranial rib of an intercostals space	Passes caudodorsally to the cranial margin of the more caudal rib of the space	Intercostal nn.	Expiratory	Lie deep to the mm. intercostales externi.
Mm. subcostales	These muscles are occasional small dorsal slips. They are disposed like the mm. intercostales interni; except that they extend over two or three intercostal spaces.		Intercostal nn.	Expiratory	Lie medial to the mm. intercostales interni.
M. retractor costae	Transverse process of the first three or four lumbar vertebrae	Caudal margin of the last rib	Costoabdominal n.	Expiratory	Lies deep to the m. transversus abdominis.
M. transversus thoracis	Body of the sternum	Medial surface of ribs 2 – 8 at the genu	Intercostal nn.	Expiratory	Cranial continuation of the m. transversus abdominis.
RESPIRATORY MUSCLES (INSPIRATORY MUSCLES) (All of the muscles listed below are inspiratory. Except for the m. rectus thoracis and diaphragm, they draw the ribs cranially and outward, enlarging the transverse diameter of the thorax. The m. rectus thoracis brings the sternum, and sternal ribs, cranially. This lowers the sternum and enlarges the dorsoventral diameter of the thorax. The diaphragm enlarges the craniocaudal dimension of the thoracic cavity.)					
M. serratus dorsalis cranialis	Supraspinous ligament at the level of thoracic vertebrae 1 – 8	Cranial margin of ribs 3 – 10	Intercostal nn.	Inspiratory	Has a broad aponeurosis of origin.
M. rectus thoracis	1st rib	Ventral ends of ribs 2 – 4 and cranial part of body of the sternum.	Intercostal nn.	Inspiratory	Cranial continuation of the m. rectus abdominis.
Mm. intercostales externi	From the caudal margin of the more cranial rib of the intercostal space	Extends caudoventrally to the cranial margin of the more caudal rib of the space	Intercostal nn.	Inspiratory	Fibers of this muscle cross the mm. intercostales interni at a right-angle.
Mm. levatores costarum	Transverse processes of the thoracic vertebrae	Cranial margin of the following rib	Intercostal nn.	Inspiratory	This muscle is the vertebral portion of the mm. intercostales externi.
Diaphragma: Pars sternalis, —costalis, —lumbalis	Sternum (sternal part), ribs 9 – 13 (costal part), cranial lumbar vertebrae (lumbar part)	Tendinous center of the diaphragm	Phrenic n.	Inspiratory	Cranially arched septum between the thoracic and abdominal cavities; with three openings: aortic hiatus, esophageal hiatus, and *foramen venae cavae*.

MUSCLE	ORIGIN	INSERTION	INNERVATION	FUNCTION	COMMENTS
VENTRAL ABDOMINAL MUSCLES: These muscles have a broad origin and wide aponeuroses of insertion (turn to pp. 34 and 36).					
M. obliquus externus abdominis	Ribs 4 – 13 (costal part), thoracolumbar fascia (lumbar part)	Linea alba (abdominal tendon); inguinal ligament, from the tuber coxae to the iliopubic eminence and pecten ossis pubis (pelvic tendon)	Ventral branches of intercostal, costoabdominal, and lumbar nn.	Altogether, the ventral abdominal muscles support the ventral abdominal wall. They function with the diaphragm in reciprocal movements of abdominal respiration: inspiration (diaphragm contracts, ventral abdominal mm. relax) and expiration (ventral abdominal mm. contract, diaphragm relaxes). With closure of the rima glottidis, the muscles contract in the movements of the abdominal press as takes place in urination, defecation, and parturition. The aponeuroses of the ventral abdominal mm. have a zone in which the fibres of their aponeuroses interweave proximal to their insertion at the linea alba.	The abdominal and pelvic tendons form the margins of the superficial external inguinal ring. The external abdominal oblique m. contributes throughout to the external lamina of the rextus sheath.
M. obliquus internus abdominis	Tuber coxae and neighboring part of the inguinal ligament (inguinal part), thoracolumbar fascia (lumbar part)	Linea alba and costal arch.	Ventral branches of intercostal, costo-abdominal, and lumbar nn.		Forms the deep inguinal ring with the inguinal ligament and m. rectus abdominis. The cremaster m. splits off from its caudal border. Cranially, its aponeurosis splits, contributing one layer to the external lamina and one layer to the internal lamina of the rectus sheath; in the umbilical region and caudally, the aponeurosis is undivided and contributes only to the external lamina of the rectus sheath.
M. transversus abdominis	Asternal ribs (costal part), lumbar transverse processes and deep leaf of the thoracolumbar fascia (lumbar part)	Linea alba	Ventral branches of intercostal, costoabdominal, and lumbar nn.		Rarely, splits off a cremaster m. Contributes to the internal lamina of the rectus sheath cranially and in the umbilical region. In the inguinal region, it contributes only to the external lamina of the rectus sheath.
M. rectus abdominis	Sternum and first rib (including its costal cartilage)	Pecten ossis pubis	Ventral branches of intercostal, costoabdominal, and lumbar nn.		Joins the thorax and pelvis ventrally; divided into segments by tendinous intersections.
SUBLUMBAR MUSCLES (turn to page 60)					
M. quadratus lumborum	Last three thoracic vertebrae and lumbar transverse processes	Transverse processes of the cranial lumbar vertebrae, spina alaris of the ilium up to its auricular surface.	Ventral branches of lumbar spinal nerves	Fixation and lateral flexion of the lumbar vertebral column	A strong muscle. It projects cranially and laterally beyond the m. iliopsoas.
M. psoas major	Vertebral ends of ribs 12 and 13, transverse processes of cranial lumbar vertebrae	With the m. iliacus (forming the m. iliopsoas), the trochanter minor	Ventral branches of lumbar spinal nerves	Flexor of the hip joint; with the hind limb extended, it draws the limb forward; supinator of the hip joint; with the limb fixed, stabilizes the vertebral column	Passes to the limb caudal to the inguinal ligament, through the *lacuna musculorum*. With the m. iliacus, forms the m. iliopsoas.
M. iliacus	Sacropelvic surface of the ilium	With the m. psoas major, forms the m. iliopsoas, inserting on the trochanter minor	Ventral branches of lumbar spinal nerves	(see m. psoas major)	(see m. psoas major)
M. psoas minor	Last three thoracic vertebrae and first four lumbar vertebrae, tendons of the m. quadratus lumborum	Psoas minor tubercle of the ilium	Ventral branches of lumbar spinal nerves	Ventral flexion of the lumbar vertebral column (*e.g.*, the posture adopted in defecation)	Its broad tendon of insertion is covered by the iliac fascia.
PELVIC DIAPHRAGM, COCCYGEUS AND LEVATOR ANI MUSCLES (turn to p. 72)					
M. coccygeus	Ischiadic spine	Transverse processes of the first four caudal (coccygeal) vertebrae	Ventral branch of the third sacral spinal n.	Draws the tail to the side of the muscle acting (*e.g.*, 'wagging' the tail); with both muscles contracting, clamps the tail down (ventroflexion)	
M. levator ani	Pelvic surface of pubis and ischium	Hemal processes of caudal vertebrae 4 – 7	Ventral branch of the third sacral spinal n.	With bilateral contraction, draws the tail **ventrally**	Its caudal border is attached by fascia to the external anal sphincter; forms the muscular basis of the pelvic diaphragm.
M. sphincter ani externus	With attachment dorsally to the proximal caudal vertebrae, forms a strong muscular ring surrounding the anal opening		Caudal rectal n. of the pudendal n.	Closes the anal opening	Voluntary muscle. The par-anal sinus lies between the internal and external anal sphincter mm.
M. sphincter ani internus	Strong sphincter m. of the last portion of the rectum		Autonomic nn.	Closes the anal opening	Smooth muscle
M. rectococcygeus	External longitudinal smooth muscle of the rectum	Ventromedian on the first caudal vertebrae	Autonomic nn.	Stabilization of anal canal and rectum	Smooth muscle
Mm. perinei	Join the external anal sphincter to genital mm.		Deep perineal branches of the pudendal n.	Muscular closure between anus and vulva/root of the penis	Anchored in the tendinous center of the perineum.
M. bulbospongiosus (M. constr. vestibuli and M. constr. vulvae of the female)	Transverse fibers crossing the bulb of the penis and attaching on either side to the tunica albuginea of the corpus cavernosum penis (male); transverse fibers covering the vestibular bulb and attaching to the vestibular wall (m. constr. vestibuli, —female), loose fibers dispersed within the labia of the vulva (m. constr. vulvae, —female)		Deep perineal branches of the pudendal n.	Evacuate the urethra (m. bulbospongiosus); compress the vestibular bulb and narrow the lumen of the vestibule, clamping the intromitted penis (m. constr. vestibuli), narrow the vulvar orifice providing apposition of clitoris and penis (m. constr. vulvae)	The muscles of the bitch are chiefly functional in coitus.
M. ischiocavernosus	Ischiadic arch	Crus of the penis (male), crus of the clitoris (female)	Deep perineal branches of the pudendal n.	Compress the root of the penis in erection (male), little apparent function in the female	
M. retractor penis s. clitoridis	Sacrum and first caudal vertebrae	Anus, rectum, tunica albuginea of the corpus cavernosum penis (clitoris)	Autonomic nn.	Retractor of the penis (clitoris)	Smooth muscle with pars rectalis, —analis, —penina or —clitoridis.

MUSCLE	ORIGIN	INSERTION	INNERVATION	FUNCTION	COMMENTS
MUSCLES OF THE HIP JOINT (turn to p. 78)					
M. tensor fasciae latae	Tuber coxae	Patella and tibial tuberosity by way of the fascia lata and patellar ligament (cranial, chief, part); lateral lip of the *facies aspera* of the femur (caudal, accessory, part)	Cranial gluteal n.	Flexor of the hip joint, extensor of the stifle joint, tensor of the fascia lata, draws the limb forward in the cranial movement of the stride	
CROUP MUSCLES					
M. gluteus superficialis	Gluteal fascia, lateral part of the sacrum, first caudal vertebra and the sacrotuberous ligament	Gluteal tuberosity	Caudal gluteal n.	Extensor of the hip joint, draws the limb caudally	An independent muscle only in the carnivores; in other species, fused with the biceps (m. gluteobiceps, — ruminants, swine) or united with a portion of the m. tensor fasciae latae (*Equidae*).
M. gluteus medius	Gluteal fascia and wing of the ilium	Trochanter major	Cranial gluteal n.	Extensor of the hip joint, draws the limb caudally and outward	Largest of the gluteal muscles of the dog.
M. piriformis	Ventral surface of the sacrum, sacrotuberous ligament	Trochanter major	Cranial gluteal n. or caudal gluteal n.	Extensor of the hip joint, draws the limb caudally and outward	'Pear-shaped' muscle between the m. gluteus medius and m. gluteus profundus.
M. gluteus profundus	Gluteal surface of the ilium	Cranial part of the trochanter major	Cranial gluteal n.	Supports the abducting action of m. gluteus medius, rotates the femur, turning the cranial face of the limb medially	Lies directly upon the hip joint, covered by m. gluteus medius.
CAUDAL THIGH 'HAMSTRING' MUSCLES, M. abductor cruris caudalis					
M. biceps femoris	Tuber ischiadicum, sacrotuberous ligament	Patellar ligament and tibial tuberosity, cranial margin of the tibia, crural fascia, tuber calcanei as the lateral calcanean tract	Muscular branch of the ischiadic n. (middle and caudal parts), caudal gluteal n. (cranial part)	Extensor of the hip, stifle, and tarsal joints in the weight-bearing limb; its attachment to the cranial margin of the tibia flexes the stifle joint in the non-weight bearing limb, abductor of the limb.	Homologous to the long head of the *m. biceps femoris hominis*.
M. abductor cruris caudalis	Sacrotuberous ligament	Crural fascia distal to the biceps femoris	Common peroneal (fibular) n.	Abductor of the limb, giving insignificant support to the m. biceps femoris	Homologous to the *caput breve m. biceps femoris hominis*.
M. semitendinosus	Tuber ischiadicum	Medial surface of the tibia; tuber calcanei with the tarsal tendon of the m. gracilis (medial calcanean tract)	Muscular branch of the ischiadic n.	Extensor of the hip, stifle, and tarsal joints in the weight-bearing limb; its attachment to the medial surface of the tibia flexes the stifle joint in the non-weight bearing limb; in the non-weight bearing limb, draws the limb medially and caudally and tends to rotate the crus, turning its cranial face medially	In human beings, the muscle is semitendinous; proximally there is an oblique tendinous intersection.
M. semimembranosus	Tuber ischiadicum	Medial condyle of the femur (cranial belly), medial condyle of the tibia (caudal belly)	Muscular branch of the ischiadic n.	Extensor of the hip, stifle, and tarsal joints in the weight bearing limb; its attachment to the medial surface of the tibia flexes the stifle joint in the non-weight bearing limb; in the non-weight bearing limb, draws the limb medially and caudally and tends to rotate the crus, turning its cranial face medially	In human beings, the muscle is semimembranous.
DEEP MUSCLES OF THE HIP JOINT (the 'Small Pelvic Association') These muscles chiefly serve to rotate the limb, turning its cranial face laterally. They thus act as antagonists to the m. gluteus profundus.					
M. obturator internus	Dorsal (internal) surface of the obturator membrane and the neighboring margin of the obturator foramen	Trochanteric fossa	Ischiadic n. (rotator n.)	Rotates the limb, turning its cranial face laterally ('outward' rotator), assist in extending the hip joint	Covers the obturator foramen on the floor of the pelvis.
Mm. gemelli	Lateral surface of the ischium at the lesser ischiadic notch	Trochanteric fossa, their tendons joining the internal obturator tendon	Ischiadic n. (rotator n.)	Rotate the limb, turning its cranial face laterally ('outward' rotator), assist in extending the hip joint	In human beings, divided forming 'twin' muscles; in the dog, the two bellies are incompletely separated by the obturator internus tendon.
M. quadratus femoris	Ventromedial surface of the ischium near the tuber	Caudal surface of the femur distal to the trochanteric fossa	Ischiadic n. (rotator n.)	Rotates the limb, turning its cranial face laterally ('outward' rotator), assist in extending the hip joint	Lies caudoventral to the caudal part of the mm. gemelli.
M. obturator externus	Ventral (external) surface of the obturator membrane and the neighboring margin of the obturator foramen	Trochanteric fossa ventral to the obturator internus and gemelli tendons	Obturator n.	Rotates the limb, turning its cranial face laterally ('outward' rotator), adducts the limb	Lies between the m. adductor and the ventral surface of the ischium.

MUSCLE	ORIGIN	INSERTION	INNERVATION	FUNCTION	COMMENTS
MEDIAL THIGH MUSCLES: Adductor Muscles. All are innervated by the obturator nerve. (turn to p. 80)					
M. gracilis	By aponeurosis with the symphysial tendon to the pelvic symphysis	Medial crural fascia, tuber calcanei by the medial calcanean tract	Obturator n.	Adductor; extensor of the tarsal joint (possibly and extensor of the stifle joint in the weight bearing limb by means of the fascia cruris)	A thin muscle. In the racing greyhound, subject to muscle rupture after a period of inactivity.
M. adductor magnus	Fleshy attachment to the lateral surface of the symphysial tendon and thus to the pelvic symphysis, neighboring pubic and ischiadic bones	Facies aspera of femur	Obturator n.	Adductor, tends to draw the limb caudally	
M. adductor brevis	Ventral pubic tubercle	Proximally on the facies aspera	Obturator n.	Adductor	Situated at the bifurcation of the obturator n.
M. pectineus	Iliopubic eminence	Medial lip of the facies aspera	Obturator n.	Adductor of the limb, flexor of the hip joint	Formed by the fusion of two muscles.
FEMORAL MUSCLES: Extensors of the stifle joint (turn to page 80)					
M. sartorius: Pars cranialis, Pars caudalis	Tuber coxae, iliac crest	Crural fascia, cranial margin of tibia	Femoral n.	Flexor of the hip joint, extensor of the stifle joint (cranial part), flexor of the stifle joint (caudal part); acting together, the two parts of the muscle draw the limb forward and adduct the limb	In the dog, this 'tailor's muscle' forms the cranial contour of the thigh.
M. quadriceps femoris: M. vastus lateralis, —medialis, —intermedius, M. rectus femoris	Craniolateral at the femur (m. vastus lateralis), craniomedial femur (m. vastus intermedius, m. vastus medialis), caudal ventral iliac spine (m. rectus femoris)	Tibial tuberosity by means of the patellar ligament (*Tendo m. quadricipitis*); the patella is a sesamoid bone in the tendon of the quadriceps; at its insertion, the tendon is underlain by the *distal infrapatellar bursa*	Femoral n.	Main extensor of the stifle joint; fixation of the limb, flexor of the hip joint (m. rectus femoris)	Lies as the large muscle mass of the cranial thigh, covered laterally by the m. tensor fasciae latae and the fascia lata; medially, by the m. sartorius.
SPECIAL FLEXOR AND ROTATOR OF THE STIFLE JOINT (see p. 82)					
M. popliteus	Lateral condyle of the femur	Proximal caudal surface of the tibia	Tibial n.	Flexor of the stifle joint; rotates the tibia on its long axis, turning the cranial face of the limb medially (pronation)	A sesamoid bone is within its tendon of origin at its junction with belly of the muscle. The tendon of origin passes between the lateral meniscus and the lateral collateral ligament.
CRANIOLATERAL LEG (CRURAL) MUSCLES: All are innervated by the common peroneal (fibular) n. (turn to p. 82).					
M. tibialis cranialis	Proximal cranial surface of the tibia lateral to its tuberosity and cranial margin	Proximally on Mt I	Common peroneal (fibular) n.	Flexor of the tarsal joint, supinator (tends to turn the cranial face of the pes laterally)	Passes beneath the crural extensor retinaculum.
M. extensor digitalis brevis	Dorsal surface distally on the calcaneus	With the m. extens. digit. longus on digits II – IV	Common peroneal (fibular) n.	Extensor of the digits	
M. extensor digit. longus	Extensor fossa of the femur	Dorsal aspect of distal phalanx of digits II – V	Common peroneal (fibular) n.	Extensor of the digits	Its belly is largely covered cranially by the m. tibialis cranialis; its tendon is held down by the crural and tarsal extensor retinacula.
M. extensor digiti I	Cranial surface of the fibula	Dorsal fascia of digits I and II	Common peroneal (fibular) n.	Extensor of digits I and II	The cranial tibial vessels pass alongside this muscle, deep to the m. tibialis cranialis.
M. peroneus (fibularis) longus	Lateral condyle of the tibia, head of the fibula	Plantar tubercles at proximal ends of Mt II – V	Common peroneal (fibular) n.	Turns the plantar surface of the pes laterally (pronation)	Its insertion tendon passes in a distinct sulcus on the lateroplantar side of the fourth tarsal bone and branches on the plantar pes.
M. extensor digitalis lateralis	Proximal cranial surface of fibula, lateral collateral ligament of the femorotibial joint	Dorsal surface of distal phalanx of digit V	Common peroneal (fibular) n.	Extensor of digit V	Passes in a caudal sulcus of the lateral malleolus, crossing under the tendon of the m. peroneus longus.
M. peroneus (fibularis) brevis	Distal two-thirds of the lateral surface of the fibula	Lateral prominence at the proximal end of Mt V	Common peroneal (fibular) n.	Flexor of the tarsal joint	Well-developed only in carnivores and human beings.
CAUDAL LEG (CRURAL) MUSCLES: All are innervated by the tibial n. (turn to p. 82).					
M. gastrocnemius	Distal femur, medial and lateral supracondylar tuberosities	Tuber calcanei	Tibial n.	Extensor of the tarsal joint, flexor of the stifle joint	A sesamoid bone is in the tendon of origin of each head.
M. flexor digitalis superficialis	Lateral supracondylar tuberosity, deep to the lateral head of the gastrocnemius	Sides of the tuber calcanei, proximal plantar aspect of the middle phalanx of digits II – V	Tibial n.	Flexor of digits II – V, extensor of the tarsal joint, assists in flexion of the stifle joint	The tendon caps over the tuber calcanei, attaching to either side. At metatarsophalangeal joint level, it forms the manica flexoria.
M. flexor digitalis profundus: M. flexor digitalis lateralis, —medialis	Caudal surface of the tibia, fibula, and the interosseous ligament between them	Plantar surface of distal phalanx of digits II – V	Tibial n.	Flexor of digits II – V, extensor of the tarsal joint	The tendons of the lateral and medial digital flexor muscles join in the proximal metatarsus to form the deep digital flexor tendon.
M. tibialis caudalis	Proximal fibula	Medial tarsal fascia	Tibial n.	No apparent function	In ungulates, the tendon joins the lateral digital flexor tendon at the tarsus.

130

MUSCLE	ORIGIN	INSERTION	INNERVATION	FUNCTION	COMMENTS
MUSCLES OF FACIAL EXPRESSION: All are innervated by the facial n. (turn to p. 94).					
M. sphincter colli superficialis	Transverse fibers in the superficial fascia of the ventral neck		Cervical branch (*R. colli*) of the facial n.	Tenses and moves the ventral and lateral skin	Sparse muscle fibers
Platysma	Arises from the dorsal median raphe of the neck, passing rostroventrally onto the face where, as the m. cutaneus faciei, it radiates into the m. orbicularis oris of the upper and lower lips.		R. platysmatis of the caudal auricular n., cervical branch (*R. colli*) of the facial n.	Tenses and moves the skin in the nuchal and masseteric regions, retracts the angle of the mouth, tenses the skin in the labial region	Two muscle layers in the cervical region
M. sphincter colli profundus					
AURICULAR MUSCLES					
M. cervicoauricularis superficialis	Dorsal median raphe of the neck	Dorsal (convex) surface of the auricular cartilage	Caudal auricular n., branch of the facial n.	Long elevator muscle of the ear	At their origin, the cervico-auricularis supf. and cervico-scutularis are fused
M. cervicoscutularis	Dorsal median raphe of the neck	Caudomedial part of scuti-form cartilage	Caudal auricular n., branch of the facial n.	Elevates the ear and tenses the scutiform cartilage	See *m. cervicoauricularis supf.*
Mm. cervicoauricularis profundus and –medius	External sagittal crest	Lateral border of the auri-cular cartilage	Caudal auricular n., branch of the facial n.	Turns the opening (conchal fissure) of the auricular cartilage caudolaterally	Covered by the m. cervico-auricularis superficialis
M. occipitalis	External sagittal crest	Superficial fascia of the head	Rostral auricular branches of the auriculopalpebral n.	Draws the scutiform cartilage caudomedially	Curved, very delicate muscle fibers
M. interscutularis	Transverse fibers passing between the two scutiform cartilages		Rostral auricular branches of the auriculopalpebral n.	Draws the scutiform cartilages medially	
M. frontoscutularis	Rostral continuation of the m. interscutularis		Rostral auricular branches of the auriculopalpebral n.	Draws the scutiform cartilages rostromedially	
M. scutuloauricularis superficialis	Scutiform cartilage	Rostral border of the auricular cartilage	Rostral auricular branches of the auriculopalpebral n.	Turns the auricular cartilage so that its opening (conchal fissure) faces rostromedially, erects the ear	
M. parotidoauricularis	Parotid fascia and superficial fascia of the cranial neck	Ventrolateral at the base of the auricular cartilage	Cervical branch (*R. colli*) of the facial n.	Draws the ear down, lays the ear 'back'	
M. mandibulo-auricularis	Caudal margin of the ramus of the mandible ventral to the condyle	Ventral at the base of the auricular cartilage	Caudal auricular n., branch of the facial n.		Sometimes absent
MUSCLES OF THE LIPS AND CHEEKS					
M. orbicularis oris	Closed, sphincter-like muscle at the border of the rima oris; there is no skeletal attachment		Dorsal and ventral buccal branches of the facial n.	Closes the rima oris (opening of the mouth)	
M. buccinator	Crossing fibers that pass in the cheek region bet-ween the maxilla and the body of the mandible; extends from the angle of the mouth to the level of the rostral border of the masseter m.; interwoven rostrally with orbicularis oris fibers.		Dorsal and ventral buccal branches of the facial n.	Forms the lateral boundary of the oral cavity; compresses the vestibule of the oral cavity, pressing the food into the oral cavity proper; compresses the buccal glands	
M. zygomaticus	Scutiform cartilage	Radiates into the orbicula-ris oris at the angle of the mouth	Dorsal and ventral buccal branches of the facial n.	Draws the angle of the mouth caudally; draws the scutiform cartilage rostroventrally.	
M. caninus	Maxilla, ventral to the infraorbital foramen	Upper lip	Dorsal and ventral buccal branches of the facial n.	Draws the upper lip caudo-dorsally	
M. levator labii superio-ris	Maxilla, rostral to the infraorbital foramen	Wing of the nostril; upper lip	Dorsal and ventral buccal branches of the facial n.	Elevates the upper lip and the nasal plane and draws them caudally, widens the opening of the nostril	
MUSCLES OF THE EYELIDS AND NOSE					
M. orbicularis oculi	A muscular ring passing within the eyelids. It arises dorsally and ventrally from the medial palpebral ligament and encircles the palpebral fissure		Auriculopalpebral n., branch of the facial n.	Narrowing and closure of the palpebral fissure (the opening between the eyelids	
M. retractor anguli oculi lateralis	Deep temporal fascia	Lateral angle of the eye	Auriculopalpebral n., branch of the facial n.	Draws the lateral angle of the eye caudally	
M. levator anguli oculi medialis	Fascia upon the frontal bone (frontal fascia)	Medially into the upper eyelid	Auriculopalpebral n., branch of the facial n.	Elevates the medial part of the upper eyelid; erects the tactile hairs	
M. levator nasolabialis	Maxilla in the region of the medial angle of the eye; frontal fascia	Lateral nostril and upper lip	Auriculopalpebral n., branch of the facial n.	Widens the opening of the nostril and raises the upper lip	
M. malaris	Deep fascia of the face	Lower eyelid	Auriculopalpebral n., branch of the facial n.	Draws the lower eyelid ventrally	

MUSCLE	ORIGIN	INSERTION	INNERVATION	FUNCTION	COMMENTS
MANDIBULAR MUSCLES (turn to pp. 94 and 96)					
SUPERFICIAL MUSCLES OF THE THROAT					
M. digastricus	Paracondylar process (the jugular process forms its base)	Ventral margin of the mandible	Ramus digastricus, branch of the facial n. (caudal belly); mylohyoid n., branch of the mandibular n. (rostral belly)	Lowers the mandible, opening the mouth	Intermediate tendon between the two bellies.
M. mylohyoideus	Mylohyoid line on the medial surface of the body of the mandible	Median raphe joining the muscles of the two sides ventral to the geniohyoideus m.	N. mylohyoideus, branch of the mandibular n.	Elevates the tongue, presses it against the palate	Like a hammock, supports the floor of the oral cavity.
EXTERNAL MUSCLES OF MASTICATION					
M. temporalis	Temporal fossa	Coronoid process of the mandible	Masticatory n., branch of the mandibular n.	Raises the mandible	Its accessory part extends dorsoparallel to the zygomatic arch.
M. masseter	Zygomatic arch	Masseteric fossa of the mandible	Masticatory n., branch of the mandibular n.	Raises the mandible	Divided into superficial and deep parts.
INTERNAL MUSCLES OF MASTICATION					
M. pterygoideus: M. pterygoideus medialis, M. pterygoideus lateralis	Pterygopalatine fossa (medial pterygoid); wing of the basisphenoid (lateral pterygoid)	Pterygoid fossa of the mandible (medial pterygoid), pterygoid fovea of the mandible (lateral pterygoid)	Pterygoid nn., branches of the mandibular n.	Synergist of the masseter m., raising the mandible; with unilateral contraction, draws the mandible toward the side of the muscle acting	The mandibular n. passes between the two muscles.
MUSCLES OF THE EYE (turn to p. 98)					
M. obliquus dorsalis	Medial margin of the optic canal	Dorsally on the eyeball, its tendon passing ventral to the tendon of the m. rectus dorsalis	Trochlear n. (IV)	Rotates the dorsal surface of the eyeball, turning it rostromedially	Hook-shaped course around the trochlea.
M. obliquus ventralis	Ventral to the lacrimal fossa	Laterally on the eyeball at the level of insertion of the m. rectus lateralis	Oculomotor n. (III)	Rotates the lateral surface of the eyeball, turning it ventrorostrally	
M. rectus dorsalis	Common tendinous ring on the pterygoid crest and around the optic canal	Rostrodorsal on the eyeball	Oculomotor n. (III)	Turns the eyeball dorsally on its horizontal axis	
M. rectus medialis	Common tendinous ring on the pterygoid crest and around the optic canal	Rostromedial on the eyeball	Oculomotor n. (III)	Turns the eyeball medially on its perpendicular axis	
M. rectus ventralis	Common tendinous ring on the pterygoid crest and around the optic canal	Rostroventral on the eyeball	Oculomotor n. (III)	Turns the eyeball ventrally on its horizontal axis	
M. rectus lateralis	Common tendinous ring on the pterygoid crest and around the optic canal	Rostrolateral on the eyeball	Abducent n. (VI)	Turns the eyeball laterally on its perpendicular axis	
M. retractor bulbi	Between the optic canal and orbital fissure	Surface of the eyeball, posterior to the equator	Oculomotor n. (III); lateral part by the abducent n. (VI)	Retracts the eyeball	Surrounds the optic n. (II) like a sleeve.
M. levator palpebrae superioris	Dorsal margin of the optic canal	By a wide tendon into the upper eyelid	Oculomotor n. (III)	Elevates the upper eyelid	Passes dorsal to the m. rectus dorsalis.
INTERNAL SMOOTH MUSCLE OF THE EYEBALL (turn to p. 118)					
M. ciliaris	Scleral ring (*Anulus sclerae*)	Lens capsule by its zonular fibers	Parasympathetic fibers in the short ciliary nn. (from the oculomotor n., III)	Accomodation, by bringing the ciliary body nearer to the lens	Composed of circular and meridional fibers.
M. sphincter pupillae	Circular fibers encircling the free border of the pupil		Parasympathetic fibers passing in the oculomotor n. (III)	Constricts the pupil	Smooth muscle of ectodermal origin.
M. dilatator pupillae	Radially outward from the free border of the pupil		Sympathetic fibers	Dilates the pupil	Smooth muscle of ectodermal origin.
PHARYNGEAL MUSCLES: Attached by the dorsal median pharyngeal raphe to the pharyngeal tubercle of the occipital bone (turn to p. 102)					
M. stylopharyngeus caudalis	Caudal contour of the stylohyoid element (stylohyoid bone) of the hyoid apparatus	Dorsolateral pharyngeal wall	Glossopharyngeal n. (IX)	Dilates the pharynx	It is the only dilator of the pharynx.

MUSCLE	ORIGIN	INSERTION	INNERVATION	FUNCTION	COMMENTS
MUSCLES OF THE SOFT PALATE					
M. tensor veli palatini	Muscular process of the tympanic part of the temporal bone	Palatine aponeurosis (aponeurosis of the soft palate)	Mandibular n. (V3)	Tenses the palatine aponeurosis	Belly of the muscle is joined by connective tissue to the medial wall of the auditory tube. As it contracts in the first stages of swallowing, it dilates the lumen of the auditory tube, assisting in the equalization of air pressure within the tympanic cavity.
M. levator veli palatini	Muscular process of the tympanic part of the temporal bone	Soft palate (palatine raphe)	Pharyngeal plexus (IX and X)	Elevates the soft palate	
ROSTRAL PHARYNGEAL CONSTRICTORS					
M. pterygopharyngeus	Hamulus of the pterygoid bone	Pharyngeal raphe	Pharyngeal plexus (IX and X)	Constricts the pharynx, drawing the roof of the pharynx rostrally	Passes lateral to the m. levator veli palatini.
M. palatopharyngeus	Palatine raphe, palatine aponeurosis	Pharyngeal raphe and dorsolateral pharyngeal wall	Pharyngeal plexus (IX and X)	Constricts the pharynx, drawing the roof of the pharynx rostrally; draws the soft palate caudally	Most of the muscle fibers pass medial to the m. levator veli palatini.
MIDDLE PHARYNGEAL CONSTRICTOR					
M. hyopharyngeus	Thyrohyoid element (thyrohyoid bone)	Pharyngeal raphe	Pharyngeal plexus (IX and X)	Constricts the pharynx	Frequently in two parts.
CAUDAL PHARYNGEAL CONSTRICTORS					
M. thyropharyngeus	Thyroid cartilage	Pharyngeal raphe	Pharyngeal plexus (IX and X)	Constricts the pharynx	Continuous rostrally with the hyopharyngeus, caudally with the cricopharyngeus.
M. cricopharyngeus	Cricoid cartilage	Pharyngeal raphe	Pharyngeal plexus (IX and X)	Constricts the pharynx	Continuous rostrally with the thyropharyngeus.
MUSCLES OF THE TONGUE AND HYOID APPARATUS (turn to p. 104)					
M. lingualis proprius	Intrinsic muscle of the tongue, having origin and insertion within the tongue		Hypoglossal n. (XII)	Intrinsic movement of the tongue	Longitudinal, transverse, and perpendicular fiber bundles.
EXTRINSIC MUSCLES OF THE TONGUE					
M. styloglossus	Stylohyoid element (stylohyoid bone)	Tongue; its fibers are lateral and extend toward the apex	Hypoglossal n. (XII)	Arches the base of the tongue caudodorsally in swallowing; unilaterally, draws the tongue toward the side of the muscle acting	Covers the lateral aspect of the stylohyoid and epihyoid elements.
M. hyoglossus	Basihyoid and thyrohyoid elements (basihyoid and thyrohyoid bones)	Tongue; its fibers pass between the styloglossus and genioglossus mm. rostrodorsally toward the apex.	Hypoglossal n. (XII)	With the styloglossus, arches the base of the tongue caudodorsally in swallowing; unilaterally, draws the tongue caudoventrally toward the side of the muscle acting	The largest part of the muscle is at the root of the tongue.
M. genioglossus	Medial aspect of the body of the mandible near the intermandibular joint	Tongue; its fibers radiate fanlike in a paramedian line to the dorsum of the tongue.	Hypoglossal n. (XII)	Depresses the central part of the tongue	
HYOID MUSCLES					
M. geniohyoideus	Medial surface of the body of the mandible near the intermandibular joint, ventral to the m. genioglossus	Basihyoid element (basihyoid bone)	Hypoglossal n. (XII)	Draws the tongue and hyoid bone rostrally	Muscular basis of the floor of the oral cavity.
M. thyrohyoideus	Thyroid cartilage	Thyrohyoid element (thyrohyoid bone)	Branch from *ansa cervicalis* (XII and C1)	Draws the larynx rostrally to the base of the tongue, draws the hyoid apparatus caudally toward the larynx	Continues cranially from the attachment of the sternothyroideus.
LARYNGEAL MUSCLES (INTRINSIC MUSCLES OF THE LARYNX)					
M. cricothyroideus	Ventrolateral arch of the cricoid	Caudal part of thyroid lamina	Cranial laryngeal n., branch of the vagus n.	Tenses the vocal ligaments, narrows the *rima glottidis*	
M. cricoarytenoideus dorsalis	Dorsal surface of the lamina of the cricoid cartilage	Muscular process of the arytenoid cartilage	Caudal laryngeal n., branch of the vagus n.	Enlarges the *rima glottidis*	
M. cricoarytenoideus lateralis	Rostral border of the cricoid arch dorsally	Muscular process of the arytenoid cartilage	Caudal laryngeal n., branch of the vagus n.	Narrows the *rima glottidis*	
M. arytenoideus transversus	Arcuate crest of the arytenoid cartilage	Median tendon joining it to the muscle of the opposite side	Caudal laryngeal n., branch of the vagus n.	Narrows the *rima glottidis*	
M. thyroarytenoideus: M. ventricularis, M. vocalis	Cuneiform process of the arytenoid cartilage (m. ventricularis), ventromedial internal aspect of the thyroid cartilage (m. vocalis)	Arytenoid cartilage rostral to the arytenoideus transversus (m. ventricularis), vocal process (m. vocalis)	Caudal laryngeal n., branch of the vagus n.	Enlarges the *rima vestibuli* (m. ventricularis); narrows the *rima glottidis*, tenses the vocal fold (m. vocalis)	

2. LYMPHOLOGY

LYMPHOCENTER (lc.) OR LYMPH NODE (ln.)	LOCATION	AREA/ORGANS DRAINED BY AFF. LYMPHATICS	EFFERENT LYMPHATICS	COMMENTS	PAGE
1) **Parotid ln.**	Beneath the rostral border of the parotid gland, ventral to the temporomandibular joint.	Chiefly the superficial head region dorsal to a line connecting the eye and ear.	To medial retropharyngeal ln.	Palpable, especially when enlarged; deep nodes, when present, lie in the parotid gland.	92
2) **Mandibular lnn.**	Rostroventral to the mandibular gl., dorsal and ventral to the facial v.	Superficial and deep parts of the face, muscles and glands ventral to the eye – ear line	To medial retropharyngeal ln.	Readily palpable	92
Retropharyngeal lymphocenter					
3) Lateral retropharyngeal ln.	Caudal to the parotid gland at the level of the wing of the atlas	Superficial and deep areas of the head, lymphatic pharyngeal ring, cranial cervical muscles	To medial retropharyngeal ln.	Inconstant	92
4) Medial retropharyngeal ln.	Deep to the sternocephalicus m., dorsolateral to the pharynx	Afferent lymphatics from the parotid and mandibular lnn.	To tracheal (jugular) lymphatic trunk		92
Superficial cervical lymphocenter					
5) Superficial cervical lnn.	Cranial to the shoulder, deep to the omotransversarius m.	Superficial parts of the head, of the neck, of the abdominal wall, and of the proximal (shoulder) extremity of the thoracic limb	To the venous angle (junction of internal and external jugular vv.) or to the large lymphatic trunks at the angle	Readily palpable	14
Deep cervical lymphocenter					
6) Cranial deep cervical ln.	Craniodorsal to the thyroid gland	Deep parts of the neck, larynx, thyroid gl., trachea, esophagus	To the next following deep cervical ln. or to the mediastinal lc.	Inconstant; danger of confusion with the parathyroid gl.	14
7) Middle deep cervical ln.	In the middle third of the neck	Visceral structures of the neck	To the next following deep cervical ln. or to the mediastinal lc.	Inconstant	14
8) Caudal deep cervical ln.	On the trachea cranial to the first rib	Shoulder and arm (brachial) region	To the thoracic duct, right lymphatic duct, tracheal lymphatic trunk, or to the mediastinal lc.	Inconstant	14
Mediastinal lymphocenter					
9) Cranial mediastinal lnn.	Precardial mediastinum	Deep structures of the thorax; in part, also neck, shoulder, pleura, thoracic viscera, afferents from 7), 8), 10), 12) – 14)	To terminal part of tracheal (jugular) lymphatic trunk or thoracic duct	Middle and caudal mediastinal lymph nodes are lacking.	40
Ventral thoracic lymphocenter					
10) Cranial sternal ln.	Cranial border of the m. transversus thoracis	Thoracic wall, shoulder girdle, diaphragm, mediastinum, cranial mammary gland complexes, ventral abdominal wall	To cranial mediastinal lnn.	Caudal sternal lnn. and cranial epigastric lnn. are lacking.	40
Dorsal thoracic lymphocenter					
11) Intercostal ln.	In the proximal 5th or 6th intercostal space	Deep parts of the dorsum, of the shoulder; abdominal muscles, aorta	To cranial mediastinal lnn.	Often absent	40
Bronchial lymphocenter					
12) Right tracheobronchial ln.	Cranial to the right primary bronchus	Lung and other thoracic viscera	To cranial mediastinal lnn.	Cranial tracheobronchial lnn. are lacking.	40
13) Middle tracheobronchial ln.	Dorsal at the bifurcation of the trachea	Lung and other thoracic viscera	To cranial mediastinal lnn.	Pulmonary lnn. lie at the hilus of the lung.	40
14) Left tracheobronchial ln.	Dorsal to the left primary bronchus	Lung and other thoracic viscera	To cranial mediastinal lnn.	Pulmonary lnn. lie at the hilus of the lung.	40

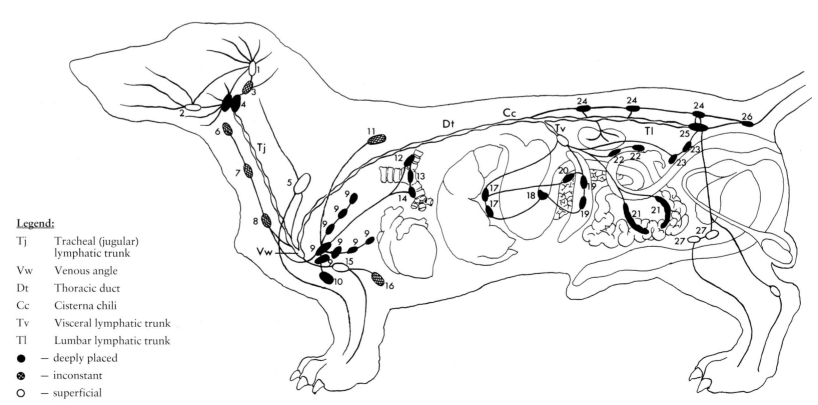

Legend:

Tj	Tracheal (jugular) lymphatic trunk
Vw	Venous angle
Dt	Thoracic duct
Cc	Cisterna chili
Tv	Visceral lymphatic trunk
Tl	Lumbar lymphatic trunk
●	– deeply placed
⊗	– inconstant
○	– superficial

LYMPHOCENTER (lc.) OR LYMPH NODE (ln.)	LOCATION	AREA/ORGANS DRAINED BY AFF. LYMPHATICS	EFFERENT LYMPHATICS	COMMENTS	PAGE
Axillary lymphocenter					
15) Axillary ln.	Caudal to the shoulder joint along the lateral thoracic vein	Superficial parts of the thoracic wall and ventral abdominal wall; thoracic and abdominal mammary gland complexes	Venous angle or terminal part of the tracheal (jugular) lymphatic trunk or thoracic duct	Cubital lnn. and axillary lymph nodes of the first rib (*Lnn. axillares primae costae*) are lacking in the dog.	18 and 22
16) Accessory axillary ln.	(2 cm caudal to the axillary ln.)	As for 15)	As for 15)	Palpable, inconstant	18 and 22
Celiac lymphocenter					
17) Hepatic (portal) lnn.	Beside the portal vein	Lymph vessels from all areas supplied by the celiac a.	To the visceral lymphatic trunk	Lymph nodes of the liver	52 and 58
18) Gastric ln.	On the lesser curvature of the stomach near the pylorus	Stomach	To hepatic lnn. or splenic lnn.	Inconstant	
19) Splenic lnn.	At the branching of the splenic a. and v.	Spleen and afferents from the gastric ln.	To the visceral lymphatic trunk	Group of small lymph nodes	52
20) Pancreaticoduodenal lnn.	Between the cranial part of the duodenum and the pancreas	Duodenum, pancreas, greater omentum, and stomach	To hepatic lnn.	Inconstant	53
Cranial mesenteric lymphocenter					
21) Jejunal lnn.	Proximal mesojejunum	Organs supplied by the cranial mesenteric a.	Visceral lymphatic trunk	Large group of lymph nodes	52
22) Colic lnn.	Mesocolon of ascending colon and transverse colon	Ascending and transverse colon	Visceral lymphatic trunk	Ileocolic and cecal lnn. are lacking in the dog.	52
Caudal mesenteric lymphocenter					
23) Caudal mesenteric lnn.	Mesocolon of descending colon	Organs supplied by the caudal mesenteric a.	Visceral lymphatic trunk	A vesical ln. is lacking in the dog.	52
Lumbar lymphocenter					
24) Lumbar aortic lnn.	Dorsal, ventral and lateral to the abdominal aorta and the caudal vena cava	Deep portions of the dorsal abdominal wall, of the abdominal and pelvic cavities; urinary and genital organs; adrenal glands; afferents of the iliosacral lymphocenter	To the lumbar lymphatic trunk or directly to the cisterna chyli	Proper lumbar, renal, ovarian and testicular lnn. are absent in the dog.	62 and 68
Iliosacral lymphocenter					
25) Medial iliac lnn.	At the origin of the deep circumflex iliac a. and v.	Pelvic wall, pelvic organs; possibly testis; primary lymphatics and afferents from lymph nodes of the pelvic limb	To lumbar lymphatic trunk or lumbar aortic lnn.	Lateral iliac, anorectal and uterine lnn. are lacking.	62 and 68
26) Sacral lnn.	Between right and left iliac arteries at their origin	Rectum, genital organs and neighboring areas	To medial iliac lnn.	Obturator ln. is lacking in the dog.	62 and 68
Supf. inguinal lymphocenter					
27) Supf. inguinal lnn.	At the division of the external pudendal a. and v. into caudal supf. epigastric and ventral scrotal/labial vessels at the level of the inguinal mamma	Skin and cutaneous structures of the ventral abdomen, scrotum, pelvic outlet, tail, pelvic limb, caudal mammary gland complexes and parts of the external genital organs.	To the medial iliac lnn.	Palpable. Epigastric, subiliac, and accessory coxal lnn. and lymph nodes of the paralumbar fossa are absent in the dog.	32 and 68
Popliteal lymphocenter					
28) Popliteal lnn.	Upon the lateral saphenous vein as it emerges caudally between the m. biceps femoris and m. semitendinosus	Pelvic limb distal to the stifle joint	To medial iliac lnn.	Palpable	83 and 84

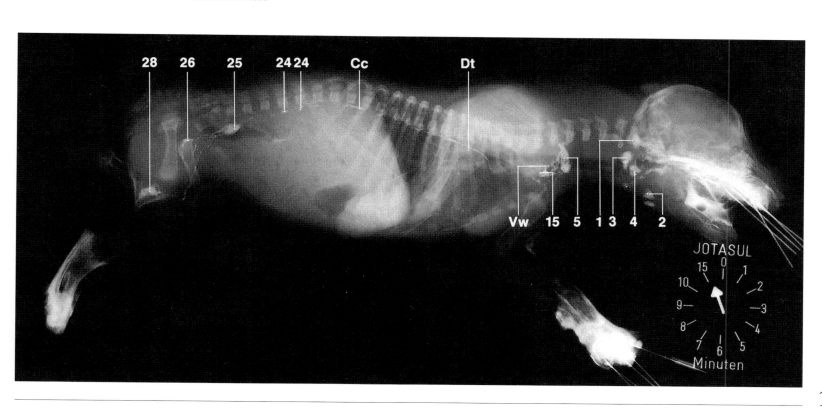

3. CRANIAL NERVES

		Classification	Origin From the Brain	Passage Through Cranium	Fiber Type (based on function and developmental origin)	Area of Innervation	Comments
I	Olfactory nerves	Sensory nerves	Olfactory bulb, tel-encephalon	Cribriform plate of ethmoid bone	Special visceral afferent	Olfactory region of the *fundus nasi* and the vomeronasal organ	The receptor cells are primary sensory cells located in the olfactory mucosa.
II	Optic nerve	Sensory nerve	Diencephalon	Optic canal	Special somatic afferent	Retina (internal coat, nervous tunic of the eyeball)	Arises as an outpouching of the diencephalon and is enveloped by the three meninges.
III	Oculomotor nerv Motor root	Motor nerve	Ventral midbrain	Orbital fissure	Special somatic efferent	External muscles of the eyeball except for the mm. obliquus dorsal, rectus lat., and lateral parts of the m. retractor bulbi	Parasympathetic preganglionic fibers synapse in the ciliary ganglion. Postganglionic sympathetic fibers pass in the short ciliary nn. to the m. dilatator pupillae.
	Parasympathetic (general visceral efferent) root				General visceral efferent	Mm. sphincter pupillae and ciliaris	
IV	Trochlear nerve	Motor nerve	Dorsal midbrain	Orbital fissure	Special somatic efferent	M. obliquus dorsalis	Smallest of the cranial nn.
V	Trigeminal nerve	Nerve of the 1ˢᵗ branchial arch	Junction of pons and medulla oblongata				Its end-branches contain parasympathetic fibers from the pterygopalatine ggl. of VII, from the otic ggl. of IX, from the mandibular and sublingual ggll. of the chorda tympani of VII. These fibers supply the salivary glands, lacrimal and nasal glands. Clinical consideration: Trigeminal neuralgia.
	Ophthalmic nerve (V1)	Sensory nerve		Orbital fissure	General somatic sensory	Caudal dorsum nasi and skin of the interorbital region, ethmoid bone and dorsal nasal mucous membrane, lacrimal gland, upper eyelid	
	Maxillary nerve (V2)	Sensory nerve		Round foramen and alar canal	General somatic sensory	Facial region including nostril and upper lip, ventral nasal mucous membrane, dorsal oral mucous membrane, teeth of the upper jaw, temporal region	
	Mandibular nerve (V3) Sensory root			Oval foramen (united with motor root)	General somatic sensory	Lateral and ventral oral cavity, temporal and auricular region, ventrolateral face, mental region	
	Motor root			Oval foramen (united with sensory root)	Special visceral efferent	Masticatory and ventral throat mm., m. tensor veli palatini, m. tensor tympani	
VI	Abducent nerve	Motor nerve	Medulla oblongata	Orbital fissure	Special somatic efferent	M. rectus lateralis and parts of m. retractor bulbi	With III and V1 in a common dural sheath.
VII	Facial nerve (N. intermedio-facialis)	Nerve of the 2ⁿᵈ branchial arch	Medulla oblongata	Facial canal from the *porus acusticus internus* to the stylomastoid foramen	Special visceral efferent (facial n.), general visceral efferent (greater petrosal n. and fibers in chorda tympani), general somatic afferent (internal auricular branches), special visceral afferent (gustatory fibers of chorda tympani)	Facial muscles, mm. stapedius, occipitohyoideus, stylohyoideus, digastricus (caudal belly); tympanic membrane and external acoustic meatus, mandibular and sublingual glands, lacrimal gland and glands of the oral and nasal cavities, taste buds of rostral tongue	Clinical: Facial paralysis. The intermediate nerve can be regarded as a '13ᵗʰ' cranial n.
	Facial n.	Motor n.			Special visceral efferent	Facial muscles, mm. stapedius, occipitohyoideus, stylohyoideus, digastricus (caudal belly); tympanic membrane and external acoustic meatus (communicating branch from X)	
	Intermediate n.: Chorda tympani			Facial canal to petrotympanic fissure	General visceral efferent, special visceral afferent	Mandibular and sublingual glands, taste buds of rostral tongue (fungiform papillae)	Joins the lingual branch of V3.
	Greater petrosal n.			Facial canal to petrosal canal to pterygoid canal	General visceral efferent (parasympathetic)	Lacrimal gland, glands of the nasal and oral cavity	Joins the deep petrosal (sympathetic) n. to form the n. of the pterygoid canal.
VIII	Vestibulocochlear nerve (N. statoacusticus)	Sensory nerve	Medulla oblongata	*Porus acusticus internus*	Special visceral afferent	Macula utriculi, macula sacculi, crista ampullaris, ductus cochlearis	In the CNS, connecting pathways to nuclei of III, IV, and VI.
IX	Glossopharyngeal nerve	Nerve of the 3ʳᵈ branchial arch (part of the vagus group)	Medulla oblongata	Jugular foramen and tympano-occipital fissure	Special visceral efferent, general visceral efferent, special visceral afferent, general visceral afferent	Pharyngeal musculature (special visceral efferent), taste buds of vallate and foliate papillae (special visceral afferent), parotid and zygomatic glands (general visceral efferent), pharyngeal mucosa (general visceral afferent)	Ramus to the carotid sinus mediates impulses from sinuosal baroceptors to the circulatory center.
	Pharyngeal branch					Pharyngeal musculature and mucosa (with X)	
	Lingual branches				Special visceral efferent (stylopharngeus m.), special and general visceral afferent	Pharyngeal mucosa (caudal third of tongue), including vallate and foliate papillae	Communicates with the lingual n. of V3.
	Tympanic n.			Tympanic canaliculus	General visceral efferent, general visceral afferent	Parotid and zygomatic glands, mucosa of tympanic cavity	Its continuation is the minor petrosal n., which synapses in the otic ggl.
X	Vagus nerve	Nerve of the 4ᵗʰ branchial arch (part of the vagus group)	Medulla oblongata	Jugular foramen and tympano-occipital fissure	Special visceral efferent (pharyngeal musculature, with IX; laryngeal mm.), general visceral afferent (thoracic and abdominal viscera), general visceral efferent (parasympathetic fibers to thoracic and abdominal viscera), special visceral afferent (taste buds of epiglottis)		The 'wandering' nerve. Its distal (nodose) ganglion is examined for rabies diagnosis.
XI	Accessory nerve	Nerve of the 4ᵗʰ branchial arch (part of the vagus group) and of the cervical spinal cord	Medulla oblongata and cervical spinal cord	Jugular foramen and tympano-occipital fissure	Special and general visceral efferent (medullary root), special visceral efferent (spinal root)	Pharyngeal and laryngeal musculature (special visceral efferent), thoracic and abdominal viscera (general visceral efferent) distributed in branches of X, (medullary root – radices encephalicae); mm. sternocleidomastoideus, trapezius, and cleidocervicalis (special visceral efferent – spinal root)	The medullary root joins (radices encephalicae) the vagus external to the jugular foramen; the spinal root supplies the superficial cervical musculature named above.
aXII	Hypoglossal nerve	In part a cervical nerve	Medulla oblongata	Hypoglossal canal	General somatic efferent	Muscles of the tongue and hyoid apparatus (m. geniohyoideus, m. thyrohyoideus)	Joined to the 1ˢᵗ cervical n. by the *ansa cervicalis*.

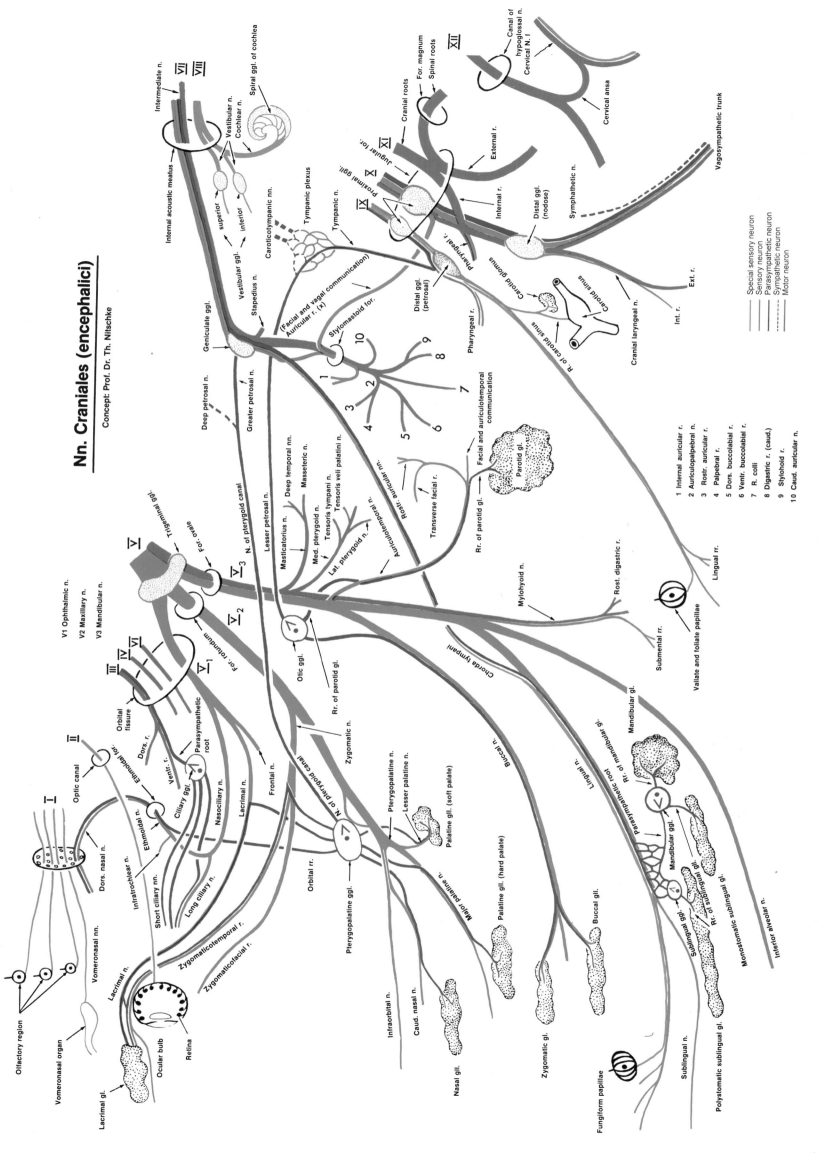

Nn. Craniales (encephalici)

Concept: Prof. Dr. Th. Nitschke

V1 Ophthalmic n.
V2 Maxillary n.
V3 Mandibular n.

1 Internal auricular r.
2 Auriculopalpebral n.
3 Rostr. auricular r.
4 Palpebral r.
5 Dors. buccolabial r.
6 Ventr. buccolabial r.
7 R. colli
8 Digastric r. (caud.)
9 Stylohoid r.
10 Caud. auricular n.

Special sensory neuron
Sensory neuron
Parasympathetic neuron
Sympathetic neuron
Motor neuron

Olfactory region
Vomeronasal organ
Lacrimal gl.
Ocular bulb
Retina
Optic canal
Ethmoidal for.
Dors. r.
Ventr. r.
Orbital fissure
Parasympathetic root
Ciliary ggl.
Nasociliary n.
Lacrimal n.
Frontal n.
Intratrochlear nn.
Short ciliary nn.
Long ciliary n.
Dors. nasal n.
Vomeronasal nn.
Lacrimal n.
Zygomaticotemporal r.
Zygomaticofacial r.
Fungiform papillae
Nasal gll.
Zygomatic gl.
Buccal gll.
Infraorbital n.
Caud. nasal n.
Sublingual n.
Polystomatic sublingual gl.

Trigeminal ggl.
For. ovale
N. of pterygoid canal
Lesser petrosal n.
Deep temporal nn.
Masseteric n.
Med. pterygoid n.
Tensoris tympani n.
Tensoris veli palatini n.
Lat. pterygoid n.
Auriculotemporal n.
Rostr. auricular nn.
Transverse facial r.
Masticatorius n.
Olitic ggl.
Rr. of parotid gl.
Zygomatic n.
N. of pterygoid canal
Orbital rr.
Pterygopalatine n.
Lesser palatine n.
Palatine gll. (soft palate)
Pterygopalatine ggl.
Buccal n.
Lingual n.
Palatine gll. (hard palate)
Major palatine n.
Mandibular gl.
Rr. of mandibular gl.
Parasympathetic root
Mandibular ggl.
Sublingual ggl.
Rr. of sublingual gl.
Monostomatic sublingual gl.
Inferior alveolar n.

Intermediate n.
VI VII
Internal acoustic meatus
Vestibular n.
Cochlear n.
Spiral ggl. of cochlea
superior
inferior
Vestibular ggl.
Carolicotympanic nn.
Tympanic plexus
Geniculate ggl.
Stapedius n.
Deep petrosal n.
Greater petrosal n.
(Facial and vagal communication)
Auricular r. (x)
Stylomastoid for.
Facial and auriculotemporal communication
Parotid gl.
Rr. of parotid gl.
Mylohyoid n.
Rost. digastric r.
Rost. digastric r.
Chorda tympani
Submental rr.
Vallate and foliate papillae
Lingual rr.

Canal of hypoglossal n.
Cervical N. I
For. magnum
Spinal roots
Cranial roots
XII
Cervical ansa
Cervical ansa
Cranial roots
XI
External r.
Internal r.
Distal ggl. (nodose)
Sympathetic n.
Vagosympathetic trunk
Jugular for.
X
IX
Proximal ggll.
Tympanic n.
Pharyngeal r.
Distal ggl. (petrosal)
Pharyngeal r.
Carotid glomus
Carotid sinus
Carotid sinus
R. of carotid sinus
Ext. r.
Int. r.
Cranial laryngeal n.

I
II
III
IV VI
V1
V2
V3
For. rotundum
V

GENERAL ANATOMY

1. OSTEOLOGY: MEMBRANOUS AND CHONDRAL OSSIFICATION; GROWTH OF BONES IN LENGTH AND DIAMETER

a) MEMBRANOUS OSSIFICATION is direct ossification. It takes place chiefly in the formation of the flat bones of the skull. In this process the **mesenchymal cells** of the embryonic mesenchyme differentiate into **bone forming cells, osteoblasts (A)**, which give rise to the **primary trabeculae of woven bone (B)**. The osteoblast synthesizes the organic osseous matrix or osteoid, that is, the fundamental osseous substance with its associated collagen fibers. The osteoblast becomes enveloped by the osteoid and, with progressive mineralization of the osteoid, is sequestered in a small chamber, a lacuna. At this stage, the osteoblast has matured to become an **osteocyte (C)**. The osteoid is mineralized by an orderly deposition of calcium phosphate crystals (hydroxyapatite) in association with collagenous fibers. This primary bone tissue is organized initially as trabeculae. The transformation of primary trabecular bone into secondary compact bone is accomplished by the layer of osteoblasts that remains apposed to the surface of the trabecular bone. The flat bones increase in circumference (girth) by the deposition of bone tissue at their margins. They increase in thickness by the deposition of bone upon the external and internal surfaces. Remodeling is accomplished by **osteoclasts (D)**, specialized multinucleated cells that are capable of resorbing bone. The apposed margins of most of the flat bones of the skull have not formed a bony union at birth and remain joined by fibrous tissue. At birth, the larger of these spaces occupied by the connecting fibrous tissue may be several centimeters in width. Such spaces occur as irregular circumscribed areas designated fontanelles. The lack of bony fusion allows for some compression of the skull as the head passes through the birth canal at parturition.

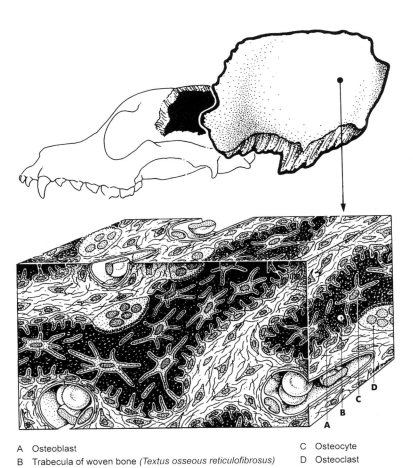

A   Osteoblast
B   Trabecula of woven bone *(Textus osseous reticulofibrosus)*
C   Osteocyte
D   Osteoclast

b) CHONDRAL OSSIFICATION is indirect ossification. It is characterized by the formation of a cartilaginous primordial skeleton that is then replaced by bone. The bones that form the base of the skull, the vertebrae, ribs, and sternum, and the bones of the limbs are formed by chondral ossification, appearing first as a cartilage model of the future bone and then being replaced by bone. Chondral ossification takes place in two stages in which a perichondral ossification precedes endochondral ossification. In the case of the long bones of the limbs, which have an **epiphysis (1)** at each end and a bone-shaft or **diaphysis (4)** between them, perichondral ossification is seen only in the diaphyseal region. The cells of the perichondrium of the diaphysis of the cartilage model differentiate into osteoblasts, transforming the perichondrium into a **periosteum (6)**. Perichondral ossification proceeds in

the manner of membranous ossification in that the osteoblasts form a **sleeve of trabecular bone (*Anulus osseus perichondralis*, −3)** around the cartilaginous diaphysis. This provides mechanical stabilization. The endochondral ossification that follows takes place within the cartilaginous diaphysis as a **primary** or **diaphysial ossification center** (see clinical-functional anatomy). It begins with the sprouting of **perforating blood vessels (21)** into the primordial cartilaginous skeleton in which the perichondral sleeve is perforated at the place that will later become the **nutrient canal (22)**. The perforating blood vessels with surrounding connective tissue form the primary bone marrow, which is located in the **primary medullary cavity (7)**. The latter arises by the activity of **chondroclasts (2)** after destruction of the hypertrophied cartilaginous cells and mineralized cartilaginous matrix in the **zona resorbens (16)**. Osteoblasts **(5)** adhere to the remnants of **cartilaginous matrix (19)** and, with the formation of **osseous matrix (20)**, differentiate into osteocytes **(8)** that lie within the **primary osseous trabeculae (18)**. Owing to their mineral content, the ossification centers of the developing long bones are readily observed in radiographs. The mineralized matrix is only a little permeable to x-rays. On the other hand, the cartilage that surrounds the ossification centers is much more permeable to x-rays. Later, blood vessels penetrate into the cartilaginous **epiphysis** and an **ossification center** is formed by mineralization. In general, this ossification center appears later and is designated a **secondary** or **epiphysial ossification centre (12)**. From the epiphysial ossification center, ossification extends peripherally, especially toward the diaphysis. In the region between the diaphysial and epiphysial ossification centers, thus between the diaphysis and epiphysis, cartilage persists for a time as the **physial cartilage (13, −growth cartilage)**. This cartilage is at first unmineralized and therefore easily recognized in radiographs. From its **reserve zone (14)**, it furnishes hypertrophied, vesicular, cartilage cells (chondrocytes) that are arranged in short **columns (15)** and compressed in the direction of the zona resorbens. Here they are destroyed by chondroclasts and replaced by osseous tissue. The ossification zone of the primary ossification center progresses from the diaphysis in the direction of the epiphysis and the secondary ossification center of the epiphysis advances toward the diaphysis. The result is that the physial cartilage becomes thinner with increasing age. The primary osseous trabeculae of primitive cancellous bone with their central remnants of cartilaginous ground matrix are transformed by the activity of **osteoclasts (9)** and osteoblasts into secondary osseous trabeculae (see p. 140). In the region of compact bone, they are formed according to the structural principle of lamellar bone and contain regularly arranged osteocytes, collagenous fibers and mineralized osseous ground substance but, different from the primary osseous trabeculae, contain no cartilaginous ground substance.

The **metaphysis (17)** is the region of diaphysial transformation of the primary into secondary osseous trabeculae. It is located at the epiphysial ends of the diaphysis where the bone begins to expand and there is an intensive mineralization process.

Apophyses (10) are processes of bone that are the insertion of many muscles (other definitions are used). Apophyses first appear as a cartilaginous process of the original cartilage model of bone, and a center of ossification develops within the apophysis in the same manner as in the epiphysis. As long as bone growth continues, part of the cartilage remains as an **apophysial cartilage (11)** between the ossification center and the main body of the forming bone.

c) GROWTH IN LENGTH OF LONG BONES is assured as long as the zone of proliferating chondrocytes remains active. When the degeneration of hypertrophic chondrocytes and their replacement with trabecular and compact bone is no longer compensated by chondrocyte proliferation, the zones of ossification approach each other, consuming the entire growth plate cartilage. The zones fuse and eliminate the possibility of further growth in length of the long bone. This osseous tissue that replaces the radiolucent growth plate cartilage appears on a radiograph as a radiopaque epiphyseal line.

d) GROWTH IN CIRCUMFERENCE of the bone results primarily from the apposition of bony lamellae produced on the inner aspect of the thin osteogenic layer of the periosteum. This external apposition of new bone tissue coupled with an internal resorption of osseous tissue at the margin of the medullary cavity results in an enlargement of the cavity while increasing the circumference of the cortical bone. At the metaphysis, growth in thickness is completed in a different manner. Here, new bone tissue is laid down internally on the perichondral bone sleeve; whereas, on the external, periosteal surface a resorption of bone takes place. (Fracture repair, see clinical-functional anatomy.)

Chondral Ossification

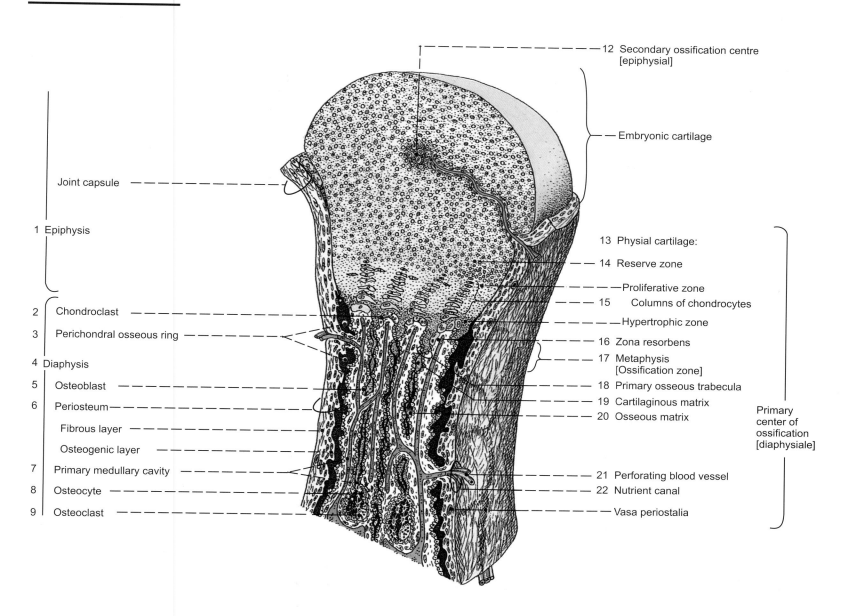

Joint capsule

1 Epiphysis

2 Chondroclast
3 Perichondral osseous ring
4 Diaphysis
5 Osteoblast
6 Periosteum
  Fibrous layer
  Osteogenic layer
7 Primary medullary cavity
8 Osteocyte
9 Osteoclast

12 Secondary ossification centre [epiphysial]

Embryonic cartilage

13 Physial cartilage:
14 Reserve zone
  Proliferative zone
15   Columns of chondrocytes
  Hypertrophic zone
16 Zona resorbens
17 Metaphysis [Ossification zone]
18 Primary osseous trabecula
19 Cartilaginous matrix
20 Osseous matrix

21 Perforating blood vessel
22 Nutrient canal
  Vasa periostalia

Primary center of ossification [diaphysiale]

Femur (juvenile dog)

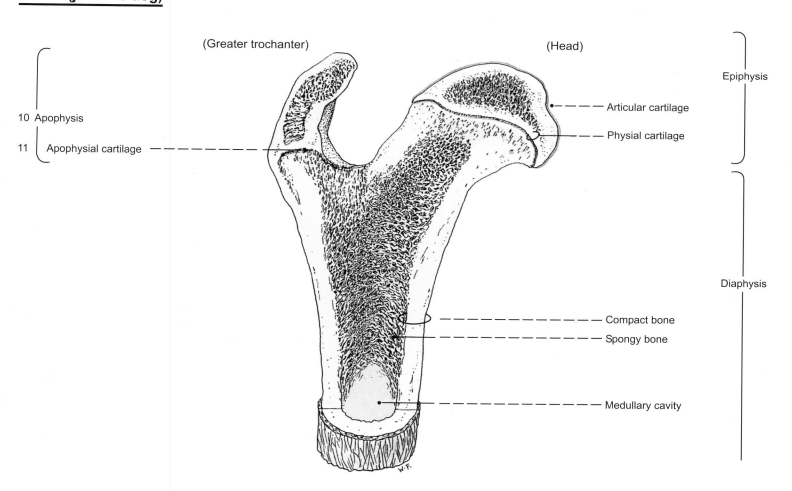

(Greater trochanter)

(Head)

10 Apophysis

11 Apophysial cartilage

Articular cartilage

Physial cartilage

Epiphysis

Compact bone

Spongy bone

Medullary cavity

Diaphysis

139

2. OSTEOLOGY: STRUCTURE AND FORM OF BONE AND CARTILAGE

Bone tissue consists of osteocytes and mineralized osseous ground substance (osseous matrix) with systems of collagenous fibers. The dry matter of a fully differentiated bone is made up of one-third organic and two-thirds inorganic constituents. After demineralization the bone retains its external form, but its rigidity is lost and it becomes flexible. In contrast, bone freed of its organic constituents is brittle and easily broken. The lamellar bone that has arisen secondarily is found particularly in the compact substance of the long bones. Tissue that will later become bone remains for a long time after birth as the sutures of the skull.

a) The **HARD PORTIONS OF THE BONE** are the compact substance that forms the wall of the medullary cavity of long bones, the cortical substance of the epiphysial surface and the surface of the short bones, and the trabecular meshwork of spongy substance in the interior of the bone.

I. The **compact substance (27)** consists of lamellar osseous tissue. **Osteons (14)** are the predominant structural units of the lamellar bone tissue. They are between the **external circumferential lamellae (26)** at the external surface of the compact substance and the **internal circumferential lamellae (28)** at the boundary to the medullary cavity and the spongy bone tissue. The osteons are up to 2 cm long and, in the vicinity of their central canal, consist of **osteonal lamellae (16)** that are adapted to one another. Osteocytes lie between these lamellae. The lamellae of the osteon contain collagenous fibers in their mineralized osseous ground substance. (A comparable structural principle is found in reinforced concrete where rigidity, the concrete or mineral salts within the bone, and flexibility, the steel rods or collagenous fibers, complement each other to make the structure functionally complete.) The **collagenous fibers (15)** alter their course of direction from one osteon-lamella to another osteon-lamella in the manner of a flat and steeply winding right-hand and left-hand screw (like the structural principle of plywood with differently directed wood grain in each of the individual glued layers). Between the osteons are **interstitial lamellae (8)**, which are the morphological result of the constant and regular restructure of bone. Remodelling of bone takes place lifelong. In the growth phase, bone formation predominates. With age, loss of bone predominates and is responsible for an increasing fragility of bone.

II. **Cortical (or compact) bone substance (12)** occurs as a superficial layer in short bones and epiphyses.

III. The **spongy substance (6)** lies internal to the compact substance and consists only in places of atypical lamellar osseous tissue. A trajectorial structure can be recognized in that the trabeculae, lamellae, or tubules of the spongy bone are arranged according to **lines of pressure and tension (11)**, leaving free medullary spaces (*Cellulae medullares*) that contain bone marrow. (This structural principle permits reduction in weight. For example, in the structure of high-voltage towers, there is a reduction of structural materials while retaining great strength. This is comparable to the structure of spongy bone.) In some cranial ones the spongy bone (diplöe) is considerably reduced or it is absent as in the pneumatic bones of the paranasal sinuses. Some bones, for example, the petrous temporal bone, or the mandible of the elephant, consist chiefly of compact bone with complete or nearly complete absence of spongy substance.

b) The **SOFT TISSUES OF BONE** are the periosteum, the articular cartilage, the vessels and the bone marrow.

I. The **periosteum (18)** consists of a superficial **fibrous layer (20)**, from which **perforating fibers (19)** radiate into the compact substance, and of an **osteogenic layer (21, —Cambium)** rich in cells and bearing numerous vessels and nerves. In the region of a joint, the periosteum is continuous with the fibrous layer of the joint capsule. **Endosteum (10)** lines the walls of the medullary cavity and the medullary spaces. It is much thinner than the periosteum and contains precursor cells capable of forming osteoblasts, as well as osteoblasts and osteoclasts.

II. The **articular cartilage (1)** consists of a non-mineralized **superficial zone (2)** from which collagenous fibers run tangential to the surface and then, by change of their course, penetrate deeply into the **intermediate zone (3)** and into the even more deeply located mineralized **deep zone (4)**. The border between the mineralized deep layer of the articular cartilage and the **osseous tissue (5)** is irregular and aids in preventing slippage of the cartilage. The free surface of articular cartilage is not covered by perichondrium.

III. The **vessels of bone** run as fine **periosteal arteries (22)** in the depth of the periosteum. **Perforating branches (24)** enter the surface of the bone (this is disputed by some authors). The vessels enter the bone by canals that lead to the **central canal (7)** of the osteon, where they are named HAVERSIAN vessels. The transverse canals connecting the osteons are **VOLKMANN'S canals (17, —Canales perforantes)**, which contain VOLKMANN'S vessels. Blood passes by slender branches from the capillaries to the **periosteal veins (23)**. Long bones are supplied by diaphysial, metaphysial, epiphysial (not illustrated) and periosteal vessels (see clinical-functional anatomy). In young individuals the blood supply of the epiphysis is totally separated from that of the diaphysis by the physial cartilage. Following closure of the physial line and completion of growth in length, anastomoses form between the diaphysial and metaphysial vessels. Periosteal nerves (23) accompany the larger vessels.

IV. **Bone marrow** is located in the **medullary cavity (13)** and in the **medullary spaces (9)** of the spongy bone. In the fetus and juvenile organism it is widespread as red bone marrow, which forms the red blood cells. With increasing age, the red bone marrow is present preferentially in short and flat bones. In long bones, yellow bone marrow predominates. In cases of severe blood loss, the yellow marrow can differentiate into red blood cell forming red marrow. With very old or emaciated animals, the yellow marrow is transformed irreversibly into a grayish, glassy, gelatinous marrow.

c) With respect to the **SHAPE OF BONES**, we distinguish **long bones** (most of the limb bones), **short bones** (tarsal and carpal bones), **irregular bones** (vertebrae) and **flat bones** (certain cranial and facial bones). In the short and flat bones, a thin layer of cortical (compact) substance surrounds the spongy bone. A marrow cavity is not present. In the long bones, the marrow cavity enlarges with increasing age. The manner of ossification is different in the different bones. Long bones ossify predominantly by endochondral ossification (epiphysis and diaphysis) and in the diaphysis also perichondrally. Short bones ossify similar to epiphyses, predominantly endochondrally. Flat bones develop by desmal (membranous) ossification or by perichondral ossification. The vertebrae ossify with three ossification centers in the body of the vertebra (two epiphyses with a center for the diaphysis in between), which is formally comparable to long bones.

d) **SESAMOID BONES** are special skeletal components on the basis of their development within tendons (sometimes in association with the joint capsule), their function in protecting the tendon, and the absence of a cambium (osteogenic) layer of the periosteum. They are located in the region of joints, usually in a tendon (*e.g.*, the patella), or as a gliding surface deep to a tendon (*e.g.*, plantar at the distal interphalangeal joint) and thus are connected to the underlying bone by ligaments. Some are present as sesamoid cartilages and for that reason are designated *sesamoides*.

e) **VISCERAL BONES** are present, for example, as the os *penis* of the male dog and the os *cordis* of the ox.

f) **CARTILAGE TISSUE** is an avascular supporting tissue that consists of chondrocytes and an intercellular matrix. The matrix contains connective tissue fibers and a more or less firm cartilaginous ground substance (in particular, chondroitin sulphate). On its surface, the cartilage is covered by a vascular perichondrium, which is lacking on articular cartilage. Cartilage tissue is structured according to the principle of vesicular supportive tissue (turgor tissue) in that, the turgor properties of the cells with the surrounding ground substance and on the other hand the tension-resistance of the collagenous fibers provides a functionally complete mechanism. Fibers of cartilage are collagenous and elastic, which characteristically differ in morphology, amount and direction in the different regions of the body and in the three different types of cartilage. Collagenous fibers are predominantly trajectorially arranged, following lines of pressure and tension. In hyaline cartilage (magnified inset on the left side of the figure on the opposite page) of the stifle joint, the collagenous fiber-bundles are arciform, running from the underlying bone toward the articular surface and returning again to the bone. In the meshes between the collagenous fiber-bundles, the cartilage cells lie in groups or territories within a lacuna surrounded by a capsule of cartilage-matrix. Collagenous fibers occur in all **three types of cartilage (hyaline, elastic, and fibro-cartilage)**.

140

Femur (Homo sapiens)

(Head)   (Greater trochanter)

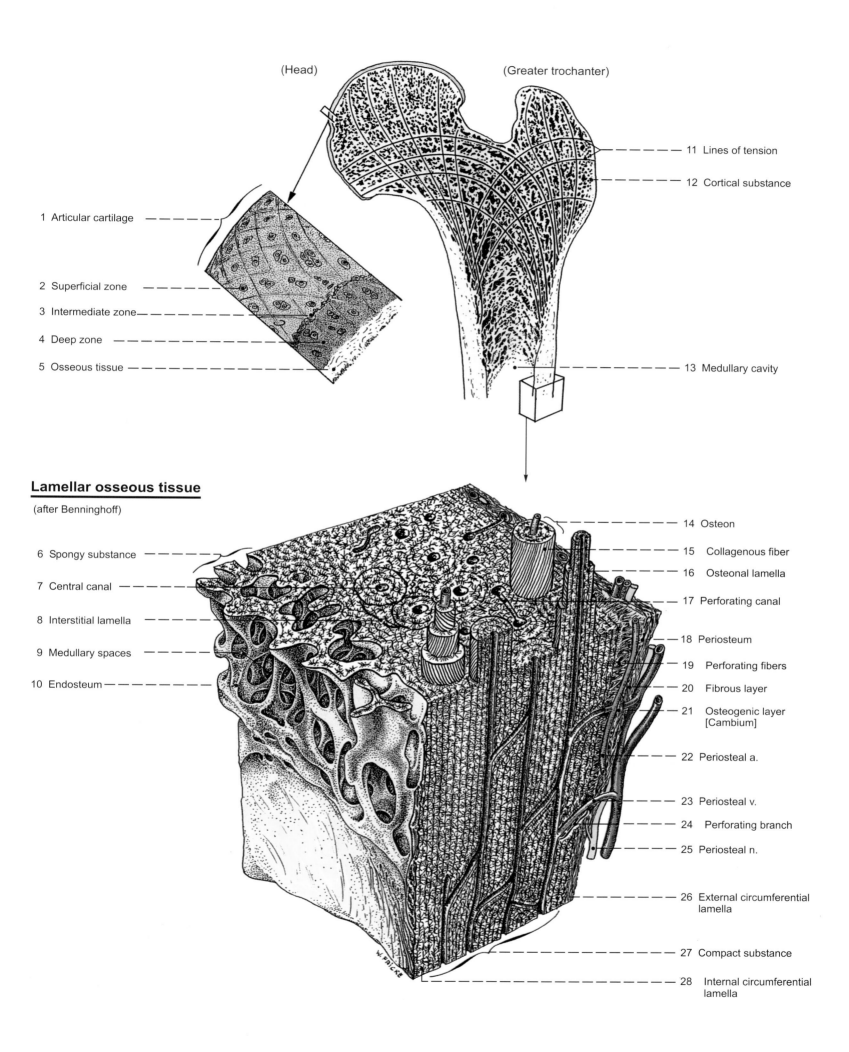

1 Articular cartilage

2 Superficial zone

3 Intermediate zone

4 Deep zone

5 Osseous tissue

11 Lines of tension

12 Cortical substance

13 Medullary cavity

Lamellar osseous tissue

(after Benninghoff)

6 Spongy substance

7 Central canal

8 Interstitial lamella

9 Medullary spaces

10 Endosteum

14 Osteon

15 Collagenous fiber

16 Osteonal lamella

17 Perforating canal

18 Periosteum

19 Perforating fibers

20 Fibrous layer

21 Osteogenic layer [Cambium]

22 Periosteal a.

23 Periosteal v.

24 Perforating branch

25 Periosteal n.

26 External circumferential lamella

27 Compact substance

28 Internal circumferential lamella

3. ARTHROLOGY: THE CONNECTIONS OF BONES AND THE FORM OF JOINTS

a) The **CONNECTIONS OF THE BONES** comprise the synarthroses: fibrous and cartilaginous joints and synostoses, which lack a joint space; and the true joints, synovial joints or diarthroses.

I. Fibrous joints are: 1. **Syndesmoses** (e.g., crural interosseous membrane); 2. **sutures** (sutures between the flat bones of the skull); and 3. **gomphoses** (the union of the cementum of the tooth to the bone of the alveolus by the periodontium (periodontal ligament).

II. Cartilaginous joints are: 1. The **synchondrosis** (union by hyaline cartilage; e.g., between the late ossifying parts of the sternum, for example, the manubriosternal synchondrosis); and 2. the **symphysis** (joint formed by fibrocartilage, e.g., the pelvic symphysis).

III. The **synostosis** is formed by fusion of two or more individual bones in which the union is made by bone (e.g., sacrum).

IV. The **synovial or true joint** has an articular space. This space is bounded by the ends of two bones (simple joint; e.g., shoulder joint) or of three or more bones (composite or compound joint; e.g., stifle joint; see also p. 87). The **articular cavity** (1) containing the synovia is surrounded by an **articular capsule** (2). Fibrous, parallel-fibered reinforcement of the joint capsule is provided by the **joint ligaments** (4, 6). The ends of the articulating bones are covered by **articular cartilage** (3). The fibrous, layer of the periosteum is continuous with the **external, fibrous, layer** of the joint capsule. The **internal, synovial, layer** of the joint capsule lines the fibrous capsule and extends to the margins of the articular cartilages. It has two types of loosely arranged synovial cells: 1. The secretory synovial cells determine the composition of the **joint fluid, synovia**, which leaves the blood capillaries as an ultrafiltrate and enters the joint cavity through the synovial layer. The synovia has a nutritive function with respect to the avascular articular cartilage. 2. Phagocytic synovial cells take up substances that are foreign to the normal synovia, e.g., blood cells following intra-articular hemorrhage (hemarthrosis) or the smallest of shed particles of cartilage in cases of arthroses and other degenerative articular changes. The joint capsule covers more or less smoothly the vertex of the joint (highest point on the extensor aspect) and is in folds and villi in the depth of the flexor aspect. This is particularly distinct in joints with great mobility. Outpouchings of the joint capsule may surround the tendons of origin of muscles as capsular vaginal sheaths. An example is the capsular sheath surrounding the tendon of origin of the long digital extensor muscle at the level of the stifle joint.

b) The structure of the wall of **SYNOVIAL BURSAE AND SYNOVIAL SHEATHS** is the same as that of the joint capsule. Synovial bursae lie between bone and an overlying, gliding tendon, e.g., the **distal infrapatellar subtendinous bursa** (7) or in areas beneath the skin that are subject to particular stress. Synovial sheaths help to guide the tendons and keep them in place where they pass for a long distance over bone (details, see p. 146).

c) **FIBROCARTILAGINOUS DISCS** occur in a few joints in three variations of form. In part, these discs function as a shock absorber:

I. Two **articular menisci** (5) project from medially and laterally into the joint cavity as semilunar discs and thus, except for the central area that is left free, subdivide the cavity. They are held in place by meniscal ligaments. Example: femorotibial joint.

II. An **articular disc** completely subdivides the joint cavity into two parts that lie one above the other. Example: temporomandibular joint.

III. **Intervertebral discs** fill completely the space between two vertebral bodies. For this reason, this joint is not considered a 'true' joint. True joints of the vertebrae are present between their articular processes, and between the atlas and axis. In these joints, no intervertebral disc is present. Intervertebral discs consist of a fibrous ring, the *anulus fibrosus*, and a centrally located, gelatinous *nucleus pulposus*. The latter is a remnant of the chorda dorsalis (notochord) of the embryo.

d) Corresponding to their **COMPOSITION** of two or several bones, the joints are classified as a **simple joint** (two bones make up the joint) or **composite (complex) joint** (more than two bones make up the joint).

e) **JOINT FORM** (see also the text-illustrations.)

I. A **plane joint** is present between the articular processes of the vertebrae, whose articular surfaces are flat and glide on each other. The tight sacroiliac joint is a special form as the irregular joint surfaces, which are fitted to one another, are held by very short joint ligaments such that play in the joint is hardly possible (*amphiarthrosis*).

II. A **spheroid or ball-and-socket joint** has a spherical articular depression, which is less than a hemisphere (e.g., the shoulder joint).

III. An **enarthrosis** is a special form of spheroid joint in which the articular socket encroaches upon the corresponding articular head beyond its equator (e.g., coxal joint of human beings). According to Henschel, E. (Berlin), the coxal joint of the dog is not an enarthrosis but a simple spheroid joint.

IV. In a **trochoid joint**, a hollow 'cylinder', the atlas, rotates around a fixed articular projection, the dens of the axis, forming, in this example, the atlanto-axial joint.

V. An **ellipsoid joint** has an ellipsoid articular elevation (*Condylus occipitalis*) and a correspondingly formed articular socket (articular cavity of the atlas), forming thus the atlanto-occipital articulation.

VI. In the **sellar (saddle) joint**, the articular elevation in lateral view appears saddle-shaped and projects into a congruent, concave articular socket. Example: distal interphalangeal joint.

VII. The **condylar joint** has either two separate condyles or a uniform, transversely situated, articular condyle that fits into a more or less congruent articular depression, e.g., temporo-mandibular joint. **Special forms** of the condylar joint are the **ginglymus, cochlear joint, spiral joint, and gliding joint (VIII — XI).**

VIII. The **ginglymus** has a perpendicularly located guiding ridge on the condyle, which limits movement to extension and flexion, e.g., the elbow joint, which has a certain 'snapping' action.

IX. The **cochlear joint** has obliquely arranged ridges on the trochlea that permit only extension and flexion, e.g., the hock joint.

X. In the **spiral joint**, the external contour of the articular condyle is an incomplete spiral. This can be observed in lateral view. The collateral ligaments are attached eccentrically and are made taut in extension or flexion, e.g., femorotibial joint with 'braking' action.

XI. In the **gliding joint**, the patella glides in an articular depression between two ridges: femoropatellar joint.

f) **JOINT FUNCTION** depends on the **form of the joint** and the laxity (ampleness) of the joint capsule as well as the length and firmness of the joint ligaments. The **amphiarthrosis** has practically no moveability because of its very short ligaments and tight joint capsule. **Uniaxial, biaxial, and multiaxial joints** are differentiated according to the degree of their **freedom of movement**. The uniaxial joint is a hinge joint, permitting extension and flexion. The angle of flexion is usually less than 1 80 degrees (only in the case of dorsal flexion or 'overextension' is it exceptionally larger). In flexion, the flexion angle is decreased. In extension, it becomes larger. The **multiaxial joint** is functionally a **free joint** as it permits several **possible movements**.

Classification of joints

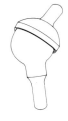 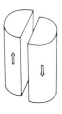 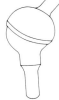 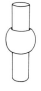 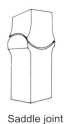 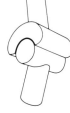 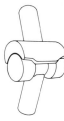 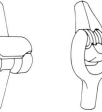

| Plane joint | Ball - and - socket joint | Enarthrosis | Pivot or trochoid joint | Ellipsoidal joint | Saddle joint | Condylar joint | Hinge joint | Cochlear joint: |

Synovial joints

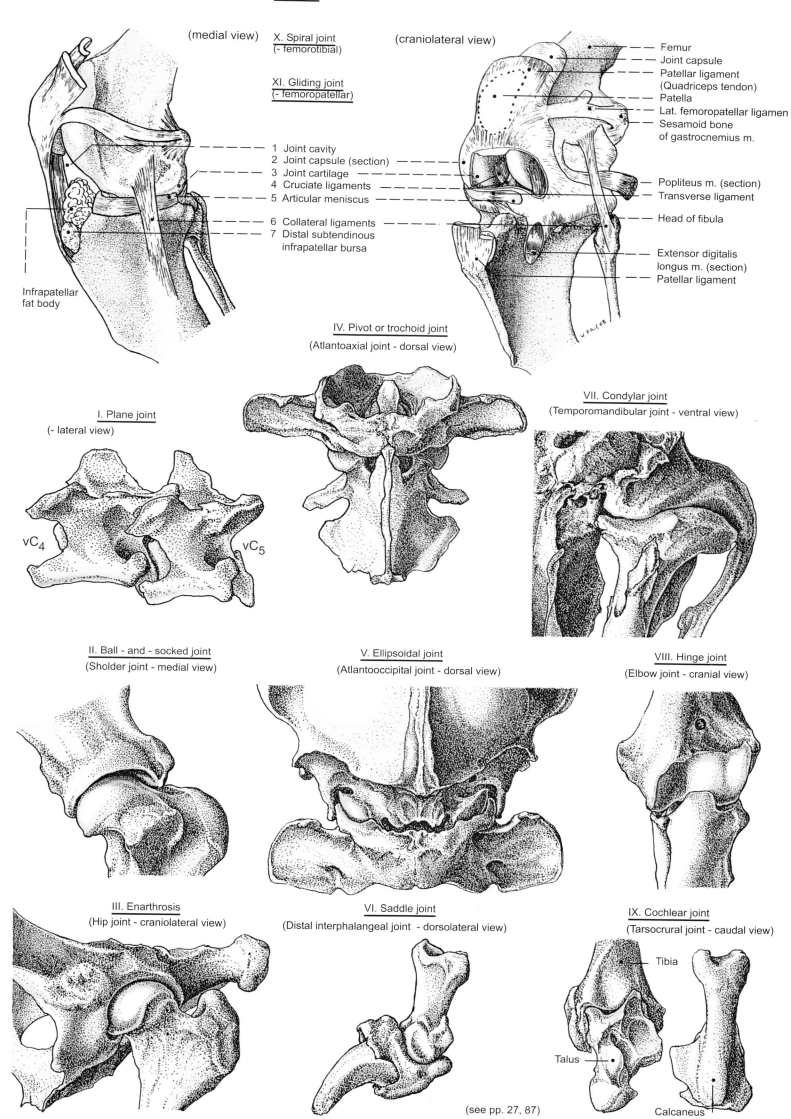

Stifle joint

(medial view)

X. Spiral joint
(- femorotibial)

XI. Gliding joint
(- femoropatellar)

(craniolateral view)

— Femur
— Joint capsule
— Patellar ligament
 (Quadriceps tendon)
— Patella
— Lat. femoropatellar ligamen
— Sesamoid bone
 of gastrocnemius m.

1 Joint cavity
2 Joint capsule (section)
3 Joint cartilage
4 Cruciate ligaments
5 Articular meniscus

— Popliteus m. (section)
— Transverse ligament

6 Collateral ligaments
7 Distal subtendinous
 infrapatellar bursa

— Head of fibula

Infrapatellar
fat body

— Extensor digitalis
 longus m. (section)
— Patellar ligament

IV. Pivot or trochoid joint
(Atlantoaxial joint - dorsal view)

VII. Condylar joint
(Temporomandibular joint - ventral view)

I. Plane joint
(- lateral view)

vC₄   vC₅

II. Ball - and - socked joint
(Sholder joint - medial view)

V. Ellipsoidal joint
(Atlantooccipital joint - dorsal view)

VIII. Hinge joint
(Elbow joint - cranial view)

III. Enarthrosis
(Hip joint - craniolateral view)

VI. Saddle joint
(Distal interphalangeal joint - dorsolateral view)

IX. Cochlear joint
(Tarsocrural joint - caudal view)

— Tibia

Talus

(see pp. 27, 87)

Calcaneus

143

4. MYOLOOGY: GENERAL MYOLOGY

The structural elements of muscle are the **muscle cells**, which are enveloped by connective tissue in an ideal manner. Muscle cells are able to contract, the result of the sliding of the muscle-filament bundles which they contain in such a way as to overlap one another. Three kinds of muscle tissue are distinguished on the basis of their fine structure and their physiological characteristics.

Muscle Type	Color	Cell Length	Cell Diameter	Innervation	Form of the Muscle
A. Cross-striated (striated or skeletal) muscle	reddish	up to 15 cm	ca. 0.1 mm	somatic nervous system	individual muscles variably shaped
B. Smooth (visceral), muscle	yellow-gray	ca. 0.1 mm	ca. 0.1 mm	autonomic nervous system	layers
C. Cardiac (heart) muscle	red-brown	ca. 0.1 mm	ca. 0.5 mm	autonomous rhythm regulated by the autonomic nervous system	layers

a) TYPES OF MUSCLE TISSUE:

The **cross-striation** of **skeletal** and **cardiac musculature** is based on the alignment of the contractile elements of the muscle cells, the myofilaments, and their different refraction of light. Cross-striation is lacking in the **smooth muscle cells** of the viscera.

I. Striated, skeletal, musculature (A) is not limited to the skeleton. A variant of cross-striated muscle of the visceral type is also present in portions of the viscera, the pharynx and esophagus. The striated cutaneous musculature also has no direct connection to the skeleton but is invested by the superficial fascia of the body and terminates in the skin where it functions to move and to tense the skin. The **smooth, visceral, musculature (B)** can also have connection to the skeleton, *e.g.*, the smooth rectococcygeus muscle passes from the rectum to the caudal vertebral column (see p. 73). The **cardiac, heart, musculature (C)** is present as the working musculature of the heart and as the impulse conducting system for cardiac contraction (see p. 47). The cardiac muscle also extends onto the first part of the pulmonary and caval veins, where they pass to the atria of the heart.

1 **II. The color** of striated skeletal musculature is more or less distinctly red. That of smooth muscle is yellowish gray and gives a typical color to the intestinal wall. The working muscle of the heart is continuously active and is of red-brown color.

III. The length of muscle cells in the three kinds of muscle is quite different. Striated skeletal muscle cells may reach a considerable length, up to 15 cm and an individual cell may possess several hundred nuclei. For this reason 2 and because of other structural peculiarities it is also called a *syncytium* (genesis by cell fusion) and a muscle *fiber*. The length of smooth muscle cells can vary considerably with change in physiological parameters; *e.g.*, in the gravid uterus, the length of cells can increase tenfold and more. The length of cardiac muscle cells is limited by the intercalated discs. The cardiac musculature can be regarded as a syncytium only in the functional view, but not morphologically.

IV. The innervation of skeletal musculature is by fast conducting myelinated 3 nerves across the motor end-plate (neuromuscular terminations). This takes place voluntarily (the striated esophageal musculature is an exception and is 4 supplied involuntarily by the vagus nerve; see p. 48). The smooth visceral musculature contracts slowly (maintenance muscle) and is supplied involuntarily by slow-conducting unmyelinated nerve fibers of the autonomic nervous system. The smooth muscle of the uterus also contracts under the influence of the hormone oxytocin that is released by the neural lobe of the hypophysis. (Stimulation and innervation of the heart, see p. 46.) Spontaneous contractions of visceral smooth muscle can be triggered by stretch-stimuli, for example, in the wall of lymph vessels. Every striated skeletal muscle cell receives its innervation at a motor end-plate. In contrast to this, smooth muscle and heart muscle cells are directly stimulated only in isolation. Stimulation is conducted from these to neighboring cells across electrical synapses *(nexus)*.

V. The form of muscles varies greatly and is dependent on topography and function. Cross-striated skeletal muscle is represented in the body with about 250 individual muscles. Smooth muscle cells and heart muscle cells are chiefly found as layers.

b) CROSS-STRIATED SKELETAL MUSCULATURE is discussed in the

following with respect to its mesoscopic-microscopic anatomy. Each muscle cell is bounded by a plasmalemma (sarcolemma), external to which is a basal lamina and fine **collagen fibrils (12)** and **reticular fibers (13)**. The latter radiate into the surrounding tissue, between neighboring muscle cells, as **endomysium (11)**. Several neighboring muscle fibers form a **primary muscle fiber bundle (10)**. A muscle fiber bundle is the 'meat fiber' that is visible to the naked eye and is invested by the **internal perimysium (9)**. Several primary bundles are united by the **external perimysium (8)** to form a **secondary bund-**

le **(3)**. Finally, all secondary bundles, the entire muscle, are invested by a **loose layer of collagenous fibers, the epimysium (7)**. The epimysium is followed by a **fascia (6)** that is a latticework of collagenous fibers chiefly and is only partially reinforced with elastic fibers.

I. The functions of the connective-tissue sheaths are multiple:

1. They serve to maintain the form of the muscle, providing a supporting function. 2. They function to permit parts of the muscle to contract while other parts remain uncontracted or less active. The muscle seldom acts with all of its contractile parts at the same time. Rather, utilizing the principle of conserving energy, only as many primary bundles are employed as are necessary to provide the required strength of contraction. The subdivision of the muscle by connective tissue sheaths makes possible the contraction of individual primary bundles in an optimal expenditure of energy. 3. The connective tissue coverings also provide a path for the vessels and nerves that supply the muscle. 4. Because the fascia is partially fused with the skeleton, it guides the direction of muscle action. 5. The connective-tissue coverings oppose a maximal contraction (thickening) of the muscle and an excessive use of strength, thus protecting the muscle from rupture. 6. The veins and lymphatic vessels in the fascia are compressed by the pressure of muscle contraction. By this, in cooperation with the valves, a proximal flow of blood and lymph is 5 fostered.

II. The myotendinous junction (14) is discontinuous (not all in one plane). The slightly undulating tendinous fibrils interweave with the sheath of reticular fibers. The attachment of the tendon-fibrils on the muscle cells takes place especially in the region of the finger-shaped muscle 'processes', which are the ends of muscle fiber bundles. This attachment is brought about by the fibrils anchoring across the endomysium and the basal lamina. The **insertion of the tendon on bone (1)** is dependent on the form of the tendon. In the case of attachment over a large area, the collagenous tendon fibers radiate into the network of collagenous fibers of the periosteum. The fibrous layer of the periosteum is anchored in the bone by Sharpey's fibers (*Fibrae perforantes*). Strong, round **tendons (2)** may perforate the periosteum with their collagenous fibers and terminate directly in the osseous tissue. In this case, strong forces are exerted on a relatively small area of the bone. In these places, avulsion fractures can occur in which a piece of bone with the tendon-attachment is torn out of the bone. The discontinuous muscle-tendon junction and the micro-undulation also serve to protect the muscle from rupture. They make possible a soft elastic pull.

III. The gross anatomical structure of a muscle, especially the mode of inser- 6 tion of its fibers on the tendon, permit conclusions as to its development of strength and its range of contraction. If the muscle has only simply formed tendons of origin and insertion that are connected by relatively few but long muscle fibers running diagonally from one tendon to another, then it is designated a **unipennate muscle (D)**. In a **bipennate (E)** or **multipennate muscle**, the tendons of origin and insertion are branched and more complex and connected by relatively many, but short, muscle fibers. The simple, unipennate muscle can carry out a large range of external, contraction; whereas, the bipennate and multipennate muscle can develop only a slight range of contraction. This is because the extent of shortening increases proportional to the length of the muscle fibers, which can shorten up to about half their length. It is the reverse situation with respect to the development of strength. Since the strength of a muscle is proportional to the number of its muscle fibers, the strength of a multipennate muscle is greater than a unipennate muscle. This is determined objectively by a comparison of the **anatomical diameter (4)** with the **physiological diameter (5)** of a muscle. The anatomical diameter cuts the entire muscle at its thickest point perpendicular to the muscle's longitudinal axis. The physiological diameter cuts the muscle fibers perpendicular to *their* longitudinal axis. In a unipennate muscle, the two diameters coincide. In a multipennate muscle, the physiological diameter is greater than the anatomical diameter.

Muscle tissue

Legend :

a Neuromuscular complex
b Neuromuscular termination

c Striated muscle cell
d Smooth muscle cell

e Cardiac muscle cell
f Intercalated disc

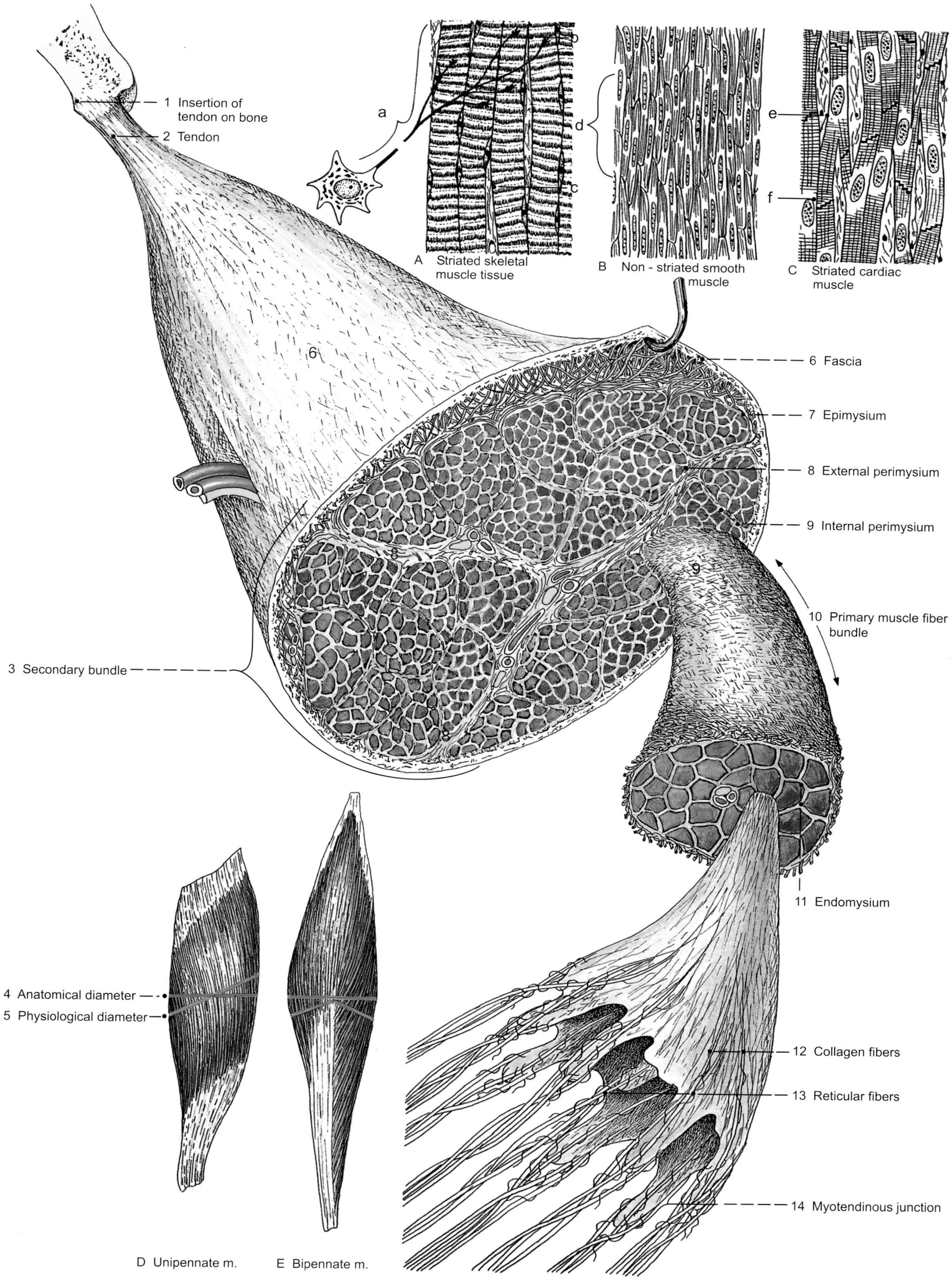

1 Insertion of
tendon on bone

2 Tendon

a

b

d

c

A Striated skeletal
muscle tissue

e

f

B Non - striated smooth
muscle

C Striated cardiac
muscle

6

6 Fascia

7 Epimysium

8 External perimysium

9 Internal perimysium

10 Primary muscle fiber
bundle

3 Secondary bundle

9

11 Endomysium

4 Anatomical diameter

5 Physiological diameter

12 Collagen fibers

13 Reticular fibers

14 Myotendinous junction

D Unipennate m.

E Bipennate m.

145

5. MYOLOGY: SKELETAL MUSCULATURE AND ITS ACCESSORY STRUCTURES

a) In the consideration of **SKELETAL MUSCULATURE**, muscle and tendons are discussed together since the two complement one another in structure and function.

I. In its typical spindle-shaped (fusiform) form, the **muscle** in respect of its shape is comparable to a small mouse and the term 'musculus' means 'small mouse.' Like the small mouse, the muscle has a head (**origin**, **−1**), a belly (**2**) and a tail (**insertion or termination**, **−4**). The tendon of origin is attached at a more fixed point on the skeleton (usually proximal on the body). The tendon of insertion ends at a more moveable point that is usually distal on the body. With some muscles, for example, on the vertebral column, origin and insertion are interchangeable. The origin and insertion of a muscle can be 'read' from the dissection specimen. With attention to both components and 'common sense' the function of a muscle can be determined in most cases. The function of different muscles may complement each other as *synergistic* muscles, *e.g.*, the powerful biceps brachii muscle is the synergist of the weaker brachialis muscle. Antagonistic muscles have opposing function. In a harmonious movement both synergists and antagonists act together. (Ventral flexion of the trunk is initiated by the abdominal muscles and 'slowed down' by the dorsal muscles to prevent a 'collapse.')

The **form of muscles**, regarded phylogenetically, is quite variable (progressive). It may go to the extent that a certain muscle in different species can appear very different so that in its form the muscle can no longer be identified with certainty.

Functionally the muscles are chiefly responsible for movement. In addition, auxiliary functions are present and serve for the maintenance of body processes such as respiration, defecation and urination. Beyond that, the muscles enable the animal to stand by stabilization and fixation of joints. In the case of shivering due to cold, the muscles produce heat for thermoregulation.

II. The **tendon (3)** is usually adapted to the form of the muscle belly. Fusiform muscles have round tendons; whereas, on the other hand, broad, parallel-fibered muscle bellies pass over into broad, parallel-fibered tendons, and the latter are called **aponeuroses (5)**. (That term should not be confused with fascia, which is formed as a lattice-like fibrous structure.) In addition to the tendon of origin and tendon of insertion, the term **central tendon** (see p. 145) is mentioned here. This tendon can be seen on the multipennate muscle. Central tendons are within the muscle, therefore in the flesh. They diminish the quality of the meat as food. The surface of a tendon glistens and has a silvery appearance. Muscle bellies that lie one behind the other are connected by a **tendinous intersection (6)**. Muscles having an extended area of origin or insertion without the obvious interposition of a well-defined tendon can in macroscopic appearance begin or end by a 'fleshy' attachment. Microscopically, however, one can ascertain that there are many very fine tendons. The form of muscles and tendons as well as their function is in many cases reflected in the name of the muscle (*e.g.*, **M. serratus, −B**, the serrate muscle; **M. digastricus, −C**, the two-bellied muscle; **M. bi- or quadriceps, −D**, the two- or four-headed muscle; **M. extensor, −A**, the extensor muscle; **M. orbicularis, −E**, the ring-shaped muscle; functional name: **M. sphincter**).

The **cutaneous muscles** are usually pale variants of skeletal muscle having little myoglobin and no direct attachment to the skeleton. They are chiefly located between layers of the superficial fascia. They end by short tendons in the cutis, thus moving and tensing the skin when they contract.

III. The **fasciae** invest individual muscles as a lattice-like structured covering (dense connective tissue covering, see p. 145). With the swelling of the belly of the muscle in contraction, the crossing fibers can be seen and a change in their rhombus-like configuration can be observed. The more extensive fasciae invest groups of muscles and separate them from neighboring groups. Insofar as the fascia has connection to underlying bones, there are formed osteofibrous compartments that establish the position and direction of individual muscles and muscle groups. Muscles may also arise or end in fascia, bringing about reinforcement of the fascial fibers in the direction of muscle pull. The large fasciae of the body form the external and internal fasciae that lie external or, respectively, internal to the outer and inner muscle layers of the trunk that have attachment to bone and invest the body cavities. The external fascia of the trunk is subdivided into the superficial and deep fascia of the trunk. The superficial fascia of the trunk corresponds to the subcutis and is in relation to the cutaneous muscles where they are developed (trunk, neck, head). The deep fascia of the trunk lies in the body wall directly upon the thoracic and abdominal muscles and separates the individual muscles

with a layer of fascia (e.g., the thoracolumbar fascia, which with its fascial layers insinuates between the muscles of the vertebral column). On the limbs, the antebrachial and crural fasciae form reinforcements, the **retinacula (8)**, for passing tendons, which in this way are held fixed in position. The fasciae are relatively impermeable to fluids as, for example, extravasates or pus that migrate along the fascia and may break through the surface of the body far from the focus of the disease.

IV. The **blood vessels** and nerve of the muscle enter together at the **hilus (7)**. The vessel branches run mostly in the longitudinal axis of a muscle, predominantly in the internal and external perimysium. Blood capillaries are chiefly observed in the endomysium. Four to eight capillaries surround a single muscle cell. The blood supply varies according to the muscle type and, in relation to the high energy requirement of muscle, is generally more intensive in the muscle belly than in the sparsely vascularized tendon. The intensive vascularization provides the drainage of metabolic end-products and temperature regulation; since the veins, utilizing the principle of a tubular water-cooling system (the automobile water-cooling system), take up the heat produced and give it off at the surface of the body by way of the cutaneous veins.

V. The **innervation** of most muscles is provided by a single nerve. Only the long muscles of the trunk (e.g., the longissimus dorsi muscle), which embryologically develop from several myotomes, are supplied by multiple nerves. Also such muscles that were formed by fusion of two individual muscles during phylogenesis have a double innervation (e.g., in the dog, the adductor longus and pectineus muscles are fused but the muscles are completely separate in the cat). The nerve of a muscle ramifies in the same manner as the blood vessels in the peri- and endomysium. It consists of myelinated, thick (alpha) and thin (gamma) motoneurons, unmyelinated autonomic fibers and myelinated sensory fibers. A thick motoneuron (large multipolar nerve cell with dendrites within the ventral column of the spinal cord and its peripheral process = axon) and the muscle fibers innervated by it form a motor unit. In muscles with finely adjusted movements (e.g., the muscles that move the eye) only a few small muscle fibers belong to a motor unit. In contrast to this, in the larger muscles of the limb several hundred (perhaps in some cases a thousand or more) muscle fibers form a single motor unit. The thin gamma motoneurons innervate the modified muscle cells of the neuromuscular spindle. The unmyelinated nerve fibers innervate the blood vessels within the muscles. The sensory fibers have their origin in pain receptors and in the neuromuscular and neurotendinous spindle receptors that provide information on the tonus of the muscle. Muscle and nerve form a unit. Each muscle is stimulated to contract by a motor nerve by way of the motor endplate. If the muscle is frequently stimulated to contract, then its fibers become physiologically thicker. The result is muscle hypertrophy. The opposite is the atrophy of inactivity. The functional-anatomical unity of muscle and its associated nerve is so intimate that it is scarcely changed in the ascending development that takes place in phylogenesis (conservative behavior). Regarded from the point of view of comparative anatomy, it is clear that a certain muscle even in a different species has its special nerve. For this reason, the nerve is utilized as an important criterion in determining the homology of muscles as only in rare case does it give up an already formed unity.

b) The **AUXILIARY STRUCTURES OF MUSCLES** including their tendons are the **synovial bursae** and the **synovial sheaths of tendons**, which like joint capsules are lined internally by **synovial membrane (10)** and contain synovia. This synovia is modified in comparison to that of the joint. The outer layer is the **fibrous layer (11)**. Like the sesamoid bones, synovial bursae and synovial sheaths have the function of protecting the tendon, which because of pressure or rubbing as it passes upon hard and pointed underlying bone can be crushed or splayed. If the mechanical insults come only from one direction, a synovial bursa is interposed. For the protection of the total surface of the tendon synovial sheaths are formed that are chiefly present at the carpus and tarsus. If the synovial bursae are subcutaneously located (**subcutaneous synovial bursa, −9**), then they are usually acquired; if subtendinous (**subtendinous synovial bursa, −15**) or submuscular, then they are usually inherited. The synovial sheath improves the gliding of a tendon upon a bony prominence. The wall of a synovial sheath consists of a **parietal part (12)**, which passes over into a **tendinous part (13)**, by way of the **mesotendineum (14)**, a mesentery-like intermediate part that conveys blood and lymph vessels and nerves. The fibrous layer of the tendinous part is thin and identical to the connective tissue cover of the tendon. Common tendon-sheaths form a gliding cover for several tendons.

Myology, synovial bursae and sheaths

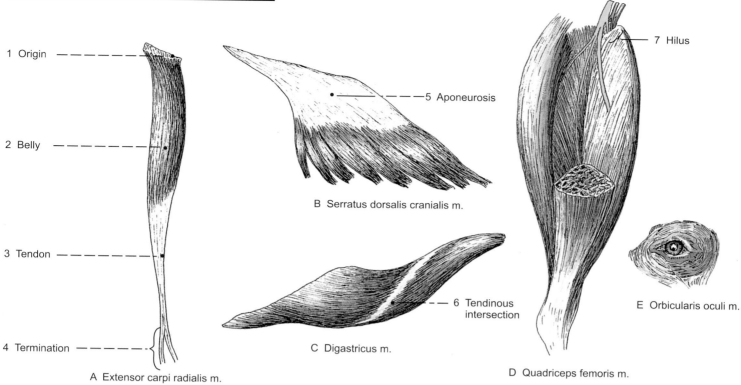

1 Origin

2 Belly

3 Tendon

4 Termination

A Extensor carpi radialis m.

5 Aponeurosis

B Serratus dorsalis cranialis m.

6 Tendinous intersection

C Digastricus m.

7 Hilus

D Quadriceps femoris m.

E Orbicularis oculi m.

Synovial sheath of tendon

Synovial bursae of calcaneus

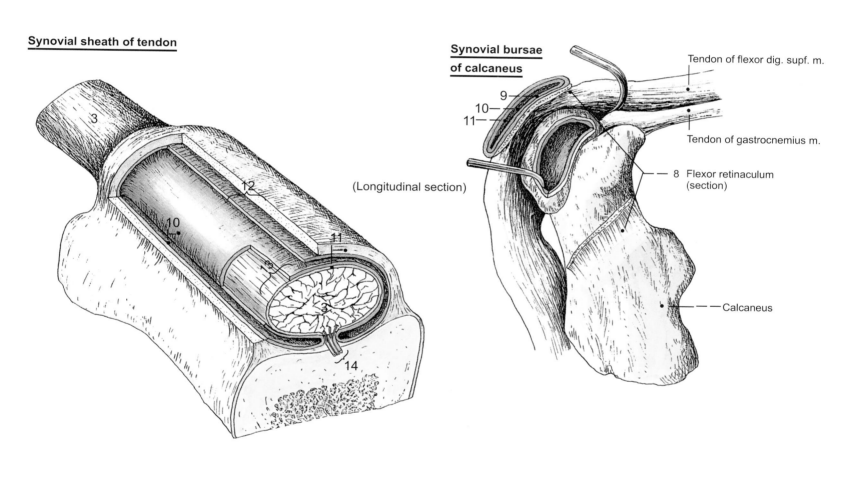

Tendon of flexor dig. supf. m.

Tendon of gastrocnemius m.

8 Flexor retinaculum (section)

(Longitudinal section)

Calcaneus

(Transverse section)

(Transverse section)

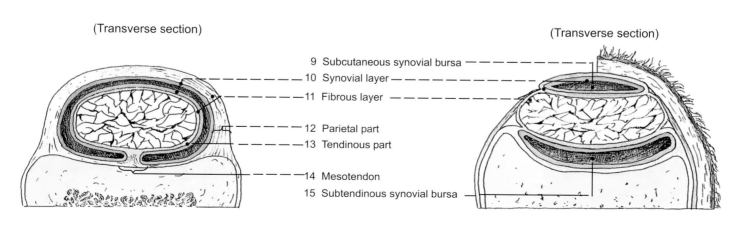

9 Subcutaneous synovial bursa

10 Synovial layer

11 Fibrous layer

12 Parietal part

13 Tendinous part

14 Mesotendon

15 Subtendinous synovial bursa

6. NERVOUS SYSTEM

Nervous tissue consists of **nerve cells** with their **processes**; nerve cells are also called **neurons** and are surrounded by neuroglial cells. Neurons are excitable and are able to receive impulses, to conduct and modify them as well as to discharge impulses in a modified form. In this way the nervous system regulates the coordination of internal body functions, especially of the internal organs, and facilitates the interaction of the organism with the environment (uptake and conduction of stimuli from the skin and sensory organs to the central nervous system) by way of the afferent part of the reflex arc as well as the response to stimuli by way of the efferent part of the central nervous system to the effectors of the body, muscle and gland.

The division of the nervous system can be according to topographical as well as functional criteria. According to **topographical criteria** it is subdivided into the **central nervous system (CNS)** and the **peripheral nervous system (PNS)**. Using **functional criteria** it is subdivided into the **somatic nervous system** and the **autonomic (vegetative) nervous system**. In both classifications, the nervous system belongs partially to the CNS and partially to the PNS.

The autonomic (involuntary) nervous system is classified according to the neurotransmitter, and according to its origin and its topography into sympathetic and parasympathetic systems, which often have opposite effects on the effector organ (heart muscle, smooth muscle, and gland). Both systems are efferent, conducting the outflow from the CNS (central nervous system) to heart muscle, smooth muscle and the glands of the body. Some consider the autonomic system to include afferent (sensory) nerves of the viscera (see p. 49); but in general the autonomic nervous system is regarded today as a strictly efferent system.

The somatic (voluntary) nervous system makes possible interaction with the environment, both external (outside the body) and internal (within the body). The activities are at least partially conscious (the organism is aware of the stimulus). Insofar as they are unconscious (the organism is unaware of the stimulus), they can nevertheless be influenced by voluntary action.

a) TOPOGRAPHICAL SUBDIVISION OF THE NERVOUS SYSTEM

I. The **central nervous system** is composed of the brain and the spinal cord. In both parts there is a **gray substance (15)** and a **white substance (16)**. Within the gray substance are the cell bodies (perikarya) of the nerve cells, which are surrounded by the neuropil (the complex of glial cells and nerve fibers). The white substance is characterized mainly of tracts or fasciculi composed of myelinated fibers, the phospholipid of which is strikingly white. In the cerebral hemispheres and cerebellum, the gray substance is located in the main peripherally as cerebral or, respectively, cerebellar cortex; whereas, the white substance is chiefly central. It is the reverse in the spinal cord. The gray substance of the cord forms the typical central butterfly-figure and is surrounded by the peripheral white substance in which the tracts and fasciculi that pass to or from the brain. Oligodendrocytes (glial cells) form the myelin sheaths that, with their enclosed axons, compose the white substance of the central nervous system. A single oligodendroglial cell regularly invests axons of several nerve cells (see clinical-functional anatomy).

II. The **peripheral nervous system** is composed of all neural parts that lie outside the superficial glial limiting membrane of the central nervous system (12 cranial, 8 cervical, 13 thoracic, 7 lumbar, 3 sacral and about 5 caudal nerves). The peripheral nervous system integrates chiefly parts of the somatic nervous system but contain also autonomic fibers.

The **peripheral nerves** are composed of bundles of **nerve fibers**. The nerve fiber (7) consists of an axon and its investment. The nerve cell body with its processes is called a **neuron (3)**. The **nerve cell body (4)** commonly gives off several **dendrites (5)**, but always a single **axon (6)** or neurite. The single axon usually branches, its branches being designated *collaterals*. The single dendrite of an **afferent (sensory) neuron** proceeds from a receptor and conducts stimuli always in one direction, toward the cell body. The impulse is then conveyed by way of the axon to the spinal cord. The **axon of motor neurons** originates at an expanded part of the perikaryon, the **axon hillock**, which is free of tigroid substance (chromatophil substance). From the cell body, the axon conducts the impulse to the effector organ (muscle or gland). In many nerve fibers, the axon can be up to 1 m in length and is invested by a myelin sheath (**myelinated nerve fiber, —25**). Between **RANVIER's nodes (8)** of the nerve fiber, the myelin sheath is formed by a single peripheral **SCHWANN (neurolemmal) cell (23)**. External to the SCHWANN cell, there is the endoneural sheath (cytoplasm of the SCHWANN cell, basal lamina and concentrically arranged fine reticular fibrils) and the **endoneurium (20**, loosely arranged fine-fibered connective tissue that lies between the individual nerve fibers). At the proximal and distal end of the SCHWANN cell, the myelin sheath ends and leaves the axon exposed in the region of the RANVIER node that is located there. The nodes are a precondition for the saltatory conduction of stimuli (the stimulus 'jumps' from node to node). The nerve fibers form bundles that are surrounded by **perineurium** (a continuation of the spinal arachnoid, see p. 109) with an external **fibrous part (21)** and an internal lining of **neurothelium (22)**. Several nerve bundles form a peripheral nerve, which is covered superficially by **epineurium (19**, — a continuation of the dura mater). From here a *paraneurium*, loose connective tissue with adipose tissue, radiates into the surrounding tissue and attaches the nerve to neighboring structures. In the case of an **unmyelinated nerve fiber (24)**, several axons are enclosed within invaginations of the plasmalemma of a peripheral glial cell (SCHWANN cell), but without forming a myelin sheath. A nerve may be composed of myelinated or unmyelinated or both types of fibers.

b) FUNCTIONAL SUBDIVISION OF THE NERVOUS SYSTEM

I. Insofar as the **spinal nerves** are concerned, the **somatic nervous system** has its nerve cell bodies (motoneurons) in the ventral column of the gray (butterfly) substance of the spinal cord and, insofar as the **cranial nerves** are concerned, ventrally in the brain stem. The conduction of impulses is from the central nervous system by way of **efferent nerve fibers** to the **ventral root (13)** of the spinal nerve and to the **motor** end-plate of skeletal muscle fibers (neuromuscular terminations).

Afferent (sensory) nerve fibers conduct impulses from receptors in the body over usually long dendrites to their nerve cell bodies. These are located in the **spinal ganglia (18)** near the spinal cord and the intervertebral foramen. From the spinal ganglion, the stimulus reaches the spinal cord by way of an axon in the **dorsal root (14)** of the spinal nerve. It reaches the dorsal column of the gray (butterfly) substance, and some axons continue cranially to the brain stem. The sensory fibers of most cranial nerves have their nerve cell bodies in ganglia near the foramina where the nerves leave the cranial cavity.

The **spinal nerves** can be subdivided into segmental and plexus nerves.

The **segmental nerves (9)** of the somatic nervous system (e.g., cranial iliohypogastric nerve) form together with neighboring nerves no plexus-like structures, but run as isolated nerves approximately parallel to each other. The segmental nerves can be classified into **dorsal (d)** and **ventral (v)** branches, and further into dorsomedial **(dm)** and dorsolateral **(dl)** branches or, respectively, ventromedial **(vm)** and ventrolateral **(vl)** branches.

The **plexus nerves** originate from **nerve plexuses (2**, —see also brachial plexus, p. 19, and lumbosacral plexus, p. 71). The nerve plexuses are formed by the communication (joining) of the **ventral branches** of several spinal nerves. The exchange of fibers between the individual ventral nerves forms the plexus from which the individual plexus nerves (e.g., **genitofemoral nerve, —1**) are formed. These are composed of nerve fibers from several spinal nerves (e.g., the genitofemoral nerve originates from nL 3 and 4). Corresponding to this, the individual spinal cord segment gives off nerve fibers to several plexus nerves (nL 3 to the lateral cutaneous femoral nerve and genitofemoral nerve, see p. 60). The **dorsal branches** of these spinal nerves take their course as typical segmental nerves.

II. The **autonomic nervous system** (see also p. 49) innervates with **efferent neurons** the heart, smooth musculature, and glands of the organs and vessels and guides and coordinates (regulates) the function of the internal organs. These activities are for the most part carried out without conscious control (the organism is not generally aware of them). The autonomic nervous system tends to form plexuses especially formed by sympathetic fibers. The autonomic plexuses are preferentially arranged around large arterial trunks and consist mainly of myelinated sensory and unmyelinated sympathetic and parasympathetic nerve fibers. In contrast to the spinal nerve plexuses, the autonomic plexuses also contain ganglia. For example, the **celiacomesenteric (solar) plexus** at the origin of the celiac and cranial mesenteric arteries also contains ganglia (celiac ganglion, cranial mesenteric ganglion) of the same name as the arteries. See p. 109. The efferent autonomic nervous system consists of a chain of two neurons that extend from the CNS to the peripheral effector. The nerve cell bodies of the proximal neurons are in the central nervous system. Their **preganglionic, myelinated fibers** pass in **white communicating rami (12)** to peripherally located **autonomic ganglia** (e.g., **ganglia of the sympathetic nerve trunk, —17**). Here, or more distal at the prevertebral ganglion (e.g., **cranial mesenteric ganglion, —10**), the synapse with the second neuron takes place. Nerve cell bodies in the abovementioned autonomic ganglia give rise to postganglionic, unmyelinated fibers. The **postganglionic, unmyelinated fibers** pass to effector organs within the viscera; or they pass in **gray communicating rami (11)** to the spinal nerves of the somatic nervous system with which they are distributed to the smooth muscle and glands of the skin and to the smooth muscle of peripheral vessels. The **afferent (visceral sensory) neurons** (regarded by some authors as a part of the autonomic nervous system) conduct impulses from the periphery to the central nervous system, for example, impulses having their origin in pain receptors of the viscera. Their cell bodies are also located in a spinal ganglion (ganglion of a spinal nerve) or a cranial ganglion (ganglion of a cranial nerve).

There is also the **intramural nervous system**, which is a constituent of the autonomic nervous system. It is in the wall of hollow organs (e.g., in the intestine, see p. 109; for details, see histology). Its nerve cell bodies belong predominantly to the parasympathetic nervous system. The intramural nervous system functions in the hollow organs as a self-regulating system for the movements of the intestine, movements which can take place even after isolation of the intestine.

Nervous system

Spinal cord (Lumbar part)

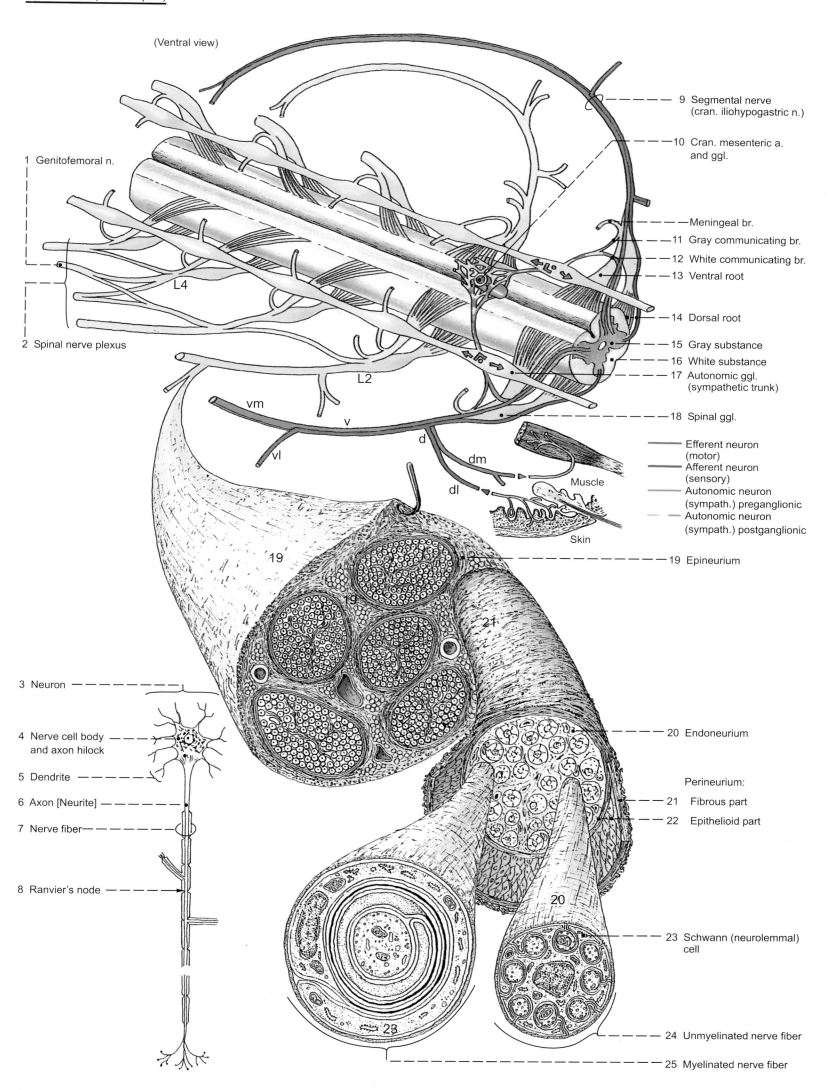

(Ventral view)

1 Genitofemoral n.

2 Spinal nerve plexus

L4

L2

vm

v

vl

d

dm

dl

Muscle

Skin

9 Segmental nerve
(cran. iliohypogastric n.)

10 Cran. mesenteric a.
and ggl.

Meningeal br.

11 Gray communicating br.

12 White communicating br.

13 Ventral root

14 Dorsal root

15 Gray substance

16 White substance

17 Autonomic ggl.
(sympathetic trunk)

18 Spinal ggl.

—— Efferent neuron
(motor)

—— Afferent neuron
(sensory)

—— Autonomic neuron
(sympath.) preganglionic

– – Autonomic neuron
(sympath.) postganglionic

19 Epineurium

20 Endoneurium

Perineurium:

21   Fibrous part

22   Epithelioid part

23 Schwann (neurolemmal)
cell

24 Unmyelinated nerve fiber

25 Myelinated nerve fiber

3 Neuron

4 Nerve cell body
and axon hilock

5 Dendrite

6 Axon [Neurite]

7 Nerve fiber

8 Ranvier's node

(see pp. 71, 109)

149

7. ENDOCRINE SYSTEM

The **endocrine system** comprises the endocrine glands (hormonal glands) and the endocrine secreting organs, which release hormones in addition to their proper function (*e.g.*, the gastrointestinal tract with its intestinal endocrine cells). The hormones belong to different chemical groups of compounds (*e.g.*, steroids, peptides, amines) and act even in very low concentration. In comparison to their effect, the endocrine glands appear remarkably small. Contrary to former opinion, a single cell type can form several hormones. The secreted hormones are messengers which influence the development of certain organs and coordinate different functions of the body in cooperation with the autonomic nervous system. The endocrine gland cells secrete their hormones usually into the intercellular space of their immediate surroundings. Here the hormone can act directly on the neighboring cells and tissues (*e.g.*, the hormones of the testicular interstitial cells, androgens, act directly on the neighboring seminiferous tubules) or, after their being taken up by the blood vascular and lymph vascular systems, the hormones are transported to distant receptor-bearing target cells (*e.g.*, the prostatic cells). To facilitate the uptake of hormones, the blood capillaries have a special structure of their endothelial wall, fenestrations. In this regard, the gonads are an exception in that they have a closed endothelial lining of their blood capillaries that assures the function of a blood-testis (gonad) barrier.

1 The **hypothalamo-hypophysial system (1)** is the central, superior endocrine regulating system that acts on peripheral endocrine glands by means of adenotropic hormones (*e.g.*, on the adrenal cortex, but not the adrenal medulla). Thus, the hypothalamo-hypophysial system with its regulating hormones acts by way of the peripheral endocrine secreting cells (*e.g.*, testicular interstitial cells) indirectly on the peripheral target cells or target organ (*e.g.*, the prostate gland). In addition, hypophysial effector-hormones are formed that act directly on peripheral cells or organs as, for example, prolactin hormone on the mammary gland.

a) The **HYPOTHALAMUS (1 g)** is a center superior to the hypophysis and intimately associated with the latter topographically, embryologically and functionally.

b) The **HYPOPHYSIS (*Hypophysis cerebri*)** develops with its **anterior lobe**, the **adenohypophysis**, from the ectoderm of the roof of the primitive stomodeum and migrates to the sphenoid bone where it attaches to the **posterior lobe** of the hypophysis, the **neurohypophysis**, which develops from the diencephalon of the brain.

I. Releasing hormones and release-inhibiting hormones are formed in the hypothalamus and act on the **adenohypophysis (1, a – c)**, controlling the release of the adenohypophysial hormones (tropins). These hypothalamic hormones are formed by nerve cells of the tuberal hypothalamic region, and transported to the median eminence within their axons. The axons form the tubero-infundibular tract (text-illustration c). The median eminence is a median, crescent-shaped prominence of the tuber cinereum that projects into the infundibulum of the third ventricle.

II. The **neurohypophysis (1, d – e)** receives its effector hormones (oxytocin and vasopressin = antidiuretic hormone) from the hypothalamus, where they are formed in the supraoptic and paraventricular nuclei. In the hypothalamus, the activity of the blood-brain barrier prevents the uptake of the hormones into the blood. They are transported from the location of synthesis, the hypothalamus, and according to the principle of neurosecretion are

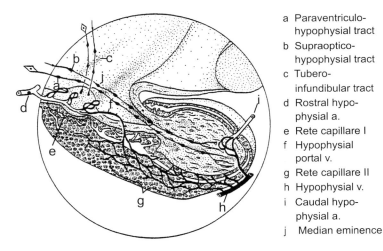

a Paraventriculo-hypophysial tract
b Supraoptico-hypophysial tract
c Tubero-infundibular tract
d Rostral hypo-physial a.
e Rete capillare I
f Hypophysial portal v.
g Rete capillare II
h Hypophysial v.
i Caudal hypo-physial a.
j Median eminence

The **venous portal system** (text-illustration, e – g) of the hypothalamo-hypophysial system facilitates the transport of the releasing hormones from the median eminence to the adenohypophysis. In association with this, the **rostral hypophysial artery (d)** in the **median eminence (j)** breaks up into a **(first) capillary net** (Rete capillare I, —e), which takes up the hypothalamic releasing hormones and transports them by way of the **hypophysial portal vein (f)** to the adenohypophysis, where they are released in a **(second) capillary net** (Rete capillare II, —g). Here, the regulating and effector hormones are also taken up into the bloodstream.

c) In dependence upon TSH (thyroid stimulating hormone) of the adenohypophysis, the **THYROID GLAND (2, a)**, with its hormones thyroxin (T4) and tri-iodothyronine (T3), in addition to others, stimulates cellular metabolism and regulates the growth of the body. The hormones are part of the thyroglobulins and are stored in the thyroid follicles (= store gland, suitable for storing hormones). In this condition the follicular epithelial cells are flattened. With increasing release of the secretion the epithelial cells become cuboidal or columnar. The parafollicular C-cells act on calcium metabolism and are antagonists of the **PARATHYROID GLAND (2, b)**. 2

d) The **ADRENAL GLAND (3)** is subdivided into an **adrenal cortex (a)** and an **adrenal medulla (b)**. The three zones of the adrenal cortex synthesize steroid hormones. In the subcapsular zone, *zona glomerulosa (arcuata)*, mineralocorticoids (aldosterone) are produced that act on the salt and water metabolism of the body. In the *zona fasciculata* (layer of cords and columns), which is central to the zona glomerulosa, glucocorticoids are produced. They function in carbohydrate metabolism. Representatives of this group of hormones are cortisone and hydrocortisone, which also have an anti-inflammatory action and are of paramount medical importance. The internal layer of the cortex is the *zona reticularis*, which produces androgens.

e) The **GONADS (TESTIS, —4A** and **OVARY, —4B)** with their **testicular interstitial cells (4A, b)**, also called Leydig's interstitial cells, and the **ovarian interstitial cells (4B, b**, also called theca interna cells) and the **corpus luteum (4B, c)** are the target cells of the adenohypophysial luteinizing hormone (LH). They synthesize androgens with testosterone and hydrotestosterone as their most important representatives. In the ovary the androgens in the follicular epithelial cells of the ovarian follicles are aromaticized to estrogens. Luteinizing hormone fosters the genesis of the corpus luteum.

Follicle-stimulating hormone (FSH) of the adenohypophysis stimulates the growth of secondary and tertiary follicles in the ovary as well as (jointly with LH) the synthesis of estrogens and androgens. In the testis it stimulates the Sertoli cells among others to produce androgen-binding proteins. Furthermore, it promotes the formation of LH-receptors on the Leydig interstitial cells.

f) In the second half of pregnancy, the **PLACENTA (4C)** takes over the formation of progesterone and estrogen, which previously were produced by the corpus luteum of the ovary. The change takes place about the middle of pregnancy. Because the production of progesterone by the corpus luteum ceases, only the placenta functions to protect pregnancy.

g) The **EPIPHYSIS CEREBRI (PINEAL GLAND) (5)** synthesizes melatonin and antigonadotropin (see clinical-functional anatomy).

h) In the **KIDNEYS** the **modified cells of the tunica media (6, a)** of the afferent glomerular arteriole, which form part of the **juxtaglomerular complex (6)**, produce renin and thus control renal vascularization, and the blood pressure of the entire body. 4

i) The **PANCREATIC ISLETS (7, a)** of human beings are 1 – 2 million in number. Their B-cells promote the formation of glycogen by synthesis of insulin and, in this way lower the blood pressure. The A-cells synthesize glucagon, which raises the blood pressure. In addition, the D-cells produce hormones that belong to the group of gastrointestinal hormones. 5

j) The **GASTROINTESTINAL ENDOCRINE CELLS (8, a)** are scattered between the epithelial cells of the mucous membrane of the gastrointestinal tract.

transported by the axons of the paraventriculo-hypophysial and supraoptico-hypophysial tract (text-illustration, a and b) to the neurohypophysis. Here the blood-brain barrier is absent and the hormones are taken up by fenestrated blood capillaries and further transported by the blood vascular system. Vasopressin (= antidiuretic hormone) fosters the reabsorption of water from the renal tubules and increases the blood pressure. Oxytocin acts on the myoepithelial cells at the periphery of the end pieces of the sweat and mammary glands and also on the smooth musculature of the uterus, where it triggers its contractions at the termination of pregnancy.

Endocrine system

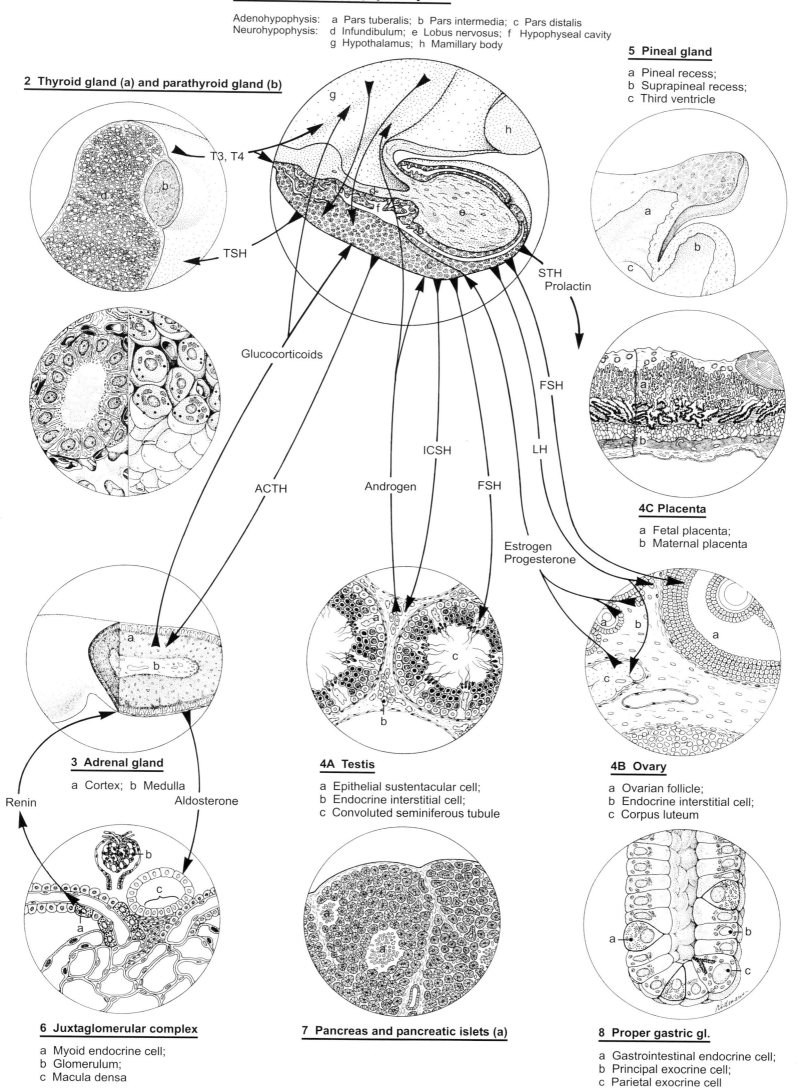

1 Hypothalamo - hypophyseal system

Adenohypophysis: a Pars tuberalis; b Pars intermedia; c Pars distalis
Neurohypophysis: d Infundibulum; e Lobus nervosus; f Hypophyseal cavity
g Hypothalamus; h Mamillary body

5 Pineal gland

a Pineal recess;
b Suprapineal recess;
c Third ventricle

2 Thyroid gland (a) and parathyroid gland (b)

T3, T4

TSH

STH
Prolactin

Glucocorticoids

FSH

LH

ICSH

ACTH

Androgen

FSH

4C Placenta

a Fetal placenta;
b Maternal placenta

Estrogen
Progesterone

Renin

Aldosterone

3 Adrenal gland

a Cortex; b Medulla

4A Testis

a Epithelial sustentacular cell;
b Endocrine interstitial cell;
c Convoluted seminiferous tubule

4B Ovary

a Ovarian follicle;
b Endocrine interstitial cell;
c Corpus luteum

6 Juxtaglomerular complex

a Myoid endocrine cell;
b Glomerulum;
c Macula densa

7 Pancreas and pancreatic islets (a)

8 Proper gastric gl.

a Gastrointestinal endocrine cell;
b Principal exocrine cell;
c Parietal exocrine cell

8. THE CARDIOVASCULAR SYSTEM

In the cardiovascular system the blood reaches all regions of the body by the pumping action of the heart. In this way, the body is supplied with resorbable nutrients, oxygen, water and hormones; and waste products are removed and heat is transferred.

a) The **CARDIOVASCULAR SYSTEM** is divided into a systemic circulation, a pulmonary circulation, and several portal circulations. The large **systemic circulation** begins in the left ventricle of the heart and passes by means of the systemic arteries to the entire body, returning by systemic veins to the right heart. The smaller **pulmonary circulation** begins in the right ventricle of the heart and transports (deoxygenated) blood by the pulmonary trunk and arteries to the alveolar capillaries of the lung for gaseous exchange. Oxygen-enriched blood passes from the alveolar capillaries to the left atrium of the heart by means of the pulmonary veins. The **hepatic portal circulation** assures the functional blood supply of the liver (see also p. 58).

Organs like the heart, liver, and lungs have a dual blood supply: a **nutritive blood supply** that supplies the organ's tissues, and a **functional blood supply** by which the organ carries out its essential body functions.

b) The **BLOOD VESSELS** are classified according to the structure of their walls, which, in turn, depends on the blood pressure. Veins with a weaker wall (*e.g.*, veins of the limbs) will, after transplantation into the arterial system, (e.g., the coronary arterial system), develop bit by bit a typical arterial wall. The vessel wall consists of three layers. There are the **internal tunic or tunica intima (2)**, which consists of an endothelial lining, a collagen-fibered subendothelial layer and, in the case of arteries, an internal elastic membrane. The second layer is the **middle tunic, tunica media (3)**, which is composed of smooth muscle cells and a network of elastic fibers and borders on the external elastic membrane with a chiefly collagen-fibered **external tunic, tunica externa or adventitia (4)**. In the blood capillaries, these three layers are lacking. Capillaries consist exclusively of an endothelium with an incomplete investment by pericytes.

I. The **arteries** carry blood from the heart and, except for the pulmonary trunk and arteries, contain blood rich in oxygen. According to the composition of the tunica media, arteries are distinguished as **elastic arteries (1)**, **muscular arteries (11)**, and arteries of mixed type. The elastic arteries (aorta, brachiocephalic trunk) are near the heart and contain in their media less smooth muscle cells, but mainly fenestrated elastic membranes, which are responsible for the yellowish appearance of this type of artery. The coronary arteries and arteries distant to the heart are muscular arteries. Their media is composed predominantly of smooth muscle cells, and there are fewer elastic fibers. **End (terminal) arteries** (*e.g.*, cerebral arteries) are of considerable medical importance because they have no **collateral arteries (7)** and no anastomoses or insufficient anastomoses with adjacent arteries. It is for that reason that they are called end or terminal arteries (*e.g.*, the cerebral arteries) or functional terminal arteries (e.g., the coronary arteries). In case of occlusion of these terminal arteries, the surrounding tissue becomes necrotic (infarction). **Convoluted arteries** are special arteries that have a distinct tortuous, sometimes corkscrew-like course. They exist as helicine arteries in the penis and uncoil and stretch out at the time of erection. In the mesovarium, their occurrence does not depend on volume differences. Certain portions of the helicine arteries of the penis are structured according to the principle of 'blocking' **arteries**. They have a bloodstream regulating function insofar as their lumen can be totally closed by **myoid intimal cushions (6)**. In that case, the entire blood stream passes through the capillary bed (erection, see clinical-functional anatomy). Arteriovenous anastomoses regulate the blood flow. Only a few organs such as the kidney and brain need an even blood supply for their function. The blood supply of most organs, *e.g.*, the gastrointestinal tract, varies and its intensity is adapted to actual functional need. This hemodynamic is maintained in the first line by simple **arteriovenous anastomoses (5)**. In their active arterial initial part they are often structured like helicine arteries. The terminal venous part is not specially differentiated. In case of their being closed off, all of the blood flows through neighboring arterioles and the neighboring capillary area. When they are open, the blood bypasses the capillary bed and selects the more 'convenient' way of the wide-lumen anastomosis. **Glomerular arteriovenous anastomoses (8)** with very complicated structure occur in the digits and skin. Also, the first part of the arterial side of the anastomosis contains blocking mechanisms. The glomerular arteriovenous anastomoses are richly supplied by autonomic nerves. Their function is still not completely clear.

II. **Arterioles (9)** are smaller than 0.1 mm in diameter and contain in their tunica media only a few layers of spirally arranged smooth muscle cells. The precapillary arteriole contains only one layer of smooth muscle cells.

An **arterial rete mirabile** is a specialty insofar as it is located within the arterial branch of the cardiovascular system and is predirected to the proper arterial capillary bed (*e.g.*, rete mirabile of the feline maxillary artery).

III. In the **capillaries (10)** the layers of the wall are reduced to the internal layer. This consists of the endothelial lining, a basal lamina and a discontinuous layer of pericytes. The capillaries are up to 1 mm long and have a diameter of 3 – 10 microns. According to their endothelial lining the capillaries are classified into three types, which are adapted to corresponding functional requirements. **Unfenestrated endothelial cells (13)** form a continuous lining of the lumen of the capillary. This type of capillary is found in the musculature, skin and connective tissue. **Fenestrated endothelial cells (12)** abut neighboring endothelial cells without spaces between them, but have intracellular fenestrae or pores. Fenestrated capillaries occur in organs with intense metabolism such as the gastrointestinal tract, endocrine glands and the kidneys. A **discontinuous endothelium with openings between the endothelial cells (intercellular apertures, —14)** and having a discontinuous or absent basal lamina is found in the sinusoids of the liver, where the presence of the fenestrae improves the passage of metabolites.

IV. **Venules (16)** are located at the beginning of the venous branch of the cardiovascular system and have a diameter up to about 50 microns. The tunica media has no myocytes but pericytes. In the collagen-fibered external tunic, white blood cells and macrophages are often found. The **postcapillary venules (17)** of some lymphatic organs are characterized by a cuboidal or columnar endothelium, which facilitates the penetration of lymphocytes from the vessel lumen into the perivascular lymphoreticular tissue.

V. **Veins** are more loosely structured in comparison to the arteries and their layers are less distinct. In the middle-sized veins, spirally arranged muscle fiber bundles with intermediate collagen-fibered connective tissue are located in the tunica media. In the large veins (for example, the caudal vena cava) the external tunic is especially distinct. It contains a lot of smooth muscle in longitudinal arrangement. In contrast to this, only a few muscle cell bundles are present in the tunica media.

The **venous valves (18)** project as semilunar endothelial duplications into the lumen. They cover a central layer of connective tissue. The valves regulate the direction of blood flow. During the initial phase of blood stasis, the semilunar valves fill and their borders approach those of neighboring valves. In this way, the lumen is occluded and a back flow of blood is prevented.

Occluding veins (*e.g.*, those in the liver) are special veins in endocrine glands, uterus, uterine tube, cavernous bodies and the liver that, by the development of intimal cushions, function as their name indicates.

Venous plexuses are venous networks and are found, for example, in the testicular vein as a pampiniform plexus. This functions in thermoregulation.

Venous sinuses are wide-lumened outpouchings of the veins (e.g., at the mouth of the caval veins). The sinuses of the dura mater of the brain are special veins with a wide lumen. They have no tunica media and outer layer in their walls and lack valves.

VI. **Vasa vasorum (15)** are nutritive blood vessels in the walls of the large arteries, veins and lymphatic trunks. On account of their size, these vessels cannot be nourished sufficiently by the blood within the vessel lumen. Smaller vessels have on the other hand a 'self-supply' from the bloodstream.

VII. The **nerves of vessels (15)** are for the most part unmyelinated and belong to the autonomic nervous system. Vasoconstriction is under control of the sympathetic nervous system. (For innervation and the action of hormones on the vessels, see textbooks of physiology.)

Cardiovascular system

Arteries

Veins

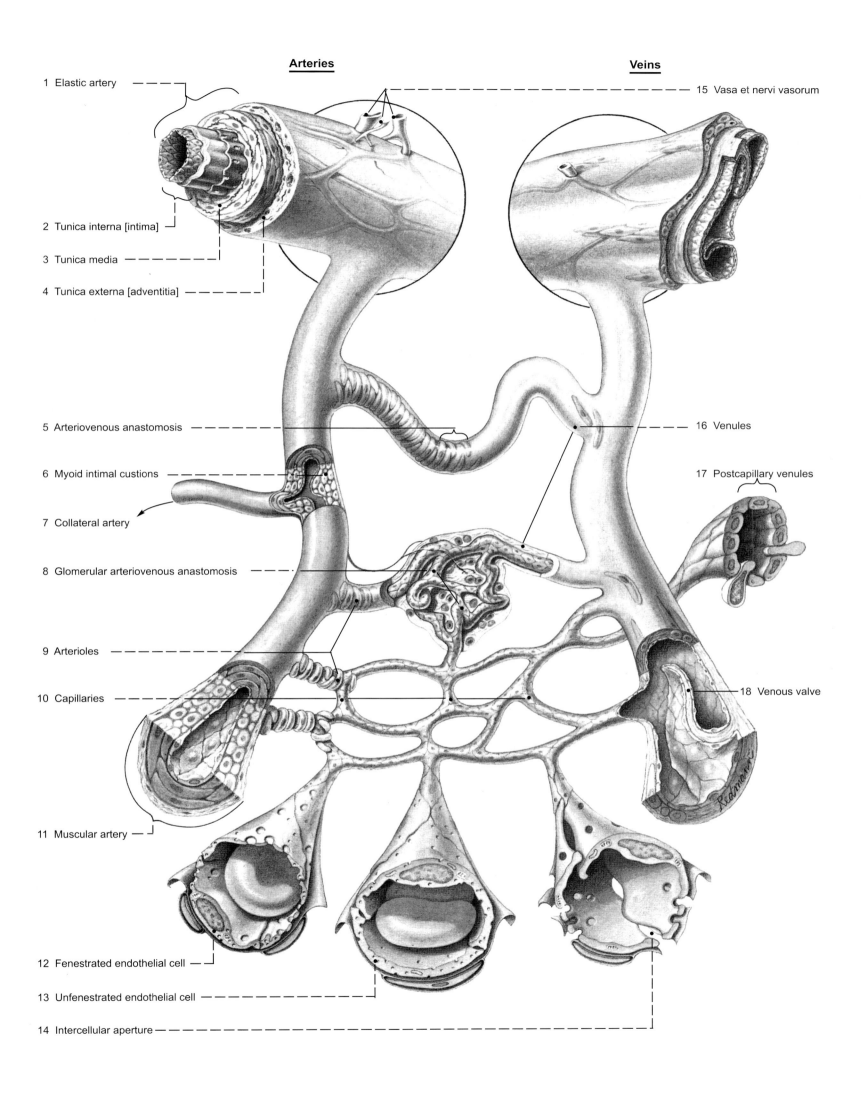

1 Elastic artery

2 Tunica interna [intima]

3 Tunica media

4 Tunica externa [adventitia]

5 Arteriovenous anastomosis

6 Myoid intimal custions

7 Collateral artery

8 Glomerular arteriovenous anastomosis

9 Arterioles

10 Capillaries

11 Muscular artery

12 Fenestrated endothelial cell

13 Unfenestrated endothelial cell

14 Intercellular aperture

15 Vasa et nervi vasorum

16 Venules

17 Postcapillary venules

18 Venous valve

153

9. LYMPHATIC SYSTEM

The **lymphatic system** is composed of a defense or immune system and a transport system (lymph vessel system), which complement each other functionally. The defense system includes the recognition and elimination of substances foreign to the body. It consists of the lymph nodes and the lymphatic organs.

a) The **LYMPH VASCULAR SYSTEM** has a drainage function to remove fluid from the tissues and a transport function to transport the lymph to the lymph nodes and finally to the venous side of the cardiovascular system. In contrast to the cardiovascular system, the lymph vascular system is not a closed circulation; as it begins peripherally by a network of blind capillaries (*Rete lymphocapillare*, −1) and ends centrally at the thoracic inlet at the so-called venous angle. The venous angle is the angle formed by the confluence of the internal and external jugular veins (see p. 15). With the absence of a central pump — lymph hearts are found only in the lower vertebrates and some avian species— the transport capacity is only 0.035% of that of the cardiovascular system. The lymph is generally a clear, yellowish fluid, but milky in color in the intestinal region owing to its fat content (chylomicrons). Lymph originates from the blood and reaches the interstitium by passing through the blood capillary wall. From here the tissue fluid flows to the venous part of the capillary bed or into the lymph capillaries, where by fluid back-flow – therefore concentration – lymph arises. A lymph drainage and therefore a lymphatic capillary network is lacking in the central nervous system, in cartilage, bone marrow, thymus and in the cornea of the eye. With the ordinary light microscope, lymph capillaries cannot be distinguished with certainty from blood capillaries. However, this is clearly possible with the electron microscope and the ultrastructure of lymph capillaries will be considered in detail here for a better understanding of their function.

I. From the endothelial cells of the **lymph capillaries (22)**, especially from their overlapping processes, very fine **fixation-fibers (24)** radiate into the interstitium and anchor to the **plexus of collagenous fibers (25)**. In spite of these fixation-filaments the lymph capillaries are often found collapsed. In case of an increased interstitial pressure (increased amounts of fluid in the tissue — lymph edema) the fixation-filaments are stretched, thus fixing the external layer of the overlapping endothelial cells. The internal layer of the endothelial cells is pushed toward the lumen by the in-streaming fluid and, in this way, interendothelial openings **(open junctions, −23)** are temporarily formed. These are very large by electron microscopic standards and considerable amounts of fluid and also macromolecules, dust, viruses, bacteria and complete tumor cells are able to enter the lymph capillaries. Also metabolic products, hormones and, in the intestine, long-chain fatty acids in the form of triacylglycerides as constituents of the chylomicrons are carried away by the lymph vessels. Summarized, it can be said that such stuff can successfully enter through the 'open junctions' of the lymph capillaries that, on account of their size, would be unable or scarcely able to pass through the blood capillary walls. An earlier concept that the processes of the lymph capillary network have openings must on closer examination be made precise insofar as such openings occur only if the intestitial pressure is increased, and that the openings are not permanently present. Quite another situation is present in the diaphragmatic pleura and peritoneum, where real stomata are found that open and close in synchrony with the respiratory rhythm by passive 'snap'-movements and promote the transport of the lymph.

II. Postcapillary lymph vessels (*Vasa lymphatica fibrotypica*, −26) are also called conducting vessels because they 'direct' the lymph flow by their valves and 'lead' it to the mouth of the myotypic lymphatic vessel that follows. Apart from the valves, the structure of the wall corresponds to that of the lymph capillaries.

III. The lymph vessels that follow the postcapillary lymph vessels have muscular walls (*Vasa lymphatica myotypica*, −27). These transport-vessels, usually accompany blood vessels and nerves and conduct the lymph to the lymph node. The transport-vessels have a three-layered wall: the lumen-sided, endothelium-containing **tunica interna** or **tunica intima (28)**, the muscle-containing **tunica media (29)** and the mainly fibrous **tunica externa** or **tunica adventitia (30)**. Valve-bearing, indented segments without muscle in their wall or poor in muscle, alternate periodically with valveless expansions with walls rich in muscle. When abundantly filled with lymph, this gives rise to the typical 'pearl- chain' appearance. The indentations at the **segmental valves (36)** bound a **lymphangion (2)**. At the mouth of the lymph vessels, where they discharge their lymph, **conjunctional valves (35)** are found.

IV. The **lymphatic vascular trunks (20)** are the thoracic duct, the cisterna chyli and the lumbar, intestinal and jugular trunks. They receive the transport-vessels. Their final parts, the thoracic and jugular ducts, open at the venous angle. The three-layered wall exhibits longitudinal muscle bundles, especially in the adventitia, and contains **vasa and nervi vasorum (21)**.

The **valves of the lymph vessels** and their musculature are the morphological basis for their proper peristalsis with proximally directed lymph flow. This is supported also by other factors such as 'massage' by adjacent striated muscles and also by the pulsations of surrounding arteries, which is carried over to the lymph vessels by figure-of-eight connective tissue bundles (see text-illustration). In the body cavities, the motor activity of the gastrointestinal tract and variations in respiratory pressure foster movement of the lymph. After the surgical removal of a lymph node, the lymph flow is at first interrupted. Peripheral to the site of interruption, the body region is devoid of its lymph drainage and by this flooded (edematous). When palpated it feels cold and 'doughy.' Skin impressions are compensated only very slowly at those parts of the body which are somewhat misshapen. Lymph flow is restored by the gradual growing together of the separated stumps.

b) The **LYMPH NODES (8)** are designated topographically (*e.g.*, axillary lymph node). Regional lymph nodes and lymph centers are distinguished.

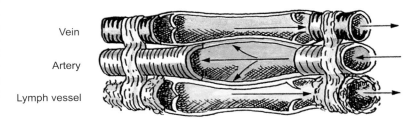

Vein

Artery

Lymph vessel

[Effect of the arterial pulse on lymphatic and venous transport]

The primary lymph of a certain tributary area flows to the regional lymph node by **afferent lymphatic vessels (9)**. Two to four **efferent lymphatic vessels (17)** leave the lymph node at its hilus and contain secondary or transitory lymph that contains about tenfold the number of lymphocytes. Lymph nodes farther on in the series, which are arranged like a chain, filter the secondary lymph and can, in addition, take up primary lymph. Adjacent lymph nodes with comparable, overlapping tributary regions are designated a lymph center. Lymph nodes have a smooth and firm surface. Their form is bean-like. They are usually embedded in fat tissue and surrounded by a **connective tissue capsule (10)**, which is penetrated at its **hilus (14)** by blood vessels and also (in the dog and most other species; *cf.* pig) efferent lymph vessels and at its convexity by afferent vessels. From the capsule, there radiate centrally directed **trabeculae (11)**. Underneath the capsule, the afferent lymph vessels open into the **subcapsular sinus (12)**, which transports the lymph by **intermediate sinuses (13)** that pass beside the trabeculae and **medullary sinuses (16)** that pass beside the medullary cords to the efferent vessels.

The **lymphatic sinuses (3)** are cleft-like lymph passages that are bounded by **endothelial cells (4)** and lumenally reinforced by a 'fish-trap-like' system of **reticular cells (6, −some authors consider these to be modified endothelial cells)** as well as by **intrasinusal reticular fibers (5)**. The 'fish-trap-like' system is able to trap particles of soot, viruses, bacteria, the body's own cells or cell detritus and thus enables their incorporation by the **intralumenal macrophages (7)**.

The parenchyma of the lymph node produces B-lymphocytes and plasma cells that function in humeral immunity. It consists of **lymphoreticular tissue (31)** with **reticular cells (32)** and **reticular fibers (33)**, which are interspersed with **lymphocytes (34)**. In the outer cortex, the parenchyma forms characteristic **lymph nodules (19)**, rich in lymphocytes, which are a main site of the B-lymphocytes. Centrally, the cortex passes over into the diffuse lymphoreticular tissue of the inner cortex (**paracortex, −18**), which is the main site of T-lymphocytes. The T-lymphocytes have their origin in the thymus, pass by way of special postcapillary venules into the bloodstream and are carried by the blood to the lymph nodes. They function in cellular immunity. **Medullary cords (15)** are in the medulla; they form a main site for B-lymphocytes and their further differentiation into plasma cells. **Lymphatic organs**, see topographical anatomy, the tabular appendix to the special anatomy, and clinical-functional anatomy.

Lymphatic system

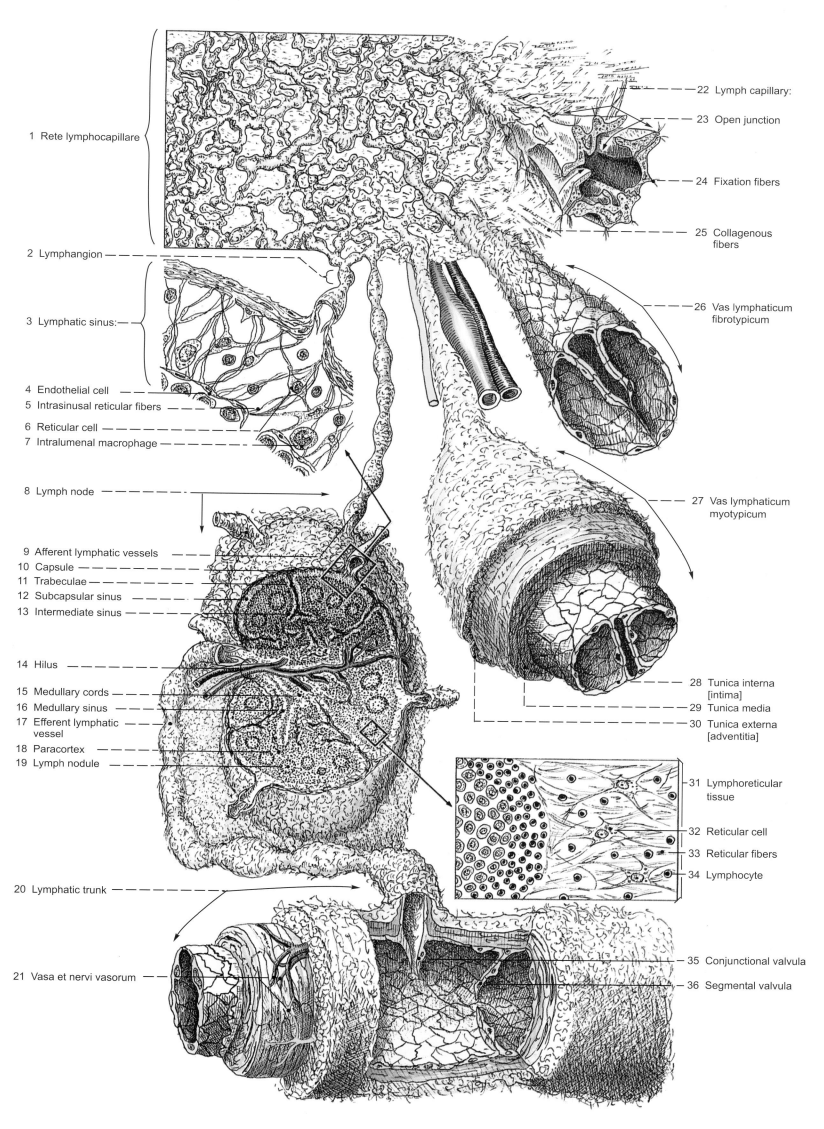

1 Rete lymphocapillare

2 Lymphangion

3 Lymphatic sinus:

4 Endothelial cell
5 Intrasinusal reticular fibers
6 Reticular cell
7 Intralumenal macrophage

8 Lymph node

9 Afferent lymphatic vessels
10 Capsule
11 Trabeculae
12 Subcapsular sinus
13 Intermediate sinus

14 Hilus

15 Medullary cords
16 Medullary sinus
17 Efferent lymphatic vessel
18 Paracortex
19 Lymph nodule

20 Lymphatic trunk

21 Vasa et nervi vasorum

22 Lymph capillary:

23 Open junction

24 Fixation fibers

25 Collagenous fibers

26 Vas lymphaticum fibrotypicum

27 Vas lymphaticum myotypicum

28 Tunica interna [intima]
29 Tunica media
30 Tunica externa [adventitia]

31 Lymphoreticular tissue
32 Reticular cell
33 Reticular fibers
34 Lymphocyte

35 Conjunctional valvula
36 Segmental valvula

10. GLANDS, MUCOUS MEMBRANES AND SEROUS MEMBRANES

a) The activity of **GLANDS** is called secretion. The secretions act external to the gland cells (*e.g.*, saliva, hormones). To produce the secretion, the gland cells take up basic materials, synthesize the secretions in the cell organelles and give them off according to a particular manner of secretion (see below). The secretion is regulated chiefly by hormones and the autonomic nervous system.

Glands are classified by different criteria.

Endocrine glands (hormonal glands) release their **secretion** into the intercellular space from which it enters the **blood or lymph capillaries**. The hormones are transported to the effector organs by the cardiovascular system. **Exocrine glands** release their **secretion** onto the **internal or external surface of the body**. They are discussed in the following (see also pp. 6 and 32).

According to the **form of their secretory end-pieces, glands** are classified as **tubular, acinar** and **alveolar**. The tubular end-pieces may be 1. simple tubular, 2. simple coiled, and 3. simple branched. The compound tubular gland has branched excretory ducts.

According to the **mode of secretion, glands** are subdivided into **eccrine** = merocrine (release of the secretion by exocytosis), **apocrine** (a part of the gland cell is shed together with the secretion) and **holocrine** (the gland cell in its entirety is transformed into the secretion).

According to the **character of the secretion**, there are distinguished **serous** (thin, watery secretion), **mucous** and **mixed** (serous and mucous constituents) **glands**.

According to their **composition**, we distinguish intraepithelial, **unicellular glands** (*e.g.*, mucus producing goblet cells) and **multicellular glands**. The intraepithelial glands lead without excretory ducts directly into the adjacent lumen. The multicellular glands lie either within the wall of the organ concerned and discharge into the lumen by way of a short excretory duct **(wall glands)**; or they are larger groups of glands that lie outside the wall and open into the lumen of the organ usually with a longer efferent duct **(associated glands)**.

b) The **MUCOUS MEMBRANE (TUNICA MUCOSA)** is the internal lining of hollow organs that bounds the lumen and is in contact with the external environment. These organs are the alimentary canal, the respiratory and urinary tracts and the passages of the genital organs that have a lumen. With the exception of the urinary passages, the lumen is covered by mucus that originates from the glands of the mucous membrane (goblet cells, wall glands or associated glands).

The **mucous membrane of the intestine** consists of a lumen-sided **columnar epithelium (7, E, E')** and a **lamina propria (lamina propria mucosae, −6)** the connective tissue layer proper. In large areas of the gut, the lamina propria contains a thin layer of smooth muscle **(lamina muscularis mucosae, −5)**. In many regions of the gut, there are layers additional to the mucous membrane: A **tela submucosa (4)**, a loose, gliding layer, is directly external to the mucous membrane. Besides the submucosa there may be a muscular layer **(Tunica muscularis, −2 and 3)** as well as on the external surface, *e.g.*, of the intestine, a **tunica serosa (Pars visceralis, −13)** or a connective tissue layer, the **tunica adventitia**, connecting the gut to its surroundings. The constituents of the mucous membrane of the different organ systems are structurally adapted to the functional needs of the individual organs.

I. In the **digestive apparatus**, which begins at the mouth and ends at the anus, functionally related differences become especially distinct. The transition to the integument is formed at both ends of the alimentary canal by a cutaneous mucous membrane with **stratified squamous epithelium (A, Cavum oris;** see also histology). In the oral cavity, at sites with maximal mechanical stress such as the hard palate and the mechanical lingual papillae, the stratified squamous epithelium is, in addition, cornified. The rapid transport of the prehended food is brought about by the striated musculature of the muscular tunic, which continues onto the esophagus. The transport is facilitated by the mucous secretions of the salivary glands of the oral cavity and pharynx. The muscularis mucosae is present as a delicate muscle layer of the mucous membrane that starts in the esophagus and increases slightly in thickness in the caudal direction. Its smooth muscle facilitates a certain mobility of the mucous membrane independent of the contraction of the predominant striated (esophagus) or smooth muscle (stomach, intestine) of the muscular tunic from which it is separated by the tela submucosa.

From the cardia of the stomach, a **tall columnar epithelium (E)** lines the lumen. It has a less protective function and more secretory and resorptive functions. This is reflected by the different epithelial cells. The **secretion of mucus** in the intestine is chiefly brought about by **goblet cells (9)** that lie scattered in the lumenal epithelium and increase in number from the duodenum to the rectum. Digestive juices are secreted by glands of the stomach and intestinal wall and by associated glands (liver, pancreas). **Resorption** requires a large area of contact with the intestinal content. The increase in the surface area is provided by **transverse, circular folds (1), intestinal villi (E' a)** and **crypts (E' b)** as well as by **microvilli (8)** on the lumenal surface of the resorptive epithelial cells.

II. In the **respiratory tract** the function of the **pseudostratified ciliated columnar epithelium (B, −trachea)** with scattered goblet cells is the production and transport of mucus by which the finest dust particles can be excreted. Respiratory mucous membrane is found in the air-conducting passages: nasal cavity, paranasal sinuses, pharynx and auditory tube including the middle ear, larynx, trachea, and bronchi.

III. The **mucous membrane of the genital tract**, like the uterine tube and uterus (see clinical-functional anatomy), is lined by a **simple columnar epithelium (C, uterine tube)** with cilia and epithelial cells bearing microvilli. The lining of parts of the male genital tract, *e.g.*, the deferent duct, is a **columnar pseudostratified epithelium (D, deferent duct)** with long, branched, immobile cellular processes, the so-called stereocilia, which are long microvilli.

IV. The **mucous membrane of the urinary tract** of the dog is aglandular. The mucosa lines the urinary passages with a transitional epithelium from the renal pelvis to the ureter and urinary bladder up to the urethra. This **transitional epithelium (F, ureter)** is a pseudostratified epithelium, whose cells all rest upon the base but do not all reach the surface (some authors classify the epithelium here as stratified; that is, not pseudostratified). In the cells that bound the lumen, the transitional epithelium has special mechanisms for protection against the aggressive action of the urine.

c) The **SEROUS MEMBRANE (G)** lines the serosal cavities and covers the external surface of many organs. It consists of a **mesothelium (14)**, a simple squamous epithelium that is developed from the mesoderm, with a connective tissue basis, the **lamina propria (15)**.

The **function of the serous membrane** consists mainly of the establishment of a smooth and moist surface by which the friction between the serosal membrane covered organs is reduced. It produces a serous fluid that is given off into the serous cavities and lends a typical character (moist, smooth and glistening) to the surface. According to the principle of equilibrium it also regulates the resorption of fluid (uptake of fluid from the serosal cavities). The serous fluid is normally kept constant by **transudation** and **resorption**. The **transudate** is formed by its 'release' from the blood capillaries into the lamina propria serosae and its passage through the mesothelium of the serosa.

A **subserosal layer (16)** functions as a gliding layer and is a primary depot for fat storage as subserosal fat tissue. It is present throughout the abdominal cavity and in particular in relation to the kidney and those organs that are subject to great variation in size as, for example, the stomach and intestine.

In the case of the **serous cavities**, we are dealing with spaces that contain only a little serous fluid. The serous cavities are the pleural cavities, pericardial cavity and the peritoneal cavity. The organs are external to the serous membrane, invaginating it and drawing with them a part of the serous membrane that is the mesentery, omentum, or ligaments of peritoneum (*e.g.*, the ligaments of the liver; the broad ligament that suspends the ovary, uterine tube, and uterus, etc.). The serous membrane lining the walls of the peritoneal cavity **(parietal peritoneum, −11)** is continuous with the serous membrane covering the surface of the organ **(visceral peritoneum, −13)**. The connecting peritoneum that extends from the parietal peritoneum of the body wall to the visceral peritoneum covering the organ is always given a particular name: mesentery, omentum, or peritoneal ligaments (*e.g.*, broad ligament of the uterus, triangular ligaments of the liver, etc.). The mesentery is shown in the figure on the opposite page **(Pars intermedia, −12)**.

The **topographical relationship** of the organs to the **peritoneum** is especially important for surgery. In the case of a surgical operation, this relationship determines whether or not the peritoneal cavity must be opened with its greater risk of infection of the peritoneum (peritonitis; see p. 50).

The **sensory innervation** of the parietal layer of the peritoneum is by the **segmental spinal nerves** (lumbar and thoracic nerves). The peritoneum covering the abdominal aspect of the diaphragm receives its sensory innervation by the phrenic nerve. The sensory innervation of the mesenteries, omenta, and peritoneal ligaments proceeds from stretch and probably other less well understood receptors, but not from ordinary pain, temperature, and touch receptors. The viscera are relatively insensitive to the sensations associated with the skin and the parietal peritoneum. If excessive stretch (tension) or pressure is avoided, the viscera can be incised and otherwise surgically manipulated without pain to the animal.

Tunica mucosa and Tunica serosa

Small intestine

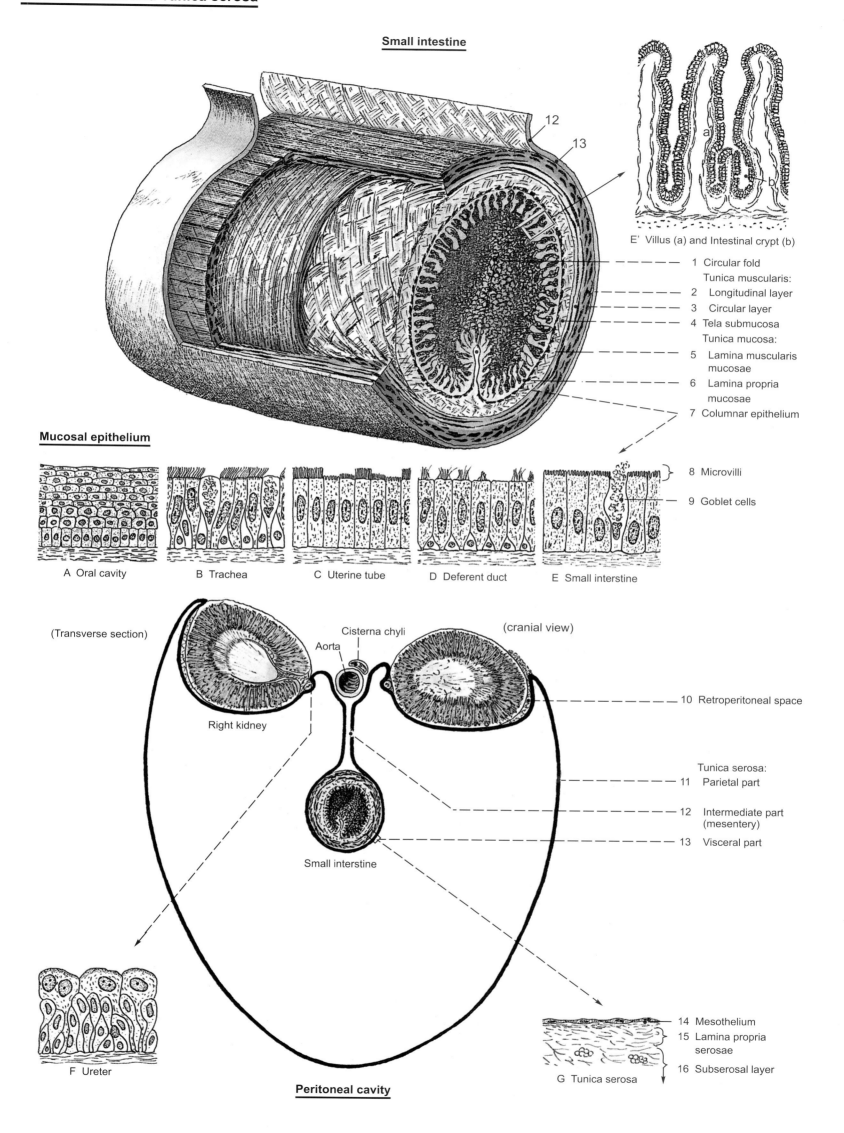

E' Villus (a) and Intestinal crypt (b)

1 Circular fold
Tunica muscularis:
2 Longitudinal layer
3 Circular layer
4 Tela submucosa
Tunica mucosa:
5 Lamina muscularis mucosae
6 Lamina propria mucosae
7 Columnar epithelium

Mucosal epithelium

8 Microvilli
9 Goblet cells

A Oral cavity   B Trachea   C Uterine tube   D Deferent duct   E Small interstine

(Transverse section)

Cisterna chyli

Aorta

(cranial view)

Right kidney

10 Retroperitoneal space

Small interstine

Tunica serosa:
11 Parietal part

12 Intermediate part (mesentery)

13 Visceral part

F Ureter

14 Mesothelium
15 Lamina propria serosae
16 Subserosal layer

G Tunica serosa

Peritoneal cavity

AN INTRODUCTION TO THE PHYSICAL-TECHNICAL BASICS OF X-RAY AND ULTRASOUND DIAGNOSTICS

CORDULA POULSEN NAUTRUP

1 CONVENTIONAL AND DIRECT MAGNIFYING RADIOGRAPHY

1.1 X-rays

X-rays are electromagnetic waves with frequencies of approximately 10^{12} to 10^{14} MHz (megahertz).

1.2 Generating x-rays

When accelerated electrons hit an anode or target, part of the kinetic energy is transformed into bremsstrahlung (a continuous radiation spectrum of various wavelengths) and characteristic x-rays (a line spectrum). Most of the energy, however, is lost in the form of heat.

The emitted x-ray radiation, which is made up mainly of bremsstrahlung and, to an extent, of characteristic x-rays, is responsible for image formation. The voltage determines the most energetic radiation with the shortest wavelength. Potential differences useful for x-ray diagnostics and the resulting energies lie between 18 and 120 kV and 1 and 120 kV, resp. Soft x-rays of long wavelengths (low kV values) are opposed by harder and more energetic radiation of short wavelengths (high kV values).

1.3 The behavior of x-rays in material and the formation of radiographs

Materials absorb and scatter x-rays. Differences in absorption in an x-rayed patient, body part, or object produce a new radiation spectrum. All planes of a three-dimensional body are thereby presented on a single plane. A radiograph is thus a summative picture, in which areas lying one above or below another are superimposed (fig. 1).

1.3.1 Absorption in relation to the irradiated material

Absorption depends on the density and valence number of the irradiated material. Air or organs containing air with their low densities and resultingly low absorptions can be easily differentiated from other soft tissues with higher densities. Due to their higher densities and higher effective valence numbers, calcified or bony areas absorb x-rays better than soft tissues and are clearly contrasted from these.

1.3.2 Absorption in relation to the radiation quality

The quality of the x-rays further influences the level of absorption. Whereas with the use of soft x-rays absorption is predominant, absorption decreases and scattering increases with increasing radiation energy levels. In soft radiation exposures the large differences in contrast allow the differentiation between soft tissues and slightly calcified or ossified structures (fig. 3). In human medicine this technique is employed in mammography for radiological tumor diagnosis of the female breast. Medium hard to hard radiation is suited for the depiction of sufficiently calcified bone tissue (fig. 2).

1.3.3 Contrast media

Contrast media are necessary for the differentiation of vessels in soft tissues and bone (figs. 4, 5, 6) as well as for evaluating certain organ regions. Such media are classed as negative (less absorption than bone) or positive (higher absorption), according to their ability to absorb x-rays. The first group includes easily absorbed gases such as air, carbon dioxide, and nitrous oxide.

These are primarily used for presenting the alimentary canal and urinary bladder, often in the form of double contrast images, in which a positive contrast medium is combined with a negative. Positive contrast media have a higher density and a large valence number. In addition to barium sulfate, a water insoluble contrast medium for controlling passage in the esophagus and digestive tract, there are many water soluble media, usually containing iodine, for the depiction of vessels (angiography – figs. 4, 5, 6; arteriography, phlebography, lymphography) and nearly all of the body cavities (urography, bronchography, arthrography, myelography).

1.4 Image formation and recording

X-rays pass through the body film (photographic effect) or energize the luminescent chemicals of an intensifying screen or image amplifier (luminescence effect).

X-ray film images are negatives; highly-absorbent regions such as bone or calcifications appear white to light gray, whereas radiolucent areas, such as air-filled and parenchymatous organs, fat, muscle, cartilage, connective tissue, or fluids (blood, urine, liquid ingesta, etc.), appear dark (fig. 7). As a positive, the monitor image shows radiodense areas as black to dark gray, and radiolucent areas as white to light gray (fig. 8).

The analogue pictures of x-ray-closed circuit TV systems or radiographs can be digitalized and then reworked with a picture processor. Typically-used methods in medical diagnostics include digital measurements, multiple image integration for improving contrast, edge enhancement to improve the depth of field, and picture subtraction to bring out or isolate vessels (DSA: digital subtraction angiography).

Experimentally, color coding and pseudo-3D presentation after object shifting have proved useful for evaluating areas of low contrast (fig. 9). All methods of digital picture processing serve to increase the quality of x-ray film images with improved and more complete possibilities of evaluation, and at the same time to reduce the dangerous levels of radiation or the amounts of contrast media necessary.

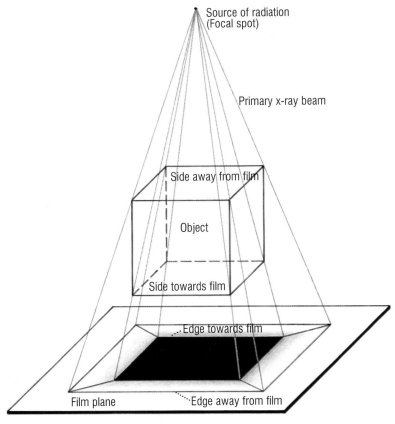

Fig. 1: Schematic drawing of the formation of a radiograph (summative picture).

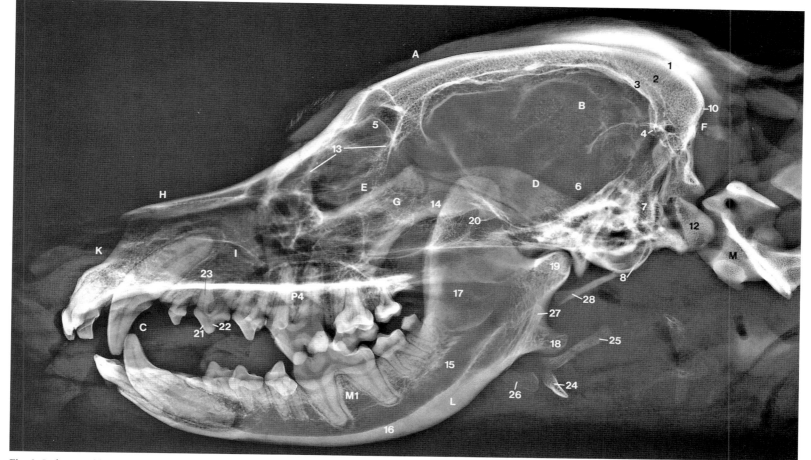

Fig. 2: Left cranial half of a adult dog. High-kV technique, 100 kV, lateromedial view – LM.

Anatomic structures (figs. 2, 3)

Cranium
1 External lamina
2 Spongy bone (diploe)
3 Internal lamina
4 Tentorial process

Neurocranial bones
A Frontal bone
5 Frontal sinus
B Parietal bone
D Temporal bone
6 Squamous part
7 Petrous part
8 Tympanic part/tympanic bulla
E Ethmoid bone
F Occipital bone
9 Squamous part
10 External occipital crown
11 Lateral part
12 Occipital condyle

Face
13 Orbits

Facial bones
G Zygomatic bone
14 Temporal process

H Nasal bone

I Maxilla
K Premaxilla
L Mandible
15 Mandibular canal
16 Mandibular body
17 Mandibular ramus
18 Mandibular angle
19 Condylar process
20 Coronoid process

Teeth
C Canine tooth
P4 Fourth premolar
M1 First molar
21 Enamel
22 Dentin
23 Dental cavity

Hyoid bone
24 Basihyoid
25 Thyrohyoid
26 Ceratohyoid
27 Epihyoid
28 Stylo and tympanohyoid

M Atlas

N Axis

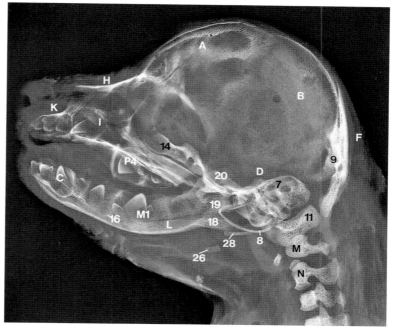

Fig. 3: Left cranial half of a six-day-old puppy. Low-kV technique, 40 kV, lateromedial view – LM.

1.5 The laws of projection

Picture formation with x-rays follows the laws of central projection; rays emanating from a more or less expansive, ideally point-formed focal spot diverge in straight lines.

1.5.1 Geometric magnification

In describing projections it differentiated must be made between the film-focal distance (FFD), focal-object distance (FOD), and the object-film distance (OFD). With a conventional image at a scale of 1 : 1 the FFD is nearly the same as the FOD, which means that with a large FFD the patient or area to be filmed is close to the film plane. Reductions in the FOD caused by raising the patient or object result in direct x-ray magnification (keep in mind the problem of geometric blurring,

chapter 1.6.1, fig. 17). The factor of magnification, V, is the quotient of FFD to FOD, i. e., FFD: FOD (fig. 10).

1.5.2 Superpositioning

Two structures lying one above the other are projected into each other and can no longer be differentiated from each other. Cracks, fissures, or fractures, which run roughly perpendicular to the path of the x-rays remain hidden, due to superpositioning (figs. 11 A, 12). Only by rotating the object do the details run parallel to the path of the rays and then appear in radiographs (figs. 11 B, 13). Disturbing superpositioning can be reduced when examining anatomical preparations by preparing thin sections (0.1 – 1.0 mm). In vivo the superposition-free radiological depiction of structures of one plane is possible with the help of tomography.

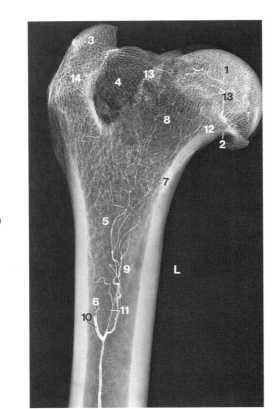

Anatomic structures

Bone structures
 1 Femur head (epiphysis)
 2 Femur neck
 3 Major trochanter
 4 Trochanteric fossa
 5 Femur shaft
 6 Nutrient canal
 7 Compact substance
 8 Spongy substance
 9 Medullary cavity

Intraosseal vessels
10 Nutritive artery
11 Diaphyseal vessel
12 Metaphyseal vessel
13 Epiphyseal vessel
14 Apophyseal vessel

Fig 4: Radiograph of the proximal intraosseal vessels of the left femur filled with contrast medium. Mediolateral view – ML.

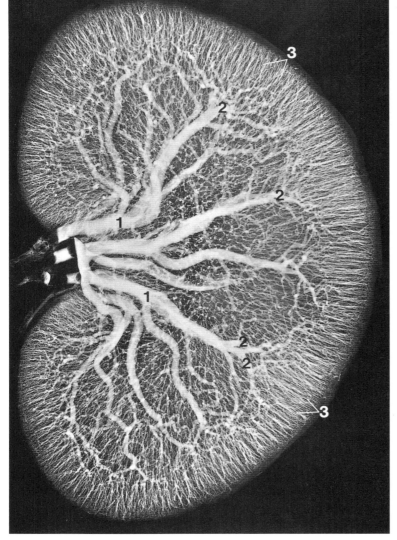

Fig. 5: Radiograph of the arterial kidney vessels filled with contrast medium.

Anatomic structures (figs. 5, 6)

Intrarenal vessels
1 Interlobar artery
2 Arcuate artery
3 Interlobular artery
4 Afferent glomerular arteriole
5 Glomerular capillaries

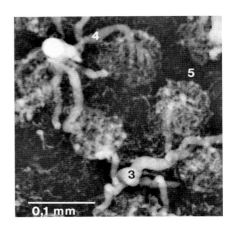

Fig. 6: Radiograph of the glomeruli in the renal cortex filled with contrast medium. (Tissue slice approximately 5 mm thick).

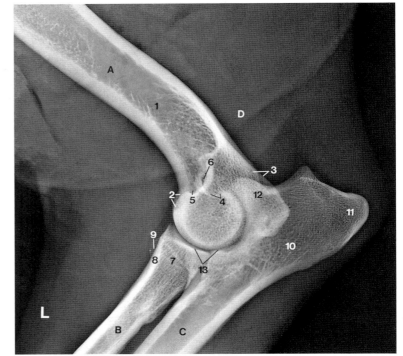

Fig. 7: Radiograph of the left elbow = negative. Lateromedial view – LM.

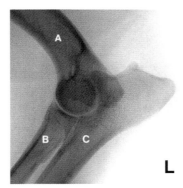

Fig. 8: Monitor image of the left elbow = positive. Lateromedial view – LM.

Fig. 9: Monitor image of the left elbow. Digital pseudo-3D-depiction after object shifting. Lateromedial view – LM.

Anatomic structures (figs. 7, 8, 9)

A Humerus
1 Humerus shaft
2 Humeral condyle
3 Epicondyles
4 Olecranon fossa
5 Radial fossa
6 Supratrochlear foramen

B Radius
7 Head

8 Radial neck
9 Radial tuberosity

C Ulna
10 Olecranon
11 Olecranon tuberosity
12 Anconeal process
13 Coronoid process

D Soft tissue

1.5.3 Geometric distortion

The higher magnification in radiographs of areas further from the film, in contrast to areas near the film, is known as geometric distortion (figs. 1, 14 A, 15). An increase in the geometric distortion can occur by placing the object in the outer area of the x-ray beam (figs. 14 B, 16). Such an effect can also be obtained by po- sitioning the object at an angle to the central x-ray beam. Geometric distortion can give an impression of three-dimensionality and simplify the categorizing of details to specific planes, especially with direct radiographic magnification. Exact measurements from radiographs, however, should only be made on images free of geometric distortion; the points to be measured should be located within the central beam and with larger FFDs should be close to the film plane.

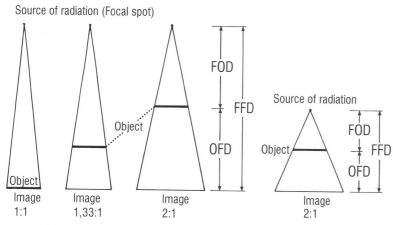

Fig. 10: Schematic drawing of a 1:1 scale image and various geometric magnifications.

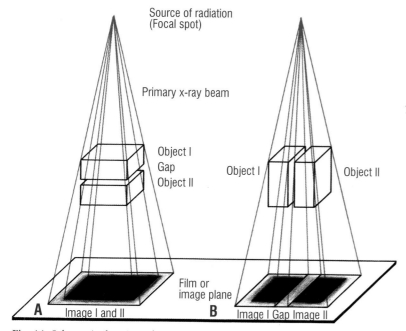

Fig. 11: Schematic drawing of superpositioning in the central projection; A: gap perpendicular, B. gap parallel to the beam.

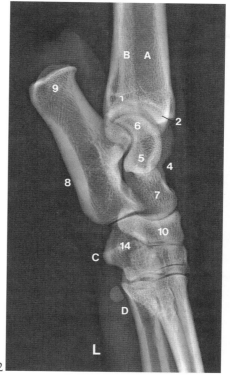
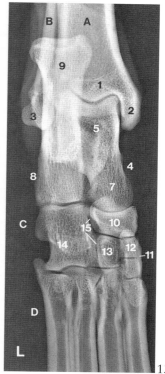

Fig. 12: Left tarsal joint. Mediolateral view – ML.

Fig. 13: Left tarsal joint. Dorsoplantar view – DPI. The typical hinge joint form of the tarsocrural joint and the intertarsal joints can be differentiated, in contrast to fig. 12.

Anatomic structures (figs. 12, 13)

A Tibia
1 Tibial cochlea
2 Medial malleolus

B Fibula
3 Lateral malleolus

C Tarsal bones
4 Talus
5 Body of talus
6 Trochlea of talus

7 Head
8 Calcaneus
9 Calcaneal tuber
10 Central tarsal bone
11 First tarsal bone
12 Second tarsal bone
13 Third tarsal bone
14 Fourth tarsal bone
15 Intertarsal joints

D Metatarsal bones

1.6 The quality of radiographs

The ability to evaluate fine structures in radiographs or with an image amplifier and monitor presuppose sufficient picture quality. The following factors are responsible for the quality of radiographs:

sharpness or blurring,
contrast,
resolution of the image formation and recording system.

The functions sharpness and contrast are dependent on a number of various parameters, which are given by the geometry of the radiation source, the radiation, the object to be depicted, and the x-ray machine.

1.6.1 Sharpness or blurring

The recognition of details in radiographs can be limited or lost with blurring due to movement, geometric blurring, or film-screen blurring.

Blurring due to movement is the result of the patient's moving when insufficiently fixed, or the movement of organs (heart contractions, breathing movements, etc.). This can be avoided by stable positioning and using shorter exposure times (for example, cardiographs under 1 ms).

Geometric blurring (GB) is determined by the diameter of the focal spot and the relationship of the FFD to the FOD. Whereas a larger focal spot leads to significant blurring of the outer edges when the patient is raised above the film/image plane, an ideally point-formed radiation source gives sharp pictures without blurred edges in every area between the focal spot and film plane (figs. 18, 20). An object lying directly on the film plane is always sharply projected, regardless of the size of the focal spot. Whereas direct magnifications of up to 2.5x are possible with focal spots of 100 μm (mammography machines), direct magnifications of up to 200x with satisfactory sharpness are possible using microfocal spots of less than 10 μm (fig. 6).

Film-screen blurring depends on the type of screen used and the contact between the screen and film. X-ray or intensifying screens contain fluorescent crystals, which convert incoming x-rays into visible light. The photographic coating of the film in contact with the screen is blackened by the light emitted by the screen. Intensifying screens serve to reduce doses. The more sensitive the screen, i. e., the larger the amplification, and the shorter the necessary exposure time needed for blackening the film, the better the sharpness (fig. 23).

The three blurring parameters described here all influence each other at the same time. Due to the low dosage levels, reducing geometric blurring by using a smaller focal spot results in long exposure times and increases the danger of blurring due to movement. All three factors have to be tuned to each other and adapted to the situation.

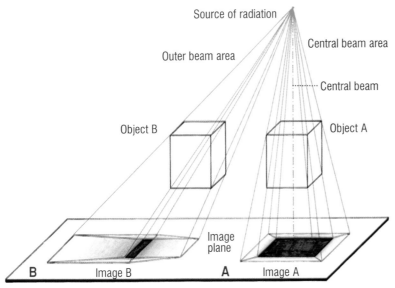

Fig. 14: Schematic drawing of geometric distortion. Geometric magnification of an object in the central beam path (A) and in the outer beam path (B).

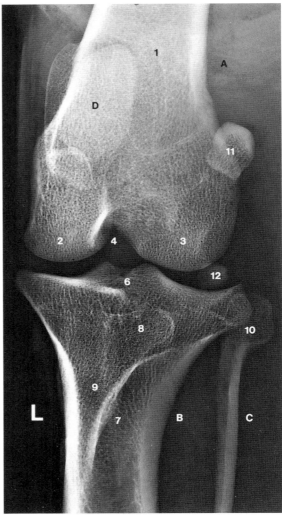

Fig. 16: Radiograph of the left knee joint in the outer beam path. Craniocaudal view, beam path 20° oblique to the craniocaudal beam path – Cr20L-CdMO.

Anatomic structures (figs. 15, 16)

A Femur
1 Femur shaft
2 Medial condyle
3 Lateral condyle
4 Intercondyloid fossa
5 Femur trochlea

B Tibia
6 Intercondylar eminence
7 Tibia shaft

8 Tibial tuberosity
9 Cranial margin

C Fibula
10 Head of fibula

D Patella
11 Sesamoid bone of the gastrocnemius muscle
12 Sesamoid bone of the popliteal muscle

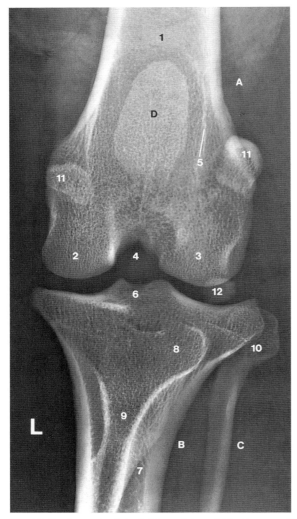

Fig. 15: Radiograph of the left knee joint within the central beam path. Craniocaudal view – CrCd = beam path.

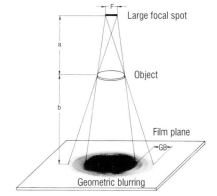

Fig. 17: Schematic drawing of geometric blurring (GB) caused by raising the object from the film plane when a large focal spot is used.

1.6.2 Contrast

Contrast means the difference between two intensities of blackening on the film or between two levels of brightness on the image amplifier. The contrast on the image recording system (x-ray film or monitor) corresponds to the differences in intensity after absorption of the primary beam by the patient or object. The contrast level depends mainly on the beam quality, the body region to be examined, and scatter radiation.

Soft x-rays give clearer differences in contrast than hard x-rays, for which the blackening gradations are smaller (see chapter 1.3.2). An area exposed with overly-hard radiation appears dull; it lacks bright whites and deep blacks.

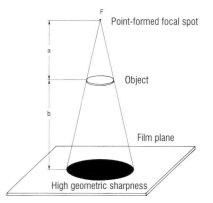

Fig. 18: Schematic drawing of sharp direct magnification when an ideally point-formed focal spot is used.

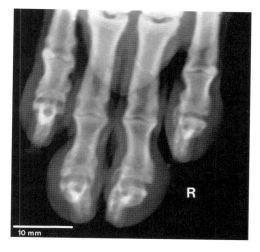

Fig. 19: Heavy geometric blurring in a 4x direct magnification made with a 400 μm focal spot (original photographically reduced for technical reasons of printing).

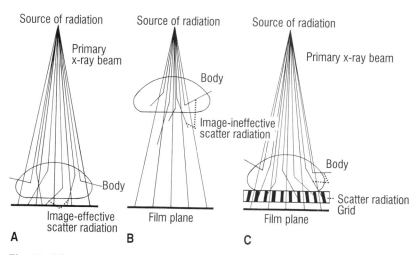

Fig. 21: Schematic drawings of the effect (A) and reduction (B, C) of scatter radiation (B- distance technique with large OFD, C-use of a grid).

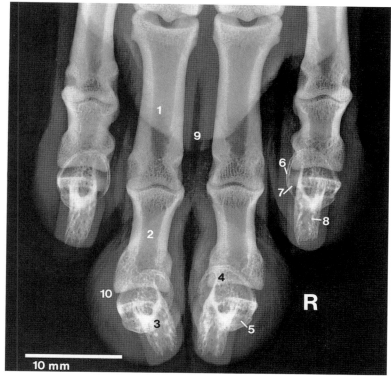

Fig. 20: High geometric sharpness in a 4x direct magnification made with a 5 μm microfocal spot. Middle and distal phalanges of the right rear paw. Dorsoplantar view – DPl. (original photographically reduced for technical reasons of printing).

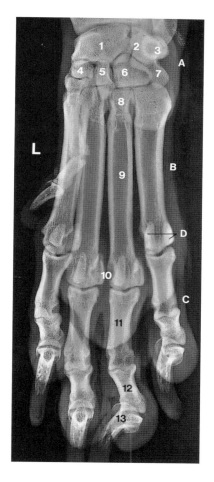

Fig. 22: Bones of the right front paw as seen with high resolution nonscreen x-ray film (Structurix D7, Agfa-Gevaert). Exposure values: 2.5 mm Al filter, FFD 80 cm, 60 kV, 50 mAs.

Anatomic structures

Digital bones
1 Proximal phalanx
2 Middle phalanx
3 Distal phalanx
4 Extensor process
5 Flexor tuberosity

6 Unguicular crest
7 Unguicular groove
8 Unguicular process

Soft tissue
9 Metatarsal cushion
10 Toe pad

Clear differences in contrast are seen between bones and soft tissues and between vessels or organs filled with contrast media and the surroundings.

Scatter radiation, which originates in the irradiated material, reaches the recording surface multidirectionally and causes a diffuse blackening of the x-ray film or diffuse energizing of the illumination crystals of an x-ray screen or image amplifier (fig. 21 A). Fine differences in contrast, i. e., small differences in absorption in tissues, are covered up. Scatter radiation increases with increasing hardness of the primary beam. It is also dependent on the properties and size of the irradiated object. To reduce the scatter radiation the primary beam can be restricted with a diaphragm, a grid can he used (fig. 21 C), or the OFD can be increased (fig. 21 B).

Scatter radiation grids are made of lead strips, which are placed parallel to the primary beam and only allow these to pass, whereas multidirectional scatter radiation is absorbed. The disadvantage is the necessary increase in power, since in addition to the scatter radiation, a part of the primary beam is lost in the grid (fig. 21 C).

1.6.3 Resolution of the image formation and recording system

The resolving ability of the image formation or recording system determines the size of details, which can just be recognized. Periodical structures, such as the lead strips of a grid, which are smaller than the silver halide grains of the film or the illumination crystals of a screen or imaging device, cannot be distinguished from one another. The local resolution of nonscreen film is approximately 50 μm (fig. 22), for screen-film systems between 80 – 200 μm (fig. 23), and using image amplifiers and closed-circuit TV systems, between 200 – 420 μm. In order to recognize such small structures, the contrast between the structures and the surroundings has to be sufficient. This is generally not the case for biological material.

With conventional standard radiographs the screen-film system used generally limits the recognition of details to 100 μm.

All of the factors mentioned, which influence the quality of the picture, interact highly with each other. Small structures at the limit of resolution, which are affected by geometric blurring or show unclear edges as a result of superpositioning, can only be

163

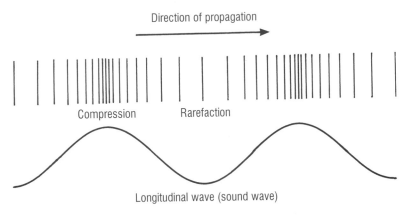

Fig. 24: Schematic drawing of the propagation of a longitudinal wave in tissue.

Anatomic structures (figs. 21, 23)

A Carpal bones
1 Radial carpal bone
2 Ulnar carpal bone
3 Accessory carpal bone
4 First carpal bone
5 Second carpal bone
6 Third carpal bone
7 Fourth carpal bone

B Metacarpal bones
8 Base
9 Shaft
10 Head

C Digital bones
11 Proximal phalanx
12 Middle phalanx
13 Distal phalanx

D Sesamoid bones

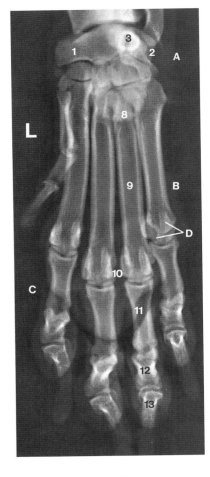

Fig. 23: Bones of the right front paw taken with a highly sensitive screen-film combination (Trimax T6 screen and XM film, 3M). Compared with fig. 22, lower resolution and increased screen blurring can be seen. Exposure values: 2.5 mm Al filter, FFD 80 cm, 60 kV, 1.5 mAs.

evaluated if the contrast is high enough. Reversely, with good sharpness and sufficient detail size the contrast is of less importance.

1.6.4 Labeling radiographs

The quality of radiographs can be further improved by comprehensive labeling, including exposure parameters, positioning, and patient identification.

Lead letters placed on the cassette at the time of exposure can be used to mark cranial, caudal, medial, lateral, right, and left. The terminology used for the views shown in radiographs generally follows guidelines set by the Nomenclature Committee of the American College of Veterinary Radiology.*) The positioning of the patient and the direction that the central ray of primary beam penetrates the body part, from the point of entry to the point of exit, are to be given using proper veterinary anatomic directional terms.

1.7 Radiation protection

In principle it can be said that x-rays exert dose-dependent, generally undesirable effects on biological tissues. Soft radiation is more likely to be damaging (especially to the skin), due to its greater absorption.

The requirements set on equipment and operation by state agencies are to be consciously followed. First and foremost is that the required image quality be obtained with the lowest amount of radiation possible.

2 PHYSICAL – TECHNICAL BASICS OF SONOGRAPHY OR ECHOGRAPHY

2.1 Ultrasound

Sound waves are longitudinal waves. The particles of a tissue are brought to vibrate by the sound. The direction of vibration corresponds to the direction of sonic propagation, which results in compression and rarefaction within the wave (fig. 24). Fre-

quencies above 20 kHz are known as ultrasound. The frequencies used in ultrasound diagnostics lie between 1–20 MHz (megahertz = 1000 kHz), and are considerably higher than the ultrasonic frequencies perceivable by animals, such as cats, dogs, or bats.

2.2 Behavior of sound waves in material

2.2.1 Wave propagation velocity and acoustic impedance

The velocity with which ultrasound travels in tissue (wave propagation velocity) depends on the ultrasound frequency and properties of the material. The speed averages 1540 m/s in soft tissues and liquids, is considerably lower in air, and distinctly higher in bone. The acoustic resistance or impedance of a tissue is the product of the speed of the sound beam in a given tissue and the density of the tissue.

2.2.2 Reflection, transmission, refraction, scattering, and absorption

When sound waves pass interfaces between two tissues with different wave propagation velocities or with different acoustic impedances (see chapter 2.2.1), a part of the sound beam is reflected (reflection – figs. 25, 26). The direction of reflection of a wave hitting an interface **perpendicularly** is the same as that of the incident wave. The nonreflected wave continues in the second medium without changing direction (transmission – fig. 25). If the interface is hit at an **angle**, the angle of reflection is the same as the incident angle. The transmitted wave is refracted (refraction – fig. 26).

Irregular acoustic interfaces cause reflection of the sound waves in all directions (scattering).

In addition, the sound beam is absorbed as it passes through tissues (absorption). The degree of absorption depends on the sound frequency and the quality of the insonated tissue. Higher frequencies are absorbed more strongly than low ones. When considering body tissues, bone and calcifications have high rates of absorption.

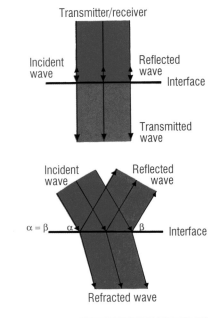

Fig. 25: Schematic drawing of the reflection and transmission of an incident sound wave hitting the interface perpendicularly.

Fig. 26: Schematic drawing of the reflection and refraction of an incident sound wave hitting the interface at an angle.

---

*) SMALLWOOD. J. E., M. J. SHIVELY, V.T. RENDANO, and R. E. HABEL: A standardized notation for radiographic projections used in veterinary medicine. Vet. Rad. 26, 2–9. (1985).

2.2.3 The effect of diagnostic ultrasound on biological tissues

The sound intensities used in the course of ultrasonic diagnostics of only a few mW/cm², as well as frequencies used, are considered safe, so that repeated pregnancy examinations are possible.

2.3 Generation and reception of ultrasound waves

The scanner head is both a transmitter and receiver. A piezoelectric crystal in the transducer or scanner is brought to vibrate by high-frequency electric pulses and converts them to ultrasound. At the same time reflected sound waves are transformed into corresponding electrical impulses, which can be made visible on a monitor. With an impulse duration of 1 – 2 μs the relationship between the times of transmission and reception is approximately 1:5 00 to 1:1000.

2.4 Resolution

The axial resolution along the path of the ultrasound beam depends primarily on the frequency used. With frequencies of 1 and 10 MHz, structures of at best 1.5 mm and 100 μm, respectively, can be made out. High frequencies not only have a higher resolution, but also less penetration, since the rate of absorption is higher. 5.0 MHz has proven to be a universal frequency for cardiac and abdominal examinations of dogs.

The lateral resolution is less than the axial and is determined primarily by the geometry of the transducer.

2.5 Formation of two-dimensional ultrasonographs

2.5.1 Transducer-dependent form of the ultrasonographs

For the presentation of anatomical or pathological structures, the two-dimensional real-time technique is almost always used today. Depending on the ultrasound field scanned, one can differentiate between the sector scan and linear or parallel scan. A compromise between these two forms is the convex scan. Whereas the sector scanner produces a triangular image (figs. 27, 28), the image produced by a linear or parallel transducer is rectangular (figs. 29, 30). Only the sector scanner is suited for examination of the heart, due to the narrow intercostal acoustic window in the area of the cardiac notch of the lung. Abdominal examinations can also be made easily in dogs with sector transducers (fig. 28). Linear or convex scanners are also used for

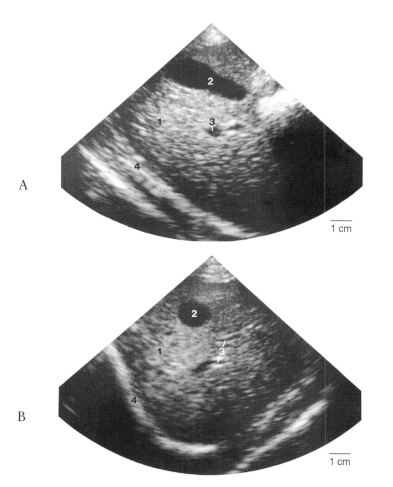

A

B

1 cm

Fig. 28: Sector sonographs of the liver with the gallbladder shown longitudinally (A) and transversely sectioned (B).

Anatomic structures
1 Liver, 2 Gallbladder, 3 Branch of the portal vene, 4 Diaphragm.

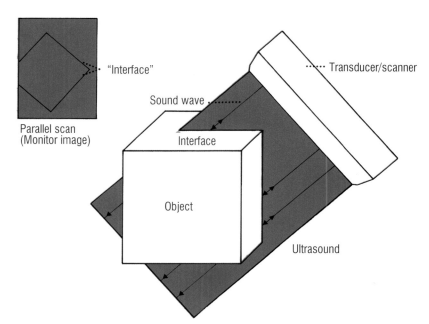

Parallel scan (Monitor image)

"Interface"

Transducer/scanner

Sound wave

Interface

Object

Ultrasound

Fig. 29: Schematic drawing of the formation of a two-dimensional sonograph (section), using a linear transducer.

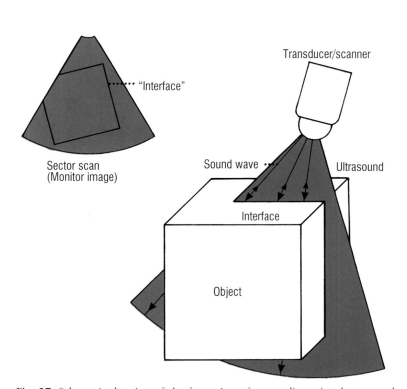

Sector scan (Monitor image)

"Interface"

Transducer/scanner

Sound wave

Ultrasound

Interface

Object

Fig. 27: Schematic drawing of the formation of a two-dimensional sonograph (section), using a sector scanner.

canine abdominal sonography, especially for diagnosing pregnancy, since they provide better resolution of structures close to the transducer (fig. 30).

2.5.2 Categorizing structures on the sonograph

In contrast to the radiograph (fig. 1), an ultrasonograph is a section, which shows the acoustic interfaces between various soft tissues (figs. 27, 29). Reflections of the ultrasound beam occur at each interface and appear on the monitor as echogenic regions, i. e., as bright areas (figs. 28, 30).

Fibrous wall structures of vessels and organs are seen as more or less hyperechogenic (white) areas, when hit perpendicularly with the ultrasound beam. Ultrasonographs of parenchymatous

165

organs (liver, spleen, renal cortex) and muscle (including the heart) are made up of numerous single echoes (white-spotted areas).

Nearly the entire beam intensity is reflected (strong white echo) at interfaces between soft tissues and structures containing air (lung), bone, or calcifications, as a result of the large difference in acoustic impedance. Since the remaining beam intensity is absorbed in penetrating bone or calcifications, tissues found behind them cannot be shown; a black anechoic area, acoustic shadowing, is seen on the monitor (fig. 30). The same is true for tissues covered by the lungs.

Homogenous tissue regions, such as renal parenchyma, or liquids, such as blood, bile, or urine, appear hypoechoic (constant dark gray) or anechoic (constant black).

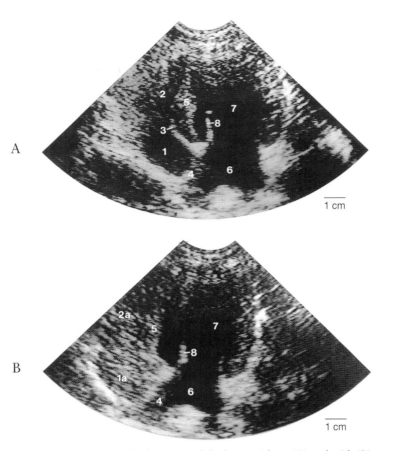

A

B

Fig. 31: Diastolic four-chainber view of the heart without (A) and with (B) contrast medium in the right atrium and ventricle.
(Tobias, R., Small Animal Clinic, Hannover Veterinary School).

Anatomic structures

1 Right atrium	4 Interatrial septum
1a Contrast medium in the right atrium	5 Interventricular septum
2 Right ventricle	6 Left atrium
2a Contrast medium in the right ventricle	7 Left ventricle
3 Opened tricuspid valve	8 Opened mitral valve

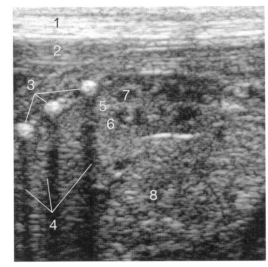

Position of the fetus

right

cranial ┼ caudal

left

1 cm

Fig. 30: Linear scan of a Cairn Terrier, 59d after conception. Horizontal section of a fetus, thorax, and intrathoracal abdomen with ribs and typical acoustic shadows.
(Grof, D., Wissdorf, H., Institute of Anatomy, Hannover Veterinary School).

Anatomic structures

1 Echos of the ribs	5 Diaphragm
2 Acoustic shadows of the ribs	6 Liver
3 Heart	7 Caudal vena cava
4 Lung (collapsed)	8 Forelimb

2.5.3 Contrast media

Ultrasound contrast media are used to improve presentations of vessels or heart chambers, or to evaluate heart defects, such as in the interventricular or interatrial septum (fig. 31). They contain extremely finely distributed gas bubbles as the echogenic substance. In addition to CO_2 or various well-mixed solutions, such as physiological saline, 5 % glucose solution, plasma expander, or patient blood, commercially prepared echocontrast media will be available in the future. The latter contain gas bubbles, which are bound to saccharide microparticles. Following intravenous injection the contrast medium can be traced to the pulmonary trunk. The presently available contrast media cannot pass the pulmonary capillaries.

2.5.4 Orientation on the ultrasonograph

By turning, tilting, or sliding the transducer, every sectional plane of the body can be reached in principle (fig. 28). The desired sonographic plane has to be correspondingly exactly selected or reproduced for measurements or repeated examinations. Regarding the localizations in ultrasonographs, areas near the transducer are seen in the upper part of the picture and areas distant to it in the lower part (figs. 27, 29). The right or left side of the picture corresponds to the left or right side, dorsal or ventral, or cranial or caudal side of the body.

2.6 Doppler echography

The waves reflected from stationary interfaces have a lower intensity, but the same frequency as the incident ultrasound waves (fig. 32 a). If, on the other hand, the waves strike a moving ob-

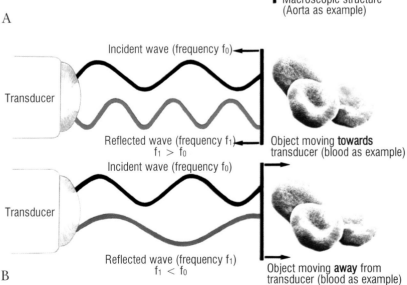

A

B

Fig. 32: Schematic representations of two-dimensional (A) and of doppier echography (B).

ject, such as an erythrocyte, the frequency of the reflected wave is altered in accordance with the direction and spaced of the moving "interface" (doppler principle – fig. 32 b).

By definition, blood flowing towards the transducer is shown above the baseline (continuous or pulsed doppler) or in red

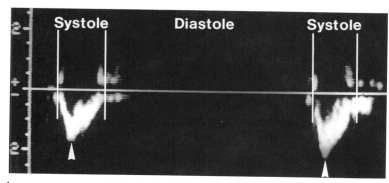

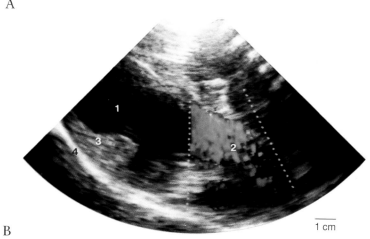

A

B

Fig. 33: Blood flow at the level of the aortic valve: pulsed doppler (A) and color-coded doppler (B).

Anatomic structures

Arrow shows maximum speed of the blood at the level of the aortic valve.
1 Left ventricle (outflow path)

2 Ascending aorta
3 Myocardium
4 Pericardium

(color-coded doppler) – Reversely, i. e., blood shown below the base line or in blue is flowing away from the transducer. This presentation of the direction of blood flow is completely voluntary and has nothing to do with the type of vessel (artery or vein) or the oxygen content of the blood. Oxygen-rich blood in the ascending aorta, for example, is shown in blue (fig. 33 b) or below the baseline (fig. 33 a), since it flows away from the transducer.

The speed of the blood flow can be read directly from the y-axis with a conventional doppler and can be estimated from the color intensity with a color-coded doppler.

If the blood velocity exceeds the reception frequency of the transducer, the so-called aliasing phenomenon occurs, which corresponds to the stroboscopic effect in film. With color-coded dopplers this results in reversing of the colors and with conventional dopplers in reversed presentation, relative to the x-axis.

2.7 Preparing the dog for ultrasonic examination

A prerequisite for quality ultrasonographs is sufficient contact of the transducer with the surface of the skin. For cardiac examination a wiping of the skin with alcohol and heavy application of contact gel is sufficient for most dogs. The same procedure can be used for abdominal sonography of dogs with little or medium amounts of hair. Animals with thick long fur and much underfur, however, have to be shaved in the area to be examined.

The positioning of the dog depends on the preference of the operator, the behavior of the animal, and the examination to be performed. Echocardiography in lateral recumbancy is proposed as well as cardial examinations made on sitting or standing dogs. Abdominal sonography is possible in lateral and dorsal recumbancy, as well as on standing animals.

SONOGRAPHIC ANATOMY

by CORDULA POULSEN NAUTRUP

AN INTRODUCTION TO SONOGRAPHIC ANATOMY

As with radiographic anatomy, sonographic anatomy has direct clinical references. Only a thorough knowledge of the normal ultrasonograph allows the successful clinical use of this method, which is relatively new to veterinary medicine. Several examples of ultrasonographs follow, showing various organs and organ systems. The most important structures in the ultrasonographs are depicted in sketches and labeled. The respective positions for the ultrasonographic examination are shown in accompanying schematic drawings.

HEART – COR

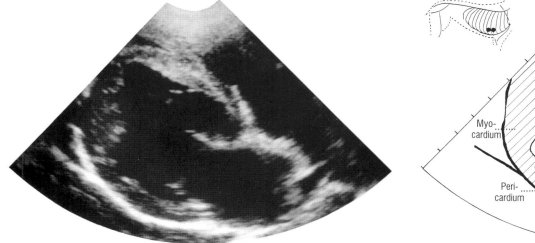

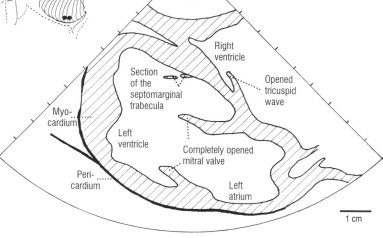

Fig. 1: Inflow tract of the left ventricle; late-diastolic longaxis section of the left ventricle.

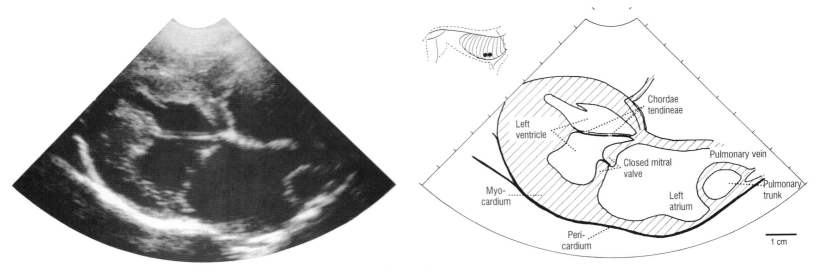

Fig. 2: Inflow tract of the left ventricle; late-systolic long-axis section of the left ventricle.

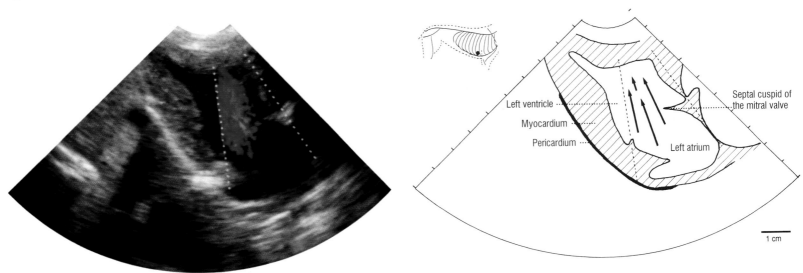

Fig. 3: Inflow tract of the left ventricle; long-axis section of the left ventricle with inflowing blood in the early diastolic phase.

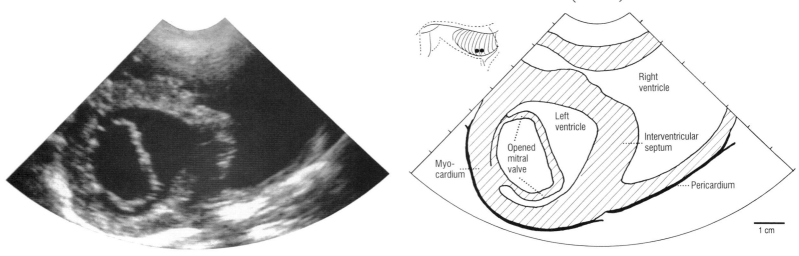

Fig. 4: Inflow tract of the left ventricle; diastolic short-axis section at the level of the mitral valve.

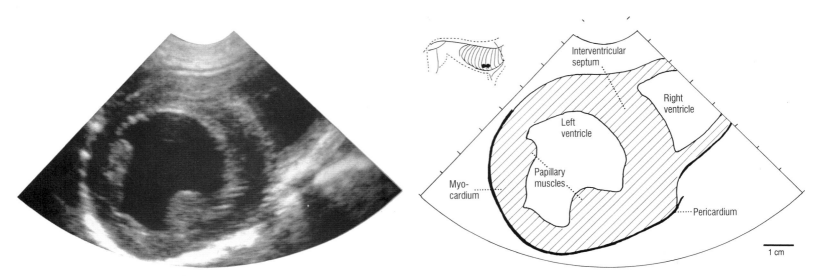

Fig. 5: Inflow tract of the left ventricle; systolic short-axis section at the level of the papillary muscles.

168

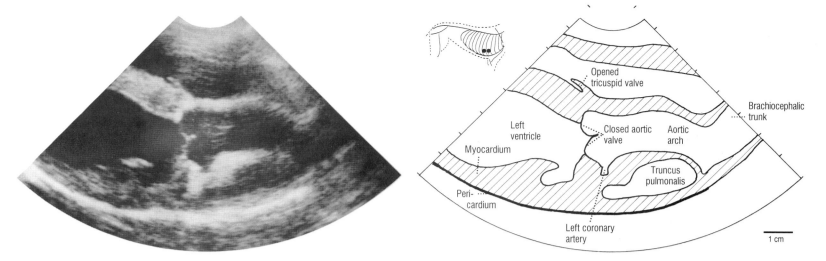

Fig. 6: Outflow tract of the left ventricle; diastolic long-axis section.

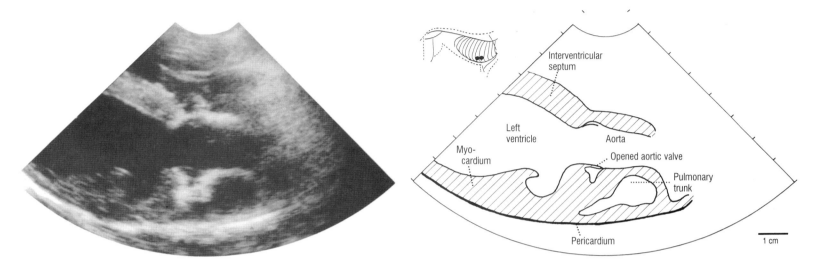

Fig. 7: Outflow tract of the left ventricle; systolic long-axis section.

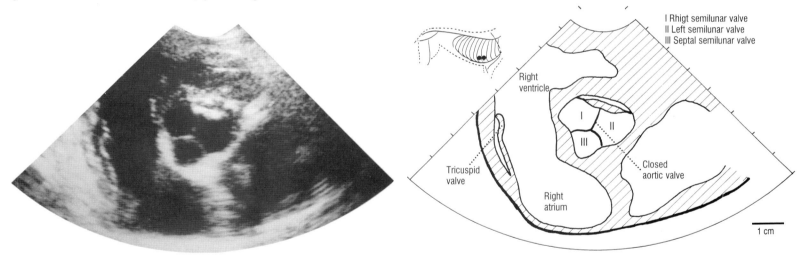

Fig. 8: Outflow tract of the left ventricle; diastolic short-axis section at the level of the aortic valve.

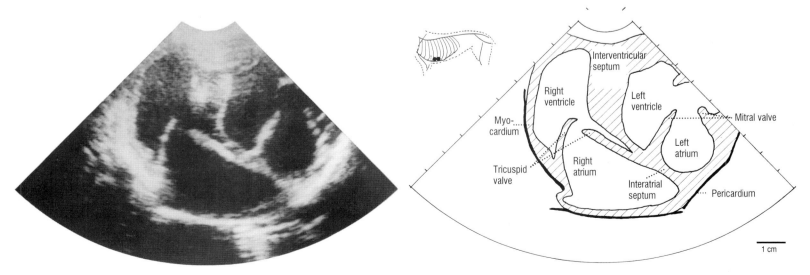

Fig. 9: Outflow tracts of the right and left ventricles; late-diastolic view of the four chambers.

STOMACH

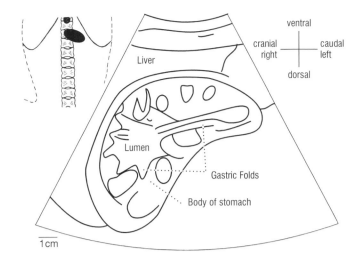

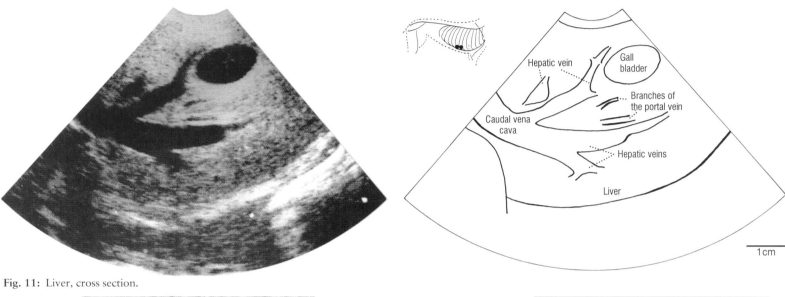

Fig. 10: Empty stomach, longitudinal section.

LIVER – HEPAR

Fig. 11: Liver, cross section.

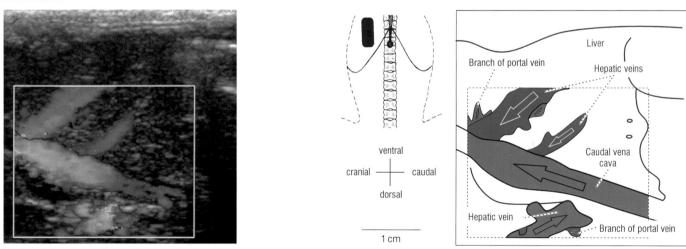

Fig. 12: Liver of 5-day-old puppy; color-coded doppler depiction of blood flow in hepatic veins and caudal vena cava during inspiration.

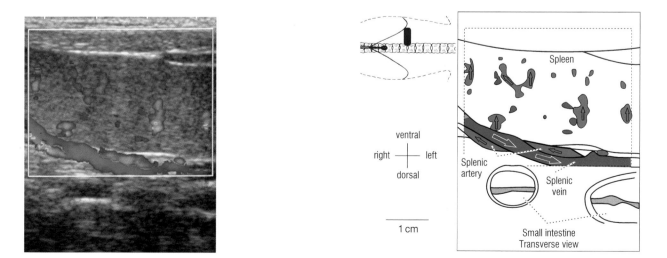

Fig. 13: Spleen and hilus of spleen, longitudinal section; color-coded doppler depiction of blood flow in the splenic artery and vein and intrasplenic blood vessels.

KIDNEY

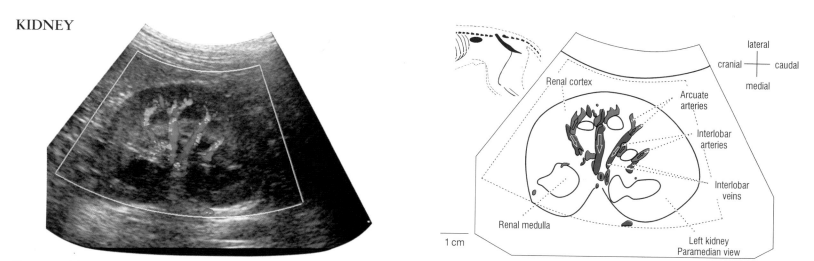

Fig. 14: Left kidney, paramedian longitudinal section; color-coded doppler depiction of blood flow in intrarenal blood vessels.

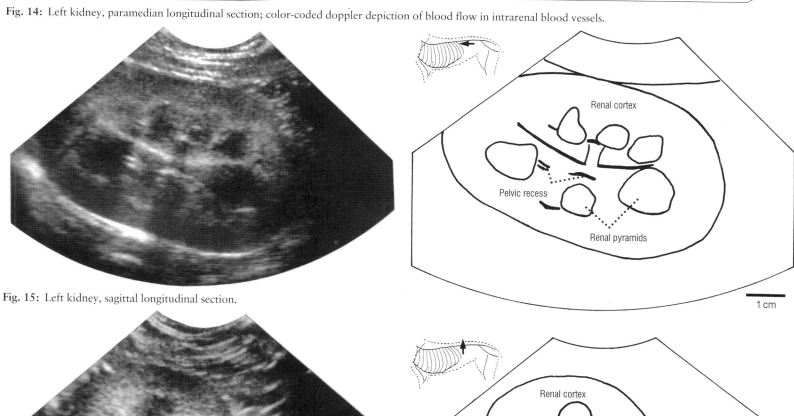

Fig. 15: Left kidney, sagittal longitudinal section.

Fig. 16: Left kidney, cross section.

OVARY

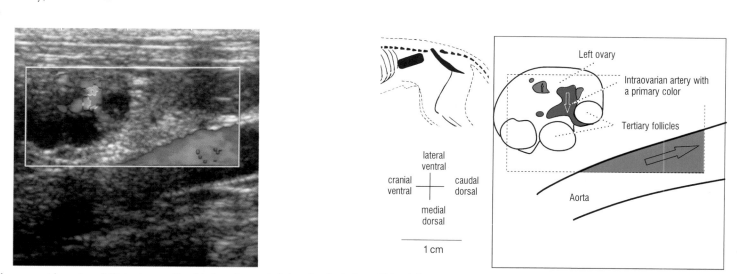

Fig. 17: Left ovary with tertiary follicles in a cycling bitch; color-coded doppler depiction of blood flow in aorta and intraovarian blood vessels.

URINARY BLADDER, UTERINE HORNS

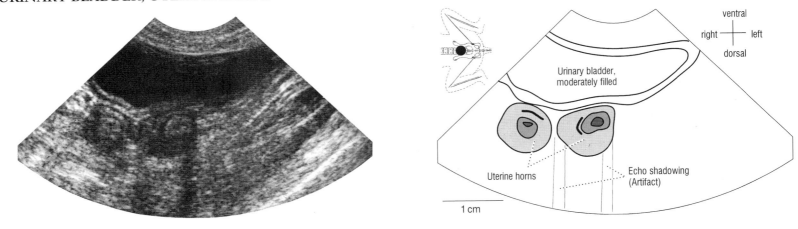

Fig. 18: Moderately filled urinary bladder and uterine horns of a cycling bitch in cross section.

PROSTATE

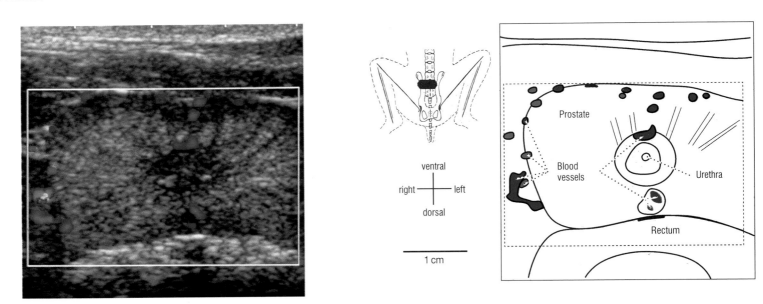

Fig. 19: Prostate and urethra in cross-section; color-coded doppler depiction of the blood flow in intra- and periprostatic blood vessels.

TESTIS

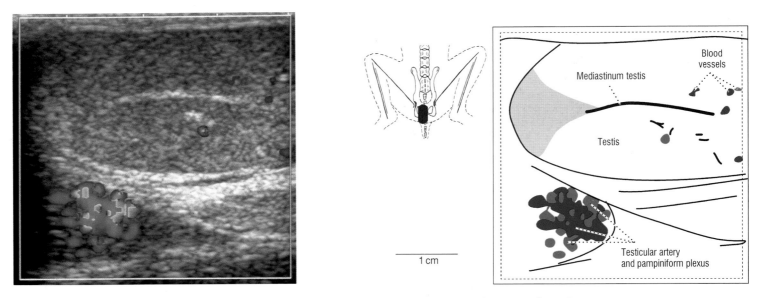

Fig. 20: Testis, longitudinal section; color-coded doppler depiction of blood flow in the testicular artery and the pampiniform plexus.

Address of the author:
PROF. DR. CORDULA POULSEN NAUTRUP
Institut für Tieranatomie
Tierärztliche Fakultät
Ludwig-Maximilians-Universität
München
Germany

Layout:
SUSANNE FASSBENDER, med. techn.
assistant

Technical drawings:
GERTRUD POULSEN NAUTRUP,
technician

I would like to thank the FEINFOCUS Röntgen-Systeme Co. for allowing the use of their Microfocus x-ray machines. For the support with various ultrasound equipment, including color-coded doppler systems, I would like to thank DR. W. KÄSTNER, Hannover, and the following companies and people: aTL Advanced Technology Laboratories, especially MR. R. FISCHER, DYNAMIC IMAGING, especially MRS. S. WILSON and MR. T. GERHARDS, as well as DIASONICS Sonotron, especially DR. H. SCHNEIDER.

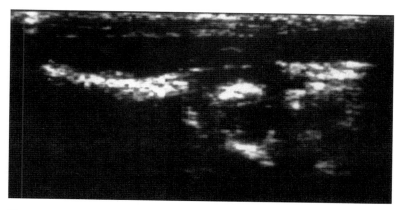

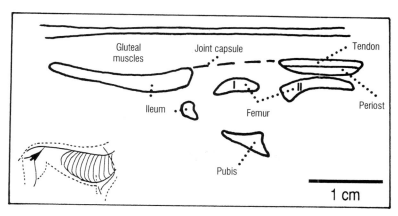

Fig. 21: Hip joint, longitudinal section.
(Kresken, J.-G., Köstlin, R.G., Clinic of Veterinary Surgery, Ludwig-Maximilian-University, Munich)

Gluteal muscles · Joint capsule · Tendon · Ileum · Femur · Periost · Pubis · Neck

I (Head, ossified epiphysis)
II Neck

1 cm

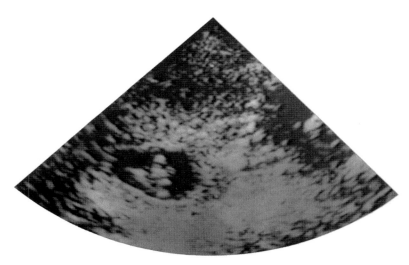

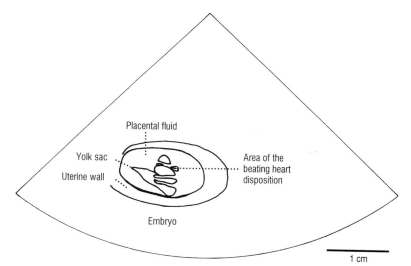

Fig. 22: Early pregnancy, embryo, 20d after conception.

Placental fluid · Yolk sac · Uterine wall · Area of the beating heart disposition · Embryo

1 cm

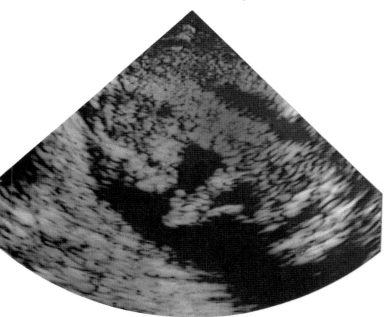

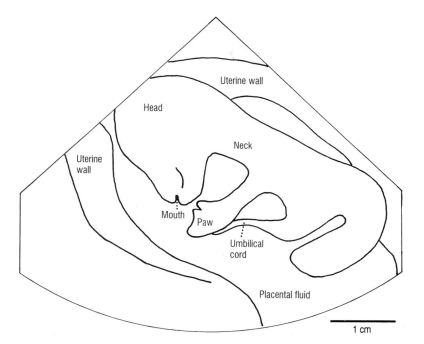

Fig. 23: Pregnancy, fetus, 38d after conception.

Uterine wall · Head · Neck · Uterine wall · Mouth · Paw · Umbilical cord · Placental fluid

1 cm

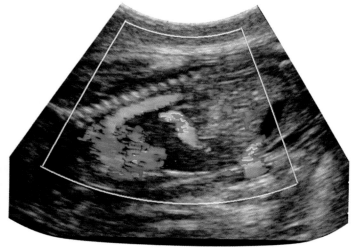

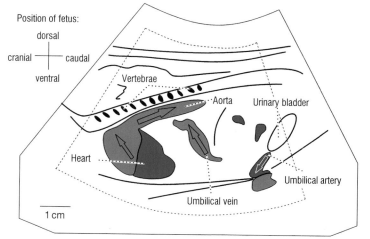

Position of fetus:
dorsal
cranial — caudal
ventral

Vertebrae · Aorta · Urinary bladder · Heart · Umbilical artery · Umbilical vein

1 cm

Fig. 24: Late stage of pregnancy, fetus 52 days after ovulation, thoracic cavity and abdominal cavity, slightly oblique paramedian section; color-coded doppler depiction of fetal circulation.

173

CONTRIBUTIONS TO CLINICAL AND FUNCTIONAL ANATOMY

4.1 EPIDERMIS constricted off during the embryonic period and displaced into the dermis forms **epidermoid cysts (true atheroma;** see also 6.1) which can assume a diameter up to 5 cm. In addition **dermoid cysts** include in their walls constituents of epidermal organ complexes (hair follicles, sebaceous and sweat glands).

4.2 The **STRATUM CORNEUM** or simple **keratin** forms the essential semipermeable barrier of the epidermis. It consists of keratinized epidermal cells which are united with one another by means of an **intercellular cement** similar to bricks in a wall united by mortar. The intercellular cement is formed in the stratum spinosum during keratinization and is secreted from so-called membrane coating vesicles in the intercellular fissures. Essential components of the intercellular cement are lipids, particularly ceramide, which are bound chemically by way of glycoprotein of the epidermal cell envelope. In the **autoimmune disease pemphigus** an autoimmune reaction against this glycoprotein leads to a detachment of epidermal cells from one another. A widening of the intercellular fissures and vesicle formation are a consequence of this. The continuous process of new growth and keratinization from epidermal cells expends energy and nutrients. These cells ultimately cornify and are detached from their epidermal association by means of **desquamation** or exfoliation. The process is regulated by a feed-back mechanism. An interruption of this dynamic balance, for example in vitamin A and zinc deficiencies, can lead to **thickening of the stratum corneum (hyperkeratosis).** In congenital (for example steroidsulphatase absence in ichthyosis congenita) or acquired (for example fatty acid deficiency) derangement of lipid metabolism, inferior intercellular cement is formed, having visible **seborrhea** as a sequel.

4.3 In different body regions at times the collagen and elastic fibers of the **CORIUM (dermis)** possess a definite orientation exhibited through so-called **cleavage or tension lines.** Surgical incisions across the lines result in dehiscent skin wounds of which the edges are wide apart. The margins of incisions made along the cleavage lines are situated together free of tension. In **intradermal (i/d) injections,** the strong connective tissue of the stratum corneum permits the application of only small quantities of liquid. Material injected intradermally comes into restricted contact with the defence mechanism of the skin so that this type of injection is employed in allergy tests.

4.4 Likewise the loose **SUBCUTIS (hypodermis)** of dogs is well adapted for **subcutaneous injections** which employ larger volumes of fluid. Ordinary or regular pressure loads can result in the formation of **subcutaneous bursae** over a solid base such as a bony prominence. These are found for example over the tuber of the olecranon in heavier dog breeds.

4.5 OUTER HAIR of the coat and **WOOL HAIR** of the undercoat pass through a regular cycle which determines **hair growth** in autumn and spring. This cycle is regulated by the epiphysis or pineal gland depending on length of daylight and environmental temperature.

6.1 SEBACEOUS GLAND SECRETION is mixed with that of the sweat glands in the excretory duct of the hair follicle and forms a **superficial lipid film** on skin and hair. This provides a strong water repellant effect particularly with a very thick hair coat. An obstruction of the follicular openings results in an accumulation of secretion and the formation of **small follicular retention cysts (false atheroma)** see also 4.1). **Acne** occurs due to an increased sebaceous secretion combined with a hyperkeratosis in the hair follicle. This can be squeezed out as a sausage shaped product from the follicle.

6.2 The secretion of the **CERUMINOUS GLANDS OF THE EAR** is mixed with desquamated epidermal cells as a yellow brownish **ear wax (cerumen).** With obstruction of the external acoustic meatus due to excessive hair growth, as occurs repeatedly in Poodles, ear wax accumulates and due to bacterial decomposition can have otitis externa ceruminosa as a consequence.

6.3 The **CIRCUMANAL (PERIANAL) GLANDS** are hepatoid glands which do not have excretory ducts. Under the influence of androgens they are disposed to **hyperplasia** which occurs 10 times more frequently in male dogs than in bitches. With more marked distension they can abscess, ulcerate or form fistulae under cover of m. sphincter ani externus and are treated surgically. The more unusual **adenocarcinomas** of the apocrine perianal sweat glands produce autonomous parathormone (pseudohyperparathyroidism). Hence in hypercalcemia of doubtful genesis, the perianal region must be examined for tumors.

6.4 PARANAL SINUS see 56.5

6.5 The **DORSAL GLANDS OF THE TAIL** are situated dorsal to caudal vertebrae 5–7. Regularly in feral canidae they are fully developed and serve for mutual olfactory recognition. Their primordia in the dog are considered atavistic, no longer possessing an apparent function, and in their histological synthesis, they correspond to hepatoid circumanal glands. In old male dogs they are disposed to **hyperplasia** eventually

combined with a local alopecia. The condition then appears as a roughly soft swelling, recognized as a callus or a hairless area.

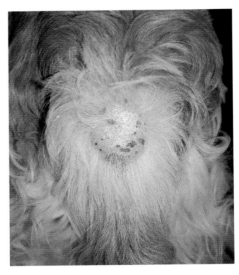

6.5 Hyperplasia of the (dorsal) glands of the tail in a male Hovawart.

6.6 In the subcutaneous cushions of the **PADS** are the incompressible fat cells – comparable to the inner sole of a running shoe – enclosed by septa of elastic connective tissue. In an elastic manner they absorb the accruing forces during foot contact with the ground and protect the bones of the phalanges from compression. The strong mechanical load borne by the epidermis of the pad necessitates a high rate of epidermal formation guaranteed due to a very good vascularization of the pad corium. Hence injuries to the pads bleed intensely.

6.7 CLAWS undergoing insufficient attrition become too long, can curl, and eventually become ingrown. Particularly is this so with the claw of the first digit which plays no part in ground contact. Therefore it should be checked regularly and shortened if necessary. With **clipping of the claws** one should observe that the claw is not at a right angle to the claw sheath; on the contrary, depending on the rate of natural wear and tear the claw should be shortened at a slightly acute angle.

8.1 The **VERTEBRAL COLUMN** is an essential element of the parabolic construction of the arched tendinous bridge which distributes load bearing to the trunk between the thoracic and pelvic limbs. Simultaneously this construction possesses a high flexibility which depends on the summation of the small increments of movement between individual vertebrae. The dynamics which the S-shaped curvature of the vertebral column permits, are demonstrated particularly in the stride of racing dogs. This is not possible in hoofed animals which have their vertebral columns essentially extended.

8.2 In anatomical colloquial usage the **TERMINOLOGY RELATING TO VERTEBRAE** is derived from the Latin 'vertebra' and in clinical usage from the Greek 'spondylos'.

8.3 HEMIVERTEBRAE have dissimilar shapes due to the fusion of vertebral bodies or of complete vertebrae based on an arrested development. They occur particularly frequently in brachycephalic or short skulled dog breeds. Hemivertebrae can cause deformation and curva-ture of the vertebral column either laterally (scoliosis), ventrally (kyphosis) or dorsally (lordosis). Due to constriction of the vertebral canal this can produce symptoms of paralysis.

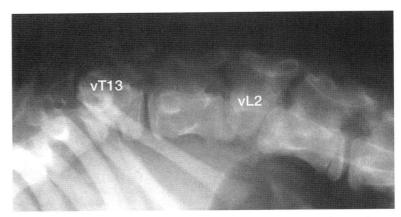

8.3 Shortened development of vT13 and vL2 producing hemivertebrae with resulting lordosis.

8.4 The **VERTEBRAL CANAL** protects the sensitive spinal cord from external influences. A congenital **partially patent spinal canal** is accompanied as a rule by clinical symptoms such as paralysis, urinary or fecal incontinence. This anomaly based on arrested development is termed spina bifida (rachischisis). The vertebrae most concerned are lumbar and sacral, more rarely those of the cervical and thoracic regions. In spina bifida aperta the meninges lie exposed at the surface while in spina bifida occulta the external skin is closed and intact and covers the defect. **Narrowing of the vertebral canal** is a frequent cause of functional derangements of the spinal cord. They can be based on discopathies (see 10.3), deformations of vertebral joints, subluxations or luxations (see 10.1 and 10.2) vertebral defects (see 8.3) and more rarely tumors and hematomas. A congenital **instability of the caudal cervical vertebrae (caudal cervical spondylomyelopathy or wobbler syndrome)** occurs particularly in large sized dogs, the Dobermann showing a predisposition. Radiographically this instability leads to an evident shortening of the intervertebral spaces and a narrowing of the vertebral canal. Chronic compression of the spinal cord with a typical neurological deficit is a sequel.

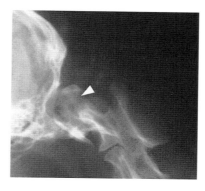

10.1 Atlantoaxial subluxation with constriction of the vertebral canal (arrow).

10.2 Alterations in the region of the **LUMBOSACRAL ARTICULATION** cause **compression of the cauda equina** which can be associated with pain, paralysis, ataxia and paresis of the pelvic limbs as well as urinary and fecal incontinence. The most frequent causes are degenerative changes at vL7 and vS1 (spondyloses see 8.6.), disc herniation (see 10.3.) and a proliferation of the ligamenta flava leading to dorsoventral stenosis of the vertebral canal.

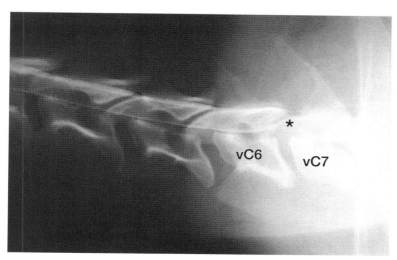

8.4 Myelographic demonstration of narrowing (*) of the vertebral canal at the level of vC6 and vC7 in a Dobermann with wobbler syndrome.

8.5 A RESECTION or **PARTIAL RESECTION OF THE VERTEBRAL ARCH (LAMINECTOMY, HEMILAMINECTOMY)** is the most frequently applied method for surgical relief of pressure on the spinal cord caused by constriction of the vertebral canal in the thoracolumbar region.

8.6 Chronic deforming bony outgrowths (osteophytes) of the **VERTEBRAL BODIES AND JOINTS (spondylosis deformans)** are a more frequent chance finding radiographically in older dogs. Especially in Boxers, the outgrowths can attain considerable dimensions and the lumbar vertebrae unite completely with one another (**spondylarthrosis ancylopoetica**). In rarer cases clinical symptoms occur where transverse processes normally coursing ventrally, compress spinal nerves at their egress from the intervertebral foramina.

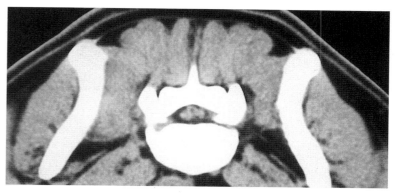

10.2 Narrowing of the vertebral canal and the intervertebral foramina between vL7 and vS1 in a dog with cauda equina compression syndrome (Computer tomography: Animal Clinic Krüger, Hamburg).

10.3 INTERVERTEBRAL DISCS undergo age dependent processes of reconstruction which progress quickly in chondroplastic dog breeds by one year of age. The nucleus pulposus and the internal connective tissue lamellae of the anulus fibrosus grow larger due to replacement cartilaginous tissue (chondroid metaplasia). Deficient nutrition due to diffusion from peripheral blood vessels, leads to degenerative alterations and dystrophic calcification both of which are evident on radiographs. The reconstructed pulp nucleus is no longer in position, axial compression forces deranging and removing it. The resultant overloading of the fibers of the anulus fibrosus produces overstretching and bulging dorsally. Or it can tear apart dorsally with herniation of the pulp nucleus in the vertebral canal as a result. A **disc prolapse** leads to compression of the spinal cord and/or the roots of the spinal nerves. This produces severe back pain as well as low to middle grade ataxia and paresis as seen frequently in 'Dachshund paralysis'. A **disc herniation** causes a high degree of damage to the spinal cord with a corresponding severe neurological deficit. The most frequent location of discopathies is the thoracolumbar transition region between vT11 and vL3. This is followed by the cervical vertebral column between vC2 and vC7. A disc prolapse is rare in the region of the thoracic vertebrae between vT2 and vT10 due to the fully developed intercapital ligaments. Generally the dorsal longitudinal ligament prevents a direct dorsal rupture or a herniation of the intervertebral disc and deflects the pulp nucleus which is pushing forwards. In herniation of the disc, associated with severe neurological symptoms a surgical decompression of the spinal cord is essential. This entails opening the vertebral canal and the removal of the prolapsed material. In the thoracolumbar region a hemilaminectomy (see 8.5) is preferred. In order to relieve pressure on the cervical spinal cord, a cleavage or 'ventral slot' is milled in the midline ventral to the vertebral bodies cranial and caudal to the affected intervertebral disc. As the case may be, this measures a third of the length or breadth of a vertebral body. The removal of prolapsed material by way of a ven-

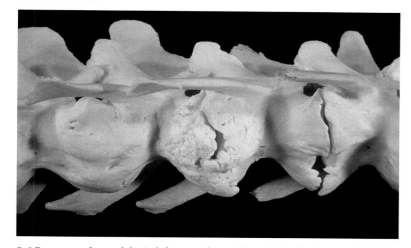

8.6 Pronounced spondylosis deformans from vL2 to vL5 with fusion of vL2 and vL3 (spondylarthrosis ancylopoetica).

8.7 Anomalies of the **CAUDAL VERTEBRAL COLUMN** occur in various forms, and from a breeder's viewpoint are desirable in individual breeds such as the French Bull Dog, and Pug. The consequent breeding of taillessness combines with numerous other vertebral defects such as spina bifida. Hence from the viewpoint of animal protection this rejects quality breeding.

10.1 An **INSTABILITY OF THE ATLANTOAXIAL ARTICULATION** brings about an excessive flexion of the articulation, leading to compression of the spinal cord and neurological deficit. The condition occurs congenitally in dwarf dog breeds and is due to a hypoplasia or aplasia of the dens of the axis. It is also caused due to trauma with fracture of the dens (breaking of the neck) or rupture of associated joint ligaments.

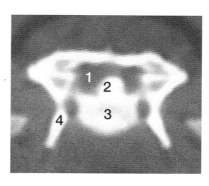

10.3 Disc hernia between vC2 and vC3.
1 Vertebral canal;
2 Prolapsing pulp nucleus;
3 Body of vC3;
4 Transverse process of vC2.
(Computer tomography: Animal Clinic Krüger, Hamburg).

tral fenestration of the anulus fibrosus can attain, but not always, an adequate release of pressure.

12.1 The **DORSAL THORACIC SERIES OF SUBCUTANEOUS NERVES** form the afferent limb of the panniculus reflex arc (cutaneous reflex). Skin irritation along the dorsal line leads reflexly to stimulation of the lateral thoracic nerve and with it to contraction of m. cutaneus trunci.

14.1 The **EXTERNAL JUGULAR VEIN** can be used for collecting larger quantities of blood for blood transfusion and is also accessible when peripheral veins are already collapsed. This vein is also the site of choice for central venous catheterization.

14.2 The **RECURRENT LARYNGEAL NERVE** lies laterally on the trachea and should be taken into consideration and preserved in absolute terms in surgery of the neck particularly involving the ventral approach to the cervical vertebral column. Damage to the nerve results in a unilateral paralysis or hemiplegia of the larynx.

14.3 The **SUPERFICIAL CERVICAL LYMPH NODE** is easily palpable and should be examined for changes during each general clinical examination.

14.4 The further transport of swallowed boluses in the **ESOPHAGUS** occurs due to contractions of esophageal musculature which are undulating, directed aborally, and are involuntary. Peristalsis takes place automatically after the initiation of the swallowing reflex but is also promoted directly or even released by mechanical stimuli. Thus a more complete transport of small components such as tablets exerting no stretch excitation is unguaranteed. **Interruption of motility** can involve the transitional region between pharynx and esophagus locally or the total esophageal musculature. **Interruption of pharyngoesophageal motility** is caused by a congenital neuromuscular derangement with paralysis of m. cricopharyngeus (cricopharyngeal achalasia see 102.1) but can also result from distemper or rabies for example. Disturbance to motility of esophageal musculature results in insufficient transport of food and a dilation of the esophagus (**megaesophagus**). The origin can be a congenital derangement of innervation, a condition to which German Shepherds are predisposed, as well as secondary neurogenic sequelae, or myogenic diseases such as polyneuritis and myasthenia gravis. In rarer cases a dilation of the caudal section of the esophagus is due to an insufficient relaxation of m. sphincter cardiae.

Foreign bodies such as swallowed bones stuck in the esophagus, block the lumen partially or completely (obturation). Narrow anatomical sites predisposed to obstruction are the cranial thoracic aperture or inlet, that at the base of the heart and the esophageal hiatus of the diaphragm. The continuous stretch excitation due to the presence of foreign bodies can lead to spasm of the esophageal musculature which in turn can result in a reduced circulation of blood, ischemic necrosis, and ultimate perforation of the esophageal wall. An extrinsic constriction of the esophagus (stenosis) is caused most frequently by anomalies in the course of the large blood vessels (right aorta see 44.4).

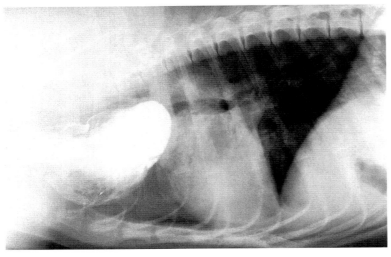

14.4 Contrast radiograph of precardial megaesophagus in a dog with a right aorta and persistent ductus arteriosus.

14.5 A CONSTRICTION OF THE TRACHEA (TRACHEAL STENOSIS) leads to dyspnea. The chief cause is a weakness and overstretching of the membranous wall and m. trachealis resulting in the dorsoventral flattening of trachea (**tracheal collapse**). The condition is diagnosed almost exclusively in dwarf dog breeds (Yorkshire Terrier, Toy Poodle, Chihuahua) and is at least partly congenital. Alterations in shape such as lateral flattening (**scabbard trachea**) or hypoplasia of the tracheal cartilages in the Bulldog, are rarely congenital. An acute life threatening dyspnea due to obstruction of the upper airway for example in laryngeal edema can be treated through an opening of the trachea (tracheotomy). After ventromedian exposure of the trachea an incision is

made through one of the annular ligaments between tracheal cartilages 2–5. Through this a T-shaped tracheal tube is introduced.

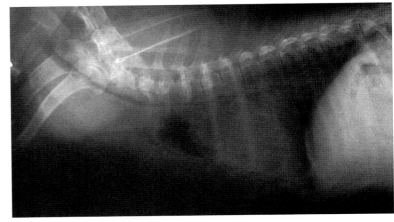

14.5 Flattening of the intrathoracic portion of the trachea (tracheal collapse) in a Yorkshire Terrier. The radiograph was taken during the expiratory phase.

14.6 The **THYROID GLAND** is an endocrine gland which, due to the controlled output of its hormones tetraiodothyronine (thyroxine) and triiodothyronine into the bloodstream, regulates the intensity of metabolism. In addition its parafollicular or C-cells produce the hormone calcitonin, the distribution of which causes a reduction in calcium level. The thyroid develops, with its main portion dorsally, from the endoderm of the root of the tongue. (The C-cells originate from the ultimobranchial bodies and initially from the neural crest). The ductus thyreoglossus descends from the tongue to the ventral laryngeal-tracheal boundary. The distal end of the ductus thyreoglossus develops into the right and left lobes of the thyroid gland as well as the isthmus glandularis which in dogs is fully developed only occasionally. Normally the remaining portions of the ductus regress completely. Individually maintained remnants differentiate into accessory thyroid glands. These can occur on all organs, which, during embryological development, have contact with the primordium of the thyroid gland namely tongue, larynx, trachea, and base of heart. Occasionally cysts of the ductus thyreoglosus can develop generally at the base of the tongue. The size of the thyroid gland is dependent on a multitude of factors such as body weight, age, sex, and season of the year, and can be determined sonographically. Any form of thyroid enlargement is known as a **goiter** and has many origins. A classical example is a goiter caused by chronic iodine deficiency present in populations in iodine deficient regions such as south Germany. In dogs, tumor related goiters are frequently malignant (struma carcinomatosa). In dogs such as Beagles which are predisposed to the condition, relatively frequent autoimmune inflammation of the thyroid (thyroiditis) can cause a reduction in size of the gland and hypofunction (hypothyroidism).

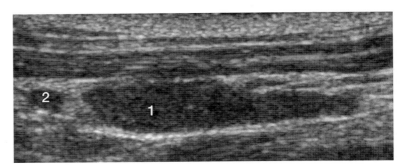

14.6 and 14.7 Sonographic longitudinal section through the thyroid gland (1) and the cranial external parathyroid gland (2).

14.7 The **PARATHYROID GLANDS** regulate calcium and phosphate metabolism. Their hormone, parathormone, functions as an antagonist of calcitonin, resulting in an increase in blood calcium levels and simultaneously a reduction in phosphate levels. Within a short time a **functional failure** of the parathyroid glands leads to a life-threatening hypocalcemic tetany; this is why parathyroid glands are preserved unconditionally in thyroid surgery. Errors in feeding, for example with the predominant feeding of meat especially in young dogs, are a frequent source of **excessive exposure to phosphate** and/or **insufficient supply of calcium**. Counter regulation results in increased distribution of parathormone (**alimentary secondary hyperparathyroidism**) and ultimately a **hyperplasia of the parathyroid glands**. The sequel is an increase calcium resorption from the bones and this is why the condition is also termed **juvenile osteoporosis** or osteodystrophia fibrosa. The demineralization of bones leads to a distortion of the long bones and a tendency for greenstick and vertebral fractures to occur. A typical cause of hyperplasia of the parathyroid glands in old dogs is a **chronic kidney insufficiency**. This, due to the interruption of enteral calcium absorption and likewise an increased distribution of parathormone (**renal secondary hyperparathroidism**) causes a hypocalcemia with corresponding consequences for the skeletal system.

Adenomas of the parathyroid glands can develop autonomous parathormone and lead to rare symptoms of **primary hyperparathyroidism** of which a direct symptom is hypercalcemia (see also 6.3).

16.1 In order to facilitate lateral access to the neck of the scapula during surgery the **ACROMION** can be detached temporarily at its base by osteotomy. In so doing one notes the close relative position of the suprascapular nerve. At the end of surgery the acromion is reattached using surgical screws and wire.

16.2 In growing dogs the **HUMERUS** possesses an epiphysis (the head of the humerus) and an apophysis (greater and lesser tubercles). Both centers of ossification fuse in the course of development and are then separated from the diaphysis by a characteristic growth plate or suture. Distally the trochlea and capitulum of the humerus each possess an individual center of ossification both of which fuse after about 2 months of age and likewise form a common epiphysis. The proximal growth plate or epiphyseal suture has an essentially higher growth potential that the distal so that longitudinal growth of the humerus takes place predominantly towards its proximal part. Hence compressions or fractures of the proximal growth plate have potentially more aggravating consequences for the further longitudinal growth of the humerus than injuries to the distal growth plate.

16.3 FRACTURES OF THE OLECRANON occur due to traumata acting laterally or originating from overextension of the elbow joint. The vigorous traction of m.triceps brachii on the tuber of the olecranon causes fracturing in a cranioproximal direction. The dislodged part of the olecranon is restored surgically using kirschner wire and plates. Additionally traction forces of m.triceps brachii must be absorbed using tension webbing.

16.4 The **ANCONEAL PROCESS** provides stability to the extended elbow joint against sideway and rotational movements. Its detachment (isolated or fragmented anconeal process) leads to slight instability and development of arthrosis. The symptoms of isolated process are included with the complex of elbow dysplasia. It is caused not only by trauma but is a probable consequence of growth and nutritional disturbances of its cartilaginous apophyseal suture. Promoted for example by deficient nutrition and poor breeding there is also a genetic predisposition as in the German Shepherd dog.

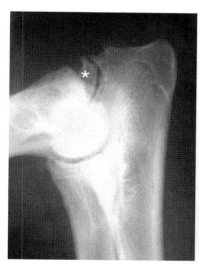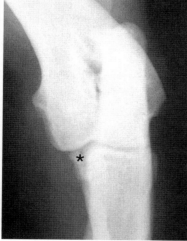

16.4 (Left) isolated anconeal process (*) in a German Shepherd and
16.5 (Right) radiograph of fragmentation of the medial coronoid process (*).

16.5 FRAGMENTATION OF THE MEDIAL AND LATERAL CORONOID PROCESSESS are likewise included in the complex of dysplasia of the elbow joint and occur predominantly in large breeds of dogs such as Berner Sennenhund and Rottweiler. One of the possible causes lies in growth retardation of the radius (short radius syndrome). The humerus no longer articulates with the shortened radius but bears particularly on the medial coronoid process which becomes deformed or fragmented as a reaction.

16.6 Eighty percent of the longitudinal growth of the ulna occurs in the distal **ULNAR EPIPHYSEAL SUTURE**. Genetic (Dachshund, Basset), traumatic or alimentary (delayed mineralization see 14.7) factors can result in a retarded longitudinal growth. The sequel is a shortening and distortion of the ulna (short ulna syndrome) and a steplike growth of the elbow joint (**distractio cubiti**) or carpal joint (**distractio carpi**). The growth of the distal radius beyond the styloid process of the ulna leads to outward rotation of the distal limb segment (**carpus valgus**). A delayed mineralization of the cartilaginous ulnar epiphyseal suture is evident

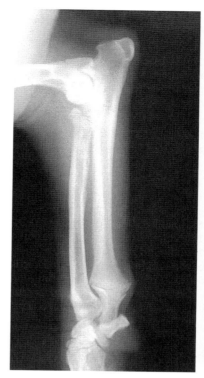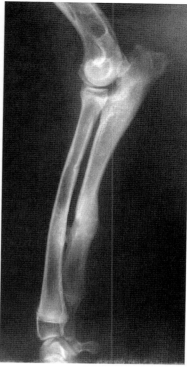

16.5 and 16.6 Short radius syndrome (left) and short ulnar syndrome (right) as a result of growth retardation after fracture of the ulna.

radiologically as a persistent conical area which is scarcely radio opaque. In very large dog breeds it is easily defined almost on a regular basis.

18.1 The nerves of the **BRACHIAL PLEXUS** can be injured through pressure, contusion or over extension but also by tumors or abscesses emanating from the axillary lymph nodes. Particularly during over extension the nerves with shorter course distances between the lacuna at the m.scalenus and entrance into the appropriate muscle/s are vulnerable. The axillary nerve is an example. Lacerations or tearing away of the roots of the plexus from the spinal cord are generally the result of extreme abduction of the limb, as in car accidents. A complete avulsion of the brachial plexus leads to paralysis of the whole of the limb musculature with drooping of shoulder and elbow and a flexed carpal joint. In addition, laceration of n TV1 causes deficit of the panniculus reflex (see 12.1) and by injury of the white rami communicantes tugging at the cervicothoracic ganglion produces an ipsilateral Horner syndrome (see 118.1)

18.2 Injuries of **M.BICEPS BRACHII** are generally concerned with its tendon of original which ruptures directly, or in young dogs can tear away from the supraglenoid tubercle of the scapula (avulsion fracture). A typical diagnostic characteristic of this rupture is that the shoulder joint can be overflexed considerably and in addition the elbow joint overextends.

18.3 Due to the effects of trauma the **RADIAL NERVE** can be easily injured in its course over the lateral supracondylar crest. The result is a **(distal) radial paralysis** accompanied by a deficit of action of digital and carpal extensor muscles leading to what has been described as the 'kiss hand position'. With injury of the radial nerve in the region of the brachial plexus there is an additional deficit of action of the m. triceps brachii (**proximal radial paralysis**). Besides a motor deficit with radial paralysis there is a deficiency of sensation on the dorsal aspect of the paw.

18.4 The **ULNAR NERVE** is palpable on the medial surface of the olecranon and with the elbow extended and the triceps musculature relaxed it can be followed proximally.

20.1 The **CEPHALIC VEIN** at forearm level is suitable for venipuncture for the taking of blood samples, for intravenous (i/v) injections and for the placement of longterm cannulae. Medially and laterally the vein is accompanied by sensory branches of the radial nerve. Therefore paravenous needle perforations produce violent defence reactions by the canine patient concerned.

20.2 The **SUPRASCAPULAR NERVE** can easily be damaged in its course around the neck of the scapula due to fractures. Its injury results in instability of the shoulder joint, abduction of the shoulder with weight bearing, as well as problems of protraction or forward movement of the limb.

20.3 An overloading of **M.INFRASPINATUS** with accompanying swelling leads to a reduced blood circulation (acute functional com-partment syndrome) from which can develop a fibrosis contingent upon ischemia and resultant contraction of the muscle. The shortening of the muscle produces an outward rotation of the limb with an adducted elbow and decreased motility. Early transection of m.infraspinatus usually leads to complete recovery of limb function (see also 146.2).

20.4 The **LONG HEAD** of **M.TRICEPS BRACHII** can rupture due to a fall or springing to a higher level. As a result the affected dog is no longer able to extend its elbow.

22.1 The strong **ANTEBRACHIAL FASCIA** encloses the **caudomedial muscles of the forearm** completely and forms fascial compartments housing the muscles concerned. On the other hand the fascial envelope of the **craniolateral muscles of the forearm** forms no distinct muscle compartments (see also 146.2).

22.2 The tendon of insertion of **M.FLEXOR CARPI ULNARIS**, due to surgical translocation to the extensor tendons of the carpus, can be used in the recovery of carpal extension in irreversible radial paralysis.

26.1 The **SHOULDER JOINT** of the standing dog forms an angle of 110°–120°. When flexed it is about 45°–70° and in extension is possibly 10°–30°. Adduction is up to approximately 30° and abduction possibly up to 40°. An **intrarticular injection of the shoulder joint** can take place a fingerbreadth distal to the acromion and above the greater tubercle of the humerus. After puncture of the skin horizontally the needle is pushed mediocaudally until synovial fluid flows out. Mechanically, the articular surface of the head of the humerus is severely stressed in its caudal section, which predisposes to injury of the articular cartilage. This condition is known as osteochondrosis dissecans (**OCD**, see 142.4).

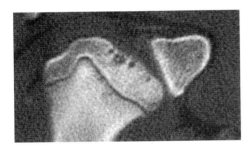

26.1 OCD of the shoulder joint (Computer tomography: Animal Clinic Krüger, Hamburg).

26.2 In the standing position the **ELBOW JOINT** occupies an angle from 125°–140°. Flexion is possibly about 90°–110° while extension results in only 5°–20°. **Puncture** of the slightly flexed joint is made from a craniolateral direction by inclining the needle mediodistally and distal to the palpable lateral epicondyle of the humerus. A series of diseases of the elbow joint (isolated anconeal and coronoid processes, distractio cubiti, and congenital luxation of the small head of the radius) is grouped under the name **dysplasia of the elbow joint**. In particular it results from a disturbance of skeletal development with asynchronous longitudinal growth of radius and ulna (see 16.6) leading to steplike development of the elbow joint (**distractio cubiti**).

26.3 In the **PROXIMAL AND DISTAL RADIOULNAR ARTICULATIONS** a pronation around 10° and a supination around 20°–30° can take place with elbow and carpal joints flexed around 90°. Following **rupture of the lateral collateral ligament of the elbow**, on the other hand, there is an inward rotation of more than around 45° and after **rupture of the medial collateral ligament** possibly an outward rotation above 90°.

26.4 The **CARPAL JOINT** in the standing dog occupies an angle from 190°–200° which is a slightly overextended position. Besides this overextension there is also a slight physiological valgus position from 12°–20°. A further extension of the carpal joint is strictly limited (maximum 5°). Flexion is up to 150°–160° and a supination possibly around 10°–20°. The flexibility of the different joints comprising the overall carpal articulation is very different. The main mobility takes place in the antebrachiocarpal joint which also permits a slight rotation of 5°–10°. On the other hand, the mediocarpal articulation can be flexed only up to 15° and the carpometacarpal articulation only 5°. A traumatic rupture of the palmar ligament apparatus results in hyperextension of the carpal joint.

26.5 The **SUBCUTANEOUS BURSA OF THE OLECRANON** can fill with synovial fluid (hygroma) as a reaction to a markedly excessive demand or strain on it. It becomes visible as a tense plump swelling up to hen's egg size at the olecranon.

28.1 Left and right **M. LONGUS COLLI** are separated from each other by blunt dissection after an incision through the deep fascia of the neck. This provides a ventral approach to intervertebral discs of the cervical vertebral column.

30.1 INSPIRATORY MUSCLES are more strongly developed than their **EXPIRATORY** counterparts. Inspiration is a more active process whereas expiration takes place largely in a passive manner, the latter due to contraction of elastic elements of the lung which become stretched during inspiration. Only in forced respiration or more difficult expiration (expiratory dyspnea) are expiratory muscles involved intensely including abdominal muscles acting as accessory expiratory muscles. Respiration with greater increased expansion of the thorax is defined as **costal in type** as distinct from **abdominal** where the diaphragm is chiefly involved. Physiologically in dogs costal respiration predominates.

30.2 DIAPHRAGMATIC HERNIAE can be congenital or acquired traumatically with displacement of abdominal viscera such as liver, stomach and small intestines, into the pleural cavity. Hence, in inspiration, expansion of the lung is more or less strongly encroached upon. Due to a reduced pressure during inspiration, abdominal organs to some extent are sucked into the pleural cavity. **Congenital diaphragmatic hernia** has its aperture of rupture mostly at the site of passage of the esophagus, namely its hiatus. The hernial sac regularly present is often the distended serosal cavity of the mediastinum. With congenitally incomplete closure of the ventral section of the insertion of the diaphragm and a similar defect of the pericardium abdominal viscera can penetrate them. **Traumatically acquired diaphragmatic hernia (rupture of the diaphragm)** occurs generally due to rupture of the muscular portion of the costal part of the diaphragm and produces no hernial sac. It always produces serious clinical symptoms.

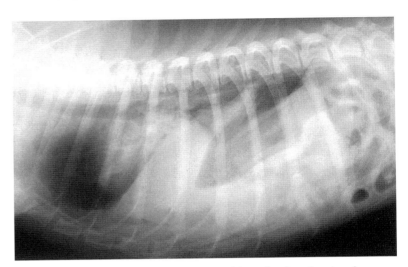

30.2 Partial displacement of liver and stomach into the pleural cavity after rupture of the diaphragm.

32.1 The **PREPUTIAL OSTIUM (ORIFICE)** can be constricted (**phimosis**) either congenitally or with wound healing after injury and then impedes extrusion of the penis. Urinary retention and a severe inflammation of prepuce and glans penis (balanoposthitis) can result. A slight bacterial balanoposthitis (preputial catarrh) develops chronically in many male dogs.

32.2 The **MAMMARY GLAND** is a skin gland, more specifically an aprocrine sweat gland modified markedly. Mammary gland tissue is imbedded in septa of superficial fascia of the trunk. Consequently its surgical removal (mastectomy) can be oriented by the surgeon due to deep fascia lying underneath it. Only in the region of inguinal and thoracic mammae do blood vessels approach the gland tissue dorsally. Dorsal to the inguinal mamma in a majority of bitches one observes a fat filled vaginal process. Its injury produces an opening into the peritoneal cavity.

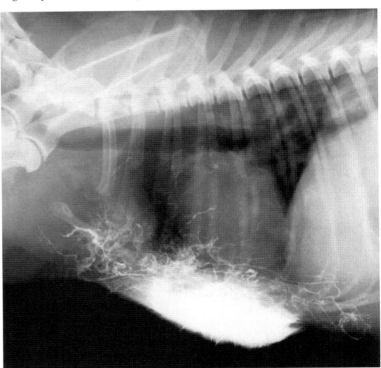

32.2 Indirect lymphography of an abnormal cancerous mammary complex adjacent to thorax, 20 minutes after application of radiographic contrast medium (iotasul-schering). Afferent lymph flow takes place cranially in the direction of the axillary lymph nodes and caudally in the direction of the superficial inguinal lymph nodes. Perforating lymphatic vessels enter through the thoracic wall to the pleural cavity within (Radiograph: Professor Dr. D. Berens von Rautenfeld, Hannover).

Lymph drainage and regional lymph nodes (axillary, superficial inguinal) determine the routes of metastases of malignant mammary tumors which occur relatively frequently in old bitches. Efferent lymphatic vessels from thoracic mammae also penetrate the thoracic wall and discharge by way of mediastinal lymph nodes. The possibility of direct drainage of lymph from abdominal mammae into medial iliac lymph nodes has also been detected in old bitches.

34.1 ABDOMINAL MUSCLES are brought into action for the active reduction of abdominal volume during which intra-abdominal pressure is raised (the abdominal press) by the **contracted** diaphragm. This 'press' is established during defecation, micturition, vomition and during parturition for the expulsion of the fetus. In difficult expiration, on the other hand, the **relaxed** diaphragm is pressed cranially by abdominal viscera due to tense abdominal musculature and thus decreases the size of the pleural cavity.

34.2 The **LINEA ALBA** in the dog is selected as the most frequent site for surgical access to the abdominal cavity (laparotomy). After incision of the linea alba for preumbilical access to the cavity, one encounters the preumbilical fat bodies within the falciform ligament; these should be detached from the body wall and flapped away from the site.

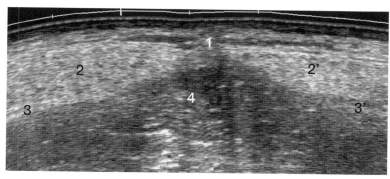

34.2 Sonographic transverse section of the ventral body wall cranial to the umbilicus. 1, Linea alba; 2, 2' right and left mm.recti abdominis; 3, 3' right and left internal laminae of the rectus sheath; 4 Preumbilical fat bodies (Sonograph: Professor Dr. C. Poulsen Nautrup, Munich).

34.3 UMBILICAL HERNIA is the most frequently occurring hernia of the dog. As a rule only fat or a section of omentum prolapses through the relatively small aperture of rupture. With the exception of inguinal hernia (see 36.1) other forms of hernia of the abdominal muscles are rare.

36.1 Essentially **INGUINAL HERNIA** occurs more frequently in the bitch than in the male dog, the complete opposite to the proportion in other domestic mammals. One differentiates 2 types of inguinal herniae, the more frequent indirect – generally congenital – and the rarely direct, which is always acquired. In the **indirect inguinal hernia** the vaginal ring

forms the aperture of rupture and the vaginal process the hernial sac. In contrast to other female domestic mammals, the sac is almost always overdeveloped in the bitch and is predisposed to inguinal hernia since it does not have to envelop the structures of the spermatic cord as in the male. In addition, in several dog breeds (Cocker, Dachshund, Golden Retriever) an abnormally wide, vaginal ring of heritable origin has been detected as the basis of an indirect inguinal hernia. In animals so disposed, due to pressure increase in the abdominal cavity (abdominal press, pregnancy) it is easy to have not only a prolapse of sections of omentum and fat, but also loops of intestine, urinary bladder, uterus etc into the vaginal process. A prolapse of portions of viscera through the vaginal ring of the male is referred to in the clinic as scrotal hernia. In **direct inguinal hernia** generally the aperture of rupture lies medially besides the inguinal ring. Consequently there is tissue laceration and abdominal viscera bursts through the abdominal wall by the shortest direct route.

36.2 In rare cases the **FEMORAL RING** is the aperture of rupture (femoral hernia) whereby peritoneum and transverse fascia are everted in the femoral space with secondary laceration.

38.1 The **FIELD OF THE LUNG** is determined by percussion. In the dog the caudal border of the lung lies approximately at the level of the tuber coxae in the 11th intercostal space, mid-thorax in the 9th intercostal space and at the level of the tuber of the olercranon in the 6th intercostal space.

38.2 LUNG FUNCTION is involved essentially with gas exchange between blood and inspired air. Air is introduced by means of a non-anastomosed bronchial system to lung alveoli involved in air exchange. These signify an enormous increase of the internal surface of the lung. Respiration is based on an alteration in volume of the thoracic cavity. With **inspiration** its increase is attained by a flattening of the diaphragmatic dome (diaphragmatic respiration) and through craniolateral displacement of the ribs (costal respiration). Due to adhesive forces in the pleural cavity, the lung must follow the movements of the wall of the thoracic cavity whereby the alveoli expand. In the first instance **expiration** is produced due to perialveolar elastic nets which contract the alveoli in a passive manner.

38.3 In radiographs the **BRONCHI** which contain air are not delineated from surrounding lung tissue also containing air. If for example, lung tissue is compressed or condensed due to inflammation air–containing bronchi in the affected region are defined (**air bronchogram**). Their artificial presentation is also possible by using a positive contrast medium (**contrast bronchogram**). Whereas the trachea has sensory innervation and releases a cough reflex as a reaction to an inhaled foreign body, no cough stimulus is produced by a similar body inhaled further into the bronchi. The display and removal of such a body can take place endoscopically (bronchoscopy).

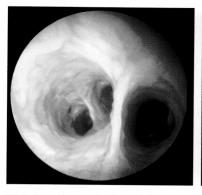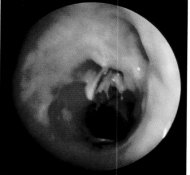

38.3 Bronchoscopic view of the primary bronchi of a healthy dog (left) and bronchoscopic display of an inhaled awn (right). (Bronchoscopic photographs: Professor Dr. W. Kraft, Munich).

40.1. The **PULMONARY ARTERY OF THE CRANIAL LOBE OF THE LUNG** always courses dorsal and parallel to the corresponding pulmonary vein lying cranioventrally. Radiographically both vessels are separated clearly from air-contained lung. In a laterolateral radiograph both vessels can be identified reliably on the basis of their characteristic positional relationship, the pulmonary artery dorsally, the pulmonary vein ventrally.

40.2 The **absent** or only **slightly developed VISCEROSENSORY INNERVATION** of the bronchial tree (see also 38.3) and lung is why pulmonary and bronchial tumors are not recognized until later or often too late, since they cause no or hardly no pain.

40.3 The **AORTA** and the large arteries ramifying in the vicinity of the heart are recognized as containing elastic tissue due to their yellowish color. The wall of the ascending aorta stretches because blood is driven out of the heart in systole. In the following diastole it contracts again and therefore transports the blood further in a passive manner. (See text book of physiology).

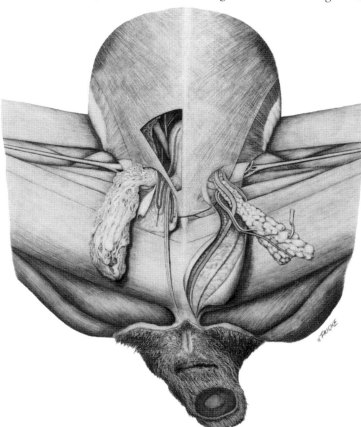

36.1 A preparation of bilateral inguinal hernia in the female cat (!), which, in principle, can be present in the same form in the bitch. Left side of illustration: direct inguinal hernia. Right side of illustration: indirect inguinal hernia with opened vaginal process (note fenestrated abdominal wall).

40.4 The **STERNAL LYMPH NODE** is not directly accessible for clinical diagnostic procedures, but with a pathological increase in size is displayed in laterolateral radiographs.

40.5 The **THYMUS** is a **primary lymphatic organ** which, on comparative anatomical grounds, has only a thoracic part with right and left lobes. Involution with accompanying fatty degeneration is never complete, functional remnants remaining even in old age. According to dominant opinion fetal stem cells migrate from bone marrow into the thymus where daughter cells differentiate into **thymocytes**. From the thymus these colonize the secondary lymph organs such as lymph nodes and spleen, and after their imprinting to T-lymphocytes are responsible for cellular immunity (undesirable activity with rejection of transplants). Thymic atrophy can occur with disappearance of lymphocytes in alimentary upsets, stress and wasting diseases. An unphysiologically **delayed regression** is present in endocrine disturbances and can be a consequence of premature castration. A **thymic hyperplasia** with **overfunction** analogous to that in humans occurs rarely in young dogs with **myasthenia gravis** (neuromuscular interruption of conduction with prompt muscle fatigue) (see 144.3). Due to **thymectomy** (removal of thymus) an improvement can be achieved in humans.

42.1 The **COSTAL PLEURA** is provided with sensory innervation from branches of the intercostal nerves. As a result inflammation of the pleura (pleurisy) is very painful. Diaphragmatic and mediastinal pleurae receive sensory nerve fibers from the phrenic nerve and viscerosensory innervation via the vagus nerve. On the other hand the **pulmonary pleura** is either not innervated or only with low grade viscerosensory fibers.

42.2 Air can penetrate the **MEDIASTINUM (pneumomediastinum)** due to injuries of the tracheal or bronchial wall and the esophagus for example with a perforating foreign body. In a pneumomediastinum those organs, blood vessels and airways not visible under normal physiological conditions are reproduced radiographically.

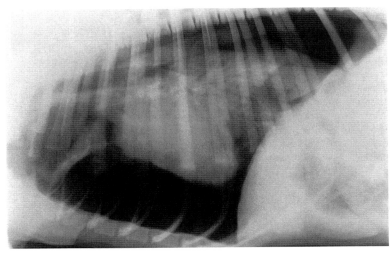

42.2 and 42.3 Bilateral appearance of a pneumomediastinum which conveys a distinct image of the large blood vessels, and a pneumothorax which has, as a sequel, the removal of the heart apex from the sternum.

42.3 In a physiological sense the **PLEURAL CAVITIES** simply exhibit a capillary wide gap filled with a serous liquid film. The limiting parts of the pleura (parietal and visceral) cling to each other across the serous gap, by adhesion, without, however, the loss of their sliding capacity during respiratory movements of the lung. In a qualitative and quantitative regard the pleural cavities can exhibit unphysiological content such as air (**pneumothorax**), an increased watery liquid (**hydrothorax**), lymph containing fluid (**chylothorax** after rupture of the thoracic duct) or blood containing fluid (**hemothorax**). A **pneumothorax** results if air penetrates through an external injury into the pleural cavity (**external pneumothorax**) or due to a laceration of the lung tissue (**internal pneumothorax**). The consequence is widening of the potential fluid filled gap and therewith a termination of the adhesive forces holding the lung to the thoracic wall. The pulmonary lobe of the affected side collapses to a fraction of its original size. A bilateral pneumothorax can occur if the mediastinum of both pleural cavities is not completely separated. This results in difficult life threatening shortness of breath (dyspnea). **Valvular pneumothorax** likewise results in a life threatening dyspnea. With this, further air at the injured site is sucked into the pleural cavity and this cannot escape on expiration since the site functions as a valve only permitting an inflow of air. During auscultation no respiratory noises are heard and heart sounds also are reduced markedly in intensity. A radiograph of a pneumothorax has characteristic features: The collapsed pulmonary lobe is displaced dorsally towards the hilus of the lung, is dense radiographically, and is separated distinctly from the pleural cavity which contains air. Likewise the heart is displa-

ced dorsally and no longer lies with its apex on the sternum. A frequent cause of **hydrothorax** is cardiac insufficiency with a damming back of blood in the pulmonary circulation. This results in an increased diffusion of liquid from the blood vascular system into the surrounding cavities.

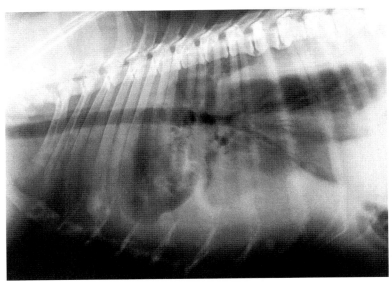

42.3 Massive effusion of liquid into the pleural cavity (hydrothorax).

42.4 The **COSTODIAPHRAGMATIC RECESSES** are complementary or reserve spaces into which the lungs do not extend during normal respiration. In large dog breeds they are 2 or 3 finger breadths wide. Cranially they are limited by the caudal border of the lung field (see 38.1) and caudally by the line of insertion of the diaphragm. Only with deep inspiration as in yawning or in pathologically increased lung size, for example in emphysema, do the caudal borders of the lung extend partly into the costodiaphragmatic recess. In lung emphysema which occurs rarely in dogs the field of the lung can extend almost up to the line of insertion of the diaphragm.

42.5 The **PERICARDIAL CAVITY** as with the pleural cavities is a capillary gap filled with serous fluid. It brings about frictionless heart movement with each action of the heart. The further filling of the cavity with fluid restricts the expansion of the ventricles of the heart and therefore limits cardiac efficiency and capacity. A chronic hydropericardium can be treated surgically by drainage into the pleural cavity. Severe hemorrhages into the pericardium after rupture of a large artery cause considerable increase in pressure in the pericardium (pericardial tamponade) and can cause heart stasis.

44.1 **SPECIAL TERMS RELATING TO HEART** are derived from the Latin 'cor cordis' or from Greek – 'cardia'. Positional designations such as right atrium relate to the heart itself and not to position in the general body.

44.2 In the realization of its **FUNCTION AS A PRESSURE AND SUCTION PUMP** the heart runs through a regular cycle of **ventricular muscle contraction(systole)** and **relaxation (diastole)** with a frequency of 80 – 120 contractions (beats) per minute.

44.3 The **LATERAL SURFACES OF THE HEART** have those portions approaching the heart apex lying in direct contact with the left and right thoracic walls. Here one can feel the apex beat at its strongest and **sonographic examination of the heart (echo cardiography)** (see pp 168 and 169) is possible. **Percussion** enables one to define this area as a dampened heart field. The direct association of heart to thoracic wall generates a severely dampened or deadened knocking sound (absolute heart dampening). Due to the sloping position of the longitudinal axis of the heart, the right heart lies more to the right and cranially and the left heart more to the left and caudally. With expiration the heart is contiguous with the diaphragm. In a laterolateral radiograph it rests on the sternum by means of the apical end of the right ventricular border.

44.4 The **LIGAMENTUM ARTERIOSUM** is the connective tissue remnant of the **ductus arteriosus** which is patent prenatally and through which the current of blood is conveyed directly from the pulmonary trunk to the aorta thus avoiding the lung. Normally the ductus arteriosus is closed completely a few weeks after birth, becoming the fibrous ligamentum arteriosum. On the basis of an altered volume ratio an abnormal persistence of the ductus leads to a severe load on the left ventricle, since a portion of the blood volume (shunt volume) arrives at the pulmonary trunk directly from the aorta (left-right shunt) and by pulmonary veins into the left atrium. The right left shunt is essentially rare and originates in humans from a shunt reversal. With auscultation of a left – right shunt typical 'machine murmurs' are audible. At times a persistent ductus arteriosus is coupled with other heart anomalies (for example ventricular defects). The ductus arteriosus is closed using different surgical techniques. During the procedure one takes note of the **left recurrent laryngeal nerve** which branches away from the vagal nerve, and at the ductus arteriosus 'copes with' rounding the aortic arch. In **abnormal persistence of the right aorta** (see embryology of the arteries of the branchial arches), instead of the normally present left aorta, the right aorta lies to the right of the esophagus whereas normally the aorta lies to its left. In this abnormality the distinctly displaced ductus arteriosus courses dorsally from the pulmonary trunk which lies continuously on the left, over the esophagus and away to the abnormal right aorta. The esophagus then becomes constricted due to the ductus arteriosus and is severely dilated precardially (causes of esophageal dilation see 14.4.). The dilation is easily seen radiographically after a barium meal.

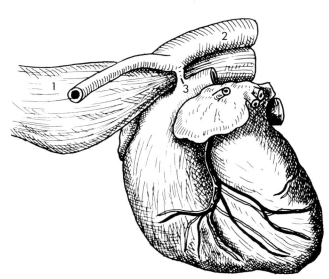

44.4 Persistent right aorta. 1 esophagus; 2 Descending aorta; 3 Ductus arteriosus. Details see p 41.

44.5 The **ENDOCARDIUM** merges into the inner lining of the large blood vessels and is constructed in a similar fashion to this.

44.6 The **MYOCARDIUM** consists of a 'working' myocardium which predominates and in addition, a myocardium which conducts stimuli. The myocardium is the thickest constituent of the heart wall by far; it consists of several layers with fibers coursing in different directions to intermingle thoroughly in a vortex-like manner at the heart apex. Just as skeletal muscle hypertrophies with increased work so too does cardiac muscle. A proportionate 'harmonic' cardiac hypertrophy exists in all myocardial areas with increased cardiac output. By comparison, in a disproportionate hypertrophy only certain myocardial portions are thickened (for example, the right ventricle in pulmonary stenosis and the left ventricle in aortic stenosis). Since a constant numerical ratio exists between heart muscle cells and capillaries provided, hypertrophy is possible only to a limited degree. When a threshold range is exceeded hypertrophy slips into heart dilation. Radiographically by employing contrast medium, the latter is differentiated by variation of heart wall thicknesses. Dilation of the heart results in an inability to expel the blood volume completely during systole so that a considerable quantity of blood remains to be mixed with the inflow of blood.

44.7. The **EPICARDIUM** is the continuation of the serosa of the pericardium on the heart surface and thus corresponds to the visceral layer of the serous pericardium. In general terms the smooth mesothelial covering brings about a sliding between serosal membranes, in this case the frictionless sliding between heart and pericardium with cardiac action.

44.8 In **TRICUSPID INSUFFICIENCY** the right ventricle is hypertrophied. By comparison the right atrium is dilated since a portion of blood drifts back by reflux flow through the atrioventricular ostium which closes inadequately.

44.9 The **VALVE OF THE PULMONARY TRUNK** often exhibits congenital stenosis (**pulmonary stenosis**) against which the right ventricle must work and consequently hypertrophy. The pulmonary valve as well as the aortic valve is a semilunar valve with 3 cusps attached to the internal wall of the vessel like swallows' nests. With blood flow through the valve during ventricular systole the margins of the cusps are pushed against the internal wall of the pulmonary trunk. In diastole the blood tending to flow backwards 'unfolds' the 3 cusps so that the borders come together tightly and hence guarantee valve closure. **Cardiac valves** are attached to the **cardiac skeleton**. This becomes partly cartilaginous and indeed partly ossified in cattle and consists of fibrous rings with a fibrous triangle lying between them. The skeleton stabilizes the shape of the heart and serves as insertion for atrial and ventricular myocardium. These approach the heart skeleton from both directions but do not go beyond its boundaries. The closure of pulmonary and aortic semilunar valves produces the second (short) **heart sound.** The (longer) first heart sound results from tension vibrations of cardiac muscle in ventricular systole. Heart murmurs are abnormal noises which can occur due to narrowing (stenosis) as well as persistent ductus arteriosus (flow murmurs) or due to defective closure (insufficiency) of the heart valves (valvular murmurs).

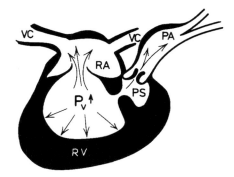

44.9 Hypertrophy of the right ventricular wall and insufficiency of the tricuspid valve as a sequel to increased pressure (Pv) in the right ventricle with a subvalvular pulmonary stenosis (PS). RA right atrium; VC cranial and caudal venae cavae; PA pulmonary artery.

44.10 The **FOSSA OVALIS** is the thinnest part of the atrial septal wall (septum). It originates due to the sudden closure of the foramen ovale with the first respiratory movement during birth, following the sudden altered pressure relationships. Due to the foramen ovale, blood flow to the as yet functionless lung is avoided. During the fetal period oxygen-rich blood flows from the placenta, through the umbilical vein and via the caudal vena cava to the right atrium. From there it flows through the foramen ovale into the left atrium and ventricle. Here it courses via aorta, brachiocephalic trunk and common carotid artery to the head where development is promoted due to the oxygen-rich blood. The blood from the cranial vena cava is poor in oxygen content – courses through the right atrium (where it intersects with the forenamed oxygenated blood) to the right ventricle. It proceeds via the pulmonary trunk, ductus arteriosus and descending aorta to the caudal part of the body which consequently retains blood poor in oxygen and lags behind in its development.

44.11 In its large apical region the **INTERVENTRICULAR SEPTUM** consists essentially of cardiac muscle. A small membranous area of connective tissue is situated in the vicinity of the atrioventricular valves. Here in the membranous portion an interventricular foramen can exist as an anomaly. In comparison foramina in the muscular portion are very rare. In septal defects, corresponding to the different pressure ratios, blood flows from the left to the right ventricle.

44.12 Insufficiency of the **BICUSPID** or **MITRAL VALVE** is the most frequent cause of cardiac insufficiency in older dogs. It is due to an ongoing fibrosis and thickening of the margins of the valve (endocardosis) with simultaneous shortening of it. Reflux blood flow leads to dilation of blood in the left atrium as well as damming back of blood in the pulmonary veins. There is an increase of blood pressure in the pulmonary circulation which has as a consequence in high grade insufficiency, the passage of fluid into the lung alveoli (pulmonary edema).

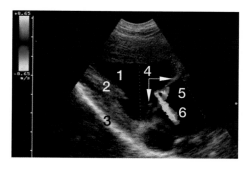

44.12 Medium level insufficiency of the mitral valve with evident systolic backflow (blue color marking, 6) from the left ventricle (1) into the left atrium (5). 2 M. papillaris subauricularis; 3 Pericardium; 4 Mitral valve.

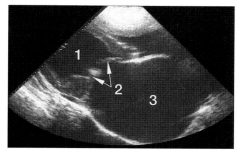

Decompensated heart insufficiency with high grade enlargement of the left atrium (3), dilated left ventricle (1) with thickening of the mitral valve (2). (Sonographic image: Professor Dr. C. Poulsen Nautrup, Munich).

44.13 Insufficiency of the **AORTIC VALVE** is rare in dogs. In contrast congenital **aortic stenosis** is frequent with Boxers a predisposed breed, and is situated mostly in a subvalvular position. The narrowing of the outflow channel from the left ventricle causes a pressure load on the latter with resultant hypertrophy of the myocardium.

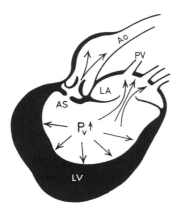

44.13 Hypertrophy of the left ventricular wall (LV) and insufficiency of the mitral valve consequent to an increase in pressure (Pv) in the left ventricle due to a subvalvular aortic stenosis. LA left atrium; PV pulmonary veins; Ao Aorta.

Valve mechanics of all heart valves are basic prerequisites for **heart action. Ventricular muscle contraction (systole)** and **relaxation (diastole)**, each always consisting of 2 phases, occur in the left and right sides of the heart synchronously. In diastole, in phase 1, the **tension release or relaxation phase**, all valves close and either lower pressure or lack there-of predominates within the ventricle. In phase 2, the **filling phase**, with higher pressure in the atrium, the A-V valves are pushed open due to blood flow just like a wind gust opens a door. (In no case does opening occur due to contraction of papillary muscles). In the first instance **ventricular filling** occurs due to **lowering** or **subsidence** of **valve level** whereby blood from the atrium is sucked into the ventricle. Additional factors involved in ventricular filling are **residual pressure in the venae cavae** and **atrial contraction.**

In the following systole ventricular muscle contracts. In phase 1, the **tension phase**, atrioventricular valves close passively because pressure in the ventricle is greater than that in the atrium. In this way the tips of the cusps of the A-V valve are pressed in the direction of the atrium (valve recoil). The chordae tendinae which are now tense, however, prevent the recoil of the valve apex into the region of the atrium. On the contrary the borders of the sail – shaped valve lie so tightly together that a leak-proof closure results. In phase 2, the **expulsion phase**, due to additional pressure increase blood is propelled into the blood vessels leaving the heart (aorta, pulmonary trunk). Thereby the semilunar valves are pushed open passively by blood flow. At the end of the expulsion phase and by the beginning of diastole, blood pressure in the ventricle falls below that in the large blood vessels. As a result the three pocket-like cusps expand or puff out due to blood flow pressing back on them. This expansion causes closure of the valve.

Due to **external heart massage** heart action may be maintained artificially for a limited space of time. In transient (temporary) heart stasis, for example with a severe shock-determined parasympathetic tonus, strong external pressure in rhythm with heart beat is exerted on the thoracic wall. Hence the heart, which, within its pericardial envelope cannot avoid external pressure, is compressed. Due to this pressure aortic and pulmonary valves are opened passively and due to relaxation blood is sucked from the venae cavae into the atrium. Without ventricular contraction therefore, a directed blood flow can be maintained artificially leading to restitution of heart beat.

46.1 Under strict anatomical criteria **CORONARY ARTERIES** are not end arteries since they produce anastomoses with narrow lumina. End arteries do not anastomose with one another and only supply completely definite areas of tissue. From the functional view-point, however, coronary arteries can be regarded as end arteries since their anastomoses are so narrow, they cannot adapt to thrombosis of a neighboring artery of which blood supply is not complete. Necroses appear in the myocardium which cause cardiac infarction. If the patient survives, heart muscle cells cannot regenerate but are replaced by scar tissue which undergoes less stress. (In contrast to humans, cardiac infarction in dogs is of minor importance).

The **danger of thrombosis** in coronary arteries is increased by endocarditis in the left ventricle because detached portions of endocardium can arrive directly in the coronary arteries at the origin of the aorta.

Impairment of blood supply in the coronary arteries causes **angina pectoris** in humans with severe cardiac pains which radiate to the left arm (see zones of Head, 48.1).

Blood supply to the heart ensues during diastole by way of the ascending aorta from which the coronary arteries arise. With an abnormal increase in heart frequency diastole in particular is shortened resulting in an under supply of blood.

46.2 The **GENERATION AND CONDUCTION OF THE CARDIAC IMPULSE** must function permanently to maintain heart action even with loss of consciousness. The conduction system consists of modified specific heart muscle cells which have largely lost their capability of contraction. As soon as the formation of the impulse does not take place in the sino-atrial node, the subsequently organized portions of the system of conduction (atrio-venticular node and the bundle of His) can assume a substitute pacemaker function, but with an essentially decreased frequency.

With **heart transplantation** a portion of the conduction system, at lease the bundle of His, is transplanted due to which heart function is maintained after the insertion of an artificial pacemaker in the recipient. Knowledge of the generation and conduction of the impulse makes possible an understanding of the electrocardiogram (ECG). In setting up an ECG one can derive, concentrate and record the electrical potentials arising from the body surface with heart action.

46.3 The **AUTONOMIC NERVOUS SYSTEM** modifies the frequency of generation of impulse (positive or negative **chronotroph**), the conduction of impulse (positive or negative **dromotroph**) as well as the contraction strength of the working muscle (positive or negative **ionotroph**). Moreover, sympathetic (positive) and parasympathetic (negative) parts of the autonomic system function antagonistically in a far reaching, exceptional manner. Baroreceptors (pressure receptors) are present in the right atrium and the sinus venosus.

48.1 AUTONOMIC NERVES and sensory cutaneous nerves of the somatic nervous system arising from the same segment of the spinal cord form viscerocutaneous reflex or conduction arcs making reciprocal effects possible. Due to cross communication, skin stimuli in certain areas **(zones of Head)** can influence the appropriate viscera and reciprocally excessive excitability in defined viscera can have consequences in the pertinent **zones of Head** namely the appertaining skin areas. The **saltation** of an impulse from autonomic to somatic nervous system and vice versa occurs in the spinal ganglion since it is there that small viscerosensory (autonomic) and large pseudounipolar (somatic) nerve cells are directly adjacent. In diseases of certain internal organs pain is noticed in pertinent skin fields; for example infarct of the heart in humans produces severe pain in the left arm. Liniments producing hyperemia in a zone of Head in humans can affect the appropriate internal organ indirectly.

48.2 Injuries of spinal cord segments T1 – T3 can reduce sympathetic tonus in the **CERVICOTHORACIC GANGLION** manifesting itself as Horner syndrome associated with the eye (see 118.1). With an injection of local anesthetic at the cervicothoracic ganglion one can interrupt temporarily, the sympathetic innervation of head, neck and the ipsilateral thoracic limb (stellate blocade). This method is used in neurotherapy to control chronic pain-producing conditions of the thoracic limb.

48.3 Injuries of the **RECURRENT LARYNGEAL NERVE** result in unilateral paralysis of the laryngeal musculature (hemiplegia laryngis). This is why, during surgical access to the cervical vertebral column, this nerve is taken into consideration at all times.

50.1 The **SURGICAL APPROACH TO THE PERITONEAL CAVITY** is termed a **laparotomy**. Most frequently access is along the linea alba. With a preumbilical approach, the fat cushion in the falciform liga-

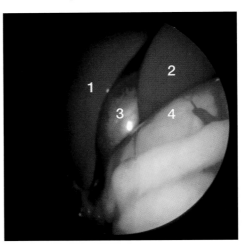

50.1 Laparoscopy:
1 Right hepatic lobe,
2 Quadrate lobe,
3 Gall bladder, 4 Greater curvature of stomach.
(Laparoscopy: Professor Dr. W. Kraft, Munich).

ment must be moved forward and detached from its insertion at the linea alba. Alternately, in specific instances, access is possible by paracostal section parallel to the costal arch or in the flank. In **laparoscopy** an endoscope is introduced through a small incision to the abdominal cavity, making possible a direct adspection of intra-abdominal organs and intended biopsy with only minimal surgical interference. Minimal invasive surgery occurs purely under laparoscopic control with the help of specific instruments introduced through a further small incision.

52.1 The **GREATER OMENTUM**, a loose expansive sliding layer, lies between the ventral abdominal wall and convolutions of intestine. It is an important defence organ of the abdominal cavity rich in macrophages and lymphocytes and moreover, it serves as a storehouse for fat. When inflammation or injuries occur at the peritoneal covering of abdominal organs or of the abdominal wall, the omentum glues to the site and thus protects it against the surroundings. This attribute can restrict pathological processes in the abdominal cavity and can delay adhesions of the bowel which restrict intestinal movement and peristalsis. This protective function of the omentum can be put to use in surgery where it lies over the surgical sutures. Fissures in the omentum (rupture, omental hernia) can lead to strangulation and ultimately to intestinal blockage (ileus), if intestinal loops push inside it. A displacement of such loops into the epiploic foramen with ileus as a sequel happens only very rarely in dogs.

52.2 **INTESTINAL LYMPH** or chyle, depending on the digestive processes, is more or less milky in color because of its fat content. With the aid of a villus pump, long chain fatty acids are transported away in the form of chylomicrons (see biochemistry) in lymphatic capillaries and in the central lymph vessel of the intestinal villus. Short chain fatty acids and the building blocks of protein and carbohydrate metabolism are conducted to the liver via a network of blood capillaries and the portal vein. **SOLITARY LYMPH NODULES** are scattered in the tunica mucosa of the mucosal membrane. (They are also present in lymphatic organs, spleen and lymph nodes). **Aggregated lymph nodules** (for example Peyer's patches) are situated in particular in the antimesenteric section of the wall of the ileum. Primary lymph nodules are spherically or elliptically shaped accumulations of the lymphocytes with a diameter of approximately 0.5 mm. Secondary lymph nodules possess a yellow germinal center and are significant in the production of B lymphocytes.

52.3 **SPLENIC FUNCTION** involves blood storage, regulation of blood pressure, metabolism through the decomposition of hemoglobin, blood processing due to phagocytosis of older erythrocytes, and the generation of immunocompetent cells. In spite of these many and varied roles, the spleen is not essential to life since the named functions, obviously, can be taken over by other organ systems. The spleen, however, is not a superfluous organ and should not be removed carelessly. Nevertheless splenectomy can be necessary in a series of conditions such as torsion of the stomach, injuries and tumors. With splenectomy in human surgery small pieces of splenic tissue a ccm in size are sutured into the greater omentum. Ruptures of the spleen after abdominal traumata and tears from splenic tumors, lead to severe life threatening hemorrhages into the abdominal cavity; these require the quickest possible surgical interference.

The spleen is adapted to its **function of blood storage**. This becomes apparent due to the different size and shape of the organ, because of the high content of **smooth muscle cells** in the splenic capsule and the trabecular system proceeding from it. Due to the storage and dispersal of blood the spleen also serves in the **regulation of blood pressure**, for example due to the easing of the load of the hepatic portal circulation into which the splenic vein discharges. With severe enlargement of the spleen on account of the increased blood storage a 'congested spleen' results. This splenomegaly can necessitate a splenectomy, rendered difficult due to the congestion. By applying adrenalin, contraction of the smooth muscle cells is attained and with it a removal of blood. In euthanasia a congested spleen can occur, supposedly caused by a paralysis of the vasomotor center of the brain (note the condition in the anatomy preparation room).

The **white splenic pulp** with its splenic corpuscles and periarterial lymphatic sheaths serves in the formation of lymphocytes. The **red splenic pulp** is so named because of its high content of red blood cells. Here blood processing takes place. According to predominant text book opinion the blood in the red splenic pulp flows partly through the splenic sinuses (closed circulation) and partly free in the lymphoreticular connective tissue (open circulation). This is not certain due to individual animal differences. **Radiographically** the spleen is demonstrated lateralaterally. The ventral end of the organ which bends towards the right and over the midline to attain the right side of the body, is described in general as a triangular shadow. The triangle corresponds approximately to the cross-sectional shape of the spleen.

54.1 **SPECIAL TERMS RELATING TO THE STOMACH** derive from the Latin – ventriculus (= a little venter or belly, for example corpus ventriculi; the term is also employed for the ventricles of heart and larynx), or from Greek – gaster (= a stomach, for example gastrosplenic ligament, or clinically gastritis = inflammation of stomach).

54.2 **STOMACH FUNCTION** involves the transient storage of food and the regulation of its further transport in smaller quantities into the small intestine. The hydrochloric acid of the stomach brings about disinfection and the activation of pepsinogen generated from the gastric glands, which, as pepsin, initiates digestion.

54.3 A direct examination of the **GASTIC MUCOUS MEMBRANE** follows the introduction of a flexible endoscope through the esophagus and into the stomach **(gastroscopy)** and makes possible the identification of stomach ulcers and tumors as well as the successful taking of biopsy material.

54.4 **TORSION OF THE STOMACH** is a dramatic progressive condition present generally in large dog breeds. It necessitates the immediate intervention of the veterinarian. The stomach is fixed cranially due only to the attached esophageal hiatus, while the dorsal mesentery of the stomach lengthened as the greater omentum is unsuited to the stabilization of the position of the stomach. The pyloric part of the stomach and the initial segment of the duodenum are freely moveable so they too cannot fix the stomach in position. Thus acute stomach dilation – mostly due to an overloading of the stomach with once daily feeding combined with an incipient accumulation of gas – lead to gastric torsion. The rotated stomach distends in a life threatening manner and as a further consequence stomach blood vessels, especially the veins, are strangulated. The gastrosplenic ligament is drawn into the rotation and the venous flow from the spleen is delayed due to obstruction or congestion of the splenic veins. This develops into massive splenic congestion. In turn torsion of the stomach leads to an acute failure of the circulation demanding urgent surgical intervention.

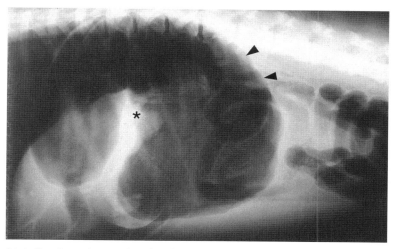

54.4 Gastric torsion combined with severe gaseous distension of the stomach. The greater curvature is situated dorsally (arrows) and the lesser curvature and angular incisure (*) are directed ventrally.

54.5 Interruption of motility of the **SPHINCTER MUSCLE OF THE CARDIA** which results in an insufficient relaxation (achalasia) or more frequently an inability to close (chalasia) can cause a megaesophagus. Affected animals are disposed to the altogether rare appearance of an invagination of the stomach into the esophagus (gastroesophageal invagination).

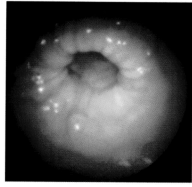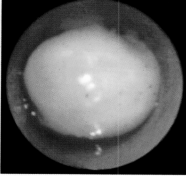

54.3 and 54.5 Endoscopic view of the pylorus of a dog (gastroscopy, left) and a gastroesophageal invagination (esophagoscopy, right). (Endoscopic photographs: Professor Dr. W. Kraft, Munich).

54.6 Narrowing of the **PYLORUS** (pyloric stenosis) leads to interruption in emptying the stomach. Its congenital shape is demonstrated after weaning and transfer to solid food. In adult dogs an hypertrophy of the pyloric mucous membrane and musculature can lead to its functional closure (spasm of the pylorus). An excessive production of gastrin is thought to be the cause. Likewise foreign bodies and tumors can produce a partial or complete closure of the outlet of the stomach.

54.7 In **GASTROTOMY** (surgical opening of the stomach) the incision is directed on the parietal surface, along the axis of the stomach midway between both stomach curvatures which convey the blood vessels. Because of muscle tonus the incised mucous membrane is always everted strongly to the outside.

54.8 The **PANCREAS** produces digestive enzymes in its **exocrine portion** for degrading proteins, carbohydrates and fats. The protein splitting enzymes are present within the pancreas as inactive precursors. Initially they are activated to trypsin and chymotrypsin after their transport through the pancreatic ducts into the intestinal lumen. If, with alterations to the pancreas due to disease, the activation occurs within the gland, this leads to self digestion with the development of pancreatic necrosis. After a dramatic course death often supervenes. Post mortem autodigestion occurs rapidly and in so doing the yellowish – pink colored pancreas is stained a dirty red followed by loss of lobule structure due to swelling. A pancreatitis can lead to an inflammatory swelling of the excretory ducts and the greater duodenal papilla. In turn closure of the bile duct, a damback of bile and icterus occur.

With acute necrosis or malignant degeneration, a partial pancreatectomy is necessary. The separation of healthy from diseased tissue takes place through the careful separation of the gland lobules in the interlobular connective tissue, while preserving pancreatic ducts and vessels (see p57). One notes the anastomosis between the cranial and caudal pancreaticoduodenal arteries in the right lobe of the pancreas.

The **endocrine portion** (islets of Langerhans) regulates carbohydrate metabolism by means of its hormones glucagon and insulin. This is interrupted by disease atrophy of the islets, the relative and absolute deficiency of insulin causing diabetes. Tumors (insulinoma) of the B cells producing insulin autonomously lead to hypoglycemia which can cause resulting loss of consciousness and convulsions (spasms).

54.9 FUNCTION OF THE SMALL INTESTINE consists essentially of the processes of secretion, digestion, resorption and transport. **Secretion** is maintained by mucous producing **goblet cells** interspersed in the surface epithelium, from tubular intestinal glands (= **intestinal crypts**, epithelial indentations with contained cells – kryptos = hidden), from **submucosal duodenal glands** and in particular from the pancreas adjacent and external to the small intestine.

Digestion, that is the degrading of nutrients into smaller resorbable, units occurs at one time in the intestinal lumen, at another bound to the cell membranes of the brush border cells of the surface epithelium.

The brush border cells situated superficially act in **resorption**. They produce an enormous increase in surface area due to very thick erect microvilli with a length of approximately one thousandth of a millimeter. Transport of resorbed nutrients occurs via blood capillaries with the exception of long chain fatty acids which are transported by lymphatic vessels.

The **surface increase** leads to the creation of a large intestinal resorption surface due to structures recognizable at macroscopic, microscopic or electron microscopic levels.

The **circular folds** (plicae circulares) recognized macroscopically are the results of a simple folding of mucosa and submucosa, but not, however, of intestinal muscle layers. The microscopic **crypts** and especially the everted fingerlike **intestinal villi** approximately 1 mm long bear the **brush border cells** with their microvilli which are detected microscopically. The microvilli are covered by glycocalyces seen with the electron microscope.

Motility of the intestine is concerned with the villous pump mechanism, pendulous movements and peristaltic waves. Parasympathetic innervation promotes and sympathetic supply inhibits motility. Interruption of nutrient transport can have different causes and leads to greater water absorption and therefore constipation (coprostasis see also 56.2).

The **villous pump** leads to a shortening of the villi due to contraction of sparse smooth muscle cells. In this way lymph transport in the central lymphatic vessels (chyle vessels) is promoted.

Pendulous movement due to contractions of the longitudinal muscle layer serves chiefly in the thorough mixing of intestinal content or chyme.

Due to **peristaltic waves** intestinal content is transported further. Initially the longitudinal muscle contracts and then above all the circular muscle layer.

In **abdominal sonography** intestinal loops are identified with certainty in a five-layered wall construction. The internal surface mucous membrane is demonstrated due to its high echogenicity (1). The wide mucosal tunic has a low echogenicity (2) and is separated by a slender echogenic line (3) from the anechoic, but narrow muscular tunic (4). Again the outer surface of the small intestine with its outer serosal covering is displayed as a narrow echogenic line (5).

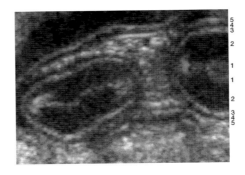

54.9 Jejunal loops in sonographic cross section.

1. Mucous membrane surface and ingesta
2. Mucosal tunic
3. Submucosal tela
4. Muscular tunic
5. Serosal tunic

54.10 The **DESCENDING DUODENUM** is identified with certainty by its characteristic straight course along the right lateral abdominal wall as a single section of small intestine. It serves as an aid for orientation of the sonographic image of the pancreas.

56.1 FUNCTION OF THE LARGE INTESTINE consists essentially in the extraction of fluid, the inspissation and concentration of intestinal content, and the admixture of mucus from very numerous goblet cells. This promotes the further transmission of content to the anus. Luminal surface increase is due only to crypts and no longer through the presence of villi.

56.2 Radiographically, the **COLON** is well represented, generally to the right, due to accumulations of gas and feces. On the other hand, alterations to the colonic wall by tumors, ulcers and stenosis are detected frequently with contrast medium. This can be applied in a retrograde manner. **Dilation of the colon** (megacolon) occurs frequently as a result of constipation (coprostatis) due to feeding errors or obstructions. The congenital form (megacolon congenitum) is rare, caused by a lack of intramural ganglion cells of the myenteric plexus (Hirschsprung's disease).

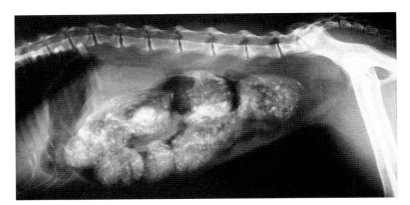

56.2 Massive obstruction of the colon due to feces (coprostasis).

56.3 ARTRESIA OF ANUS, RECTUM AND BOTH are anomalies which occur during ontogenesis (atresia = absence of opening of the as yet closed embryonic anus or rectum). The anomaly is often accompanied by fistulae between ano-rectal and urogenital systems.

56.4 CIRCUMANAL GLANDS see 6.3.

56.5 The **ANAL SACS** (more correctly termed paranal sinuses) store secretion from glands situated in their walls. Due to adhesion onto deposited feces this serves in demarcating the hunting territory and alluring partners. Normally the sacs empty with fecal deposition due to the pressure of m. sphincter ani externus, normally formed feces serving as an abutment or site of resistance. A soft unformed feces resulting from a defective diet cannot serve as a resistance site and delays the discharge of the anal sacs. The decomposition of contained secretion can cause inflammation and secondary infection. Subsequent abcesses can develop. The abnormally filled anal sac is expressed manually. Rinsing of the sacs is possible via their excretory ducts which open along the anocutaneous line at the 4 and 8 o'clock positions. Extirpation of the chronically inflamed sacs must preserve the m. sphincter ani externus.

56.6 Under the term **PORTAL VENOUS SYSTEM** one understands the insertion of a second capillary bed in the venous limb of the circulatory system. The connecting vein between the arteriovenous capillary bed and the venovenous capillary bed is defined as a portal vein. Here extra arterial blood can be introduced to form mixed arterial – venous blood. To distinguish the different portal veins, one appends the name of the organ to which the portal vein supplies blood (hepatic portal vein, hypophyseal portal vein).

58.1 The **LIVER** lies within the intrathoracic part of the abdominal cavity with the exception of the ventromedial portion which, however, cannot be palpated. With pathological enlargement the liver reaches further caudally beyond the costal arch. This can be established using palpation, percussion (duller liver sound) and radiographic as well as sonographic examination. The size of the liver which normally constitutes 3.4% of body weight, is correlated with its multiplicity of functions: 1 Function as an endocrine gland (synthesis of blood plasma protein such as albumen, globulin and fibrinogen): 2 Function as an exocrine gland (bile and cholesterol): 3 Intermediary metabolism of fat, protein and carbohydrate: 4 Storage of fat, glycogen and iron: 5 Glycogenolysis and glyconeogenesis as well as the maintenance of a physiological glucose level: 6 Detoxification of drugs and medicine. In the fetal stage the liver is relatively larger and occupies a dominant part of the abdominal cavity, the size being connected with blood formation. Pathological atrophication due to pronounced pitting and accompanying shrinkage can occur as in cirrhosis of the liver.

The 'classical' **liver lobules** are functional units detectable macroscopically with a diameter of approximately 1mm and a height of up to 2mm. The lobules possess a central vein, appearing macroscopically as a dark point, with radially discharging liver capillaries or sinusoids. As well there are liver cell trabeculae arranged radially and a fibrous tissue limiting capsule peripherally (Glisson's capsule see histology text).

Pathological fatty degeneration of the liver due to the effects of toxins or lack of oxygen and leading to yellowish discoloration is recognized macroscopically in its advanced stages. Since blood flows in the liver sinusoids from the periphery of the lobule to its center, the cells situated peripherally are affected firstly and thus undergo fatty degeneration. On the other hand with oxygen deficiency (hypoxia) fatty degeneration begins generally at the center of the lobule.

58.2 The intramural architecture of the **PORTAL VEIN** is adapted to high blood pressure. This high blood pressure is necessary for the perfusion of the second (hepatic) capillary bed of the portal venous system. The pressure is maintained due to arteriovenous anastomoses in the region of the intestine as well as the effect of rising blood pressure in the spleen of which the venous blood reaches the portal vein. Characteristic of the wall structure are muscle fasciculae lying externally and oriented longitudinally which are also termed adventitial subserosal musculature. In sonographic examination of the portal vein and its branches it has a characteristically distinct echogenicity caused by the relatively thick wall. On the other hand hepatic veins show no wall structure which is evident sonographically.

In the **portal vein** due to arteriovenous anastomoses and the spleen, an adequate blood pressure is attained for perfusion of the hepatic capillary bed. The large part of the blood already at the commencement of the venous limb (for example in the intestinal wall) flows through a capillary bed. The limited decrease in blood pressure caused by this is equalized by the blood pressure regulating function of the spleen (see 52.3) and numerous arteriovenous anastomoses at the source of the portal vein thus avoiding the capillary bed. Due to this a sufficient oxygen content is guaranteed for the supply of the liver since the thin hepatic artery cannot supply this gigantic organ alone. The portal vein collects blood of unpaired veins from unpaired organs.

The **venous outflow from the caudal section of the rectum** occurs extraportally by way of paired medial and caudal rectal veins. This blood does not arrive at the liver by way of the portal vein but flows through the body circulation. This circumstance is exploited with the application of treatments in suppository form, the drug so absorbed being efficient due to its full concentration.

In the fetal circulation the portal venous blood is conducted directly past the capillary bed of the liver via the **ductus venosus** into the caudal vena cava. If this short circuit persists after birth a diagnosis of **congenital portocaval shunt** is applied. Avoiding the liver, the central organ of metabolism, has as a consequence that its essential detoxification function is inefficient. The blood concentration of toxins such as ammonia results in injury to the central nervous system, leading in turn to development of **hepatoencephalopathy**. Congenital shunts can be ligated surgically. Since various forms of this defective vessel development can crop up, the position of the shunt must be established by administration of a contrast medium directly into a vessel in the drainage area of the portal vein (**portography**).

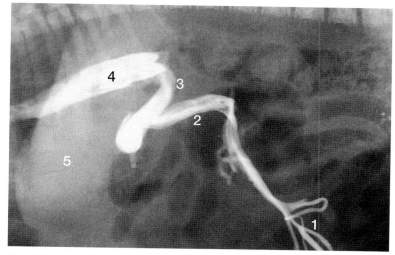

58.2 Contrast radiography (portography) of an extra-hepatic portocaval shunt. After injection the contrast medium flows into a jejunal vein (1) into a portal vein (2) and from there, by avoiding the liver (5) through a portocaval shunt (3) directly into the caudal vena cava (4). (Photography: Prof. Dr. Gravel, Leipzig)

58.3 Bile is concentrated in the **GALL BLADDER** by water resorption. A sphincter muscle at the opening of the bile duct regulates bile flow into the duodenum. Bile serves as an emulsifier of fat, the surface of which consequently increases in size thus improving the effectiveness of enzymes. Bile acids and bile pigments are resorbed again in the small intestine (enterohepatic circulation) and accordingly secreted anew in the bile. An excessive content of bile pigment in the blood becomes evident as **icterus** (pre-,intra-, and posthepatic). In prehepatic icterus increased bile pigment results from an increased destruction of erythrocytes. Intrahepatic icterus is caused by injury of hepatic cells and posthepatic icterus occurs due to obstructions within the bile duct systems. Post mortem, an autolysis of gall bladder and bile ducts sets in prematurely, with adjacent tissues exhibiting a bile colored imbibition observed during autopsy.

60.1 The **SACRAL PART OF THE PARASYMPATHETIC SYSTEM** arrives by different routes at its effector organs about which there exists no agreement in the literature. Different statements exist also about its radius of influence and region of supply, which are based perhaps, on species specific peculiarities. According to the opinion of several authors of texts on veterinary medicine its radius of influence or range is supposed to be limited to the rectum, the nerves extending to the mesenteric attachment of the rectum and to the boundary with the descending colon. (According to that therefore the hypogastric nerve would be purely sympathetic). In human anatomy the transverse colon is indicated as the boundary of supply between the parasympathetic part of the sacral spinal cord and the vagus nerve. The newest conclusions from research speak of a larger area of supply by the sacral parasympathetic system which is supposed to include the entire colon.

60.2 Because of its protected position essentially the **LUMBAR PLEXUS** is rarely affected by traumatic injuries in contrast to the brachial plexus. In contrast functional disorders are caused relatively frequently due to a narrowing of the intervertebral foramina. Causes are, for example discopathies (see 10.3) or massive spondyloarthroses (see 8.6).

62.1 Regarding the **KIDNEY** the **adipose capsule** of live animals has a soft consistency so that kidneys, to some extent, swim in their own fat.

On **radiographs** where contrast medium is not employed, the kidneys are not always shown satisfactorily, particularly the left (caudal) kidney. In better radiological display a compatible contrast medium is employed to detect urinary pathways (urography see 62.2). On the other hand sonography makes a detailed representation possible (see ultrasound anatomy pp170 – 171).

Congenital anomalies – manifest in a failed joining of the nephron to the canaliculus system, lead to cyst formations in the kidney. This defect is promoted due to the different origin of the nephron (from the metanephrogenic blastema) and the canaliculus system (from the ureteric bud). The **blood vessels of the kidney (renal artery and vein)** penetrate the kidney via the interlobar arteries and veins and finally the arcuate aa and vv. These vessels play a part in urine formation and besides provide blood supply to the renal parenchyma and play a part in the resorption of the non-urinary constituents from the loops of Henle.

The afferent glomerular arterioles from the arcuate artery rarely contribute to the primary formation of urine which is produced predominantly by interlobular aa. Within the kidney lobules these course radially to the kidney capsule. In the **renal corpuscle** the afferent glomerular arterioles branch into the glomerular capillary loops. The efferent glomerular arterioles of the **subcapsular renal corpuscles** accumulating from the glomeruli open into a (cortical) **capillary net** which entangles the **loops of Henle (renal tubules)** of the renal cortex and unite with the **interlobular veins**. The renal medulla is supplied by **arteriolae rectae (spuriae)** which come from a **juxtamedullary renal corpuscle** as well as from **arteriolae rectae (verae)** which radiate from interlobular arteries or more rarely from arcuate arteries. The blood flow out of the renal cortex is via the **interlobular veins** and from the renal medulla via **venulae rectae** which conduct blood via **arcuate veins** and **interlobar veins** into the renal vein.

62.2 The **URETER** penetrates the urinary bladder wall, with the section associated with its opening taking a long oblique course. In this way a reverse or reflux flow of urine to the renal pelvis is prevented. With an increase of internal pressure in the urinary bladder during micturition, the orifice section of the ureter is closed by compression. A unilateral duplication of the ureter is present as a congenital anomaly if the ureteric bud is distributed prematurely before reaching the renal sinus. This can also proceed to a duplication of the renal pelvis. Ectopic openings of the ureters with on-going urinary incontinence can be present caudal to the sphincter muscle of the urethra. The closure of a ureter can have many causes such as urinary stones (uroliths), tumors, scar tissue or anomalies. This leads to damming back of urine, a dilation of the ureters (hydroureter) and finally of the renal pelvis. With a chronic retention there is pressure atrophy of the common renal papilla and finally the whole renal parenchyma with complete loss of function. The residuum of the erstwhile kidney remains as a large sac filled with urine.

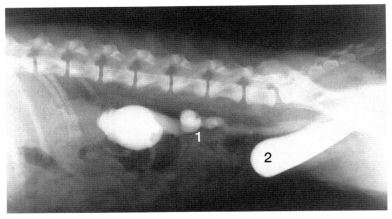

62.2 Urography: Contrast medium has concentrated in the left ectopic ureter (1) which is distended, and in the regularly filled urinary bladder (2).

64.1 The MUCOUS MEMBRANE OF THE URINARY BLADDER

is folded and with filling of the bladder the folds are eliminated, conferring on it an enormous potential volume. Obtuse abdominal trauma can lead to rupture of the full bladder. Essentially male dogs are more frequently affected than bitches. In the latter the short wide urethra makes possible an easier, fast emptying of the bladder with excessive increase in pressure.

64.2 The **URETHRA** is short and wide in bitches, and long and narrow in male dogs. Hence a blockage of the urethra by bladder stones (urolithiasis) occurs almost exclusively in the male. Predilection sites for blockage of the male urethra are the narrowing of the urethra adjacent to the os penis and the curvature of the urethra at the ischial arch.

64.3 MUSCULATURE OF THE URINARY BLADDER takes its course in an internal and an external muscle layer with a circular layer between them. The layers are not exactly separated from one another and here and there change over, one layer with another. Muscle fasciculae shear off and change over from the neck of the bladder to the initial section of the urethra. With contraction of the urinary bladder the initial section of the urethra dilates. Contraction is initiated by parasympathetic fibers originating from pelvic nerves. Sympathetic fibers reach the bladder by way of the hypogastric nerve. Neuro – and myogenic derangement can cause an uncontrolled urinary outflow (incontinence) or a retention of urine. Urinary incontinence occurs frequently after speying in bitches. The loss of estrogen appears to cause a diminution of

sphincter response to sympathetic innervation. This can be counteracted with estrogen substitution and/or sympathomimetic drugs. A variety of causes from discopathies (see 10.3) to chronic inflammation of the urinary bladder can produce paralysis with urinary retention and ultimately massive bladder distention. From the viewpoint of differential diagnosis, with bladder distention an interruption of urinary outflow caused by urolithiasis (see 64.2) has to be ruled out of the question.

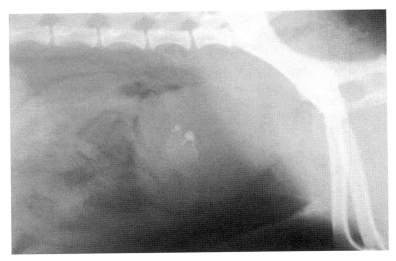

64.3 Urinary bladder stones in a male dog.

64.4 In particular the **SUSPENSORY LIGAMENT OF THE OVARY** of the left side is relatively short and with speying of the bitch (ovariectomy) impedes the forward positioning of the ovary. The ligament is palpated as a tense cord directed cranially and one differentiates it from the ovarian artery coursing dorsally. Since the ligament contains no blood vessels it can be penetrated safely without prior ligation.

64.5 The **TESTICULAR TUNICS** – the peritoneum and the continuations of the layers of body wall – are treated differently depending on the different methods of castration. In castration (orchidectomy), with covering vaginal process, the unopened process together with the enclosed spermatic cord is transected distal to the ligation site. In castration with an opened vaginal process the 'naked' deferent duct is removed together with nerves and blood vessels.

64.6 Due to **DESCENT, THE TESTES** are displaced from their site of origin into the scrotum by a continuous process occurring pre- and postnatally. The testes enter the inguinal canals from the abdominal cavity 3 – 4 days postnatally and migrate into the scrotum over the following weeks. On average the descent is complete after 1.5 months and at the latest should be complete after 3.5 months. If testicular descent is incomplete and the testis remains in the abdominal cavity or remains stuck in the inguinal canal, hence concealed, the condition is spoken of as cryptorchidism (cryptos = hidden, orchis = testis).

The **retained testis** exhibits an abnormally long proper ligament of the testis and ligament of the tail of the epididymis. Such a testis is predisposed to neoplasms. Its internal temperature approaches that of body temperature and spermiogenesis is generally interrupted while sex hormones are produced in an almost uninterrupted manner. For normal spermiogenesis an essentially lower temperature is needed and the internal temperature of the testis lying normally in the scrotum approaches that of the skin.

With the physiological site of the testis in the scrotum several factors regulate testicular temperature which is approximately $2^{0}c$ below body temperature. Two factors may be named: 1. Venous outflow from the testis occurs via the pampiniform plexus. Through the vascular loops of this venous plexus passes the testicular artery the blood of which is cooled slightly before its perfusion of the testis due to the somewhat cooler blood of the pampiniform plexus (Varicose changes of the pampiniform plexus can cause sterility in man and animals). 2. The cremaster muscle (external) and the smooth muscle of the tunica dartos cause the testis to be drawn upwards, approaching the warmer body or – with relaxation of this muscle – to glide into the bottom of the cooler scrotum. Of course this might be more efficient in species with a pendulous scrotum such as the bull or ram – than in the male dog.

66.1 The **OVARY** has a dual function comparable to that of the testis, furnishing egg cells or oocytes for fertilization and the production of sex hormones.

In the **ovarian cortex** are situated the egg cells (oocytes I) which are enveloped postnatally and depending on the stage of development are arranged in follicles of different sizes. In primordial follicles the oocyte has a diameter of 20 μm and is surrounded by flat squamous epithelial cells which become cuboidal. First of all with puberty individual primary follicles grow into secondary follicles, of which the oocyte has a diameter of 1/10 mm surrounded by the zona pellucida and a multi-layered follicular epithelium as well as a connective tissue envelope (theca externa and interna). The resultant bladder-like tertiary follicle containing follicular fluid has a detectable follicular antrum (cavity) between the follicular epithelial cells which are soft and separating from one another. The oocyte, with a diameter of about 2/10 mm is supported by a mound of follicular epithelial cells, the cumulus oophorus, and surrounded by a corona radiata, a single layered stratum of follicular epithelial cells. A few individual tertiary follicles grow into mature follicles which have a diameter of about 2 mm. The greater number of follicles do not reach ovulation but die due to follicular atresia (atresos = without light or opening).

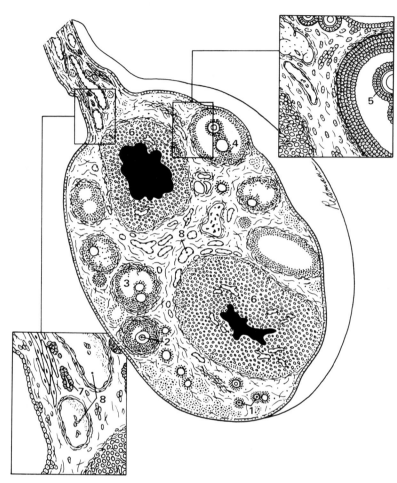

66.1 Longitudinal section through the ovary. 1 Primary follicle; 2 Secondary follicle; 3 Tertiary follicle; 4 Cumulus oophorus; 5 Corona radiata; 6 Cycling corpus luteum; 7 Medullary cords; 8 Blood vessels.

After rupture of the follicle, an endocrine gland, the **corpus luteum**, develops from the epithelium and connective tissue of the follicular envelope. In the bitch this remains in existence for around 75 days independent of pregnancy. During this time the corpus luteum produces progesterone of which the concentration during the cycle gradually diminishes. This occurs in a similar manner during pregnancy. In the pregnant bitch post partum, consequently after 63 days, there is an abrupt decrease in the concentration of progesterone. Under the influence of this in both the cycling and gravid bitch, there is a rise in blood concentration of prolactin preparing the mammary gland for lactation. Consequently in cycling bitches after regression of the corpus luteum there is frequently a **false lactation** also known as **pseudo-pregnancy**.

Interruptions of ovarian function with the formation of cystic degenerative and/or persistent follicles in the bitch are frequently a cause of delayed cycles.

Continuing sonographic examination makes a direct record of the ripening follicle, ovulation and formation of the corpus luteum possible and can be consulted for the control of ovarian function.

66.2 With ovulation the **UTERINE TUBE** collects the ovum. If the fertilized ovum arrives in the abdominal cavity there is an abdominal pregnancy. In the peritoneum surrounding the extrauterine nidation there are vascular rich proliferations which are insufficient for the fetus; therefore this dies prematurely. Hence, in comparison with abdominal pregnancy in human medicine extrauterine gravidity, which can also begin in the ovarian bursa is of minor veterinary importance.

66.3 The **UTERUS** (metra in Greek) with its **endometrium** rich in glands and blood vessels makes the nidation of the fertilized ovum possible. Uterine epithelium consists of cilia-free secretory cells and ciliated cells which change in shape depending on the phase of the cycle. During

follicular maturation the outpouring of estrogen produces a proliferation of uterine glands and a physiological edema of the endometrium. A diapedesis of erythrocytes through the endometrium leads to the development of a sanguinous discharge during this phase of the cycle. After ovulation a rising progesterone level produces secretion of uterine glands and the closure of the cervix of the uterus. Frequently in the bitch this course of events is deranged through infection and/or ovarian dysfunction and this causes different forms of endometritis. Towards the end of estrus, even before the closure of the cervix, bacteria can penetrate into the uterus, producing endometritis and filling the uterine lumen with purulent secretion **(pyometra)** which cannot discharge since the cervix is closed. With **persistence of follicles** estrogens are produced on a permanent basis, keeping the endometrium edematous over a long period, leading to chronic sanguino-serous – and after secondary bacterial infection – purulent discharge **(chronic endometritis)**. Mostly **follicular luteal cysts** develop which produce estrogen and progesterone. Continuing hormonal stimulation of uterine glands leads to continuing proliferation as well as secretion and ultimately to a very frequent development of **glandular cystic endometritis**.

The **myometrium** produces the contractions at parturition until the fetus is expelled and the **perimetrium** guarantees the ease of displacement of the organ. During pregnancy smooth muscle cells of the myometrium can lengthen perhaps 10 times (up to 1 mm) and at birth they contract due to the influence of the hypothalamic/hypophyseal system (oxytocin).

66.4 In the male genitalia the **PROSTATIC UTRICLE** or **UTERUS MASCULINUS** is present as a blind-ending pocket in the vicinity of the colliculus seminalis. (It is a remnant of the caudal end of the Muellerian ducts).

66.5 The **CERVIX OF THE UTERUS** has a mucus plug in its canal which hinders ascending infection, its consistency depending on the phase of the estrus cycle. At the time of breeding it liquefies and is expelled to make the passage of sperm through the cervical canal possible.

66.6 The **EPITHELIUM OF THE VAGINAL MUCOUS MEMBRANE** undergoes alterations depending on the phase of the estrus cycle. Hence the microscopic examination of a vaginal smear makes an estimation of the status of the cycle of the bitch possible. In anestrus large nucleated epithelial cells dominate. In the course of proestrus they are replaced increasingly by large keratinized non-nucleated epithelial cells which degenerate in estrus and towards the end of estrus and in metestrus they disappear under the influence of progesterone. Under the impact of estrogen in proestrus and estrus the mucous membrane, predominantly in young bitches of the larger dog breeds, becomes edematous. This can lead to a prolapse of the membrane. With this seasonal prolapse, in contrast to a true vaginal prolapse, the urethral orifice is not included.

66.7 In the bitch the **URETHRAL ORIFICE** lies in the ventral midline on the floor of the vagina, 2–5 cm cranial to the commissure of the lips of the vulva. To obtain urine, with the aid of a vaginal speculum and the sense of sight, one can introduce a stiff catheter and it can be passed into the urinary bladder.

66.8 The **CLITORIS** can be enlarged considerably with hormonal imbalance derived predominantly from gonads and adrenal cortex. Therefore it is often termed a miniature penis. Nevertheless this analogy has important limitations. Other than at the penis, the urethra in no case ends at the clitoris and a section of corpus spongiosum is displaced into the wall of the vaginal vestibule as bulbus vestibuli.

68.1 Concerning the **TESTIS** the anatomical terminology is derived chiefly from the Latin 'testis' with some exceptions such as epi- meso- and periorchium. Clinical usage is derived from the Greek word 'orchis orchios', for example orchiectomy for castration. The testis is an endocrine gland, besides producing sperm, which together with secretion from epididymis and prostate makes up the ejaculate. In old male dogs testicular tumors are the most frequent type. Estrogens produced from sertoli cells emanating from the neoplasm lead to feminization (gynacomastia, penile atrophy) and the attraction of other males.

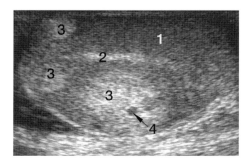

68.1 Sonographic longitudinal section through a testis with echogenic neoplasms (3) and a cyst (4).
1 Testicular parenchyma;
2 Mediastinum of testis (Sonography: Professor Dr. C. Poulsen Nautrup, Munich).

68.2 The **EPIDIDYMIS** (epi-upon; didymos – twin in a metaphorical sense) with its efferent ductules is developed from the transverse canaliculi of the mesonephros, and its epididymal duct from the Wolffian duct of the mesonephros. From the divisions into head, body and tail of the epididymis one can deduce the underlying sections of testis as head and tail extremities. The long duct of the epididymis is a place of storage and maturation of sperm which attain motility and fertilization capacity here. Damaged sperms will be eliminated by phagocytosis.

68.3 The **DEFERENT DUCT** is the direct continuation of the epididymal duct. The surgical removal of a section of the former resulting in sterilization is known as vasectomy since the duct was previously called the vas deferens. In most cases the surgical reunification of both stumps does not lead to an intended reattainment of male fertility. With the original surgical transection, autonomic nerves are severed by necessity. This is detrimental to testicular function and distal to the transection site there is deficient peristalsis of the deferent duct which is indispensable to semen transport.

68.4 With ejaculation, the **COLLICULUS SEMINALIS** closes the commencement of the urethra at the urinary bladder due to its erectile tissue. Hence semen is diverted distally.

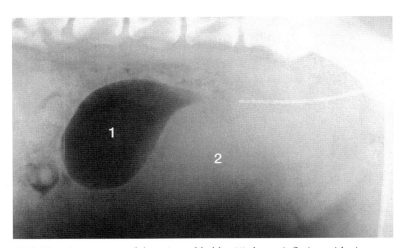

68.5 Negative contrast of the urinary bladder (1) due to inflation with air to differentiate it from a paraprostatic cyst (2) which lies caudally and is homogeneous radiographically.

68.5 In young male dogs the **PROSTATE** lies within the pelvis and is displaced incrementally in a cranial direction with age until at about 5 years of age it lies completely within the abdomen. Prostatic hyperplasia is the result of an uncalibrated hormonal effect. Androgens are responsible for glandular hyperplasia while estrogens cause squamous metaplasia. The transition to pathological prostatic hyperplasia in old dogs is a smooth one and mostly combined with intraparenchymatous cyst formations. The enlarged prostate can constrict the adjacent rectum leading to difficult defecation. By contrast, a constriction of the urethra and difficult urination are rare in male dogs. Elimination of androgenic effects through treatment with antiandrogens or by castration results in a decrease of prostatic size within a short time. In addition to frequent parenchymatous prostatic cysts, rarely do large uni- or multichambered cysts occur, as retention cysts. These are connected to the prostate or as paraprostatic cysts of unknown origin only lie adjacent to the gland. Cysts of this type

can assume extreme dimensions and occupy a considerable proportion of the abdominal cavity before producing clinical pain or annoyance.

68.6 ERECTION is controlled by the parasympathetic and ejaculation by the sympathetic divisions of the autonomic system. Erection of the penis is attained by swelling of the solid arterial erectile body, the corpus rigidum (cavernosum) penis and the spongy venous erectile body, the corpus spongiosum penis.

Erection is realized in the arterial erectile body (corpus rigidum penis) due to the following factors: 1 The cushions of intima within the helicine arteries in the quiescent state occlude these vessels. Therefore blood diverts through arteriovenous anastomoses and avoids the cavernae of the corpus rigidum (cavernosum) penis. With erection the intimal cushions flatten out and blood flow is conducted in the helicine arteries to the cavernae. 2 Due to closure of the forenamed arteriovenous anastomoses an intense blood flow is conducted in the cavernae which thereby are filled in a tense distended manner. 3 The cavernae are 'opened' due to relaxation of surrounding smooth muscle cells. 4 The veins with their oblique passages are pinched off due to stretched trabeculae. 5 Engorgement or damming back of blood in the venous limb is intense due to contraction of m. ischiourethralis and the compressing effort of the erectile bodies in the vaginal vestibule of the bitch. The m. ischiourethralis arises at the ischial arch and inserts jointly with that of the other side at a fibrous ring situated medially. Due to its contraction the blood flow from the dorsal vein of the penis which traverses this ring, is throttled or cut off. Due also to intimal cushions in the veins, drainage of blood is delayed. In the most recent investigations, however, the existence of erection promoting arterial and venous intimal cushions is doubted.

In the first phase of coitus the paired corpus rigidum penis becomes erect first of all and not until vaginal penetration occurs does complete erection of the unpaired corpus spongiosum penis occur, more specifically the corpus glandis penis. Ejaculation begins within a minute of the commencement of coitus. In the second phase the male turns itself through 180⁰ and initially cannot detach itself from the bitch. An S-shaped twist of the penis delays further the venous outflow of blood in particular from the glans penis, due to which the phenomenon of 'locking' has its origin. (Blood supply of penis see p71).

Innervation of the penis occurs via parasympathetic, sympathetic and sensory neurons. Parasympathetic supply stems from the pelvic plexus and causes erection. Sympathetic supply innervates smooth muscle as well as helicine arteries and is responsible for ejaculation. Sensory nerve endings are numerous in the glans penis and prepuce.

68.7 Due to its roof shaped superposition the **OS PENIS** restricts the ability of the penile urethra to dilate. Therefore urinary stones from the bladder can be impounded and accumulate directly caudal to the penile bone (urethrolithiasis).

68.8 An enlargement of the **MEDIAL ILIAC LYMPH NODES** is demonstrated radiographically as shadow ventral to the last lumbar vertebra and can cause a ventral displacement of the rectum.

70.1 The ovary is supplied with blood by **OVARIAN AND UTERINE ARTERIES AND VEINS** respectively and these anastomose each with the other. With speying both vascular tributaries have to be ligated.

70.2 The **LUMBOSACRAL TRUNK** and its roots in the spinal cord segments L6 to S1 can be injured and functionally so, due to a multiplicity of causes. The most frequent problems are lumbosacral constrictions (see 10.2), lateral spondyloses with narrowing of intervertebral foramina (see 8.6), but also fractures, subluxations and luxations of the caudal part of the lumbar vertebral column.

70.3 The **ADRENAL GLANDS** just as the kidneys and large blood vessels (aorta and caudal vena cava) are located in the retroperitoneal space.

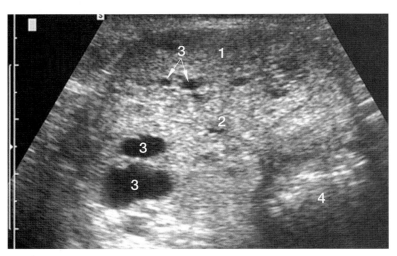

68.5 Sonographic cross section of a hyperplastic prostate with numerous intraparenchymatons cysts 1 Prostate parenchyma; 2 urethra; 3 Cysts; 4 Rectum. (Sonography: Professor Dr C Poulsen Nautrup, Munich).

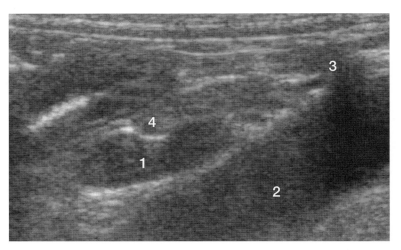

70.3 Sonographic longitudinal section through the dumb-bell shaped left adrenal gland (1); 2 Abdominal aorta; 3 Renal artery; 4 Cranial abdominal artery.

They are situated at the cranial extremity of the kidneys. These close relationships decided the terminology suprarenal glands. The constriction of the left adrenal due to the presence of the cranial abdominal vein confers on it the characteristic dumb-bell shape seen in sonographic longitudinal section, while the right adrenal is comma shaped. As an endocrine gland the adrenal has a completely divergent function to that of the kidney. Its medulla develops from ectoderm (sympathicoblasts) and produces adrenalin as well as noradrenalin. Its cortex develops from embryonic mesoderm and produces steroids. Hyperplasia and tumors (adenoma and adenocarcinoma) of the adrenal cortex are relatively frequent in dogs. The characteristic appearance of the cortex is due to the excessive production of adrenocortical hormones (see 150.1). With surgical removal perhaps due to neoplasms, the presence of the greater splanchnic nerve on its dorsal surface and its blood supply, resulting from cranial, middle and caudal adrenal blood vessels should be taken into consideration.

72.1 Today, contrary to older definitions **PERINEUM** is denoted as the entire cutaneous muscular closure of the pelvic outlet in the environs of the anal and urogenital canals. An atrophy of the pelvic diaphragm, specifically of the m. levator ani, often leads to perineal hernia present in older male dogs. Hormonal influences are considered the cause. Prostatic hyperplasia (see 68.5) at least is attributed an increasing role since this leads to increased pressure during defecation and with it increased stress on the perineum. The hernial sac contains mostly retroperitoneal fat, rarely small or large intestine. At times also, a caudally directed urinary bladder and/or prostate can occur. Surgical closure of the hernia can be effected after detachment of the tendon of m. obturatorius internus (see illustration p78) and its transposition and union with the mm sphincter ani externus and m. coccygeus which are sutured to each other. Cogent is simultaneous castration which counteracts the tendency towards hypertrophy of the prostate.

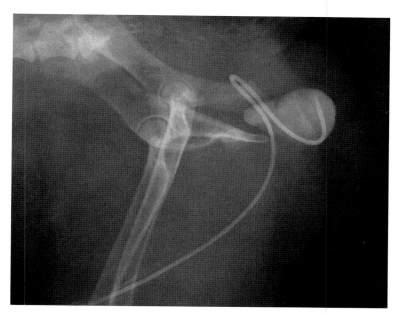

72.1 Radiograph of a perineal hernia in a male Collie. The urinary bladder, filled with contrast medium via a catheter, is displaced into the hernial sac (retroflexion of the urinary bladder). (Radiograph: Prof. Dr. E Henschel, Berlin).

An **incision of vagina-perineum (episiotomy)** is undertaken to alleviate parturition by the enlargement of the vulvar cleft, or for the removal of vaginal neoplasms. The cleft is incised dorsally but not as far as the m. sphincter ani externus.

74.1 The **OSSEOUS PELVIC GIRDLE** is often fractured in car accidents. In **fractures** with minimal displacement of the fractured parts spontaneous recovery can occur in a quiet calm situation without surgical interference. The adjacent **muscles** attached on all surfaces can promote healing due to their stabilizing effect, but also due to their contraction, they can increase the displacement of the fractured parts. In this case spontaneous healing can have serious consequences for example narrowing of the birth canal. Injuries of intrapelvic organs are often combined with pelvic fractures involving, for example urinary bladder, urethra, rectum, and branches of the lumbosacral plexus (see 78.2).

74.2 At the **PELVIC SYMPHYSIS** the os coxae of one side can be separated from the other on account of trauma, occasionally accompanied by simultaneous separation of the iliosacral articulation. Such separations affect young animals in particular since the pelvic symphysis is still cartilaginous and ossifies firstly in adulthood. The tight iliosacral articulation also becomes stronger or more compact with increasing age. In young individuals the symphyseal union which is still cartilaginous, brings about an insignificant widening of the osseous birth passage.

76.1 Aseptic necrosis of the **HEAD OF THE FEMUR** (Legg-Calvé-Perthes disease) occurs in growing dogs between 4 and 12 months of age. An insuf-

ficient blood supply is presumed as a causal agent (see 84.1); as well a breed predisposition (Terrier, Toy Poodle) exists. Radiographically at progressive stages of the disease the following are recognizable: a deformation of the head of the femur, an indentation of the head as well as reparative reactions such as compression of the substantia spongiosa and fibrous development in the endosteum. In the progressive disease, morphological alterations can encroach upon the neck of the femur with the development of endosteal connective tissue. Good therapeutic results are attained with resection of the head of the femur. In young dogs the blood supply of the femoral head takes place by way of a vascular plexus in the joint capsule and the epiphyseal artery which courses in the ligament of the head of the femur. Not until after the closure of the epiphyseal (growth) plate is it supplied in addition, by intraosseous vessels (diaphyseal arteries) (see illustration).

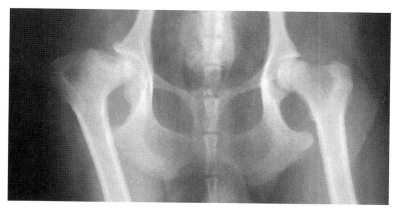

76.1 Deformation of the right head of the femur resulting from an aseptic necrosis of the head of the femur.

76.2 Fractures of the **NECK OF THE FEMUR** are important and detrimental to the blood supply of the head of the femur. Therefore they must be paid attention to quickly in a surgical and anatomically correct manner.

76.3 The **TIBIAL TUBEROSITY**, the site of insertion of the m. quadriceps femoris is an apophysis, which is united to the remaining tibia by an apophyseal cartilage during the growth period. The apophyseal cartilage consists of a caudoproximal approximately perpendicular portion and a craniodistal approximately horizontal portion. The craniodistal portion of the cartilage, on account of the tension of m. quadriceps femoris via the patellar ligament, which is continued on, attaching to the cranial border of the tibia distally has a capacity for traction. An apophysiolysis is rare and mostly due to trauma (see illustration 138.5). It occurs almost exclusively in young dogs between 4 and 6 months of age. This is before the final ossification of the apophyseal cartilage which is closed after 1 year of age. Because of its different pathogenesis, fracture of the tibial tuberosity in the dog is not equated with Osgood – Schlatter disease in humans.

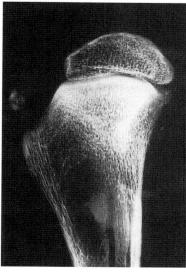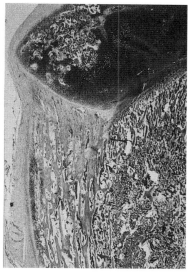

76.3 Radiograph (left illust.) and histological section (right illust.) of the tibial tuberosity of a young dog with initial ossification of the apophyseal cartilage (Radiograph Frau Dr. von Ruedorffer, Berlin).

76.4 DEWCLAWS are particularly well developed in large dog breeds (Mastiff, St. Bernard) and can also be duplicated. In individual dog breeds such as the Briard, they are a requisite breed standard.

78.1 In dogs the most common site for intramuscular injection is the **ISCHIAL MUSCULATURE**.

78.2 The **SCIATIC NERVE** is injury prone in its course over the greater sciatic notch, due to pelvic fractures. With defective injection technique intramuscular injections of irritant drugs in the long ischial muscles can lead likewise to irreversible damage of the nerve.

80.1 The **M. GRACILIS** can rupture due to intense action causing trauma. As a result the knee joint can no longer be extended actively. A shortening of m. gracilis can occur in extremely active or rigorously trained German Shepherd dogs as a result of a chronic functional compartment syndrome. In the affected dog at a walk and more intensely at the trot, the hock or tarsal joint is over extended and positioned outward while the paw is directed inward. Surgery consists of a complete resection of the muscle.

80.2 The **M. PECTINEUS (ET ADDUCTOR LONGUS)**, in addition to its action as an adductor, draws the femur proximally, pressures the head of the femur at the dorsal border of the acetabulum and therefore stabilizes the normally shaped hip joint. In hip dysplasia (HD, see 86.1) on the other hand, this pressure increases symptoms of pain on the reduced acetabular margin and accelerates joint wear and tear. Therefore with hip dysplasia, pectinomyotomy can lead to a temporary improvement of symptoms without, however halting the process of the condition.

80.3 A shortening of the **m. quadriceps femoris** generated traumatically, leads to stiffness and hyperextension of the knee joint combined with an abduction or dragging of the pelvic limb. The affected muscle is yellowish-white, atrophied and ultimately fibrotic with local degeneration and necrosis.

82.1 The **LATERAL SAPHENOUS VEIN** can be used for venipuncture prior to the subtraction of blood or for intravenous injections.

82.2 The **COMMON FIBULAR NERVE** is also termed the common peroneal nerve in the clinic. With a functional deficit the tarsal joint is maintained in an extended position and no longer can it be flexed actively (fibular paralysis). Deficit of the digital extensors leads to knuckling of the fetlock. There is also a loss of sensation on the dorsal aspect of the paw.

82.3 The **CRANIOLATERAL AND CAUDAL TIBIAL MUSCLES** are isolated into a closed compartment by crural fascia and fascia of the knee as the case may be. After oblique tibial fractures or injuries caused by biting, a severe pressure increase can occur in these locations (Compartment syndrome see 146.2).

82.4 Bone laceration at the tendon of origin of the **M. EXTENSOR DIGITALIS LONGUS** occurs rarely and this most frequently in young dogs. With the tendon displaced distally splinters of bone injure the knee joint leading to high degree lameness. Digital extension is not really restricted.

82.5 Partial or complete rupture of the **COMMON CALCANEAL TENDON** is caused mostly by trauma. Only the Dobermann breed is predisposed to spontaneous rupture. After complete rupture there is plantigrade **POSITIONING** of the **PES**. In general partial ruptures affect only the superficial digital flexor tendons.

82.6 The **CALCANEAL 'CAP'** can luxate laterally or more rarely medially. Luxation occurs particularly in overweight dogs and is combined with a severe swelling of the **subtendineal calcaneal bursa.**

82.7 Tearing away of the tendon of origin of **M. POPLITEUS** leads to a dislocation of the contained sesamoid bone, which is detected radiologically.

84.1 The **LATERAL AND MEDIAL CIRCUMFLEX FEMORAL ARTERIES** develop a vascular plexus in the capsule of the hip joint from which the main blood supply to the head of the femur results.

86.1 The **HIP JOINT** in the standing position occupies an angle of 85^0–100^0. Flexion is around 45^0–79^0 and extension 30^0–75^0. Adduction and abduction can take place at times to 70^0–80^0. For an **intraarticular injection** of the hip joint a needle 5–7 cm long must be advanced 4–6 cm horizontally from the craniodorsal border of the greater trochanter. **Luxations of the hip joint** are caused mostly by a severe external blow or impact and, as a rule, take place craniodorsally. The affected limb appears shortened and with luxation an imaginary triangle between coxal tuber, ischial tuber and greater trochanter of femur is flatter dorsally and by contrast wider ventrally (triangle test). **Hip dysplasia (HD)** is the most frequent condition of the hip joint in dogs. It is familial chiefly in many middle and large sized dog breeds and is inherited as a polygenetic trait. With HD it is a question of a postnatal retardation of the development of the hip joint. Possibly due to an unsatisfactory developmental stimulus through the head of the femur, the acetabulum remains flat or beveled. The head of the femur is held in an unsatisfactory manner in the acetabulum and can subluxate or luxate. Instability in the hip joint leads to overstress on the joint cartilage and the formation of subchondral bone which causes secondary degenerative changes of the hip joint (coxarthrosis). Diagnosis is by radiography, a classification of examined dogs being undertaken in groups A and E. (Group A = HD free, Group E = severe HD). A criterion for the depth of the acetabulum is the angle of Norberg. This angle between a line through the mid point of both femoral heads and a line projected from here to the cranial border of the acetabulum in healthy, large sized dog breeds should amount to not less than 105^0. With mid- and small sized dogs, one refers to varying specific angles for each breed to make an evaluation. In severe cases different surgical procedures are at one's disposal. Pectineomyotomy is the simplest, providing symptomatic palliative relief (80.2). With the different surgical techniques employed one attempts to improve the congruency between acetabulum and head of femur. This is attained after osteotomy of ilium, ischium and pubis with a triple swivel osteotomy whereby the acetabu-

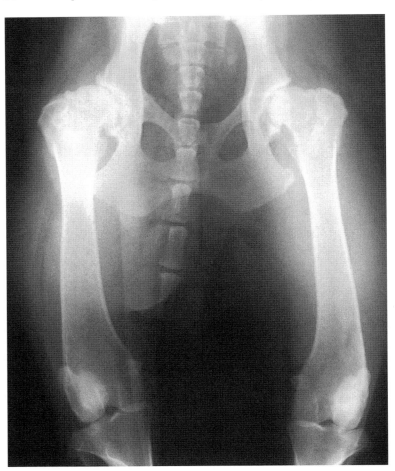

86.1 Healthy hip joint with the head of each femur fitting deeply into the acetabulum.

86.1 Severe hip dysplasia. The head of each femur is not surrounded sufficiently by the beveled or flattened acetabular margin. On the right a hip arthrosis (coxarthrosis) is fully developed.

lum is tilted over the head of the femur. With variation osteotomy the head of the femur is tilted further into the acetabulum by removal of a wedge of bone from the proximal shaft of the femur. The total replacement of the hip joint by a prosthesis has also been carried out for some years.

86.2 The **KNEE JOINT** in the standing dog occupies an angle from 105⁰ to 160⁰ on its popliteal aspect. Flexion ranges between 65⁰–90⁰ and extension between 35⁰–60⁰. With a knee joint angle of 90⁰ the tibia can be rotated 10⁰–20⁰ inwards and 35⁰–40⁰ outwards. By comparison, in extension the tense collateral ligaments permit no rotation. With intrarticular injection a needle is advanced in the slightly flexed joint medial to the patellar ligament half way between tibial tuberosity and patella. The needle is then directed caudoproximally and into the joint cavity. **Rupture of the cranial cruciate ligament** of the knee joint is among the most frequent orthopedic conditions of dogs. Average sized breeds are affected between 5 and 8 years of age, large sized breeds already in their first year, and dwarf breeds not until after 12 years. The reason for the susceptibility of the cranial cruciate ligament to rupture is the progressive differentiation of fibrous cartilage in the mid-section of the ligament with increasing age, thus reducing its tensile strength. The basis for the differentiation of fibrous cartilage is the twisting of the cranial cruciate ligament around its own long axis. This increases with each flexion of the joint producing an increase in pressure within the ligament. Usually rupture does not occur suddenly. With stages of overstretching, there is an imperceptible disintegration of ligamentous structure, ruptures within the ligament and partial rupture including the surface of the ligament. Ultimately this results in total rupture after low grade trauma. The 'drawer test' provides diagnostic proof of the condition. With the femur fixed in position the tibia can be displaced cranially. In a majority of cases of cruciate ligament rupture the rotational instability in the knee joint leads to damage of the medial meniscus. Very different surgical techniques have been developed for stabilizing the knee joint: A strip of femoral fascia or a section of patellar ligament can be pulled through the joint cavity as an intra-articular substitute for the ligament. By comparison synthetic materials are employed as extra-articular substitutes for the ligament. These are wound around the sesamoid bones of m. gastrocnemius (fabellae) medially and laterally and pulled through a hole bored through the tibial tuberosity.

In addition to the classical methods of ligament substitution a biomechanical surgical method has also been developed: The removal of the head of the fibula moves the insertion of the lateral collateral ligament cranially so that this can take over the function of the cranial cruciate ligament. With another method the tibial plateau is tilted craniodistally due to a wedge osteotomy of the proximal tibia and its slide forward is prevented. The traumatized meniscal portion, generally the caudal horn of the medial meniscus, is resectioned.

Further conditions of the knee joint occurring relatively frequently are osteochondrosis dissecans (see 142.4) which is localized as a rule in the lateral condyle of the femur, and rupture of the caudal cruciate ligament.

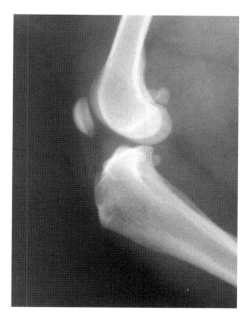

86.2 Radiograph of the drawer test with cruciate rupture. In relation to the femur the tibia is displaced cranially.

86.3 With luxation of **THE PATELLA** the latter is displaced further medially seldom laterally. Toy breeds are mostly affected and it is treated as a congenital condition. In congenital patellar luxation, the trochlea of the femur remains flat or is lacking completely because of absence of formative pressure stimulus through the patella. Frequently employed surgical techniques are the displacement of the tibial tuberosity with the insertion of the patellar ligament laterally and/or the deepening of the trochlea of the femur.

86.4 In the standing position the **TARSAL JOINT** occupies an angle from 110⁰–135⁰. Flexion is approximately 60⁰–80⁰, and extension 20⁰–35⁰. Only in the flexed joint is there a slight possibility of rotation around 10⁰–15⁰. A sidewards motility is an indication of fracture of the medial or lateral malleolus or rupture of the collateral ligaments. For an arthroscopic examination of the tarsocrural articulation an endoscope can be introduced lateral to the tendon of m. extensor digitorum longus. Arthroscopy is performed particularly to recognize lesions of osteochondrosis dissecans of joint cartilage at the trochlea of the talus.

88.1 In its original form in cartilaginous fish the **PRIMORDIAL CRANIUM** is a tubular cartilaginous brain capsule. In the course of phylogenesis the roof becomes more and more defective so that finally only a basal cartilaginous cranium remains. The connective tissue defects are filled up by osseous laminae arising directly from the connective tissue of the desmocranium and later fusing with the remaining cartilaginous primordial cranium at the base of the skull. Due to ossification emanating from numerous foci, the cartilaginous primordial cranium divides into several individual endochondral or replacement bones. These fuse partially with the membranous or connective tissue bones of the roof of the cranium to give **bones of a mixed nature** for example the temporal bone. In adults the only parts of the primordial cranium remaining are the nasal cartilages and the cartilaginous growth sutures at the base of the skull.

Fonticuli or fontanelle are connective tissue fissures which develop prenatally between the bones of the cranium. On account of the palpable pulse detected in them they are given the Latin name fonticulus meaning a source. Due to peripheral growth of the defining bones of the cranium the fonticuli unite prematurely to give cranial sutures. This process varies in a breed dependent manner. In toy breeds with strongly rounded or dished crania (see 88.2) the fonticuli can disappear with complete closure.

88.2 A marked curvature of the **CRANIUM** with simultaneous shortening of the facial part of the skull is characteristic of brachycephaly which is typical of many chondrodystrophic dog breeds (English and French Bulldogs, Chihuahua, Pugs, Pekingese, Yorkshire Terrier etc). This skull shape leads to various health defects in affected animals and is therefore rejected as bad breeding.

88.3 The **HYOID APPARATUS** unites the root of the tongue and larynx. With swallowing, the tongue is arched upwards, the larynx is drawn craniodorsally under the root of the tongue and the epiglottis is closed. Strangulations can fracture the apparatus generally involving the stylohyoids. Subsequently food intake, chewing and swallowing are severely impaired or rendered impossible.

90.1. The **WALL OF THE CRANIUM** (roof of cranium = calvaria) consists of 5 layers:

I. The **external periosteum or pericranum** is fused with the connective tissue of the skull sutures, while it can be detached from the large interjacent osseous surface (therefore subperiosteal hemorrhage cannot pass to the outside by way of the sutures of the cranium).

II. The **lamina externa** is a cortical (compact) osseous layer of the bones of the cranium.

III. The **diploë** is a reduced layer of spongy bone which nevertheless exhibits structural peculiarities. Its small cavities contain diploic veins which serve in temperature regulation. Due to the intense flow of blood through the diploë, temperature differences are equalized between the scalp and brain (an over demand of the temperature regulation mechanism results in sunstroke).

IV. The **lamina interna** is the internal cortical (compact) osseous layer of the bones of the cranium.

V. The **internal periosteum or endocranium** is fused with the solid dura mater.

90.2 The **PARANASAL SINUSES** are osseous cavities between the internal and external laminae of the bones of the skull into which respiratory nasal mucous membrane extends. In neonates they are very small and increase considerably in size with age. In long skulled dog breeds all 3 frontal sinuses are always well developed while in extremely short skulled breeds they can be completely lacking. Infections of the upper air passages and also neoplasms can lead to accumulations of mucus and pus in the frontal sinuses. With resistance to treatment the frontal sinuses must be opened surgically (trepanization) for direct local treatment. The maxillary recess is an outpocketing of the maxilla directed laterally and is bounded medially by ethmoid, lacrimal and palatine bones. The roots of the upper carnassial tooth are next to the maxillary recess so that with root emphyema it and the contained lateral nasal gland are affected.

90.3 The **SELLA TURCICA** is occupied completely by the hypophysis and the surrounding subarachnoid space. Therefore with indirect radiography, the size of the hypophysis which cannot be displayed itself, can be deduced.

90.4 A growth disorder of the **MAXILLA** with shortening as a consequence results in upper brachygnathia, and is typical of different chondrodystrophic breeds such as Bulldog, Pekingese and Pugs.

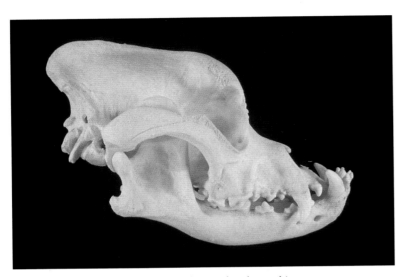

90.4 Skull of Boxer with pronounced upper brachygnathia.

90.5 With lower brachygnathia the **MANDIBLE** is too short in relation to the maxilla. Periosteal bony over-development on the mandible and in the region of the bulla tympanica is characteristic of **craniomandibular osteopathy**. This is a proliferative bone disease of young dogs occurring in West Highland White Terriers. Limited mobility of the temporomandibular articulation leads to problems of food and fluid intake. Alterations appear bilaterally symmetrical and can therefore be differentiated from bone tumors.

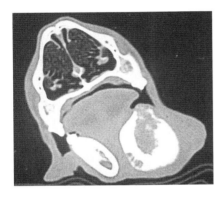

90.5 Bone tumor of ramus of mandible (Computer tomography: Animal Clinic Krüger, Hamburg).

92.1 In the narcotized dog, the **SUBLINGUAL VEIN** is situated on the ventral side of the tongue and is easily accessible for intravenous injections in emergency situations.

92.2 After exposure to injury **FACIAL PARALYSIS** always leads to different pathological deficiencies appearing either uni- or bilaterally. With **central facial paralysis** the lesion lies in the medulla oblongata of the brain in the vicinity of the facial nucleus. With deficit of the mimetic muscles, the musculature of eyelids and forehead remain entirely intact because the nuclei only of these muscles preserve impulses from both cerebral hemispheres. With **peripheral facial paralysis** lesions are present along the course of the facial nerve generally due to a blow around the border of the mandible ventral to the manibular condyle.

In **complete peripheral paralysis**, nerve branches leaving the petrous temporal bone can be injured with appropriate grades of damage. (Derangement of taste sensation due to damage of the chorda tympani, interruption of auditory sensation through damage of the stapedial nerve, faulty secretion of the lacrimal glands due to changes of preganglionic nerve fibers in the greater petrosal nerve, an injury to saliva formation due to injury of the chorda tympani which is significant in man). The mimetic muscles (of facial expression) are paralyzed in a flaccid manner as for example with drooping of the lips. With a deficit of m. buccinator, food collects in the oral vestibule adjacent to cheeks and cannot be pressed between the series of teeth. With a deficit of the muscles of the eyelid, the lids can neither be completely closed (m. orbicularis oculi) nor completely opened (m. levator anguli oculi medialis). The intact m. levator palpebrae superioris (oculomotor nerve) and smooth musculature (m. tarsalis) prevent the upper eyelid from falling down completely. Due to a loss of ability to blink, tears are not distributed over the cornea and this leads to its desiccation and cloudiness, and eye infection. (Similar injury with changes to the greater petrosal nerve results in impairment to the

formation of tears). The eyelid-cornea reflex (see 118.1) is diminished with facial paralysis.

94.1 With plastic surgery the **M. SCUTULOAURICULARIS SUPERFICIALIS** is displaced dorsomedially for the elevation of ear muscles where there is a drooping pendant ear. The muscle is sutured to the m. interscutularis, together with the scutiform cartilage.

94.2 The **MUSCLES OF MASTICATION** are paralyzed in a spastic manner with tetanus so that opening of the mouth and food intake are not possible. An inflammation of masticatory muscles of unknown origin (eosinophilic myositis) leads to a chronic, complete atrophy and causes a distinct prominence of bone contours.

96.1 PARALYSIS OF THE MANDIBULAR NERVE leads to a deficit of muscles of mastication and with bilateral paralysis to a drooping of the mandible. In addition to inflammation and trauma, one must also consider infectious diseases such as rabies and distemper as causal agents.

96.2 The **MENTAL NERVES** are blocked with local anesthetic at their palpable exit sites from the mental foramina. The nerves provide sensory innervation of the lower lip.

96.3 To eliminate pain the **INFRAORBITAL NERVE** is anesthetized during surgery to lips, nose, incisor and cheek teeth by the injection of local anesthetic into the infraorbital canal.

98.1 The **LACRIMAL GLAND AND THE GLAND OF THE THIRD EYELID** secrete serous lacrimal fluid. This provides nutriment and moisture to the cornea maintaining its tumescent state. The secretion cleanses cornea, conjunctiva and conjunctival sac as well as affording protection from inflammation due to contained effective antibacterial substances.

A **pathological drying up** of lacrimal fluid results in keratoconjunctivitis sicca (dry inflammation of cornea and conjunctiva).

98.2 With obstruction of the **NASOLACRIMAL DUCT** lacrimal fluid is discharged over the margin of the lower lid (epiphora). With the introduction of a fine catheter into the upper or lower lacrimal punctum one can irrigate the duct. Particularly in toy breeds of dogs the nasolacrimal duct is not constructed completely. Chronic lacrimal flow from the medial angle of the eye results in chronic skin irritation and brownish discoloration of the hair.

98.3 ANESTHESIA OF THE EYE is attained by injection into the periorbita or into the orbital fissure. The (sensory) ophthalmic nerve (V1) and the motor nerves of the eye (III, IV, VI) are blocked and one avoids retraction of the orbit during surgery.

98.4 In brachycephalic dog breeds such as Pekingese, the **NOSTRILS** show a tendency to develop stenoses, because the cartilaginous supports of the nostrils are insufficient. According to the functional principle of a one way valve, with inspiration there is closure of the nostrils and severe dyspnea. Surgical correction occurs with wedge shaped sectional resection of the lateral nasal cartilages. In brachycephalic breeds the bones of the facial skeleton are short proportionately and do not cover the nasal cartilages at the level of the tip of the nose. By keeping the muzzle closed during a clinical examination of the deformed nasal cartilages one can interrupt the airflow unintentionally.

100.1 The **NASAL CAVITY** belongs to the 'upper airway' in which the respiratory air in its passage alters its temperature and humidity and is cleansed of foreign particles. The equalization of breath temperature and body temperature is attained due to turbulence and the very good blood supply of the nasal cavity. For example inspired air at -30°c in winter is warmed to 37°c. The warm moist nasal mucous membrane assures the extensive saturation of inspired air. Foreign bodies such as fine particles and insects can be held up by the hair covering of the nostrils. The finest particles, bacteria and spores remain adherent to the moist mucus. These are transported away with associated mucus due to sneezing or in the first instance due to movement of cilia. The nasal cavity fulfils a further important function in the regulation of body temperature, due to heat emission with panting.

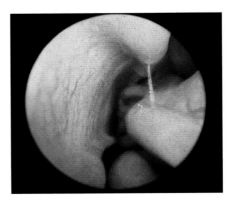

100.1 Endoscopic view of the nasal cavity (rhinoscopy) and the nasal septum.

With conditions of the nasal cavity diagnosis is centered around radiology and microbiology together with mycology, histopathology, computer tomography and magnetic resonance imaging. Among these processes endoscopy plays a prominent part. Not only are structural changes understood but biopsy material can also be taken for on-going microbiological and histopathological examination. With radiography and more profitably with computer tomography, not only can one differentiate changes in the turbinates and nasal septum but also soft tissue changes as in neoplastic tissue or mycotic infiltration. One is tempted to use magnetic resonance imaging due to its very detailed imaging of soft tissue.

For the surgical removal of neoplasms as an example, surgical access to the nasal cavity takes place over the bridge of the nose after osteotomy and nostril flap of the nasal bone (rhinotomy) have been made. (Oronasal fistula see 104.11).

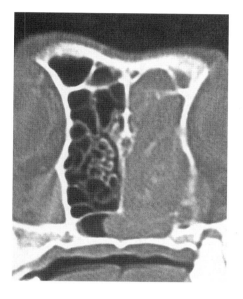

100.1 Purulent rhinitis and sinusitis with destruction of bone in the right nasal cavity and frontal sinus with discharge of pus into the nasopharyngeal meatus (Computer tomography: Animal Clinic Krüger, Hamburg).

100.2 One can advance a nasal tube through the **VENTRAL NASAL MEATUS** into the stomach. After fixing it to the head the tube can be left in place for several days to permit artificial feeding.

100.3 The **LARYNGEAL MUCOUS MEMBRANE** can swell markedly in the region of the vestibule as in allergic reactions, due to which the airway is blocked to an extreme extent. The popular notion 'edema of the glottis' is incorrect because the glottis, adjacent to the vocal folds is not swollen but rather the edematous epiglottis. Regarding the **mucous membrane** folds of the larynx, beside the ventricular and vocal folds the **aryepiglottic fold** extending from epiglottis to arytenoid cartilage forms the lateral boundary of the aditus of the larynx. Lateral to the aryepiglottic fold and the aditus lies the **piriform recess** of the pharynx.

The cuneiform and corniculate processes of the arytenoid cartilage form the cartilaginous supports of the aryepiglottic fold. A 'collapse' of the cuneiform process occurs in small brachycephalic dog breeds and is often associated with stenosis of the nostrils. This can cause serious inspiratory shortness of breath, since, during inspiration the cuneiform process is displaced into the lumen of the larynx, which is narrowed down as a result.

100.4 The **GLOTTIS** is formed ventrally by the vocal folds (the intermembranous part) and dorsally by the arytenoid cartilage (the intercartilaginous part). The glottis functions in sound formation or phonation due to vibrations of the vocal folds. The tension of the vibrating vocal folds can be altered voluntarily due to the laryngeal muscles. With the force of the airflow this affects vibration frequency and amplitude jointly thus regulating pitch and intensity of sound. Age, sex and testosterone level affect length and thickness of the vocal folds and with this the pitch. With castration the longitudinal growth of the vocal ligament ceases. Sound is modified due to resonance chambers such as nasal cavity, paranasal sinuses, and oral cavity. The glottis also participates functionally in **coughing**. In connection with this, first of all the glottis is closed. Then through an expiratory impulse the glottis is pushed open under greatly elevated pressure so that air is literally jerked forwards. Coughing drains and cleans the airways because with the impact of air, foreign bodies and mucus are expelled.

100.5 The **VOCAL LIGAMENT** extends from the vocal process of the arytenoid cartilage to the internal surface of the thyroid cartilage ventrally. It consists predominantly of elastic fibers and in common with the m. vocalis, belongs to the vocal fold.

100.6 In brachycephalic dog breeds the **LATERAL VENTRICLES** can prolapse into the laryngeal lumen which occurs due to negative pressure ratios. Surgical treatment involves their excision.

100.7 The **LARYNGEAL CARTILAGES** form the skeleton of the larynx. The **elastic epiglottic cartilage** is situated over the laryngeal entrance protecting it with swallowing. The remaining laryngeal cartilages are wholly or partially (arytenoid) hyaline and in old age there is a tendency to calcification detectable on radiographs. The cartilages are united mutually by articulations thereby having a certain freedom of movement. The **cricothyroid articulation** lies between the caudal process of the thyroid cartilage and the cranial border of the cricoid cartilage. The **cricoarytenoid articulation** lies between the arytenoid cartilage and the cranial border of the cricoid cartilage.

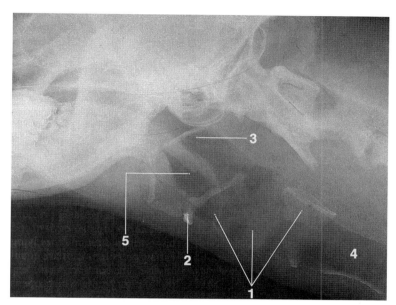

100.7 Laryngeal cartilages (1) with the Basihyoid bone (2), Nasopharynx (3) Trachea (4) Oropharynx (5). Details of basihyoid see p88. (Radiograph: Professor Dr. E. Henschel, Berlin).

100.8 The **LARYNGEAL MUSCLES** unite thyroid, cricoid and arytenoid cartilages with one another. According to their function one differentiates 'positional muscles' which attach to the arytenoid cartilage and through its change of position alter the breadth of the glottis and 'tension muscles' which alter the tension of the vibrating walls of the larynx. M. cricoarytenoideus dorsalis is a positional muscle. It draws the muscular process of the arytenoid caudodorsally and medially and with it the vocal process laterally thus widening the glottis. Likewise the m. crico-aytenoideus lateralis is a positional muscle and functions as an antagonist of the first muscle. It draws the muscular process of the arytenoid cartilage ventrally and laterally and thereby swivels the vocal process of the arytenoid cartilage medially. Thus the vocal folds lie together. The **m. cricothyroideus** innervated by the cranial laryngeal nerve is one of the 'tension muscles'. After injury to the recurrent laryngeal nerve (see 14.2) the laryngeal muscles innervated by it are paralyzed and flaccid (laryngeal hemiplegia), and atrophy. This results in a loss of tension in the ipsilateral vocal fold, over-development of an inspiratory noise and eventually dyspnea under stress.

100.9 By way of suggestion the **ORAL VESTIBULE** is divided rostromedially into 2 halves by the upper and lower frenula of the lips. The philtrum (philtron gr – love spell) courses in the midline to the **nasal plate**. A lateral **cleft lip** (or harelip in humans) is a congenital defect in the formation of the lip which lies between the embryonic nasal and maxillary processes. A **maxillary cleft** is directed through the maxilla between the canine tooth and the incisors.

100.10 In the **HARD PALATE** a cleft palate is present as an embryonic defect or after trauma; a median **cleft plate** is often seen after accidents in cats. A median congenital cleft palate originates as a defective or incomplete union of the embryonic lateral palatine processes. The separation between oral and nasal cavities due to a secondary palate ceases and so swallowing is impaired considerably. A combination of several defects can occur in the shape of a **labiomaxillary cleft**. Hereditary, toxic, hormonal as well as environmental factors such as hyper- and hypovitaminoses, are cited as the cause of the defects.

The soft palate in contrast to the hard palate, has no osseous foundation but is supported by striated muscle and the palatine aponeurosis. The mucous membrane coating the soft palate of which the side adjacent to the oral cavity and that adjacent to the nasal cavity consist of cutaneous and respiratory mucous membrane respectively, is moveable and swells severely with inflammation. In a majority of brachycephalic dog breeds a lengthening of the soft palate as a malformation is combined usually with stenosis of nostrils and larynx. Surgical correction involves shortening of the soft palate at its free border.

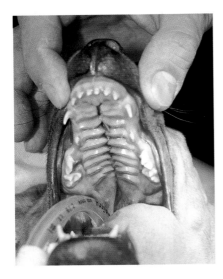

100.10 Congenital median cleft palate in a young Rhodesian Ridgeback.

100.11 The **AUDITORY TUBE** extending from the nasopharynx is surrounded by a pad which develops partly from supportive cartilage and partly from limiting muscle. The auditory tube serves as a pressure equalizer between the middle ear, occupying the tympanic cavity, and the external acoustic meatus; the ear drum (tympanic membrane) lying between them can only oscillate optimally if air pressure ratios are equal in both spaces. This is established by swallowing. The contracting m. tensor veli palatini inserts onto the wall of the auditory tube which opens due to this. In pharyngitis with tubal catarrh the opening mechanism fails on account of severe swelling of the soft palate. Due to the closure of the auditory tube higher or lower pressure in the tympanic cavity can no longer be adjusted. Sequelae are earache and a derangement of hearing since the eardrum can no longer vibrate freely.

100.12 **TONSILS** belong to the lymphatic organs. The palatine tonsil is the most important tonsil of the lymphatic 'pharyngeal ring'. It is classified on comparative anatomical principles as fossular, namely housed in a fossa, and not having crypts and follicles.

Formally it is characterized by a stratified squamous epithelium. Lymphoreticular tissue, characterized by typical primary and secondary lymph modules in close relationship with glands of the mucous membrane, is situated in the lamina propria mucosae under the epithelium. Numerous lymphocytes penetrate into the epithelial covering from the lymphoreticular tissue which in this manner becomes 'reticulated'.

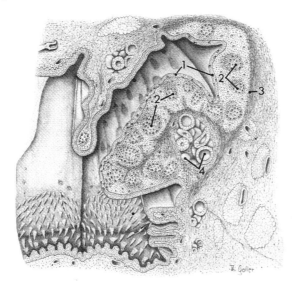

100.12 Palatine tonsil in tonsillar sinus. 1 Surface epithelium; 2 Lymph nodules; 3 Tonsillar capsule; 4 Mucous glands.

Deeply the lymphoreticular tissue is limited by a distinct connective tissue tonsillar capsule.

Functionally tonsils take part in the defence against infections which penetrate nose and mouth. The penetrating infection trigger is detected and organized specific antibodies released. Just as other lymphatic tissue is particularly well developed in the young animal so are tonsils. This is necessary since it must endure infections to which the adult animal has become immune already. With increasing age tonsils undergo regression. With chronically residing tonsillitis or pharyngitis or in squamous cell carcinoma of the tonsil a **tonsillectomy** is indicated, with the tonsillar tissue completely shelled out of its underlying tonsillar capsule. Complications can result from hemorrhage since the palatine tonsil is richly supplied by numerous branches of the lingual artery. Tonsils should not be removed thoughtlessly since they fulfill important functions of the immunity process, yet an excessive outpouring of antigen – antibody – complexes can lead to important renal and cardiac injury in the course of recurring tonsillitis.

102.1 Of the **PHARYNGEAL MUSCLES**, the pharyngeal constrictors take origin from skull, hyoid bone and larynx. The slings so formed and opening ventrally end in the dorsal midline of the pharynx along its raphe. This is a tendinous strip directed longitudinally, which in turn attaches the pharynx to the skull. The muscles of the soft palate radiate in the palatine aponeurosis forming the connective tissue skeleton of the soft palate. Their organized interplay is essentially geared to swallowing.

With **swallowing** or deglutition the moistened food from the oral cavity is conducted through the pharynx into the esophagus during which the airways namely nasopharynx and the laryngeal aditus are closed. During the **initial voluntary phase** of swallowing the muscles of the floor of the mouth become tense and the tongue like a piston, becomes pressed against the hard palate. In this way the food is pushed caudally, arriving in the oropharyx and, by an upward arching of the base of the tongue, into the vicinity of the intrapharyngeal ostium. The **involuntary end phase** of swallowing commences here with contraction of the pharyngeal constrictor muscles. The chyme, as a result, slides directly to left and right past the epiglottis and through the left and right piriform recesses into the esophagus. By peristalsis it then arrives at the stomach. In the narrow oropharynx the food path must be guaranteed from going 3 'wrong ways'. 1 **Retrogression** into the oral cavity is prevented due to the pressure of the tongue against the palate. 2 **Access to the nasopharynx is** removed due to the elevation and tension of the soft palate. 3 With regard to the **covering of the laryngeal aditus**, the larynx is displaced rostrally, the elastic epiglottis is deflected due to upward arching of the base of the tongue and lies passively over the laryngeal entrance, thus closing it. The passage of boluses through the esophagus and into the stomach is promoted by peristaltic contractions.

Deficient relaxation of **m. cricopharyngeus** contracts the entrance to the esophagus and interrupts deglutition (cricopharyngeal achalasia).

102.2 The **GLOSSOPHARYNGEAL AND VAGAL NERVES** provide sensory innervation to the pharyngeal mucous membrane and motor innervation to pharyngeal musculature respectively. Consequently they form afferent and efferent limbs of the swallowing reflex mediated by contact of food with the pharyngeal mucous membrane.

102.3 The **SYMPATHETIC PART** of the autonomic supply to the head, by way of postganglionic nerve fibers, courses to the effector organs in company with the large blood vessels, particularly the internal carotid artery (as the internal carotid plexus), the jugular vein (as the jugular nerve), and the external carotid artery (as the external carotoid plexus). **Stimulation of the sympathetic part** causes a dilation of the pupil (mydriasis) due to strong contraction of the m. dilator pupillae, and a widening of the rima of the eyelids due to powerful contraction of the smooth m. tarsalis. With **Horner syndrome** sympathetic nerve conduction can be deranged on its long path to the head (for example by goiter, enlarged lymph nodes, tumors of the mediastinum, and vertebral disc prolapse). The syndrome is conspicuous due to ptosis (narrow palpebral rima), miosis (narrow pupil), prolapse of the nictitating membrane, and enophthalmus (a more deeply situated ocular orbit).

102.4 The **PARASYMPATHETIC PART** of the autonomic nervous system of the head is connected to cranial nerves III, VII, IX and X. The preganglionic parasympathetic neurons of the **oculomotor nerve** III course in the orbit to the ciliary ganglion and from there postganglionic neurons extend to the m. ciliaris (accommodation) and m. sphincter pupillae (miosis). The parasympathetic fibers of the facial nerve VII are directed in the nerve of the pterygoid canal to the pterygopalatine ganglion and from there, after synapsing with postganglionic fibers, to meninges, nasal and lacrimal glands, and nasal mucous membrane. Another parasymphathetic portion supplies the salivary glands via the chorda tympani. The **parasympathetic part** of the **vagus nerve** extends predominantly into the larger body cavities and synapses firstly in the intramural ganglia of the effector organs. The proximal ganglion lying in the jugular foramen contains the nerve cell bodies of the sensory (afferent) neurons. The nerve cell bodies of the viscerosensory neurons lie in the distal (nodose ganglion). Synapsing does not occur in the proximal and distal ganglia as is generally true for sensory ganglia. The cell bodies of the autonomic motor neurons are located in the rhombencephalon.

102.5 **EXTERNAL AUDITORY MEATUS** see 120.2

104.1 The **ROOT OF THE TONGUE** is conspicuously large and torulose in brachycephalic breeds of dog and can therefore reduce the airflow and impede breathing.

104.2 The **TIP OF THE TONGUE** contains the **lyssa** rostromedially which was identified erroneously with rabies also knows as 'lyssa'. The lyssa is a morphological specialization in the tongue of carnivors and can be detected slightly on a cross section through the tip of the tongue. This connective tissue tube, some 4 cm long, contains adipose tissue, striated muscle and cartilage cells.

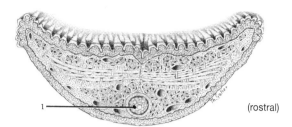

104.2 Cross section of the rostral part of the tongue with its median lyssa (1).

104.3 The **TASTE RECEPTORS** are constituents of the taste buds which are present mainly in the circular furrows of the vallate papillae, on the foliate papillae with fewer on the fungiform papillae. In humans and possibly our domestic mammals, taste buds are also present at the base of the tongue and epiglottis, which are innervated by the vagus nerve. The taste buds are barrel shaped and each consists of about 30 cells (taste cells, supporting cells and basal cells). The 'open end of the barrel' that is the taste pore, lies on the surface of the mucous membrane. Taste cells are secondary sense cells which contact synaptic nerve fibers. The circular furrow of a vallate papilla contains about 150 taste buds. In the floor of this furrow open the **serous taste glands** which possibly dissolve the material to be tasted and besides this, after taste perception washes it away. Moreover in the caudal one third of the tongue serous and seromucous glands are present which belong to the scattered salivary glands.

104.4 The **INTRINSIC TONGUE MUSCLES**, on account of the 3-dimensional arrangement of longitudinal, transverse and perpendicular muscle fiber bundles demonstrate structural characteristics which are organ specific. The otherwise typical envelopment of the fiber bundles due to endo-, peri- and epimysium as well as muscle or deep fascia is modified to a marked degree. The striated muscle bundles also show occasional ramifications in an untypical manner.

Functionally the three dimensional arrangement of longitudinal transverse and perpendicular muscle bundles permits an enormous mobility which is of particular benefit to the uptake of food. With suckling the tongue is formed into a tube. Due to contraction of perpendicular and transverse muscle fibers the tongue becomes even longer, estimably a unique muscle function.

104.5 The **HYPOGLOSSAL NERVE** can be damaged due to trauma or inflammation in the mandibular space. With unilateral paralysis, the tongue is curved towards the healthy side and atrophied on the paralyzed side. With bilateral derangement of the hypoglossal nerve there is complete paralysis of the tongue which hangs flaccidly from the mouth.

104.6 The **SALIVARY GLANDS** secrete saliva into the oral cavity or its vestibule. The appendicular glands are grouped into the **large salivary glands**. Of these in the dog, the parotid gland secretes a serous, the mandibular and sublingual glands a seromucous secretion. The **regulation** of salivary flow takes place via parasympathetic and to a lesser extend sympathetic fibers.

Parasympathomimetic drugs stimulate secretion of saliva, its flow stimulated reflexly beforehand, and by the uptake of food. **Salivary concrements** and **dental tartar** are salivary sediments, with tartar containing decomposable and foul smelling cell detritus. Molar teeth in the vicinity of the openings of parotid and zygomatic glands are particularly disposed to accumulations of tartar. Salivary concrements are situated in the excretory ducts and can obstruct them, leading to secretion dam-back, retention cysts and pressure atrophy of the gland.

104.7 Within its substance the **PAROTID GLAND** is crossed by blood vessels and the facial nerve. Pathological changes such as inflammation and neoplasms can therefore cause facial paralysis. The parotid duct which courses over the m. masseter can be redirected surgically into the lateral commissure of the eye to provide substitute tears with pathological 'drying up' of lacrimal flow.

104.8 The **SUBLINGUAL GLANDS** are significant clinically because injury to their excretory ducts can cause formation of salivary cysts. A sublingual cyst lies on the floor of the oral cavity and is known as a ranula on account of its similarity to a frog's abdomen. With a cervical position one speaks of a honey cyst or mellicerus, because of its honey like content. With contrast radiography after injection of the medium via the sublingual caruncle one can guarantee a diagnosis of left or right side damage. Since the monostomatic sublingual and mandibular glands

bound each other tightly and surgery on the sublingual gland without impairment of the neighboring gland is not possible, both organs are removed jointly.

104.9 An **EXCESS NUMBER OF TEETH (POLYDONTIA)** results from a surplus of primordial dental organs. **A fewer number (oligodontia)** is observed in brachycephalic breeds, where, as a rule, the last (caudal) teeth of the dental series are lacking. With a deficit of dental primordia, unphysiological **gaps** appear between the teeth **(diastasia)**. With tooth loss through trauma or extraction the osseous alveolus is already closed after a few weeks. This is not true, however, for the alveolus of the canine tooth of the old dog. After food particles accumulate in the alveolus, inflammation of the nasal cavity can result. Within the dental series there is self-regulation with a tendency to re-establish continuity of dentition. With **normal tooth position** the maxillary incisor teeth are situated somewhat rostrally in front of those of the mandible (a physiological shearing dentition). With faulty sectorial dentition upper and lower dental arches lie exactly one over the other. **Anomalies of position** are present due to twisting of teeth around the long axis (torsion) and transverse axis particularly with brachycephaly.

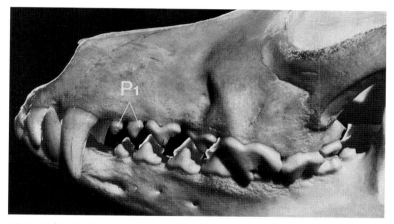

104.9 Polyodontia showing a doubling of the wolf tooth (P1) of the maxilla (Preparation: Professor Dr. E. Henschel, Berlin)

104.10 INCISORS are three cornered in shape and their wear and tear is subject to feeding and behavior patterns.

104.11 In the dog the **CANINE TOOTH** is used as a weapon. The very long root makes extraction difficult. As a complication with extraction the very thin osseous wall leading up to the nasal cavity can fracture and cause the development of an oronasal fistula.

To close the opening of the fistula tissue flaps from neighboring mucous membrane of palate and connecting mucous membrane of cheek are moved, fitted over the defect and sutured.

104.12 Premolar and molar **CHEEK TEETH** mince up and crush food. In contrast to the other premolar teeth the first premolar (P1) or wolf tooth always has 1 root and can therefore be identified radiographically. Phylogenetically in the dog this tooth is in regression thus making a place for the large root of the canine tooth.

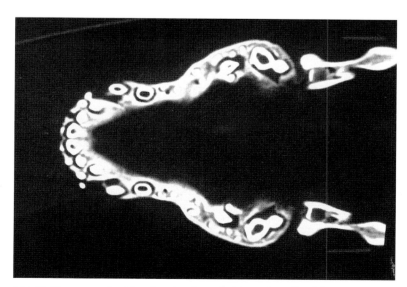

104.13 Temporary dentition showing the underlying primordia of the permanent dentition in a sectional computer tomograph taken through the mandible of a puppy (Photograph: Dr. Fahrenkrug, Quickborn, and Animal Clinic Krüger, Hamburg).

104.13 **NUMBER OF ROOTS** of the teeth can show considerable variation finally due to the fusion of several roots; with extraction these are observed at a glance on remaining portions of the root. Positional anomalies of the roots particularly those divergent and pressing outwards from one another make tooth extraction considerably difficult.

104.14 The **CARNASSIAL TEETH** possess 3 roots in the maxilla and 2 roots in the mandible. Inflammation and purulence of the upper carnassial can radiate into its surroundings. From its caudal root the openings of emanating fistulae are found ventral to the orbit under the eye.

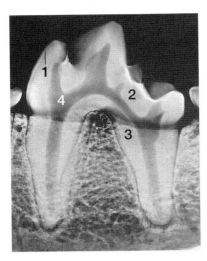

104.14 Carnassial tooth (M1) of the mandible. Enamel (1), Dentin (2), Cement (3) and Pulp Cavity (4). (Microfocus radiograph: Professor Dr. C. Poulsen Nautrup, Munich).

104.15 **DENTAL ENAMEL** is the hardest substance of the organism, essentially harder than food ingredients. The enamel forming cells also form the enamel epithelium, capping over the enamel. After tooth eruption the enamel forming cells and the epithelium are soon worn away. Enamel cannot regenerate if for example it undergoes demineralization, and disintegrates with dental caries caused by acid forming bacteria. Enamel hypoplasia with the formation of troughlike enamel defects and therewith an accompanying predisposition to dental caries occurs particularly on the incisor teeth with distemper (distemper dentition). Caries without linkage to infection attacks the last premolar and first molar of the upper dental arch. Due to disintegration of enamel the exposed dentin is stained dark brown. Tooth cavities can communicate with the pulp cavity. In dogs caries generally begins on the occlusal surface of the tooth, rarely on the enamel-cement boundary. In humans this site poses the chief risk of caries. The pulp cavity contains blood vessels and nerves enveloped by connective tissue, which is suggestive of mesenchyme.

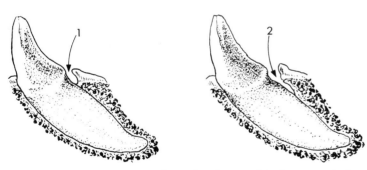

104.16 Pocket in the gingiva (1) due to detachment of the inner marginal epithelium and bone (bone pocket–2) from the tooth.

104.16 The **GINGIVA** or gum is the section of oral mucous membrane which protects the alveolar sockets of the bones involved in mastication. It projects upwards in a collar shaped manner with its external marginal epithelium then with its internal marginal epithelium it sinks deeply, attaching itself to the neck of the tooth. By means of this the peridontal membrane is protected superficially. With the detachment of the inner marginal epithelium from the tooth, **gingival pockets** form. With tooth extraction the affected tooth is exposed from the gingiva and in doing so one pays attention to the innervation thereof by buccal and sublingual nerves.

104.17 On account of the **PARADONTIUM** the tooth is suspended in the alveolus. The pressure of chewing is transmitted by oblique collagen fibers as an impulse load on the pressure susceptible bone of the alveolus. Generally inflammation of the paradontium (paradontitis) originates in gingival pockets infected with bacteria. With the progressive course of the infection there is loosening and ultimately the loss of the affected tooth.

106.1 The **TEMPOROMANDIBULAR JOINT** is important first of all as the primary joint of mastication developed from derivatives of Meckel's cartilage (cartilage of branchial arch 1.) In the course of evolution this underwent an alteration of function with its transformation into auditory ossicles and construction of the secondary (remaining) temporomandibular joint. The joint is classified as condylar, with a large angle of opening affording greater mobility simultaneously. Luxations are rare in the dog and take place only as subluxations in conjunction with jaw fractures. In the Basset and Cocker Spaniel temporomandibular luxations can take place spontaneously due to defective development of the socket and a shortening of the mandibular condyle (**temporomandibular dysplasia**). This should be taken into account with breeding.

106.2 Fractures of the **INTERMANDIBULAR SYMPHYSIS** are frequent in dogs. After repositioning, the fragments can be fixed either by wire loops around both canine teeth or by pins.

108.1 The **DURA MATER** can ossify (pachymeningitis ossificans) in older males of larger breeds (Mastiff, Saint Bernard). Only rarely does ossification cause clinical symptoms.

108.2 **EPIDURAL ANESTHESIA** involves a local anesthetic suited to blocking nerve conduction, which is injected into the epidural space. The injection site is chosen in principle so that injury to the spinal cord and injection into the subarachnoid space are avoided. The anesthetic diffuses through the meninges covering the roots of the spinal nerves leaving the cord, and, in a reversible manner, blocks the nerve stimulus-impulse transmission. Corresponding to the quantity of anesthetic applied (and dependent on the site of injection) segments situated cranially (= high) from the sciatic nerve or caudally (= low) are desensitized. Accordingly one differentiates a high or a low epidural anesthesia. With high epidural anesthesia the motor nerves of the pelvic limb, femoral, obturator and sciatic nerves, are anesthetized and the animal is incapable of standing. With low epidural anesthesia, one desensitizes predominantly sensory nerves (pudendal and caudal cutaneous femoral nerves) and motor nerves to the muscles of the tail and the pelvic diaphragm. Furthermore the patient is capable of standing which is important in large animal surgery.

As an injection site for high epidural anesthesia one generally chooses the interarcuate lumbosacral space (lumbosacral injection). The injection is made perpendicularly into the vertebral canal between both sacral tubers and caudal to the spinous process of the last lumbar vertebra. With aspiration one estimates that the needle is situated neither in the subarachnoid space (aspiration of cerebrospinal fluid) nor in the venous vertebral plexus (aspiration of blood). Otherwise the needle is retracted slightly and aspirated once again as a further check. The sacrococcygeal interarcuate space or the interarcuate intercoccygeal spaces I to III are chosen as the injection sites for low epidural anesthesia.

108.3 By means of injection of contrast medium into the **SUBARACHNOID SPACE**, the contours of the spinal cord are displayed radiographically (myelography). Constrictions and lesions of the spi-

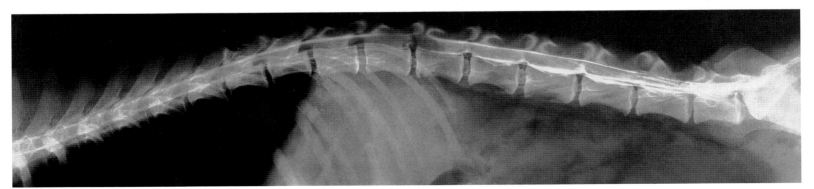

108.3 Myelography after the application of contrast medium into the subarachnoid space through the atlanto-occipital space (cranially into the cerebellomedullary cistern) and through the lumbosacral space (caudally into the subarachnoid space). Between the thoracic and lumbar vertebral column at the interruption to filling with contrast medium, an unphysiological increase in circumference is demonstrated leading to compression of the subarachnoid space. (Radiograph: Professor Dr. K. Hartung, Berlin).

nal cord are caused by alterations to vertebrae (see 8.4, 10.2), discopathies (see 10.3) and for example neoplasms, and can be displayed with myelography. The injection of contrast medium takes place either through the atlanto-occipital space into the cerebellomedullary cistern or between lumbar vertebrae 5 and 6 into the subarachnoid space. Both injection sites are suitable also for obtaining cerebrospinal fluid.

108.4 Functionally the nerve fibers coursing within the **SPINAL CORD** are fasciculated in common (mutual) tracts. The **ascending sensory tracts** can be subdivided into tracts for conscious proprioception (dorsal funiculus), unconscious proprioception (spinocerebellar tract) and deep pain (spinothalamic tract). A typical symptom for a lesion of the spinal cord is a retardation or deficiency of conscious proprioception. During this a paw of the affected animal placed passively on its dorsal aspect, either cannot or only after some delay be returned to its original stance. The **descending motor tracts** as upper motor neurons from the cerebral cortex are directed caudally in the ventral funiculus (extensors) and the lateral funiculus (flexors). After synapsing at the nerve cells in the ventral horn of the gray substance (lower motor neuron) information is conducted to the corresponding muscles. Not only injury to the upper but also to the lower motor neurons leads to paralysis; with injury to the lower neurons ipsilateral muscle tone and reflexes are lost simultaneously which is not the case with injury to the upper motor neurons. As a peculiarity in the dog there are ascending neurons from the lumbar spinal cord which impede the lower motor neurons of the extensors of the thoracic limb. Damage to these obstructing neurons due to lesions in the thoracic spinal cord leads to excessive muscle tone of the extensors of the thoracic limb (Schiff - Sherrington reaction). With regard to the resultant motor symptomatology lesions of the spinal cord are well localized.

A degeneration of the white substance in the thoracic spinal cord (degenerative myelopathy) leads to progressive ataxia, weakness of the hindquarters and finally paralysis. This is observed predominantly in old German Shepherd dogs.

110.1 An inflammation of **CEPHALIC AND SPINAL MENINGES** (meningitis) occurs rarely by itself in dogs but is generally a sequel to a primary illness such as endocarditis which results in a bacteremia. The most diverse virus infections lead to encephalites (see 110.3) which can extend to the cephalic meninges (meningoencephalitis).

110.2 CEREBELLO MEDULLARY CISTERN see 116.3

110.3 INFLAMMATION OF THE BRAIN (ENCEPHALITIS) can occur as a result of numerous infectious diseases. Of greater significance are viral infections such as rabies, distemper, Aujesky's disease and protozoal infections such as toxoplasmosis.

Rabies generally gains admission through a bite into the tissues and then proceeds along the nerves to the central nervous system. There it causes inflammation of the nerve cells, ultimately proving fatal.

With **distemper** at first the white substance of the brain and spinal cord shows inflammatory changes (Brainstem symptoms: motor derangement, disturbances of consciousness; Cerebellar symptoms: ataxia; Spinal cord symptoms: paresis).

Toxoplasmosis often causes inflammation of spinal cord and nerves as well as lesions of cerebrum and cerebellum.

Brain tumors can begin from glial cells (ectodermal portion) and from cephalic meninges together with associated blood vessels (mesodermal portion). As metastases they can stem from other organ systems and arrive at the brain by way of the vascular system. Tumors injure the brain tissue through compression or transformation into neoplastic tissue. Increased pressure on the brain leads to disturbance of permeability and to edema of the brain (swelling) owing to an unphysiological accumulation of fluid. In the diagnosis of brain tumors imaging processes especially 2 film imaging procedures, computer tomography, and magnetic resonance are of great significance. They make possible an unimpeded (free of overlay) image of soft tissue structures including those within the cranium.

110.4 With lesions of the brain stem the **RETICULAR FORMATION** mediates alterations in muscle tone and derangement of movement to impairment of consciousness ranging from apathy to coma (deep unconsciousness).

110.5 The **CEREBELLUM** regulates and coordinates voluntary movement due to sensory linkage with motor conduction. It receives information from the ascending tracts of the spinal cord and receives impulses from centers of balance, sight and hearing as well as from motor areas of the cerebral cortex. A progressive heritable degeneration of the cerebellar cortex, leads to a clinical picture of **cerebellar ataxia**. There is an increase in tone of the extensor muscles of the pelvic and finally the thoracic limbs and in the final stages of the condition the affected animal can no longer stand.

110.6 The ventral portion of the **MIDBRAIN** serves as a conduit for the long nerve tracts communicating between cerebrum and spinal cord. Important autonomic centers are situated in the tegmentum such as respiratory and vascular centers. Complex motor output is mediated for example via nerves to the eye muscles. The rostral colliculus, situated dorsally contains the optical reflex center facilitating the pupillary reflex. In the caudal colliculus lies a subcortical integration center for auditory function.

110.7 The **THALAMUS** is a subcortical integration center for sensation such as the perception of temperature and pain as well as deep sensation. It also contains a coordination center for sight function. In conditions which cannot be treated with analgesics, severe pain results.

110.8 The **EPIPHYSIS** (pineal body), due to its output of the neurosecretory hormone melatonin exerts a retarding influence on the development of the gonads (antigonadotrophin). A deficit causes sexual prematurity. According to the disputed opinion of several authors the epiphysis is supposed to regulate circadian rhythm.

110.9 In the **HYPOTHALAMUS** are situated the supraoptic and paraventicular nuclei which synthesize the hormones of the caudal lobe of the hypophysis (oxytocin, adiuretin). Other hypothalamic nuclei synthesize releasing hormones which regulate the secretion of the rostral lobe of the hypophysis (pituitary gland) (see 150.1). The hypothalamus also contains important autonomic centers for regulating body temperature, water economy, hunger and thirst.

110.10 The **ADENOHYPOPHYSIS** is the production site of numerous hormones which modulate the activity of most of the endocrine glands of the body (see p150). Tumors of the adenohypophysis are relatively frequent in dogs. Generally they extend dorsally leading to injury of the hypothalamus. As a consequence there is insufficient adiuretin and the development of diabetes insipidus. A tumor of the adenohypophysis is hormone producing, the clinical picture being connected, as the case may be, with the hormone produced. For example, an excessive ACTH production leads to the development of a hyperadrenocorticoidism (Cushing syndrome).

112.1 The **CEREBRUM** is organized into lobes (frontal, parietal, temporal and occipital lobes as well as the insula). Functionally the cerebral cortex is arranged somatotopically. Defined parts of the body are represented by fixed areas of the cerebral cortex. A 'map' with its reciprocal action between brain and the connected parts of the body is perceived as an homunculus which is illustrated lying on the brain surface. The form of the homunculus is disproportionate and severely distorted. Biologically important functions and the pertinent parts of the body such as hand and head are shown proportionately oversized and represented on correspondingly large areas of the brain.

112.2 The **INTERNAL CAPSULE** contains the strongly compressed initial segment of the pyramidal tract, about 4/5 of it changing to the opposite side of the body at the pyramidal chiasm which lies between medulla oblongata and spinal cord. Lesions of the internal capsule emanate from neighboring blood vessels and in humans cause the symptom complex of apoplexy. In dogs this illness is very rare.

112.3 The **BRAIN STEM** controls vital body functions (respiratory, cardiac) and likewise micturition, defecation, deglutition and vomition. Besides, the brain stem includes centers for control of body posture and mobility and harbors the nuclei of cranial nerves III – XII, the reflex centers for all motor and sensory – viscerosensory functions in the head region. Functional derangement of the brain stem makes itself apparent in a corresponding set of serious symptoms which can be combined with deficits of movement, postural and positional reactions, disturbances of consciousness ranging to coma, and deficits of vital functions.

112.4 The **BASAL NUCLEI** are synapsing centers for voluntary movement, particularly for slow movements (comparable to cerebellar function).

114.1 Tissue samples are taken from the **AMMONIC HORN** in the pathohistological diagnosis of rabies, leading to the detection of virus antigen and inclusion bodies using immunofluorescence.

114.2 The **ARTERIES OF THE BRAIN** are end arteries with sharply defined areas of end flow, that is to say they produce no anastomoses with adjacent parallel arteries. In general a deficient supply due to reduced blood flow (vascular spasm or emboli) or massive hemorrhage due to rupture of blood vessels causes sharply defined infarcts with continuous scarring.

The **blood brain** barrier is situated in the region of the capillary bed (morphological substrate see histology texts). Due to the barrier the capillaries in particular, are rendered impervious. Many substances in the blood do not reach the central nervous system. In this way, on the one hand, brain tissue is protected from dangerous blood constituents, on the other, certain drugs reach the brain tissue only in severely reduced concentrations. Due to the blood brain barrier, a suitable cerebral milieu is maintained in the interstitial fluid indispensable for brain function, specifically for the synaptic communication between nerve cells. On the one hand the brain must be protected from the metabolic fluctuations in the composition of the blood and on the other must be responsible for the supply of nutrients and the disposal of waste materials with the blood in indirect contact. The blood brain barrier makes the complete task possible. For the manufacture and application of neuro-drugs it is essential to develop strategies for the transport of effective materials through the blood brain barrier. Lipophilic substances overcome this semipermeable membrane easier than other materials, and can diffuse easier from the blood to the brain tissue.

The **blood-fluid barrier** can be conceived as a strongly modified variant of the blood-brain barrier.

116.1 The **CEREBRAL SINUSES** serve overall for the thermoregulation of the head ('keeping a cool head'). The blood of the diploic veins is cooled at the calvaria or roof of the cranium. In the nasal cavity blood is also cooled due to inhaled or exhaled air. From both regions blood flows in the cerebral sinuses, establishing consequently a cooling system for the brain.

The clinical significance lies in the fact that venous blood out of the nasal cavity is taken up by the ophthalmic plexus into the ventral cerebral sinus system. With neoplastic changes in the nasal cavity, cells can be spread and sediment out in the sinuses with their slow to absent blood flow. Brain tumors can result.

Sinus venography is a radiographic procedure for the display of the venous sinuses of the brain. A contrast medium is applied in the angular vein of the eye and via the ophthalmic plexus reaches the cerebral sinus system. Interruptions to the flow of contrast medium can be caused due to the space demand of the pathological process in the region of the brain. One can speak of a space occupying lesion.

116.2 With **ENCEPHALOGRAPHY** the contrast material can be dispensed in the cerebellomedullary cistern so that an opinion can be formed of the surface configuration of the brain. A specific method is ventriculography whereby a lateral ventricle of the brain (see text illustration p 116) is punctured through the cerebrum. The contained cerebrospinal fluid is withdrawn and the brain ventricles filled with air which serves as a contrast material (pneumoencephalography). Ventriculography is a means of estimation of size and symmetry of the ventricles of the brain. With the entry of computer tomography into veterinary medical diagnosis the significance of encephalography has decreased.

116.3 **CEREBROSPINAL FLUID** is formed in considerable quantities, approximately 350ml/day being quoted for the dog. Since the overall quantity of fluid in the ventricles of the brain together with that in the central canal and subarachnoid space remains constant, there must be a balance between formation and resorption. The arachnoid granulations (see p117) are considered sites of resorption as well as the offshoots of the subarachnoid space at the initial segments of the spinal nerves, and blood vessels to and from the brain. With an imbalance between formation and resorption, with increased formation or interrupted discharge, an internal hydrocephalus results. Moreover, the ventricles are dilated and increasingly brain tissue is displaced. The head is disproportionately large and the bones of the cranium are thin. Pathological increases of circumference come into question as the cause especially in the narrow regions of the 'internal' fluid spaces (interventricular foramen, mesencephalic aqueduct and the lateral aperture into the fourth ventricle of the brain communicating between the 'internal' and 'external' fluid spaces). In dwarf dogs with disproportionately large skulls (Chihuahua, Yorkshire and Manchester Terriers, Miniature Poodle) as well as brachycephalic breeds, an internal hydrocephalus occurs frequently as a consequence of congenital interruption to the discharge of cerebrospinal fluid.

In addition to nutritive and thermoregulatory functions, the cerebrospinal fluid in healthy animals is principally mechanical in that it forms a protective envelope. With blows to the head, brain movement is inhibited due to the presence of cerebrospinal fluid. This occurs at the site of impact and after some delay at the site opposite. With intense rotation, shearing forces occur at the passages of vascular and nervous structures from the skull leading to hemorrhages at the openings of the cerebral veins into the sinuses of the brain. With many infections causing inflammation of brain and meninges, cerebrospinal fluid changes its composition. First of all this relates to an increase of protein content and cell content (lymphocytes and macrophages). In some infections the agent can be detected directly. Cerebrospinal fluid, therefore, is obtained for diagnostic purposes. Using a specific spinal cannula one enters the cerebellomedullary cistern (cisterna magna) through the atlantooccipital space and aspirates the cerebrospinal fluid.

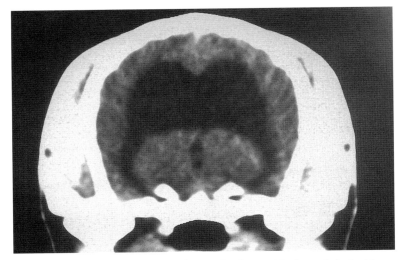

116.3 Severe dilation of both lateral ventricles (internal hydrocephalus) with displacement of cerebral hemispheres (Computer tomography: Animal Clinic Krüger, Hamburg).

118.1 The **UPPER** and **LOWER EYELIDS** limit the palpebral rima which in rare congenital cases remains closed. The eyelids are fibromuscular tissue laminae with an epithelial covering. The inner surface of the eyelid supports a stratified non-keratinized squamous epithelium. This becomes cuboidal in the conjunctival sac, finally extending onto the sclera and then cornea. Both lid surfaces merge with each other at the free border of the eyelid. The free border of the eyelid, approximately rectangular on cross section, supports the eyelashes along its outer and inner edges. The 'internal' skeleton of the eyelid, the tarsus, is a curved lamina of collagen fibers adapted to the curvature of the orbit.

The **muscular basis** of the eyelid is formed by m.orbicularis oculi (innervation: facial nerve), m.levator palpebrae superioris in the upper eyelid (oculomotor nerve) as well as the smooth m.tarsalis (sympathetic supply). A drooping of the upper eyelid can have different origins such as injury to the oculomotor nerve, facial paralysis (see 92.2) and paralysis of the sympathetic supply. With injury to sympathetic fibers, one discerns Horner syndrome with ipsilateral miosis (narrowing of the pupil), a narrowing of the palpebral rima due to drooping of the upper eyelid (ptosis), extrusion of the nictitating membrane and enophthalmus (abnormally deep position of the orbit in the orbital cavity). Of the **glands of the eyelid** the tarsal glands (sebaceous glands of Meibom) open on the border of the lid; with obstruction of their excretory ducts a painful nodule formation is produced known as a stye. Similarly the glands of the eyelashes (ciliary glands, glands of Moll – apocrine sweat glands) when blocked can become inflamed.

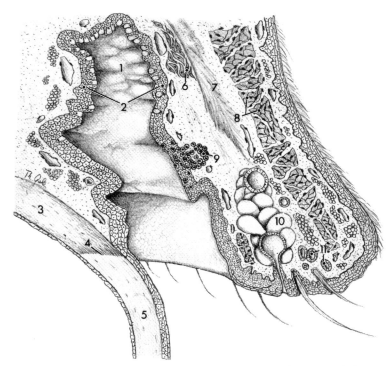

118.1 1 Fornix of the superior conjunctiva; 2 Conjunctival tunic (epithelium with goblet cells); 3 Sclera; 4 Limbus of cornea; 5 Cornea; 6 M.tarsalis superior; 7 Superior tarsus; 8 M. orbicularis oculi; 9 Conjunctival lymph nodules; 10 Tarsal glands; 11 Ciliary glands.

With **blinking**, tears (lacrimal fluid) are distributed on to the cornea. Closure of the eyelids is initiated reflexly by contact with the cornea (corneal reflex). The afferent nerve fibers of the reflex arc are contained in the long ciliary nerves (V1 see p98) and the efferents in the facial nerve to the m.orbicularis oculi. In dog breeds with markedly protruding eyes, a complete closure of the eyelids is no longer possible in individual cases. A central horizontal strip of the cornea is not kept sufficiently moist and becomes increasingly cloudy or turbid.

Deformity of the free border of the eyelid is present as an inturning or entropion due to which the cornea is irritated mechanically; an outturning or ectropion exposes the conjunctival sac. Without surgical correction abnormal positioning of the free borders of the eyelids leads to corneal and conjunctival inflammation.

118.2 The **THIRD EYELID** (nictitating membrane) lies at the medial angle of the eye supported by the cartilage of the third eyelid. With the application of pressure it comes across the orbit, and with contraction of m.retractor bulbi, as for example in tetanus, and with specific inflammation of m.temporalis in German Shephard dogs (eosinophilic myositis) it falls forward passively over the cornea. On the outer side and particularly on the inner surface of the third eyelid there are numerous lymph nodules (so called lymph follicles) which increase in size with follicular conjunctivitis and then are removed through rubbing.

The **conjunctiva** extends from the inner surface of the eyelid at the **fornix of the conjunctiva** (the conjunctival sac) to the rostral surface of the sclera and its border with the cornea.

The **cuboidal** epithelium of the fornix is adapted to resorption hence the application of eyedrops into the conjunctival sac. The sac also produces a mucous secretion from its goblet cells which decreases friction during blinking.

118.3 The **CORNEA** retains its transparency due to a precise state of tumefaction or swelling maintained externally by lacrimal fluid and internally by aqueous humor. Light is refracted at the outer surface of the cornea but not at the inner; therefore the cornea can be compared with the stiff front lens of a camera.

The healthy cornea is non-vascular. Since it is nourished by diffusion, metabolic diseases such as diabetes mellitus can cause a turbidity or cloudiness of the cornea. Moreover, with inflammation such as keratitis, blood vessels sprout into the cornea reducing sight. With superficial inflammatory processes conjunctival vessels sprout from the periphery of the cornea and with inflammation of the deeper corneal layers capillaries penetrate from the major arterial circle of the iris. Scar tissue and unphysiological curvatures of the cornea cause distortions. Cloudiness of the cornea follows soon after death because the normal tumefied state is lost due to alterations of the outer (membrane of Bowman) and inner (membrane of Descemet) limiting membranes.

118.4 Adspection of the **SCLERA** is an integral part of each general examination of an animal. Thus the faulty self-coloring of the sclera makes the recognition of, for example jaundice (icterus) possible at an early stage.

118.5 Inflammation of the **UVEA** is spoken of as uveitis.

118.6 On the **INNER SURFACE OF THE IRIS** is the shimmering pigment epithelium responsible for the blue or green color of the eye present for example in Siberian Huskies. If, in addition, pigments are present in larger quantities in the iridic stroma, a brown eye color results. Connective tissue concentrations of the iris, which are pigmentless, appear white. A partially white iris is a characteristic of heterochromasia where iris colors differ between right and left eyes, while a 'wall eye' is diffusely white. Both are seldom present in dogs. The **smooth muscles** of the iris are developed from ectoderm according to the dominant view. The m.sphincter pupillae is innervated by parasympathetic fibers. A narrow pupil (miosis) can be produced by myotic drugs, through parasympathetic stimulation (states of fear) or in sympathetic paralysis. The m.dilator pupillae is induced to contract with sympathomimetic drugs due to which the pupil is dilated (mydriasis). Net- or stroma-like formations lying on the outer surface of the iris and drawing over the pupil are indicative of a persistent pupillary membrane. This is a question of remnants of the embryonic anterior vascular tunic of the lens which, in the normal course of events has regressed completely by 3 – 5 weeks of age. Tissue interstices in the iris (iris kolobom) are due to an arrested development with incomplete closure of the choroid fissure.

118.7 The **RETINA** can be examined with an ophthalmoscope. Furthermore the pupil is dilated with a mydriatic and a beam of light thrown onto the fundus of the eye by a mirror. The examiner inspects the fundus through a central aperture in the mirror. Conditions of the retina such as inflammation, atrophy and detachment can be detected. Increased pressure within the cranium for example hydrocephalus, causes abnormal swelling of the optic disc over the retinal surface. Of the photoreceptors the rods predominate clearly over the cones, the ratio being

95:5 in dogs whereas in humans it is 50:50. Since cones are responsible for the perception of color in dogs there is probably only slight expression of this. Cones of the yellow macula are responsible for acuity of vision. Since the macula is underdeveloped by comparison acuity of vision is probably less well defined. The rods are purely for the appreciation of light intensity. Electroretinography permits a functional test of the retina even with extensive cataract of the lens. Action potentials (visually induced potentials) are recorded after the appearance of a light flash on the retina.

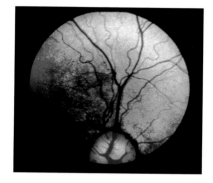

118.7 Fundus of a dog's eye with branching of the central artery and view of the retina. The tapetum lucidum is light blue. (Ophthalmoscopy: Dr. I. Allgöwer, Berlin).

118.8 **CATARACT OF THE LENS** can have very diverse origins being differentiated into those of congenital, inflammatory, traumatic or toxic causes. For example, hypoglycemia can bring about a metabolic (diabetic) cataract. In progressive cataract with restricted sight one possible treatment is the extraction of the nucleus of the lens while maintaining its capsule. The implantation of an artificial lens within the capsule is routine surgery in the dog. After rupture of the zonular fibers, a luxation of the lens can occur into the anterior chamber of the eye or onto the floor of the posterior chamber. In Terriers luxations of the lens take place cumulatively on account of an hereditary weakness of the zonular fibers.

118.9 The **PRODUCTION AND DRAINAGE OF AQUEOUS HUMOR** are in a state of flow equilibrium. Derangement of outflow at the iridocorneal angle of the anterior chamber interrupts this balance and causes an increase of intraocular pressure leading to glaucoma. The pressure rise results in pressure atrophy of the retina and ultimately in blindness. The view within the iridocorneal angle (gonioscopy) is possible after the setting of a contact lens on the cornea. Gonioscopy is an important method of clarifying the origin of glaucoma.

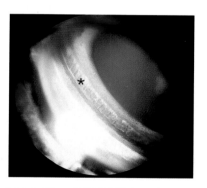

118.9 A view of the iridocorneal angle showing the pectinate ligament (Goniscopy: Dr. I. Allgöwer, Berlin).

120.1 The **AURICULAR CONCHA** produces extensive **hematomas (othematomas)** on its inner concave side and rarely on its outer surface. They are caused by different factors in some cases not yet clarified, such as shaking of the head with otitis externa or due to a blunt blow or impact. This causes hemorrhage from the small branches of the auricular vessels which course through small apertures in the auricular cartilage to the concave inner surface of the concha. Treatment is through drainage or surgical resection and must be repeated once or twice because of high return rates.

120.2 The **EXTERNAL AUDITORY CANAL** shows a sharp bend along its course. In order to examine the tympanic membrane (ear drum) otoscopically the canal must be stretched caudodorsally by traction on the auricular concha. Chronic inflammation of the external auditory canal (otitis externa see also 6.2) is a frequent condition of dogs. In difficult cases a surgical opening of the perpendicular section of the canal is necessary to provide drainage of the secretion and better access for local treatment. In addition to this a strip of cartilage is excised from the lateral wall of the canal after which the external skin is sutured to the skin of the external auditory canal lining its inner surface. Fundamental pathological changes such as neoplasms at the horizontal part of the canal can demand, in rare cases, the removal of the perpendicular and horizontal parts of the entire canal while preserving the free part of the auricular concha.

120.3 The **MIDDLE EAR** is in communication with the pharyngeal cavity by means of the auditory (Eustachian) tube. Infections can ascend from the pharynx into the tympanic cavity and cause inflammation of the middle ear (otitis media). Affected animals show a typical obliquity of the head to the infected side. Local treatment and cleaning of purulence caused by middle ear inflammation takes place through the external auditory canal after the tympanic membrane is perforated otoscopically. The defect so caused in the membrane heals up without complications. In difficult cases the tympanic cavity must be opened from its ventral aspect (bullaosteotomy).

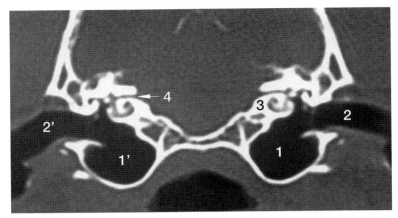

120.3 Computertomographic section of the left (1) and right (1'). Tympanic cavities. 2, 2' External acoustic meatus; 3 Cochlea; 4 Internal acoustic meatus (Computer tomography: Animal Clinic Krüger, Hamburg)

120.4 INFLAMMATION OF THE LABYRINTH (LABYRINTHITIS) is generally a consequence of middle ear inflammation passing to inner ear. Affected animals undergo considerable disturbance of balance, vomition and obliquity of head carriage.

120.5 A paralysis of the **VESTIBULOCOCHLEAR NERVE** can be caused by inflammation or tumors of the middle and the inner ear. Typical effects are movements in a circle, falling to the affected side and ataxia.

122.1 MUSCLE AND TENDON SPINDLES are receptors of involuntary deep sensation. The information relating to the state of tension of individual muscles, tendons and ligaments is conducted further. Firstly constant information regarding the state of tension of individual components of locomotion make the course of smooth motion possible. Neurological examination tests involuntary deep sensation, due to muscle reflex. Conscious deep sensation, on the other hand facilitates information for example, on the position of a limb in space. It is examined by checking the position reflex (see also 108.4).

138.1 The intrauterine stasis of **ENDOCHONDRAL OSSIFICATION** by uninterrupted **PERICHONDRAL OSSIFICATION** leads to a stoppage of the longitudinal growth of bones. This heritable condition termed chondrodystrophy (chondros -cartilage, dys- defective, trophia – nutrition), is established in many breeds of dogs consciously to attain definite breed characteristics. (for example Bulldog, Boxer, Dachshund, Pekingese, West Highland White Terrier, Sealyham Terrier, Welsh Corgi).

138.2 To permit **CHONDROCLASTIC ACTIVITY**, mineralization of cartilage ground substance during bone growth is an essential prerequisite. Unmineralized cartilage cannot be disintegrated by chondroclasts and thus cannot be replaced with bone. With vitamin D deficiency, calcium deficiency, or by a shift of optimal Ca/P ratio, mineralization is restricted in the **cartilage resorption zone**. The penetrating chondroclasts cannot degrade the cartilage and on account of the continuing proliferation, a thickening of the **epiphyseal cartilage** (growth plate) is detected radiographically. This then no longer is adequate to support the static load.

138.3 A congenital interruption of **OSTEOBLASTIC FUNCTION** including the synthesis of collagen causes defective bone development **(osteogenesis imperfecta congenita)**, an hereditary affliction occurring in Poodles, Collies and Shelties. Already in utero this causes fractures and skeletal deformations. In large and fast growing dog breeds a further form of osteoblastic insufficiency can occur between 3 and 8 months of age – hypertrophic osteodystrophy – which perhaps has an infectious or diatetic origin. Animals are afflicted with painful swelling of the metaphyses of radius, ulna and tibia which can be combined with periosteal overdevelopment.

138.4 OSSIFICATION CENTERS are defined distinctly and well recognized radiographically from the background due to mineralization of the spongy substance. Ossification centers appearing on different bones at very definite times can be used to estimate age.

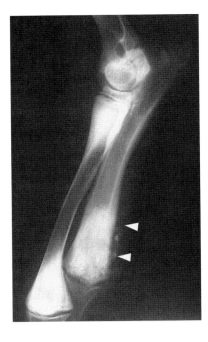

138.3 Increased radiographic density of the metaphyses of radius and ulna combined with overdevelopment of periosteum (arrows) in a young dog with hypertrophic osteodystrophy.

138.5 Longitudinal growth of bones takes place in the **(EPIPHYSEAL) GROWTH PLATE**. Genetic, traumatic and alimentary factors (see 14.7 and 16.6) can cause interruptions of longitudinal growth. Epi- and apophysiolysis caused by trauma occur particularly in young dogs, if the growth plate, still cartilaginous and weaker, is not capable of sustaining stress. Quick response and fixation of the ends of the fracture are aimed at maintaining the ability of the growth plate to grow. Within certain limits decreased longitudinal growth in the epiphyseal plate of one limb bone can be compensated for by an intensified longitudinal growth of other bones. Closure of the growth plate is well demonstrated radiographically and is referred to for estimation of age. In the dog almost all growth plates are closed at the end of the first year.

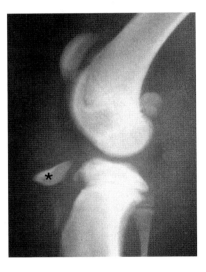

138.5 Avulsion of the tibial tuberosity (*) with subsequent dislocation due to traction of m. quadriceps femoris.

138.6 LONGITUDINAL GROWTH ceases with the beginning of puberty under the influence of sex hormones. With castration before puberty longitudinal growth continues for a longer time, early castration producing a more than average body size (large eunuchoid growth). Longitudinal growth is promoted by thyroid and growth hormones. A congenital deficiency of growth hormone as a consequence of hypofunction of the adenohypophysis, is present as a recessive genetic defect in German Shepherd dogs and leads to hypophyseal dwarfism. An increased production of growth hormone causes gigantism. The extreme growth of very large breeds depends on the temporary oversupply of growth hormone in the prepubertal period.

138.7 GROWTH IN THICKNESS of bones proceeds from peri- and endosteum. Adenomas of the adenohypophysis connected to a hypersecretion of growth hormone in adult animals causes an excessive growth in bone thickness especially to limb extremities (acromegaly) and skull. There is also folding of the skin of the face. In mild form this aspect of the condition is desired as the typical breed characteristic in Newfoundland and Saint Bernard dogs. Tumors in the thoracic cavity can cause overdevelopment of periosteal bone in the limb bones. This leads to a massive increase in thickness of all long bones (acropachy, osteopulmonary syndrome) which is visible externally.

The **repair of bone fractures by secondary intention or healing** begins from periosteum, perivascular connective tissue of blood vessels associated with bone, and from the endosteal covering of the medullary cavity which stabilizes the fracture initially through formation of a callus. Leading to callus formation connective tissue cells differentiate into osteoblasts. A primary callus is formed from cancellous bone if, by secondary healing of the fracture, an extensive fixation of the fragments is attained through osteoblastic activity. If the fracture ends are fixed insufficiently and succumb to traction and pressure fluctuations, connective tissue followed by cartilaginous replacement tissue develops before a secondary callus can arise from cancellous bone. Bone fracture repair is concluded when the callus is replaced by lamellar bone tissue. After healing and with remodeling of the bone thickness at the site of callus formation, the fracture is barely recognizable.

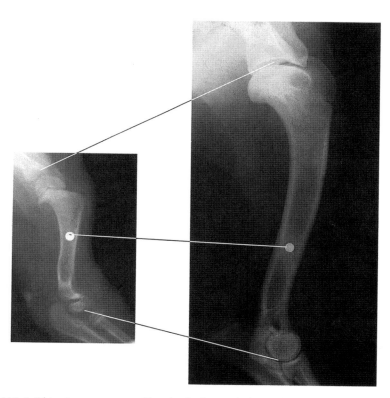

138.6 Objective assessment of longitudinal growth due to labeling of the diaphysis of a puppy (left), and after conclusion of longitudinal growth (right). The proximal humerus growth plate cartilage possesses a distinctly greater growth potential (Radiograph: Professor Dr. E. Henschel, Berlin).

138.8 Bone **REGENERATION** is promoted due to surgical union of previous repositioned bone fragments. Osteosynthesis is undertaken using different techniques such as pinning or the use of surgical screws. Healing time is thus shortened. Regeneration growth is by primary healing if, after exact repositioning, the stable fracture ends are fixed together, one on the other, without any movement. In the ideal case regeneration takes place along the fissure free fracture line according to

the principle of physiological bone reconstruction. In this instance one arrives at a situation involving either no or nonessential development of osseous replacement tissue (callus).

140.1 The continually occurring **RECONSTRUCTION OF BONE** makes possible permanent adjustment to its functional load of which the expression is the trajectorial system of bone. With degenerative processes predominating local **atrophy** occurs which can be initiated through continuous pressure. A general atrophy of one or more bones can be an expression of a defective functional load. For example this appears after prolonged lameness with complete loss of capacity of an affected limb.

Physiological bone reconstruction is effected also with autologous bone chip implants to compensate for bone damage after bone fractures. Above all, the implant serves as stabilization and disintegrates gradually but its surviving blood vessels prepare a connection to the surrounding implantation bed and cause a proliferation of osteoblasts.

140.2 Muscle attachments are anchored in the **PERIOSTEUM**. They occupy a large surface because the tendon fiber bundles spread out at the site, (periosteal- diaphyseal attachment type). With excessive muscle contraction bone fragments can be torn away to give what is termed an avulsion fracture. With continuous local mechanical insult, periosteum reacts by developing cartilage or bone tissue. In this way bony protrusions known as exostoses originate.

140.3 ENDOSTEUM which lies at the boundary of the medullary cavity and in places covers the medullary cells, is essentially thinner than periosteum. During bone growth, osteon disintegration due to osteoclasts proceeds from the endosteum. Hence the thickening of compact substance induced by the periosteum is kept within limits and the medullary cavity is enlarged continuously (Principle: external construction, internal destruction).

140.4 BLOOD VESSELS of the long bones belong to 4 different systems of supply which anastomose with one another and guarantee an intense blood supply. Hence the anastomoses and their collateral blood vessels provide for the maintenance of the blood supply after multiple bone fractures, therapeutic osteosynthesis and ligation of individual blood vessels. The 4 supply systems are described consecutively according to size.

I. The largest of the blood vessels are the **nutrient vessels** which, in the midsection of the diaphysis, penetrate through the **nutrient foramen** (foramina) and the connecting **nutrient canal** into the medullary cavity. Ultimately they ramify in the sinusoids of the bone marrow and supply the compact substance from the internal to the external side. The capillaries course along continuing **central canals (Haversian canals)** in the osteons and supply the bone tissue. Cross communications between the osteons, the **perforating canals (of Volkmann)** are drained via particular venules to periosteal veins.

II. The **metaphyseal artery and vein** begin adjacent to the epiphyseal line in the metaphyseal section of the diaphysis.

III. The **epiphyseal artery and vein** supply the extremity of the bone with its covering of articular cartilage. (In the femur the blood vessels reach the femoral epiphysis from the pelvis through the round ligament of the head of the femur). Before the end of longitudinal growth the epiphyseal vessels are separated from the meta- and diaphyseal vessels due to the cartilage of the growth plate. After epiphyseal closure – according to prevailing opinion-anastomoses form.

IV. The thin **periosteal vessels** which also course from the joint capsule along the bone approach it everywhere but supply solely the superficial sections of the compact stratum. The branches infiltrate the periphery of the compact stratum whereas the above named large vessels belong to a centrifugal supply system.

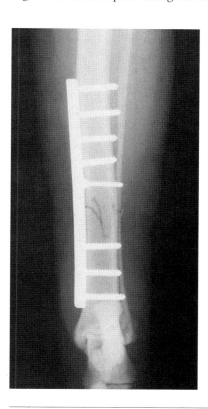

138.8 Maintenance of a fracture of the tibia with a surgical plate.

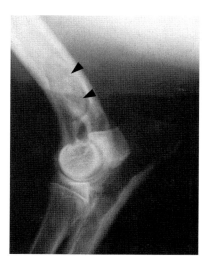

140.4 Radiograph of a circumscribed area (arrows) in the shaft of the humerus with eosinophilic panostitis.

Growth derangement of bone can cause a narrowing of the interosseous blood vessels causing an interrupted venous outflow. This produces edema in the medullary cavity which leads to an increase in interosseous pressure and compression of further blood vessels. The affected long bones are susceptible to pressure and show characteristic shadowing with radiography. This so called **eosinophilic panostitis** appears in large growing breeds and German Shepherd dogs from 6 to 8 (18) months of age.

140.5 As an additional **BONE SHAPE** the international nomenclature commission of 1983 introduced the term irregular bone (os irregulare). According to the new classification a vertebra belongs to this category and is no longer regarded as a short bone. As a basis for this, it is a question of the mode of ossification which takes place in short bones through endochondral ossification and in long bones and vertebrae through endochondral and perichondral ossification.

140.6 SESAMOID BONES function as 'pressure – slide' bodies generally associated with tendons directed over the external side of a joint.

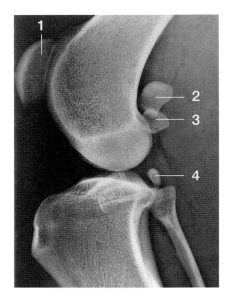

140.6 Sesamoid bones of the knee joint.

1 Patella; 2 and 3 Sesamoid bones of the m.gastrocnemius; 4 Sesamoid bone of the m.popliteus (microfocus radiograph: Professor Dr. C. Poulsen Nautrup, Munich).

140.7 CARTILAGE in contrast to bone is highly resilient to pressure, so that articulation extremities are coated with cartilage. Cartilage tissue is not or only poorly infiltrated with blood vessels and consequently is provided with its nutrition through diffusion from the surroundings. The poor vascularity delays the continuity of wound healing and promotes autoimmune processes.

142.1 A PSEUDOARTHROSIS ("FALSE JOINT") arises due to absence of fracture repair on account of instability or defective repositioning of fracture extremities. These unite by connective tissue or cartilage. There remain an unphysiological mobility and instability of the joint.

A **NEARTHROSIS** results if after luxation, tissue similar to articular cartilage and joint capsule develop at the site of deformity (for example development of a new acetabulum). Formation of a new joint is desirable after a resection of the head of the femur (see 76.1) and makes satisfactory function of the pelvic limb possible.

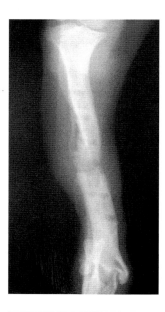

142.1 Formation of a pseudoarthrosis after unsatisfactory stabilization of a fracture of the tibia.

142.2 The **JOINT CAPSULE** is situated in folds particularly on the flexion aspect of a joint and these disappear with joint extension. Joints with great freedom of movement have wide joint capsules. In contrast, tight joints with scarcely any or no freedom of movement exhibit very tight appressed joint capsules. Joint instability leads to an increased load on the joint capsule, with thickening of the fibrous stratum. Inflammatory stimuli cause synovitis which, in chronic cases, leads to thickening and villous formation of the synovial layer.

142.3 LIGAMENTS are overstretched with strains and can be torn with luxations causing degenerative alterations of the joint (arthroses). By far the most frequently affected is the cranial cruciate ligament in the dog which ruptures (see 86.2).

142.4 ARTICULAR CARTILAGE serves as a sliding cushion, elastically compressible and capable of being deformed reversibly. It has a high water content which decreases with age. On the smooth surface of hyaline cartilage, perichondrium is lacking, and therefore capacity for regeneration is limited. Joints are never completely congruent with light loads. Not until joint cartilage is deformed under a load is congruency improved and the load distributed over a larger surface. Due to movement the regular deformation of avascular articular cartilage promotes liquid currents in the cartilage therefore essentially improving supply of nutrients. In the case of an (osteo) chondrosis dissecans (OCD) the articular cartilage is distinctly thickened in places and is not nourished adequately in its deeper parts which exhibit necrosis. The section which is altered pathologically is not capable of bearing a load statically and the superimposed intact cartilage loses its base and can break or cave in. OCD occurs in dogs particularly in the shoulder joint but also in the elbow, knee and tarsal joints.

Body load is taken up by articular cartilage and transmitted onto the subchondral compact bone plate of which the thickness is connected to the functional load. The exact thickness of the subchondral bone plate can be ascertained by computer tomographic osteoabsorptiometry (CTOAM). Symbolized in color the thickness is projected upon the joint surface which is reconstructed three dimensionally from the CT database. Absence and excess of load on a joint caused local increase of thickness (hardening) of the subchondral bone plate.

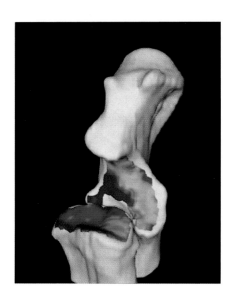

142.4 CTOAM: Color labeling of the subchondral bone thickness in the trochlear notch of the ulna and on the head of the radius.
Red = high bone thickness
Blue = slight bone thickness
(Photograph: Dr J Maierl, Munich)

142.5 BURSAE react to chronic pressure stress with increased formation of synovia (hygroma see 26.5).

142.6 INTERVERTEBRAL DISCS see 10.3

144.1 According to differences in muscle **COLOR**, one can deduce its function. 'White' essentially anerobic muscle consists of 'white' fiber type which is larger than red. White type fibers can contract faster than the red type but also fatigue quicker. The former are associated with posture, the latter with movement. The red aerobic muscles of movement have a high content of myoglobin in their predominantly red (smaller) muscle fibers and are better supplied with blood than their white counterpart. Not only contraction but also rate of fatigue are slower than with white muscle.

144.2 MYOGENESIS begins in large part from the myotome of the primitive vertebra (see Embryology). From here the primary myoblasts differentiate in 2 directions. The numerically predominant (primary) myoblast type develops with cells of the same kind into a long orderly series to form a 'myotubus'. It includes cell nuclei arranged centrally but there is no lumen; therefore the nomenclature myotubus or muscle tube is misleading. Within the myotubes the plasmalemmata disappear between the secondary myoblasts to produce a very long cell, a syncitium, which is characterized by numerous nuclei located in the periphery. The smaller portion of (primary) myoblasts differentiates into a few satellite cells lying between the muscle cells and the outer ensuing basal lamina.

With **muscle regeneration** the significance of the satellite cells becomes clear. In so far as the basal lamina remains intact with muscle cell injury, cell debris is removed by macrophages. The dormant satellite cells divide by mitosis and bridge over the defect. With further differentiation of these bridging sections proceeding from satellite cells, due to synthesis of myofilaments, discontinuity between defective ends of muscle cells is gradually closed. Hence continuity is established once again. With greater defects such as tears in the muscle fiber bundles healing occurs with the production of scar tissue.

144.3 The stimulus for transmission at the **MOTOR END PLATES** takes place due to acetylcholine. Due to formation of antibodies against acetylcholine receptors, neuromuscular excitability is interrupted. This disease, myasthenia gravis, is either congenital or acquired (see 40.5) and is characterized by rapid muscle fatigue. Very often the striated muscle of the esophagus is so affected due to which it dilates (megaesophagus).

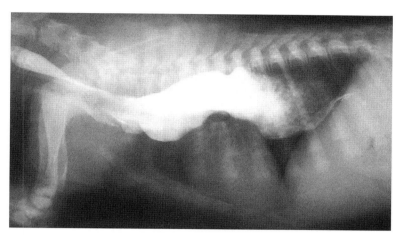

144.3 Contrast radiography of a severe dilated esophagus (megaesophagus).

144.4 The **CONTRACTION OF SMOOTH MUSCLE** is initiated due to the stimulus of stretching and spontaneous discharge at the neuromuscular junction (for example in lymphatic vessels and in the intestinal wall).

144.5 MUSCLE TEARS occur by abrupt traction of a contracted muscle or by additional over extension in an already extreme position of extension for example after a jump or fall from a greater height. The most frequently affected muscles are m.gracilis and m. triceps brachii.

144.6 The **INTERNAL STRUCTURE OF A MUSCLE** can be established in vivo using ultasonography. With this one can also diagnose hematomas, abcesses or fibroses.

146.1 TENDONS change their course of direction at joints. In general an osseous groove or a retinaculum serve as a 'steerage pulley'. Fibrocartilage is imbedded in the normal tendon with its parallel fibers to remove pressure and shearing forces. These so called regions of tendon slide have a lower tensile strength than those tendon sections with purely parallel fibers associated with movements. Therefore, tendon rupture takes place, almost exclusively in the sections of tendon slide, for example in the tendon of origin of m. biceps brachii (see 18.2).

146.2 OSTEOFIBROTIC SITES develop completely enclosed compartments which cannot expand with contained structures. Therefore extensive bleeding after a fracture, or swelling of muscles after intense stress, lead to a considerable increase in pressure, known as compartment syndrome. Sequelae therefore are reduced vascularity and derangement of neuromuscular function with attacks of pain which can cause massive ischemic injury of affected musculature without punctual treatment. (see 20.3, 22.1, 82.3).

146.3 INNERVATION OF SKELETAL MUSCLE can be checked using electromyography.

148.1 NEUROGLIA envelop nerve cell bodies and processes and separate these from blood vessels with enclosing connective tissue. Peripheral neuroglia (Schwann cells and satellite or capsule cells) are differentiated from central glial cells (ependymal cells, astrocytes, oligodendrocytes and microgliocytes). Glial cells develop a supporting framework or stroma and are significant for the nutrition of nervous tissue. They maintain an optimal perineural milieu by eliminating neurotransmitter substances in the central nervous system and protect nerves by synthesizing the myelin sheath (importance for nerve regeneration see 148.3). Benign or malignant tumors (glioma) originate from glial cells. In common with myelinated and unmyelinated fibers the neuroglia, which constantly nar-

row the intercellular gaps, form the **neuropil**. In the gray substance of the central nervous system this separates the nerve cell bodies from one another.

148.2 MYELIN FORMATION begins prenatally and continues postnatally (maturity of myelin), important functional units developing faster than those less important. As it were, the lamellated myelin sheath encloses the axon as an insulator. In cooperation with the nodes of Ranvier, this brings about a saltatory excitation transmitter. The impulse jumps from one node to another due to which the speed of conduction is essentially increased compared to that of the unmyelinated fiber. As a rule of thumb it is approximately true that the thicker the axon or dendrite, the thicker the myelin sheath, and the longer the internode the faster the conduction of the impulse.

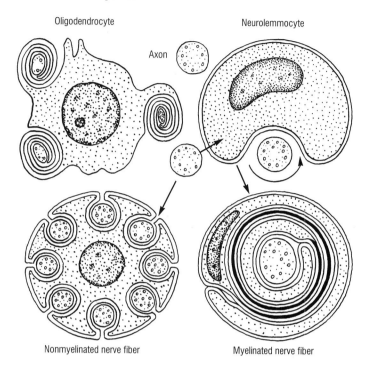

148.2 Schema of formation of the myelin sheath.

148.3 NERVE REGENERATION (restoration of neuroconductivity) begins after transection or after a lesion at the proximal and above all at the distal nerve stump involving **degeneration**. Only a few internodes degenerate proximally, as in most cases the nerve cell bodies remain intact. The axons of the distal nerve stump degenerate to the end formations. Regeneration occurs proximally with budding or sprouting of the cells of Schwann which with the likewise budding of the cells of Schwann of the distal nerve stump develop a continuum bridging over the defect. The band shaped series of Schwann cells act as conductivity 'splints' for the axons budding out of the proximal stump which regenerate as far as the effector organ. Regeneration progresses very slowly at about 3 mm per day. The prerequisite for nerve regeneration is among others, a relatively short distance between the proximal and distal nerve stumps. Regeneration is promoted by approximating and suturing the nerve stumps. (On the other hand, with a **neurectomy** to block pain, a sufficiently long piece of nerve is ablated to prevent the stumps growing together – a disputed method of treatment of sports horses less frequently used nowadays).

148.4 ENDO-, PERI-, EPINEURIUM protect the nerves from excess tension and paraneurium anchors the nerves to their surroundings.

148.5 NODES OF RANVIER are situated at breaks in the myelin sheath where the axon (dendrite) is slightly thickened. Between 2 nodes is the internode. Because of a lack of myelin, local anesthetic has its initial effect at the nodes of Ranvier and extends from there.

150.1 HORMONE SYNTHESIS IN THE HYPOTHALAMUS – HYPOPHYSIS – SYSTEM

Peripheral endocrine glands (thyroid, adrenal cortex, gonads) act by a 'feed back' mechanism on the hypothalamus – hypophysis system. An example of negative feed back is as follows: A stress situation causes the release of ACTH – RH in the hypothalamus and an increase of ACTH incretion in the adenohypophysis. This is followed by an increased output of glucocorticoids in the adrenal cortex. Finally through negative feed back on the hypothalamus this in turn causes a reduction in the release of ACTH – RH, ACTH and glucocorticoids. With a positive feed back due to a high rate of hormone synthesis of peripheral glands (for example estrogen in the interstitial cells and follicular epithelial cells) the release of hypothalamus – hypophysis hormones (for example LH – RH and LH) is still increased to ovulation term. (see also 110.10, 138.6 and 7)

203

HYPOTHALAMUS	POSTERIOR PITUITARY – EFFECTOR-HORMONE	TARGET ORGAN OR CELL	MAIN FUNCTION
Oxytocin Vasopressin = Adiuretin	Neurosecretory transport to the posterior pituitary	Myoepithelium Smooth musculature, Kidney, Blood Vessels	For example – labor pains, milk flow, water resorption in the kidney, increased blood pressure
	ANTERIOR PITUITARY – EFFECTOR-HORMONE		
RH and RIH	Somatotrophic Hormone (STH)	Growing cell association	Body growth
RH and RIH	Prolactin	Mammary gland	Milk secretion
	ANTERIOR PITUITARY – REGULATING-HORMONE		
RH	Thyroid stimulating hormone (TSH)	Thyroid Gland	Metabolism
	Gonadotrophin: Follicle stimulating hormone (FSH)	Sertoli and follicular epithelial cells	Testicular and follicular maturation
RH	Luteinizing hormone (LH = female ICSH = male)	Ovarian and testicular interstitial cells Corpus luteum	Androgen, Estrogen and Progesterone synthesis
RH	Adrenocorticotrophic hormone (ACTH)	Adrenal cortex	Steroid hormone synthesis
RH and RIH	Melatrophin of pars intermedia Melanocyte stimulating hormone (MSH)	Pigment cells	Pigmentation

RIH = Release Inhibiting Hormone; RH = Releasing Hormone
ICSH = Interstitial Cell Stimulating Hormone

150.2 THYROID AND PARATHYROID GLANDS see 14.6 and 7

150.3 ADRENAL GLANDS see 70.3

150.4 RENIN is released by a fall in blood pressure of the kidney. It converts angiotensinogen of the blood plasma into angiotensin I. In different organs, for example the lung this is then transformed to angiotensin II which stimulates the cells of the glomerular zone of the adrenal cortex to synthesize aldosterone. This mineralocorticoid produces an increase in the intravascular fluid volume through a resorption of sodium and water. With this there is a rise in blood pressure due to which renin synthesis is retarded again.

150.5 An insufficient outpouring of **INSULIN** leads to hyperglycemia and the secretion of glucose in the urine whereby the condition derives its name diabetes mellitus.

152.1 On the basis of numerous morphological and structural characteristics **VEINS** are clearly defined from arteries. Generally they have a wider lumen and are more numerous. Several collateral veins can accompany one artery in a common blood vessel – nerve – pathway. The wide lumened venous system of individual organs such as liver, lung, spleen and skin, functions in blood storage. Considerable quantities of blood can be withdrawn temporarily from the blood stream and thus cardiac requirements are reduced by an economic maintenance of function.

Venous blood return is promoted in several ways:

1. Due to the sucking action of the heart, blood is sucked from the orifices of both venae cavae and from the right atrium due to displacement of valve levels.

2. With body movements sections of the body such as parts of joints and digital pads are compressed repeatedly. Pressure is exercised on the associated veins and blood flow is directed towards the heart due to the venous valves. Due to muscle contraction blood flow is also 'propelled onwards'. This is true particularly for such veins which lie within muscle fascia.

3. The pulse wave can be transmitted with rhythmic pressure vibrations to the closely adjacent accompanying veins.

4. With respiratory rhythm and changing negative pressure in the pleural cavity blood is sucked towards the heart. (With injury to the veins near the heart, air can be aspirated because of negative pressure with the resultant danger of emboli).

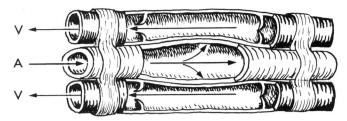

152.1 Outward action of the arterial pulse on venous return.

154.1 'OPEN JUNCTIONS' are the morphological basis for **direct** and **indirect lymphography** (radiography of the lymphatic system). With indirect lymphography, initially a colored dye (patent blue violet) is injected into the interstitial tissue. The particles of dye (diameter approximately 0.1 μm) reach the lymph capillaries via the open junctions labeling these and the proximally ensuing lymph vessels and lymph nodes. Due to this labeling the lymphatic vessels, formerly insignificant, can be identified easier and punctured to inject contrast medium. With direct lymphography a suitable contrast medium is injected into the lymphatic vessel. Radiographically then, one can recognize lymphatic channels and perhaps pathological interruptions to lymph flow (for example with lymph node changes and with obliterating lymphangiopathy following degenerative dystrophic endothelial changes).

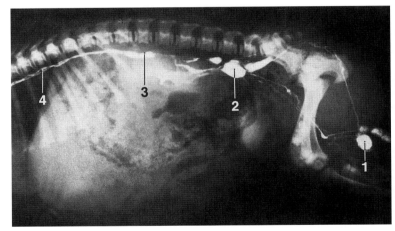

154.1 Lymphography of the caudal regions of a puppy. 1. Popliteal lymph nodes; 2 Medial iliac lymph node; 3 Cisterna chyli; 4 Thoracic duct. (Radiograph: Professor Dr. Berens von Rautenfeld, Hanover).

154.2 LYMPH NODES are of medical significance since they are affected by **inflammation** in their areas of drainage. Consequently such areas should be known. Inflamed lymph nodes are enlarged, painful, and radiate increased heat. Regarding **clinical diagnoses** such lymph nodes are easier to palpate; normally only superficial lymph nodes are more or less distinct. With lymph flow, floating malignant tumor cells are deposited in lymph nodes and can be a starting point for **daughter tumors (metastases)**.

154.3 LYMPHOCYTES, according to size, are classified as small, average and large cells. From the functional viewpoint one differentiates B- and T- lymphocytes which of course are differentiated morphologically and by special methods. **B-lymphocytes** originate in the bone marrow, are imprinted in the cloacal bursa or equivalent organs and discharge into the bloodstream and lymph nodes. B stands for bursa cloacae of birds. The **bursal equivalent** in mammals is not known or defined exactly. According to many authors bone marrow is in this category, hence, in an incorrect sense B could be employed for bone marrow. B-lymphocytes are responsible for **humoral immunity**. This is based on the ability of B-lymphocytes, which transform themselves into plasma cells, to produce immunoglobulins (antibodies). The **T-lymphocytes** originate in bone marrow, differentiate in the thymus (T stands for thymus) and after that are discharged into the thymic dependent areas of lymph node (paracortex) and the spleen. From the functional viewpoint one can differentiate helper, killer, suppressor and memory cells. The short lived **killer cells** are responsible for cellular immunity. They kill cells (for example bacteria or transplanted cells – transplant rejection) and perish spontaneously (suppuration, pus formation). **Helper**

cells regulate the transformation of B-lymphocytes to plasma cells and with it control humoral immunity. **Suppressor cells** inhibit killer and helper cells and due to this retard excessive immune reactions. The long living **memory cells** (more than a year) allow the defence system, by repeated confrontation with a specific antigen, to react quickly with a secondary immune response.

REFERENCES

Adams, D. R., 1986: Canine Anatomy. Iowa State University Press, Ames

Amman, E., E. Seiferle und G. Pelloni, 1978: Atlas zur chirurgisch-topographischen Anatomie des Hundes. Paul Parey, Berlin, Hamburg.

Anderson, W. D. and Anderson, G. B., 1994: Atlas of Canine Anatomy. Lea and Febiger, Philadelphia, Baltimore

Barone, R., 1976: Anatomie Comparèe des Mammiferes Domestiques; T.1 - Osteologie; T. 2 - Arthrologie et Myologie; T. 3 Splanchnologie, Foetus et ses Annexes. Viget Freres, Paris

Baum, H., 1917: Die im injizierten Zustand makroskopisch erkennbaren Lymphgefäße der Skelettknochen des Hundes. Anat. Anz. 50:521-539

Baum, H., 1917: Die Lymphgefäße der Haut des Hundes. Anat. Anz. 50:1-15

Baum, H. und O. Zietzschmann, 1936: Handbuch der Anatomie des Hundes, 2. Aufl., Paul Parey, Berlin

Berg, R., 1982: Angewandte und topographische Anatomie der Haustiere. 2. Aufl., Gustav Fischer, Jena

Böhme, G., 1967: Unterschiede am Gehirnventrikelsystem von Hund und Katze nach Untersuchungen an Ausgußpräparaten. Berl. Münch. Tierärztl. Wschr. 80:195-196

Bojrab, M. J., 1981: Praxis der Kleintierchirurgie. Enke, Stuttgart

Bolz, W., 1985, Hrsg.: O. Dietz: Lehrbuch der Allgemeinen Chirurgie für Tierärzte. 5. Aufl., Enke, Stuttgart

Bonath, K. H. und W. D. Prieur, 1998: Kleintierkrankheiten Bd 3 Orthopädische Chirurgie und Traumatologie. Ulmer Verlag, Stuttgart

Boyd, J. S., Paterson, C. and A. H. May, 1991: A Colour Atlas of Clinical Anatomy of the Dog and Cat. Wolfe Publ. Ltd., London

Bradley, O. Ch., 1948: Topographical Anatomy of the Dog. 5. Ed., Oliver and Boyd, Edinburgh, London

Bucher, O., und H. Wartenberg 1997: Cytologie, Histologie und mikroskopische Anatomie des Menschen, 12. Aufl., Hans Huber, Bern, Stuttgart, Wien

Budras, K.-D., 1972: Zur Homologisierung der Mm. adductores und des M. pectineus der Haussäugetiere. Zbl. Vet. Med., C, 1:73-91

Budras, K.-D., F. Preuß, W. Traeder und E. Henschel, 1972: Der Leistenspalt und die Leistenringe unserer Haussäugetiere in neuer Sicht. Berl. Münchn. tierärztl. Wschr. 85:427-431

Budras, K.-D. und D. Seifert, 1972: Die Muskelinsertionsareale des Beckens von Hund und Katze, zugleich ein Beitrag zur Homologisierung der Lineae glutaeae unserer Haussäugetiere. Anat. Anz. 132:423-434

Budras, K.-D. und A. Wünsche, 1972: Arcus inguinalis und Fibrae reflexae des Hundes. Gegenbaurs morph. Jb. 1 17:408-419

Chandler, E. H., J. B. Sutton and D. J. Thompson, 1984: Canine Medicine and Therapeutics. 2. Ed., Blackwell, Oxford, London

Christoph, H.-J., U. Freudiger und E.-G. Grünbaum, 1997: Klinik der Hundekrankheiten. 2. Aufl., Fischer, Stuttgart

Dämmrich, K., 1981: Zur Pathologie der degenerativen Erkrankungen der Wirbelsäule bei Hunden. Kleintierpraxis 26:467-476

Dahme, E. und E. Weiss, 1999: Grundriß der speziellen pathologischen Anatomie der Haustiere 5. Aufl., Enke, Stuttgart

Dellmann, H.-D. and E. M. Brown, 1976: Textbook of Veterinary Histology. Lea and Febiger, Philadelphia

De Lahunta, A., 1983: Veterinary Neuroanatomy and Clinical Neurology. 2. Ed., W. B. Saunders Comp., Philadelphia

De Lahunta, A. and R. E. Habel, 1986: Applied Veterinary Anatomy. W. B. Saunders Comp., Philadelphia

Donat, K., 1971: Die Fixierung der Clavicula bei Katze und Hund. Anat. Anz. 128:365-374

Donat, K., 1972: Der M. cucullaris und seine Abkömmlinge (M. trapezius und M. sternocleidomastoideus) bei den Haussäugetieren. Anat. Anz. 131:286-297

Done, St. H., Goody, P. C., Evans, S. A. et al., 1996: Color Atlas of Veterinary Anatomy. Vol.3: The Dog and Cat. Mosby-Wolfe, London

Dyce, K. M., Sack, W. O. und C. J. G. Wensing, 1991: Anatomie der Haustiere. Enke, Stuttgart

Ellenberger, W. und H. Baum, 1943: Handbuch der vergleichenden Anatomie der Haustiere. 18. Aufl., Springer, Berlin

Evans, H. E. and A. de Lahunta, 1988: Miller's Guide to the Dissection of the Dog. 3. Ed., W. B. Saunders Comp., Philadelphia, London, Toronto

Evans, H. E., 1993: Miller's Anatomy of the Dog. 3. Ed., W. B. Saunders Comp., Philadelphia, London, Toronto

Faller, A., 1980: Anatomie in Stichworten. Ferdinand Enke, Stuttgart

Franke, H.-R., 1970: Zur Anatomie des Organum vomeronasale des Hundes. Diss. med. vet., Freie Universität Berlin

Frewein, J. und B. Vollmerhaus, 1994: Anatomie von Hund und Katze. Blackwell Wissenschafts-Verlag, Berlin

Getty, R., 1975: Sisson and Grossman's Anatomy of the Domestic Animals. Vol. 2 - Porcine, Carnivore, Aves. 5. Ed., W. B. Saunders Comp., Philadelphia, London, Toronto

Getty, R., H. L. Foust, E. T. Presley and M. C. Miller, 1956: Macroscopic anatomy of the ear of the dog. Amer. J. Vet. Res. 17: 364-375

Grandage, J., 1972: The erect dog penis. Vet. Rec. 91:141-147

Habel, R. E., 1985: Applied Veterinary Anatomy. Pub. by author, Ithaca, N. Y.

Habel, R. und K.-D. Budras, 1992: Anatomy of the praepubic tendon in horse, cow, sheep, goat and dog. Am. J. Vet. Res. 53: 2183-2195

Henning, Ch., 1965: Zur Kenntnis des M. retractor ani et penis s. clitoridis et constrictor recti (M. retractor cloacae) beim Hund. Anat. Anz. 117:201-215

Henning, P., 1965: Der M. piriformis und die Nn. clunium medii des Hundes. Zbl. Vet. Med., A, 12:263-275

Henschel, E. und W. Gastinger, 1963: Beitrag zur Arteriographie der Aa. carotis und vertebralis beim Hund. Berl. Münchn. tierärztl. Wschr. 76:241-243

Henschel, E., 1971: Zur Anatomie und Klinik der wachsenden Unterarmknochen mit Vergleichen zwischen der Distractio cubiti des Hundes und der Madelungschen Deformität des Menschen. Arch. Experim. Vet. med. 26:741-787

Henschel, E., 1983: Das Hüftgelenk von Hund und Katze - eine Enarthrosis? tierärztl. Prax. 11:345 -348

Hoerlein, B. F., 1978: Canine Neurology. Diagnosis und Treatment. 3..Ed., W. B. Saunders Comp., Philadelphia, London, Toronto

Hyrtl, J., 1880: Onomatologia Anatomica. Braumüller, Wien

International Committee on Gross Anatomical Nomenclature, 1994: Nomina Anatomica, 4. Ed., Nomina Histologica, 2. Ed., Ithaca, N. Y.

Jacoby, S., 1968: Über einige Abkömmlinge des M. sphincter marsupii beim Hunde. Anat. Anz. 122:234-338

Kadletz, M., 1932: Anatomischer Atlas der Extremitätengelenke von Pferd und Hund. Urban und Schwarzenberg, Berlin, Wien

Kealy, J. K., 1991: Röntgendiagnostik bei Hund und Katze. 2. Aufl., Enke, Stuttgart

King, A. S., 1978: A Guide to the Physiological and Clinical Anatomy of the Thorax. 4 Ed., Dept. Vet. Anat., University of Liverpool, Liverpool

King, A. S. and V. A. Riley, 1980: A Guide to the Physiological and Clinical Anatomy of the Head. 4. Ed., Dept. Vet. Anat., University of Liverpool, Liverpool L69 3BX

Koch, T. und R. Berg, 1981 - 1985: Lehrbuch der Veterinär-Anatomie. Bd. 1-3, Gustav Fischer, Jena

König, H. E., 1992: Anatomie der Katze. Gustav Fischer, Stuttgart, Jena, N.Y.

Kraft, W., 1993: Tierärztliche Endoskopie. Schattauer, Stuttgart, N.Y.

Krölling, O. und H. Grau, 1960: Lehrbuch der Histologie und vergleichenden mikroskopischen Anatomie der Haustiere. Paul Parey, Berlin, Hamburg

Krstic, R. V., 1978: Die Gewebe des Menschen und der Säugetiere. Springer, Berlin, Heidelberg, New York

Krstic, R. V., 1984: Illustrated Encyclopedia of Human Histology. Springer, Berlin, Heidelberg, New York, Tokyo

Krüger, G., 1961: Veterinärmedizinische Terminologie. 2. Aufl., Hirzel, Leipzig

Leonhardt, H., 1990: Histologie, Zytologie und Mikroanatomie des Menschen. 8. Aufl., Thieme, Stuttgart

Liebich, H.-G., 1999: Funktionelle Histologie 3. Aufl., Schattauer, Stuttgart, N.Y.

Lippert, H., 1999: Lehrbuch Anatomie. 5. Aufl., Urban und Fischer, München

Morgan, J. P. , A. Wind und A. P. Davidson, 2000: Hereditary Bone and Joint Diseases in the Dog. Schlütersche, Hannover

Nickel, R., A. Schummer und E. Seiferle, 1991-1996: Lehrbuch der Anatomie der Haustiere. Bd. 1-4, Paul Parey, Berlin, Hamburg

Niemand, H. G., und P. Suter, 1994: Praktikum der Hundeklinik. 8. Aufl., Paul Parey, Berlin, Hamburg

Nitschke, Th., 1970: Diaphragma pelvis, Clitoris und Vestibulum vaginae der Hündin. Anat. Anz. 127:76-125

Pierard, J., 1972: Anatomie Appliquèe des Carnivores Domestiques, Chien et Chat. Sornabec, Quebec

Preuß, F., 1967: Anleitung zur topographischen Ganztierpräparation des Hundes. Selbstverlag, Berlin

Reese, S., 1995: Untersuchungen am intakten und rupturierten Lig. cruciatum craniale des Hundes. Diss. med. vet., Berlin

Ruedorffer, N. v., 1996: Morphologische Untersuchungen zur Orthologie und Pathologie der Tuberositas tibiae bei Hunden bis zum Alter von 2 Jahren. Diss. Med. vet., Berlin

Schaller, O., 1992: Illustrated Veterinary Anatomical Nomenclature. Enke, Stuttgart

Simoens, P., 1985: Morphologic study of the vasculature in the orbit and eyeball of the pig. Thesis Fakul. Vet. Med., State Univ. Ghent

Wünsche, A. und K.-D. Budras, 1972: Der M. cremaster externus resp. compressor mammae des Hundes. Zbl. Vet. Med. C, 1: 138-148

INDEX

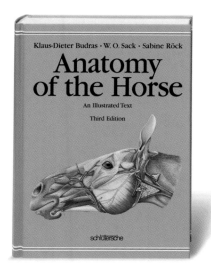

Klaus-Dieter Budras / W. O. Sack / Sabine Röck

Anatomy of the Horse

An Illustrated Text

3rd edition 2001. 136 pages, large-sized color plates
including several illustrations, radiographs,
drawings and photographs,
9³/₄ x 13¹/₂", hardcover
ISBN 3-87706-620-8

This atlas is superbly illustrated with color drawings, photographs, and radiographs providing the reader with detailed information on the structure, function, and clinical application of the parts of the body and their interactions in the live animal.

- Fully illustrated with color drawings based on new dissections, with osteology photographs and with radiographs.

- Includes topographic anatomy of the entire body; detailed information in tabular form on muscles, lymph nodes, and peripheral nerves; and clinical and functional aspects of selected structures.

Already acknowledged by students and teachers as an essential resource for learning and revision, this book will also be a valuable reference for veterinary practitioners and for those who own and value horses.

Content

Thoracic Limb – Pelvic Limb – Head – The Central Nervous System – Axial Skeleton and Neck – Thoracic Cavity – Abdominal Wall and Cavity – Pelvis, Inguinal Region, and Urogenital Organs – Selected Body Systems in Tabular Form – Contributions to the Clinical and Functional Anatomy of the Horse

---

Joe P. Morgan / Alida Wind /
Autumn P. Davidson

Hereditary Bone and Joint Diseases in the Dog

Osteochondroses – Hip dysplasia – Elbow dysplasia

Announcing an unprecedented new source of unique content that goes far beyond a description of bone and joint disorders alone. Every chapter provides information on the history, pathogenesis, diagnosis (physical and radiographic), therapy and prognosis of particular canine skeletal diseases as well as what the diseases will mean to the dog's life.

Expert authors with years of professional experience detail basic and advanced information.

This book addresses the importance of selection of dogs for breeding, including changes in breed appearance and disease predilection and the effect of high-energy diets in fast-growing animals.

As a small animal clinician, client questions about skeletal disorders are routine in your practice day. This remarkable, instructional text will give you answers, incidence figures, advice about surgery and timing, and honest analyses of treatment failures and successes. Here is a fresh look at the way we treat OCD, dysplasias and other bone diseases. With realistic assessments and positives directives for pet care and client support.

2000. 314 pages, 271 radiographs, 85 b/w photos, 38 drawings,
8 ¹/₂ x 11", hardcover
ISBN 3-87706-548-1

"The book will be helpful tool in everyday companion animal practice, especially in radiographic diagnostics. Questions given by breeders and owners are answered. The book is recommended as a contribution to the bookshelf in all veterinary clinics using radiography."
The European Journal of Companion Animal Practice

Frans C. Stades / Milton Wyman /
Michael H. Boevé / Willy Neumann

Ophthalmology for the Veterinary Practitioner

Here is a useful new reference volume that identifies and masterfully illustrates common ophthalmologic disorders of small domestic animals, such as dogs and cats, as well as horses, cattle, sheep, goats, pigs, rabbits and birds. The text emphasizes diseases that can typically be difficult to diagnose without specialised experience or specific instruments. Rare signs are also described to complete the range of possible ophthalmic disorders – making differential diagnosis easier for the veterinarian.

This book encourages and helps equip a practitioner to attempt treatment of veterinary ophthalmologic cases. Description includes preliminary measures that can be taken before referral as well as potential professional errors.

Each chapter begins with an introduction to specific anatomy and physiology of the eye and supporting structure, noting pathogenesis, etiology, clinical course and therapy. Systemic congenial disorders are discussed, especially ophthalmologic conditions brought about by external influences, such as trauma, intoxication or deficiency.

1998. 204 pages, 394 illustrations,
8 ¹/₂ x 11", hardcover
ISBN 3-87706-488-4

"I like this book. In a world of both computer screens and text, a comfortable textbook that feels nice and looks good demonstrates that this method of spreading information remains a viable option."
Journal of Small Animal Practice